ANNALS OF THE NEW YORK ACADEMY OF SCIENCES

Volume 949

EDITORIAL STAFF

Executive Editor
BARBARA M. GOLDMAN

Managing Editor
JUSTINE CULLINAN

Associate Editors
MARION L. GARRY
STEFAN MALMOLI
RICHARD STIEFEL

The New York Academy of Sciences
2 East 63rd Street
New York, New York 10021

THE NEW YORK ACADEMY OF SCIENCES
(Founded in 1817)

BOARD OF GOVERNORS, September 2001–September 2002

TORSTEN N. WIESEL, *Chairman of the Board*
JOHN F. NIBLACK, *Vice Chairman of the Board*
BILL GREEN, *Past Chairman*
RODNEY W. NICHOLS, *President and CEO* [ex officio]

Honorary Life Governors
WILLIAM T. GOLDEN   JOSHUA LEDERBERG
JOHN T. MORGAN, *Treasurer*

Governors

ELEANOR BAUM	D. ALLAN BROMLEY	KAREN E. BURKE
LAWRENCE B. BUTTENWIESER	PRAVEEN CHAUDHARI	
JOHN H. GIBBONS	MICHAEL GOLDEN	RONALD L. GRAHAM
JACQUELINE LEO	WILLIAM J. McDONOUGH	SANDRA PANEM
RICHARD RAVITCH	RICHARD A. RIFKIND	JOHN J. ROCHE
SARA LEE SCHUPF	JAMES H. SIMONS	LEE VANCE

HELENE L. KAPLAN, *Counsel* [ex officio]   NANCY B. EISENBERG, *Interim Secretary* [ex officio]

SELECTIVE ESTROGEN RECEPTOR MODULATORS (SERMs)

ANNALS OF THE NEW YORK ACADEMY OF SCIENCES
Volume 949

SELECTIVE ESTROGEN RECEPTOR MODULATORS (SERMs)

Edited by Marietta Anthony, Barbara K. Dunn, and Sherry Sherman

The New York Academy of Sciences
New York, New York
2001

Copyright © 2001 by the New York Academy of Sciences. All rights reserved. Under the provisions of the United States Copyright Act of 1976, individual readers of the Annals are permitted to make fair use of the material in them for teaching or research. Permission is granted to quote from the Annals provided that the customary acknowledgment is made of the source. Material in the Annals may be republished only by permission of the Academy. Address inquiries to the Permissions Department (editorial@nyas.org) at the New York Academy of Sciences.

Copying fees: For each copy of an article made beyond the free copying permitted under Section 107 or 108 of the 1976 Copyright Act, a fee should be paid through the Copyright Clearance Center, Inc., 222 Rosewood Drive, Danvers, MA 01923 (www.copyright.com).

♾ The paper used in this publication meets the minimum requirements of the American National Standard for Information Sciences—Permanence of Paper for Printed Library Materials, ANSI Z39.48-1984.

Library of Congress Cataloging-in-Publication Data

Selective estrogen receptor modulators (SERMs) / edited by Marietta Anthony, Barbara K. Dunn, and Sherry Sherman.
    p. cm. -- (Annals of the New York Academy of Sciences, ISSN 0077-8923 ; v. 949)
"This volume is the result of a National Institutes of Health workshop entitled Selective estrogen receptor modulators (SERMs) held April 26–28, 2000 in Bethesda, Md."--Contents p.
Includes bibliographical references and index.
ISBN 1-57331-358-0 (cloth : alk. paper) -- ISBN 1-57331-359-9 (pbk. : alk. paper)
1. Selective estrogen receptor modulators--Congresses. I. Anthony, Marietta. II. Dunn, Barbara K. III. Sherman, Sherry. IV. Series

Q11 .N5 vol. 949
[RM295]
500s--dc21
[615'.366]   2001051416

GYAT/BMP
Printed in the United States of America
ISBN 1-57331-358-0 (cloth)
ISBN 1-57331-359-9 (paper)
ISSN 0077-8923

ANNALS OF THE NEW YORK ACADEMY OF SCIENCES

Volume 949
December 2001

SELECTIVE ESTROGEN RECEPTOR MODULATORS (SERMs)

Editors
MARIETTA ANTHONY, BARBARA K. DUNN, AND SHERRY SHERMAN

This volume is the result of the **NIH Workshop on Selective Estrogen Receptor Modulators (SERMs)** held April 26–28, 2000 in Bethesda, Maryland.

CONTENTS

Preface. *By* SHERRY SHERMAN xi

Part I. Basic Biology of SERMs

The Basic Biology of SERMs: Introduction. *By* RONALD MARGOLIS 1

Nuclear Receptors, Coregulators, Ligands, and Selective Receptor Modulators: Making Sense of the Patchwork Quilt. *By* NEIL J. MCKENNA AND BERT W. O'MALLEY 3

Structure-Function Relationships in Estrogen Receptors and the Characterization of Novel Selective Estrogen Receptor Modulators with Unique Pharmacological Profiles. *By* BENITA S. KATZENELLENBOGEN, JUN SUN, WILLIAM R. HARRINGTON, DENNIS M. KRAICHELY, DESHANIE GANESSUNKER, AND JOHN A. KATZENELLENBOGEN 6

Capitalizing on the Complexities of Estrogen Receptor Pharmacology in the Quest for the Perfect SERM. *By* DONALD P. MCDONNELL, CHING-YI CHANG, AND JOHN D. NORRIS 16

Developing Animal Models for Analyzing SERM Activity. *By* JUDITH M.A. EMMEN AND KENNETH S. KORACH 36

Androgen Receptor: Structural Domains and Functional Dynamics after Ligand-Receptor Interaction. *By* ARUN K. ROY, RAKESH K. TYAGI, CHUNG S. SONG, YAN LAVROVSKY, SOON C. AHN, TAE-SUNG OH, AND BANDANA CHATTERJEE 44

Tissue-Specific Estrogen Biosynthesis and Metabolism. *By* EVAN R. SIMPSON, COLIN CLYNE, CAROLINE SPEED, GARY RUBIN, AND SERDAR BULUN 58

Part II. Cancer Treatment and Prevention

Cancer Treatment and Prevention: Introduction. *By* BARBARA K. DUNN AND BARRY KRAMER 68

The Past, Present, and Future of Selective Estrogen Receptor Modulation. *By* V. CRAIG JORDAN 72

Use of SERMs for the Adjuvant Therapy of Early-Stage Breast Cancer. *By* ANTONIO C. WOLFF AND NANCY E. DAVIDSON 80

Breast Cancer Prevention with Selective Estrogen Receptor Modulators: A Perspective. *By* KATHLEEN I. PRITCHARD 89

The Role of Tamoxifen in Breast Cancer Prevention: Issues Sparked by the NSABP Breast Cancer Prevention Trial (P-1). *By* NORMAN WOLMARK AND BARBARA K. DUNN 99

The Royal Marsden Hospital (RMH) Trial: Key Points and Remaining Questions. *By* TREVOR J. POWLES 109

The Italian Breast Cancer Prevention Trial with Tamoxifen: Findings and New Perspectives. *By* ALIANA GUERRIERI-GONZAGA, ARIANNA GALLI, NICOLE ROTMENSZ, AND ANDREA DECENSI 113

A Brief Review of the International Breast Cancer Intervention Study (IBIS), the Other Current Breast Cancer Prevention Trials, and Proposals for Future Trials. *By* J. CUZICK 123

The MORE Trial—Multiple Outcomes for Raloxifene Evaluation: Breast Cancer as a Secondary End Point—Implications for Prevention. *By* MAURA N. DICKLER AND LARRY NORTON 134

Quality of Life and Tamoxifen in a Breast Cancer Prevention Trial: A Summary of Findings from the NSABP P-1 Study. *By* RICHARD DAY 143

Part III. Cardiovascular Disease

Selective Estrogen Receptor Modulators and Cardiovascular Disease: Introduction. *By* DAVID J. GORDON 151

Cardiovascular Trials of Estrogen Replacement Therapy. *By* DAVID M. HERRINGTON AND KAREN POTVIN KLEIN 153

The Effects of Estrogen and Selective Estrogen Receptor Modulators on Cardiovascular Risk Factors. *By* BRIAN W. WALSH 163

Selective Estrogen Receptor Modulator Effects on Serum Lipoproteins and Vascular Function in Postmenopausal Women and in Hypercholesterolemic Men. *By* ARNON BLUM AND RICHARD O. CANNON, III 168

Effects of Estrogen and Selective Estrogen Receptor Modulators on Hemostasis and Inflammation: Potential Differences among Drugs. *By* MARY CUSHMAN 175

Rationale and Overview of the Raloxifene Use for the Heart (RUTH) Trial. *By* LORI MOSCA 181

Part IV. Osteoporosis

Prevention and Treatment of Osteoporosis: Introduction. *By* SARALYN MARK AND JHUMKA GUPTA 186

Preventing and Treating Osteoporosis: Strategies at the Millennium. *By* SHERRY SHERMAN 188

The Paradox of Small Changes in Bone Density and Reductions in Risk of Fracture with Raloxifene. *By* STEVEN R. CUMMINGS 198

Part IV. Cognitive Function

SERMs, Estrogen, and Cognitive Function: Introduction. *By* ANDREW A. MONJAN 202

Effects of Hormone Replacement Therapy on Cognitive and Brain Aging. *By* SUSAN M. RESNICK AND PAULINE M. MAKI 203

Estrogens, Selective Estrogen Receptor Modulators, and Dementia: What Is the Evidence? *By* KRISTINE YAFFE 215

Estrogen Replacement Therapy for the Potential Treatment or Prevention of Alzheimer's Disease. *By* MARILYN M. MILLER, ANDREW A. MONJAN, AND NEIL S. BUCKHOLTZ 223

Part V. Reproductive and Related Endocrine Considerations

Reproductive and Related Endocrine Considerations: Introduction. *By* ESTELLA C. PARROTT 235

The Effect of SERMs on the Endometrium. *By* STEVEN R. GOLDSTEIN ... 237

Effect of Selective Estrogen Receptor Modulators on Reproductive Tissues Other Than Endometrium. *By* SUSAN L. HENDRIX AND S. GENE MCNEELEY 243

The Effect of Selective Estrogen Receptor Modulators on Parameters of the Hypothalamic-Pituitary-Gonadal Axis. *By* LEO PLOUFFE, JR. AND SURESH SIDDHANTI 251

Part VI. Addressing the Benefit/Risk Ratio in Taking SERMs from Laboratory to Clinic

Translation of Basic Research—Finding the Perfect SERM: Introduction. *By* FRANCIS L. BELLINO AND LORETTA FINNEGAN 259

What Would Be the Properties of an Ideal SERM? *By* MARIETTA ANTHONY, J. KOUDY WILLIAMS, AND BARBARA K. DUNN 261

Weighing the Benefits and Risks in Clinical Trials and Practice: Introduction. *By* WORTA MCCASKILL-STEVENS 279

Benefit/Risk Assessment of SERM Therapy: Clinical Trial versus Clinical Practice Settings. *By* JOSEPH P. COSTANTINO 280

The Estimation and Use of Absolute Risk for Weighing the Risks and Benefits of Selective Estrogen Receptor Modulators for Preventing Breast Cancer. *By* MITCHELL H. GAIL 286

SERMs, Ethnicity, and Clinical Trials: Opportunities and Challenges. *By* ANNE L. TAYLOR 292

Raloxifene: Risks and Benefits. *By* ELIZABETH BARRETT-CONNOR 295

Defining Benefits and Risks for SERMs in Clinical Trials and Clinical Practice. *By* SUSAN R. JOHNSON, BARBARA K. DUNN, AND MARIETTA ANTHONY 304

Part VII. SERM Development in Industry, Academia, the NIH, and the FDA

Roles of Industry, Government, and Academia in SERM Development: Introduction. *By* MARIETTA ANTHONY AND KAREN JOHNSON 315

Developing a SERM: Stringent Preclinical Selection Criteria Leading to an Acceptable Candidate (WAY-140424) for Clinical Evaluation. *By* BARRY S. KOMM AND C. RICHARD LYTTLE 317

The Breast Cancer Continuum: Insights from the Tamoxifen Trials Impact Future Drug Development Strategies. *By* JERRY P. LEWIS 327

The Cancer Therapy Evaluation Program (CTEP) at the National Cancer Institute: Industry Collaborations in New Agent Development. *By* SHERRY S. ANSHER AND RAMI SCHARF 333

FDA Review Practices and Priorities for Drugs Used in Cancer Treatment. *By* KEN KOBAYASHI AND ROBERT J. DELAP 341

Tamoxifen for the Reduction in the Incidence of Breast Cancer in Women at High Risk for Breast Cancer. *By* SUSAN FLAMM HONIG 345

Negotiating Industry-Sponsored Clinical Trial Agreements: A View from the Trenches. *By* NIKKI J. ZAPOL 349

* * *

Conclusions: Considerations Regarding SERMs. *By* BARBARA K. DUNN, MARIETTA ANTHONY, SHERRY SHERMAN, AND JOSEPH P. COSTANTINO 352

Opportunites for Future Research. *By* SHERRY SHERMAN AND BARBARA K. DUNN 366

Everything You Wanted to Know about SERMs

Timeline of Key Events in SERM Development 377

Estrogen Receptor–Active Compounds, Estrogens, and SERMs, of Historical and Current Interest 381

Model of Estrogen Receptor (ER) Action 382

Action of SERMs in Target Tissues 383

* * *

Glossary of Abbreviations 385
Index of Contributors 389

Financial assistance was received from:
- **NATIONAL INSTITUTE ON AGING, NIH**
- **NATIONAL CANCER INSTITUTE/DIVISION OF CANCER PREVENTION, NIH**
- **NATIONAL HEART, LUNG AND BLOOD INSTITUTE, NIH**
- **NATIONAL INSTITUTE OF DIABETES, DIGESTIVE AND KIDNEY DISEASES, NIH**
- **NATIONAL INSTITUTE OF ARTHRITIS AND MUSCULOSKELETAL AND SKIN DISEASES, NIH**
- **NATIONAL INSTITUTE OF DENTAL AND CRANIOFACIAL RESEARCH, NIH**
- **NATIONAL INSTITUTE OF ENVIRONMENTAL HEALTH SCIENCES, NIH**
- **NATIONAL INSTITUTE OF CHILD HEALTH AND HUMAN DEVELOPMENT, NIH**
- **THE NIH OFFICE OF RESEARCH ON WOMEN'S HEALTH**
- **THE DEPARTMENT OF HEALTH AND HUMAN SERVICES/OFFICE ON WOMEN'S HEALTH**
- **THE AMERICAN FEDERATION FOR AGING RESEARCH**

> The New York Academy of Sciences believes it has a responsibility to provide an open forum for discussion of scientific questions. The positions taken by the participants in the reported conferences are their own and not necessarily those of the Academy. The Academy has no intent to influence legislation by providing such forums.

Planning Committee

MARIETTA ANTHONY, Ph.D.,[a]
  Office of Research on Women's Health,
  NIH

JOANNA BADINELLI, M.Ed.,
  Clinical Endocrinology and
  Osteoporosis Research, National
  Institute on Aging, NIH

FRANK L. BELLINO, Ph.D.,
  Biology of Aging Program, National
  Institute on Aging, NIH

STEVE CUMMINGS, M.D.,
  Department of Epidemiology and
  Biostatistics, University of California,
  San Francisco

PATRICE DAVIS, B.B.A.,
  Clinical Endocrinology and
  Osteoporosis Research, National
  Institute on Aging, NIH

BARBARA K. DUNN, M.D., Ph.D.,
  Basic Prevention Science Research
  Group, Division of Cancer Prevention,
  National Cancer Institute, NIH

LORETTA P. FINNEGAN, M.D.,
  Office of Research on Women's Health,
  NIH

LESLIE FORD, M.D.,
  Clinical Research, National Cancer
  Institute, NIH

DAVID GORDON, M.D., Ph.D.,
  Division of Heart and Vascular
  Diseases, National Heart, Lung, and
  Blood Institute, NIH

KENNETH GRUBER, Ph.D.,
  Chronic Diseases Branch, National
  Institute of Dental and Craniofacial
  Research, NIH

JERROLD HEINDEL, Ph.D.,
  National Institue of Environmental
  Health Sciences, NIH

KAREN JOHNSON, M.D., Ph.D., M.P.H.,
  Breast and Gynecologic Cancer
  Research Group, Division of Cancer
  Prevention, National Cancer Institute,
  NIH

RONALD MARGOLIS, Ph.D.,
  Molecular Endocrinology,
  National Institute of Diabetes and
  Digestive and Kidney Diseases, NIH

SARA LYNN MARK, M.D.,
  Office on Women's Health,
  Department of Health and Human
  Services

WORTA MCCASKILL-STEVENS,
  M.D., M.S., Division of Cancer
  Prevention, National Cancer Institute,
  NIH

JOAN A. MCGOWAN, Ph.D.,
  Musculoskeletal Diseases Branch,
  National Institute of Arthritis and
  Musculoskeletal and Skin Diseases,
  NIH

ANDREW MONJAN, Ph.D., M.P.H.,
  Neurobiology of Aging Branch,
  National Institute on Aging, NIH

ESTELLA PARROTT, M.D., M.P.H.,
  Reproductive Medicine Gynecology
  Program, Center for Population
  Research, National Institute of Child
  Health and Human Development,
  NIH

VIVIAN PINN, M.D.,
  Office of Research on Women's Health,
  NIH

LINDA POTTERN, Ph.D., M.P.H.,
  Women's Health Initiative,
  National Heart, Lung, and Blood
  Institute, NIH

SHERRY SHERMAN, Ph.D.,
  Clinical Endocrinology and
  Osteoporosis Research,
  National Institute on Aging,
  NIH

CYNTHIA WHITMAN, B.S.,
  Basic Prevention Research Group,
  Division of Cancer Prevention,
  National Cancer Institute,
  NIH

[a]Present affiliation: Women's Health Research, Georgetown University Medical Center.

Preface

The value of postmenopausal therapy with estrogen (ERT for hysterectomized women) or estrogen/progestin (HRT for women with a uterus) in the prevention and treatment of menopause-related symptoms and accelerated bone loss is well established. Furthermore, observational studies have demonstrated that ERT/HRT users have a reduced risk of age-associated diseases or conditions such as osteoporotic fractures, cardiovascular disease, and Alzheimer's disease. However, despite the potentially profound benefits indicated in epidemiologic studies, recent randomized controlled trials have found an absence of benefit in reducing the risk of myocardial infarctions and stroke, or in preventing or reversing Alzheimer's disease. Importantly, ERT/HRT use has been associated with serious adverse events on the cardiovascular system in both primary and secondary cardiovascular disease prevention studies. Thus, the use of ERT/HRT for even its approved indications is, and probably will remain, limited. In addition, adherence is poor, with the overwhelming majority of women discontinuing treatment because of unwanted bleeding and other side effects and/or fears of cancer of the breast or uterus. Last, estrogen therapy is a specific agent and has limited usefulness as a preventive or treatment strategy in men because of its potential feminizing effects.

A selective estrogen receptor modulator (SERM) is a molecule that binds with high affinity to the estrogen receptor (ER) but has tissue-specific effects distinct from estradiol, acting as an estrogen agonist in some tissues and as an antagonist in others. The development of SERMs that selectively interact with specific receptors and specific coactivators and corepressors in specific organ systems offers the possibility of improving the risk/benefit profile relative to hormone replacement therapy and perhaps even extending the use of these analogues to men.

Several SERMS are under development, and four—clomiphene, tamoxifen, raloxifene, and toremifene—are already in clinical use. Clomiphene citrate was introduced in the early 1960s for the purpose of ovulation induction and, while limited to premenopausal women, has remained the most widely used medication in the management of anovulatory infertility. Tamoxifen and toremifene are approved for treatment of breast cancer in both pre- and postmenopausal women. Broadly used throughout the world to treat breast cancer, tamoxifen received FDA approval in 1997 for risk reduction in women 35 years and older who are at high risk for breast cancer. Raloxifene was approved in 1997 for the prevention and, subsequently, for the treatment of osteoporosis and has been shown to substantially reduce the risk of invasive breast cancer in three years of follow up in the Multiple Outcomes of Raloxifene Evaluation (MORE) Study, which enrolled women at high risk of osteoporosis. Raloxifene is now being tested for equivalence to tamoxifen in breast cancer risk reduction in the Study of Tamoxifen and Raloxifene (STAR).

Although approved SERMs like tamoxifen and raloxifene have great present or potential clinical utility in the breast cancer and/or osteoporosis prevention settings, widespread use in risk reduction for currently approved indications has been limited by an increased risk of adverse events or side effects. Disadvantages of tamoxifen include an increased risk of endometrial cancer and venous thromboembolic disease as well as detrimental effects on quality of life (such as hot flashes) and potential unknowns about the risk/benefit equation vis-à-vis other tissues and physiologic systems. While raloxifene has an improved safety profile in that it does not increase the risk of endometrial cancer like tamoxifen, it also increases the risk of hot flashes and venous thromboembolic disease, and its cardiovascular and cognitive effects are uncertain.

The NIH Workshop on the Selective Estrogen Receptor Modulators (SERMs), convened April 26–28, 2000, was a multidisciplinary workshop that sought to (1) address the role of the estrogen receptor in physiologic and pathologic processes involving multiple organ systems; and (2) determine the potential for, and utility of, continued development/refinement of pharmacologic approaches to the selective modification of estrogen receptor action in the prevention and treatment of disease. The content of this workshop encompassed ongoing SERM research ranging from basic science to clinical trials in disease areas supported by multiple institutes of the National Institutes of Health. The overarching goals were to bring together multidisciplinary aspects of SERM research with an eye to identifying pivotal questions and formulating future projects that cross disease boundaries and potentially, at the outset, incorporate multiple disease end points.

The presentations and panel discussions were designed to (1) summarize key state-of-the-art basic and clinical findings on the role played by the estrogen receptor and its modulation in multiple physiologic systems; (2) explore the potential for future innovations in the selective modification of estrogen receptor action(s) to prevent chronic diseases in older individuals and promote healthy aging; and (3) identify pivotal issues, research gaps, and a potential agenda for future NIH research on estrogen receptor action and related intervention strategies to extend the beneficial clinical outcomes.

Putting together this workshop was a strenuous, but gratifying, experience for all of us on the Planning Committee. Each member brought to the program diverse, yet complementary, perspectives; and together we developed the intertwining, multidisciplinary architecture of the workshop and its proceedings. We thank the members of the Planning Committee for their generous contribution of time, for their participation in the many conference calls and meetings, and for their commitment to making this workshop a thought-provoking, multidimensional, and productive happening. The enthusiastic involvement of, and thoughtful exchanges between, the participants were essential to achieving the workshop's aims, and we are grateful for the skillful leadership of the session chairs and panel moderators for their success in stimulating discussion and helping identify new opportunities for future research. We wish to acknowledge Steve Cummings for all his energetic and insightful contributions to the design and implementation of this workshop. Craig Jordan receives our thanks for his valuable assistance in developing a concise historical orientation and timeline of SERM research and development. Patrice Davis is to be commended for her diligent efforts in facilitating the extensive communications and logistics underlying our ambitious workshop and these proceedings. We heartily thank Joanna Badinelli for all her logistic and moral support in this very complex endeavor. The authors owe much gratitude to Maryetta Lancaster for the superb graphic representations of important scientific information that she prepared for these proceedings. Importantly, this volume could not have been produced without the ready cooperation of the contributors, and we are indebted to them for their scholarly manuscripts.

Last, it is impossible to adequately acknowledge the indefatigable efforts of my co-editors, Marietta Anthony and Barbara Dunn, whose commitment to produce a workshop proceedings of excellence will ensure that the substance and spirit of this remarkable conference will be gloriously captured in these pages.

Support for the wide diversity of ideas and approaches enriching this multidisciplinary workshop was made possible by the National Institute on Aging; National Cancer Institute/Division of Cancer Prevention; National Heart, Lung and Blood Institute; National Institute of Diabetes, Digestive and Kidney Diseases; National Institute of Arthritis and Musculoskeletal and Skin Diseases; National Institute of Dental and Craniofacial Research; National Institute of Environmental Health Sciences; National Institute of Child Health and Human Development; the NIH Office of Research on Women's Health; the Office of Women's Health (Department of Health and Human Services); and the American Federation for Aging Research.

SHERRY SHERMAN, Ph.D.
National Institute on Aging
National Institutes of Health

The Basic Biology of SERMs
Introduction

RONALD MARGOLIS

National Institute of Diabetes and Digestive Diseases, National Institutes of Health, Bethesda, Maryland 20892, USA

Major conceptual and technological advances in biomedical science, fueled by advances in molecular biology, proteomics, and bioinformatics, have provided hope that enhanced basic understanding can lead to new treatments in the clinic. Nowhere is that more apparent than in the area of molecular endocrinology and the study of the nuclear receptor superfamily. These important ligand-dependent and independent transcription factors are responsible for modulating tissue and cellular responses to a host of hormones and metabolites. Examples include the orphan receptors such as the peroxisome proliferator-activated receptor (PPAR), which mediates responses to lipid substrates in fat, and other, cells, as well as the steroid receptors such as the estrogen receptor (ER), androgen receptor (AR), and glucocorticoid receptor (GR). Their involvement in development, metabolism, and reproduction has been well documented, with new roles emerging often as the result of targeted gene knockout models in the mouse and the unraveling of genomes of model organisms and humans. It has long been known that nuclear receptors play important roles in diseases, including cancer, heart disease, diabetes, obesity, and osteoporosis. A great deal of attention has been directed to key systems, such as the role of PPARs in obesity and diabetes and steroid receptors in breast (ER) and prostate (AR) cancer, as well as osteoporosis. The emphasis on these systems has spurred research efforts designed to fully understand the responses of specific tissues to these receptors, as well as to develop ligands designed to modulate those responses.

Whereas once the state of the art suggested that hormone binding to a receptor resulted in activation of the receptor and subsequent cellular response, more recent understanding has revealed a picture that is far more complex. Several classes of cytoplasmic and nuclear accessory proteins have been discovered that regulate the appearance of the receptor in the cytoplasm and/or nucleus, and modulate nuclear localization, DNA binding, and ultimately activation or repression of gene expression. The identification of some nuclear accessory proteins as coactivators and corepressors has opened a pathway to greater understanding of hormone action. The need now is to define how these various factors are integrated to establish tissue and cellular specificity.

Address for correspondence: Ronald Margolis, Ph.D., Senior Advisor, Molecular Endocrinology, National Institute of Diabetes and Digestive Diseases, National Institutes of Health**,** 6707 Democracy Boulevard, Room 6107, Bethesda, MD 20892. Voice: 301-594-8819; fax: 301-435-6047.

rm76f@nih.gov

While hormone replacement therapy (HRT), both estrogen and estrogen/progestin, has long been used to delay or reverse some of the changes attendant to menopause, epidemiologic and clinical research have elucidated potential long-term risks associated with such therapy. The result has been an outgrowth of research to develop compounds that elicit important and tissue-specific functions of many of the steroid receptors without unneeded or deleterious effects. This, in turn, has led to the definition and investigation of an entirely new class of compound: the selective receptor modulator (SRM). Selective estrogen receptor modulators (SERMs), such as tamoxifen, were the first to be used in the clinic. SERMs, with tamoxifen as the prototype, have undergone their major development in relation to their application to breast cancer. When positive effects were also noted in bone, further development of second, and later, generations of SERMs and SRMs accelerated. The operative concept has been to develop compounds that drive the targeted receptor to a form that allows for tissue- and gene-specific action. Indeed, when it was understood that tissue-specific metabolic conversion of the ligand (e.g., estrogen) is an important part of normal physiology as well as disease development/progression, it became clear that compounds that could affect this conversion, such as selective aromatase modulators (SAMs), could also be useful in the clinic.

What this research on the basic structure and function of nuclear receptors has shown us is the great promise they hold for development of new interventions to prevent or treat major diseases. The prime example set by the development of early generations of SERMs (e.g., tamoxifen) has set the tone for future developmental work. The task now before us is to better define where SRMs may be useful, how best to use them, and how to develop even more specific compounds with important therapeutic applications.

Nuclear Receptors, Coregulators, Ligands, and Selective Receptor Modulators

Making Sense of the Patchwork Quilt

NEIL J. McKENNA AND BERT W. O'MALLEY

Department of Molecular and Cellular Biology, Baylor College of Medicine, Houston, Texas 77030, USA

ABSTRACT: Nuclear receptors are ligand-inducible transcription factors that specifically regulate the expression of target genes involved in metabolism, development, and reproduction. Their primary function is to mediate the transcriptional response in target cells to hormones such as the sex steroids (progestins, estrogens, and androgens), adrenal steroids (glucocorticoids and mineralocorticoids), vitamin D_3, and thyroid and retinoid (9-*cis* and all-*trans*) hormones, in addition to a variety of other metabolic ligands. More than 100 nuclear receptors are known to exist and, together, these proteins comprise the single largest family of metazoan transcription factors, the nuclear receptor superfamily. Their natural ligands, as well as synthetic ligands (selective receptor modulators, or SRMs), are known to influence the interaction of these receptors with accessory molecules called *coregulators*.

KEYWORDS: nuclear receptors; coactivators; SERMs

The tripartite structure of nuclear receptors (NRs) is defined by a central sequence-specific DNA binding domain, an N-terminal constitutive activation function (AF-1), and a distinct C-terminal ligand-dependent activation function (AF-2). NR coregulators are defined as cellular factors recruited by the AF-1 and AF-2 domains of NRs for efficient transcriptional control of promoters regulated by their cognate DNA response elements. Intensively studied coactivators include members of the SRC-1 (steroid receptor coactivator) family (SRC-1/NCoA-1, GRIP-1/TIF2/SRC-2, and p/CIP/ACTR/AIB-1/RAC-3/SRC-3), PBP/TRAP220, and CREB-binding protein (CBP), while the functions of NCoR and SMRT have been well characterized in the case of corepressors.[1] Generally speaking, coactivators mediate the functions of activated receptors, whereas corepressors mediate the repressive effects of inactive receptors.

Natural ligands for NRs have been historically well characterized, particularly so in the case of the estrogen receptor (ER). More recently, it has been appreciated that synthetic selective receptor modulators (SRMs) can influence NR function in a manner that has profound pharmacological and clinical consequences. Tamoxifen is

---

Address for correspondence: Bert W. O'Malley, M.D., Department of Molecular and Cellular Biology, Baylor College of Medicine, One Baylor Plaza, Houston, TX 77030. Voice: 713-798-6205; fax: 713-798-5599.

berto@bcm.tmc.edu

the most popular prototype for a new arsenal of drugs, termed selective ER modulators (SERMs), which elicit a complex array of tissue-specific effects. Many of these compounds share the beneficial effects of estrogen on bone density and plasma levels of atherogenic lipoproteins like low-density lipoproteins and lipoprotein A. The elaborate pharmacology of the SERMs, however, presents obstacles to their broader clinical applications. Consider as an example the use of tamoxifen in breast cancer treatment. ER expression earmarks a primary breast tumor for an initially positive prognosis and the probability of a good response to hormone ablation therapy. Of the ER-positive breast tumors selected for tamoxifen treatment, roughly 70% will respond initially. As treatment progresses, however, a considerable proportion of tumors will acquire hormone resistance and fail to respond to tamoxifen. To compound matters, tamoxifen, while opposing estrogen activity in the breast, is an estrogen mimetic in the uterus, an important consideration in its prophylactic use against breast cancer. Conversely, raloxifene, an FDA-approved second-generation SERM, while estrogenic in its reduction of the severity of postmenopausal osteoporosis, is, broadly speaking, antiestrogenic in the breast and uterus.

Clearly, SERM effects are determined to a considerable extent both by intertissue differences in the expression of specific factors as well as by changes in the levels of these factors in a single tissue over time. The recent characterization of NR coregulators has provided clues to discern the puzzling patchwork pharmacology of SERMs. To more clearly understand the potential role of NR coregulators in determining SERM effects, attention has focused upon the AF-2 in the C-terminal ligand-binding domain of NRs. The hormone-dependent recruitment of coactivators by NRs has been attributed principally to the interaction of their NR boxes with a ligand-induced hydrophobic surface in AF-2 of NRs. The SERMs, tamoxifen and raloxifene, appear to oppose the action of estrogen by sequestering a critical AF-2 helix, helix 12, in a conformation sterically inhospitable to coactivator binding.[2] However, recent evidence suggests that antiestrogens may function not only by preventing coactivator binding, but by promoting corepressor binding (silencing). This indicates that the activity of ER bound to a specific SERM may be sensitive ultimately to the competing pool of coactivators and corepressors in that tissue. Intuitively, this equilibrium is itself a function of the tissue expression fingerprint of coregulators and their intrinsic affinity for that SERM-bound receptor. It can be appreciated then that SERM-specific manipulation of ER AF-2 topography, particularly in the case of helix 12, is an important determinant of coregulator selectivity. (See FIG. 1.)

In light of these observations, the challenges for endocrinologists and clinicians are twofold. First, how can the opposing effects of SRMs in different tissues in the body be reconciled and how can these characteristics be manipulated in order to improve prospects for their future therapeutic applications? Second, can novel SRMs be synthesized whose tissue-specific effects can be accurately predicted? A primary goal will be the establishment of an *in vivo* model system in which the effects of these candidate therapeutics can be evaluated in terms of their toxicity and overall physiological impact. Crossing of null mutants of coactivators into these models will permit the construction of comprehensive microarray databases of tissue expression fingerprints of coregulators. Such databases will be of great benefit in predicting tissue-specific responses to individual ligands and SRMs. Information gleaned from these sources would find application not only in the classic hormone-dependent cancers of the breast, ovary, and prostate, but also in disorders of carbo-

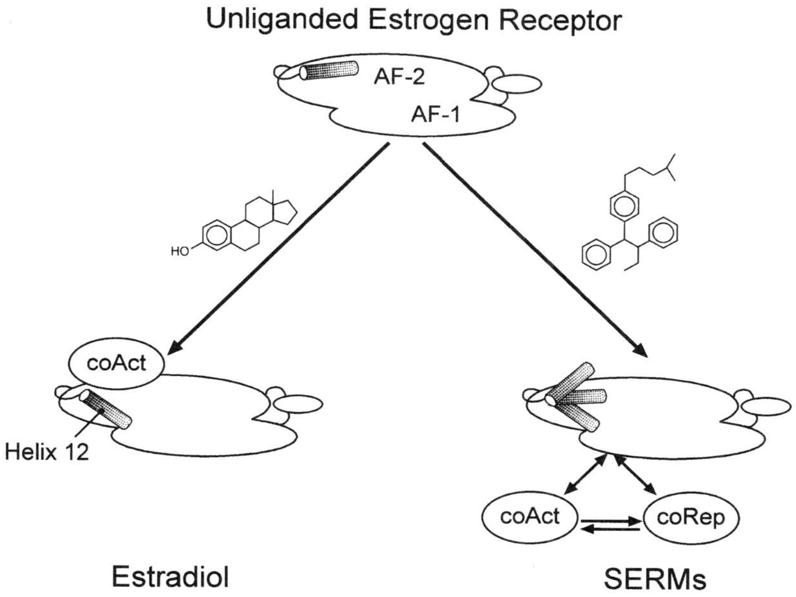

FIGURE 1. NR coregulators modulate the transcriptional potential of ER activated by estradiol or SERMs. SERM-specific variation in the topography of AF-2, particularly in the case of helix 12, appears to be an important influence on the selectivity of ER coregulator interactions. A variety of intermediate conformations of helix 12 elicited by binding of different SERMs is likely to contribute to the spectrum of tissue-specific effects of these molecules. In addition, tissue-specific differences in steady state coactivator/corepressor levels may also be key factors in SERM pharmacology. coAct = coactivator; coRep = corepressor.

hydrate and lipid metabolism, key players in which (cytokines and JAK/STATs) are known to interface with NR signaling pathways. We anticipate that this field will continue to be a rich vein of scientific and clinical revelations, whose exploration will be of the greatest benefit to therapeutic approaches in a host of diseases well into this century.

ACKNOWLEDGMENTS

N. J. McKenna is a recipient of a Department of Defense Breast Cancer Research Program Postdoctoral Award.

REFERENCES

1. MCKENNA, N.J., R.B. LANZ & B.W. O'MALLEY. 1999. Nuclear receptor coregulators: cellular and molecular biology. Endocr. Rev. **20:** 321–344.
2. SHIAU, A.K., D. BARSTAD, P.M. LORIA *et al.* 1998. The structural basis of estrogen receptor/coactivator recognition and the antagonism of this interaction by tamoxifen. Cell **95:** 927–937.

Structure-Function Relationships in Estrogen Receptors and the Characterization of Novel Selective Estrogen Receptor Modulators with Unique Pharmacological Profiles

BENITA S. KATZENELLENBOGEN,[a] JUN SUN,[a] WILLIAM R. HARRINGTON,[a] DENNIS M. KRAICHELY,[a] DESHANIE GANESSUNKER,[a] AND JOHN A. KATZENELLENBOGEN[b]

Departments of [a]Molecular and Integrative Physiology and [b]Chemistry, University of Illinois and College of Medicine, Urbana, Illinois 61801, USA

ABSTRACT: This article summarizes recent research on the development of estrogen receptor alpha (ERα) and estrogen receptor beta (ERβ) subtype-selective ligands based on our understanding of structure-activity relationships in these two estrogen receptors and differences in their ligand binding domains and activation function domains. The use of these ligands should enable greater understanding of the unique biologies mediated by ERα versus ERβ and may, as well, provide selective estrogen receptor modulators having unique biological and pharmacological profiles optimal for prevention and treatment of breast cancer, for menopausal hormone replacement, for prevention of osteoporosis, and for potential cardiovascular benefit.

KEYWORDS: ERα; ERβ; SERMs; coactivators

This has been an exciting time for research on selective estrogen receptor modulators (SERMs),[1–3] ligands that bind to the estrogen receptor, yet differ markedly in their stimulatory and/or inhibitory effects in different tissues. The intriguing tissue-selective actions displayed by SERMs are of great biomedical importance because they portend the development of novel pharmaceutical agents having optimal pharmacological profiles for prevention and treatment of breast cancer, for menopausal hormone replacement, for prevention of osteoporosis, and for potential cardiovascular benefit.

SERMs can demonstrate remarkable differences in activity in the various estrogen target tissues, functioning as estrogen agonists in some tissues, but as antagonists in others. Underlying this important biology are two estrogen receptors (ERα and ERβ) encoded by different genes, numerous coregulators that modulate the activity of the ERs, and the realization that different SERM compounds can have not only

---

Address for correspondence: Dr. Benita S. Katzenellenbogen, Department of Molecular and Integrative Physiology, University of Illinois, 524 Burrill Hall, 407 South Goodwin Avenue, Urbana, IL 61801-3704. Voice: 217-333-9769; fax: 217-244-9906.
katzenel@life.uiuc.edu

dramatic, but also distinct effects on the pharmacologies and biologies of ER-mediated events. These recent advances elucidating the tripartite nature of the actions of estrogens provide a good basis for understanding these tissue-selective actions of SERMs.[4–6]

As discussed in this article, the development of optimal SERMs must be viewed in the context of two ER subtypes that have differing affinities and responsiveness to various SERMs and differing tissue distribution and effectiveness at various gene regulatory sites. In addition, cellular, biochemical, and structural approaches have shown that the nature of the ligand markedly affects the conformation assumed by the ER-ligand complex, thereby regulating the recruitment of different coregulator proteins and receptor modifications by various protein kinases and growth factors that can greatly affect the activity of the receptor. These interactions and subsequent changes in the receptor, which determine the magnitude of the transcriptional and other responses and the potency of different SERMs, are all determined by the chemical nature of the particular SERM and its induction of different receptor conformations that establish all of the subsequent receptor interactions and activities.

EXQUISITE PRECISION IN ER REGULATION BY LIGAND

Recent studies highlight the exquisite precision that characterizes ER regulation by ligand, demonstrating that small changes in ligand structure can have major effects on the biological character of the ligand-receptor complex (FIG. 1). Thus, different ligands working through the two ER subtypes, ERα and ERβ, can exhibit very distinct pharmacologies at different target genes. The pharmacology of nuclear receptors is tripartite, involving not just the interaction of ligand with receptor, but also the recruitment by this ligand-receptor complex of a variety of coregulators, allowing differential interactions with different response elements to generate the complex and distinctive pharmacology of SERMs.[4]

The recent appreciation of this tripartite nature of estrogen action has spawned two major approaches to the regulation of ER activity, with the goal of obtaining SERMs having optimal profiles of tissue selectivity for medical therapeutic uses (FIG. 2). The first approach, on which we have focused predominantly, involves

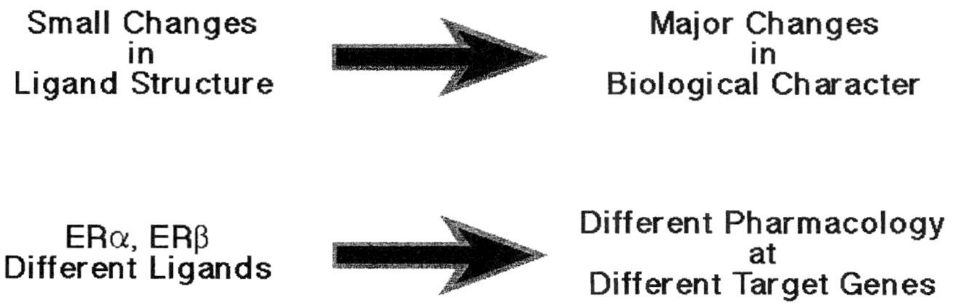

Small Changes
in
Ligand Structure
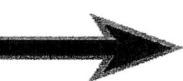
Major Changes
in
Biological Character

ERα, ERβ
Different Ligands
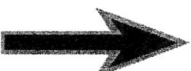
Different Pharmacology
at
Different Target Genes

FIGURE 1. Schematic depicting the exquisite precision in estrogen receptor regulation by ligand.

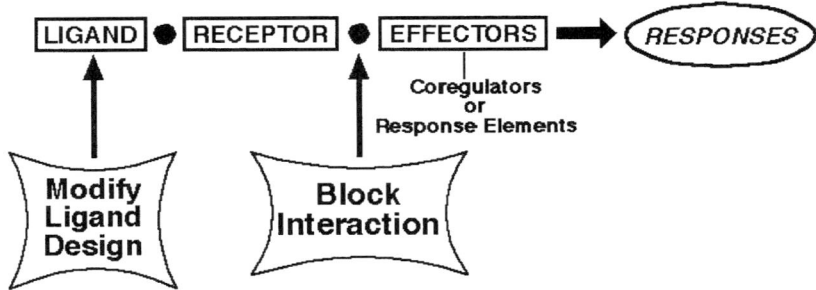

FIGURE 2. Approaches to the selective regulation of estrogen receptor activity based on the tripartite nature of hormone receptor biology involving the ligand, the receptor, and coregulator and response element effector sites. See text for details.

modifying the design of the ligand because it is the ligand that determines all subsequent receptor interactions. Indeed, structural, biochemical, and cellular analyses have shown that the nature of the ligand is the critical determinant of the conformation assumed by the liganded ER complex. A second important approach involves blocking or modulating the interaction of the ligand-receptor complex with coregulators.[7–9]

DEVELOPMENT OF ER SUBTYPE-SELECTIVE LIGANDS: STRUCTURE-ACTIVITY RELATIONSHIPS

Recent research in our laboratories has focused on the development of tissue-selective and ER subtype-selective ligands that strongly discriminate between ERα and ERβ, on the basis of either affinity/potency or efficacy (i.e., agonist versus antagonist activity). The observations that small changes in ligand structure can result in major changes in biological character of the ligand-receptor complex and that the activity of different ligands via ERα or ERβ shows distinct pharmacology at different target genes no doubt underlie the cell-specific and promoter-specific activities of estrogens in different target cells and at different gene sites.

The estrogen receptor, like other steroid hormone receptors, is a modular protein (FIG. 3), with distinct, largely autonomous domains having specific functions such as ligand binding, dimerization, DNA binding, and transactivation. In addition to a centrally located DNA binding domain, domain C, the ER contains two distinct activation functions: (i) an N-terminal A/B domain containing activation function 1 (AF-1) and (ii) a hormone-dependent activation function (AF-2), located in the E domain along with the hormone binding function of ER. Activation functions 1 and 2 work in a synergistic manner and are required for full ER activity in most cell contexts.[10–13]

As shown in FIGURE 3, ERα and ERβ differ most markedly in the N-terminal A/B domain, having only 18% amino acid identity in this region. They also differ substantially in the hormone binding domain, showing there only 56% amino acid

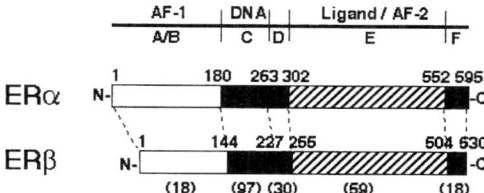

- **Different tissue/cell distributions**
- **Different affinity for ligands**
- **Different gene activations**

FIGURE 3. Schematics of the human estrogen receptor alpha and human estrogen receptor beta. The structural domains of these receptors (A/B, C, D, E, and F), as well as the hormone binding, DNA binding, and transactivation (AF-1, AF-2) functional domains, are shown, as is the percent amino acid identity of each domain between the two estrogen receptors (numbers in parentheses). AF: activation function.

identity. The great differences in the A/B domains suggest that the transcriptional activation of different estrogen-responsive genes by ERs α and β might show distinctly different patterns, a prediction that has now been documented in several cases.[14–18]

Studies by Kraus et al.[12] documented a ligand-dependent, transcriptionally productive association of the amino- and carboxyl-terminal regions of the ER, as now has also been demonstrated for the androgen[19] and progesterone receptors.[20] It is notable that the activity of each of the two activation functions of the ER varies in different cellular contexts, and different regions in AF-1 are required to support the antiestrogen-dependent and estradiol-dependent transcription activation of human ERα.[21] Region F of the receptor, the most carboxyl-terminal domain, is not essential for hormone binding or transactivation, but does play an important role in the transcriptional activity of the receptor and in the effectiveness of antiestrogens as estrogen antagonists.[22]

The receptor, in the absence of ligand, can be thought of as being in a "soft" conformation. Upon binding agonist ligand, the receptor is shifted into a conformation that is effective in recruiting a variety of coactivators, whereas other ligands that act as antagonists engender a different receptor conformation that recruits corepressor proteins and does not allow coactivator binding. It should be noted, however, that there is a spectrum of stable conformations and that the structure of the ligand critically determines the receptor conformation and thereby the balance between coactivator versus corepressor binding, a balance that will be different for these different conformational states of the receptor. The critical element in modulating this spectrum of conformational/activity states of the receptor-ligand complex is the nature of the ligand.

To understand how the two ER subtypes discriminate among different ligands, we undertook studies in which we mapped the ligand binding domain of ERα by affinity labeling and by mutational and deletion analyses, from which we identified regions in the ER critical for hormone binding and discrimination among SERM

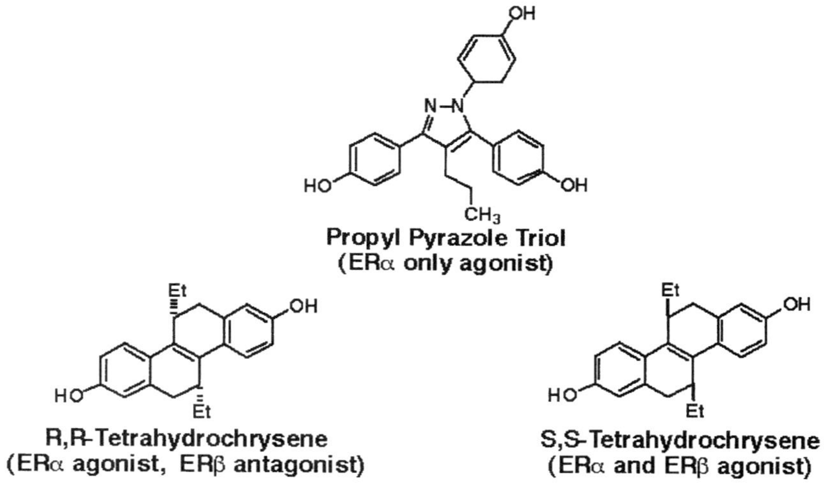

Propyl Pyrazole Triol
(ERα only agonist)

R,R-Tetrahydrochrysene
(ERα agonist, ERβ antagonist)

S,S-Tetrahydrochrysene
(ERα and ERβ agonist)

FIGURE 4. Structures of estrogen receptor subtype-selective ligands.

ligands.[5,23–29] Further, we showed that different ligands contact a distinct set of amino acids in critical portions of the ligand binding domain.[30,31]

ERα and ERβ differ significantly in their tissue distribution and ligand binding characteristics, thereby affording interesting potential for optimization of tissue-selective estrogen action. Because ERα and ERβ have only 56% amino acid identity in their hormone binding domains, it should be possible to identify ligands that have different levels of potency or efficacy through the two ER subtypes. In this manner, one should be able to selectively stimulate the gene sets that are distinctly regulated by these two ER subtypes.

We have developed compounds of novel structure that show remarkably high potency and/or efficacy selectivity on ERα and ERβ (FIG. 4). For example, we found that a propyl pyrazole triol, which has nearly a 500-fold binding affinity preference for ERα, could fully activate genes through ERα, whereas there was no gene activation through ERβ.[32–34] We also developed a series of substituted tetrahydrochrysenes that were nearly full to full agonists on ERα, but complete antagonists on ERβ (FIG. 5).[33–35] Studies with these compounds demonstrated that minor changes in the size and stereochemistry of the ligand substituents dramatically affected their activity as ERβ agonists or antagonists.[35]

These compounds are being used to help define the respective biological roles of ERα and ERβ in the actions of estrogens in different target tissues. They are also being used to study by X-ray crystallography the ligand-induced conformation of the ER subtypes that mediate agonist versus antagonist activity. These investigations further substantiate the observation that all agonists (or antagonists) do not contact an identical set of amino acids within the binding pocket of the receptor, nor induce identical receptor conformations.[5,34] This is consistent with prior observations of differences in ligand-receptor proteolysis profiles,[36–38] as well as more recent studies

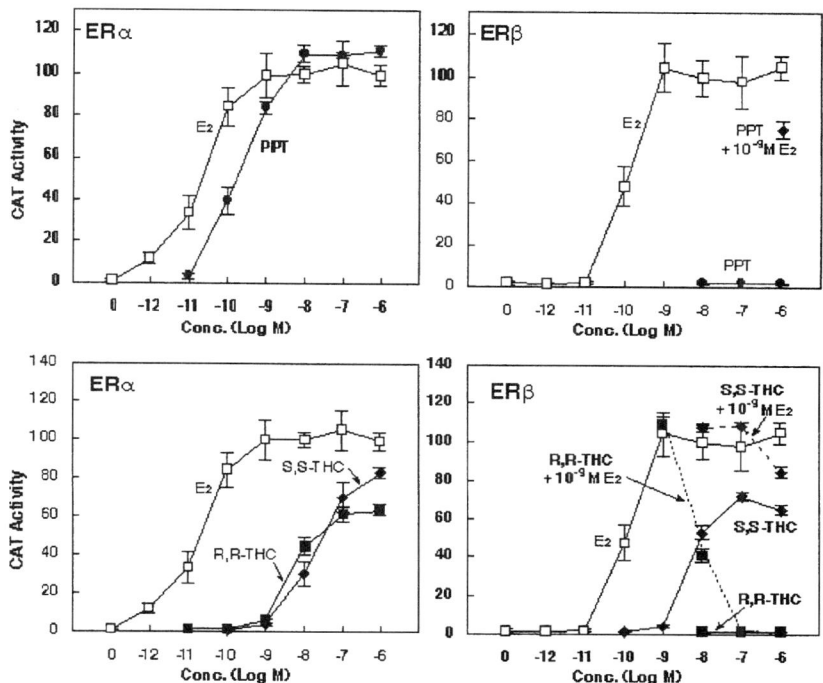

FIGURE 5. Transcription activation by ERα and ERβ in response to estradiol (E_2) and propyl pyrazole triol (PPT) **(top)** and in response to estradiol (E_2) and the R,R- and S,S-enantiomers of tetrahydrochrysene (THC) **(bottom)**. Human endometrial cancer (HEC-1) cells were transfected with expression vectors for ERα or ERβ and an $(ERE)_3$-pS2-CAT reporter gene and were treated with the indicated concentrations of estradiol (E_2), PPT, or R,R-THC or S,S-THC for 24 h. CAT activity was normalized for β-galactosidase activity from a cotransfected internal control pCMVβ plasmid. Values are the mean ± SD for three or more separate experiments and are expressed as a percent of the response with 10 nM E_2. From Ref. 34.

using phage display peptide probes, through which differences in the conformation of ERα and ERβ complexes with agonists and antagonists can be distinguished.[7-9]

These studies clearly demonstrate that it is possible to develop antagonists and agonists that are selectively effective on one of the two ER subtypes. Also, these ligands can have structures quite different from current SERMs, such as tamoxifen and raloxifene. By modulating the design of the ligand, these findings also indicate that we can amplify estrogen action through either ERα or ERβ, or in certain cases reduce ERα activity with a selective ERα antagonist while activating ERβ with a nonselective agonist such as estradiol.

Intriguingly, X-ray crystallographic studies in conjunction with Andy Shiau, Geof Greene, and David Agard have shown that R,R-tetrahydrochrysene has a split personality, being an ERα agonist and an ERβ antagonist (FIG. 4). Thus, R,R-

TABLE 1. Coactivator binding by ERα and ERβ with subtype-selective ER ligands[34]

	SRC-1		SRC-2 (GRIP-1/TIF-2)		SRC-3 (ACTR/AIB-1/RAC3/pCIP)	
ER ligand	ERα	ERβ	ERα	ERβ	ERα	ERβ
Unliganded	—[a]	—	—	—	—	—
Estradiol (E_2)	100[b]	100	100	100	100	100
ICI182,780	—	—	—	—	—	—
R,R-THC	74 ± 6[c]	—	55 ± 10	—	42 ± 3	—
S,S-THC	64 ± 3	65 ± 11	52 ± 6	79 ± 14	35 ± 4	68 ± 12
PPT	112 ± 6	—	101 ± 11	—	102 ± 7	—

[a]Denotes no interaction observed.
[b]The magnitude of interaction of coactivator with E_2-occupied ER is set at 100% in all cases.
[c]Values are the mean ± range of the yeast 2-hybrid and GST pull-down data; $n = 3$ for 2-hybrid and $n = 2$ for GST pull-down assays. The range of the five assays is shown.

tetrahydrochrysene puts ERα into a conformation very similar to that attained with the agonists, estradiol or diethylstilbestrol, whereas it engenders the antagonist structure, similar to that achieved with hydroxytamoxifen, in the ERβ ligand binding domain, particularly in the conformation of the helix 12 region, which is known to be critically important in coregulator recruitment.

Estrogen receptor protease digestion sensitivity assays and assessment of the ability of ER subtype-selective ligands to promote the recruitment of representatives of the three SRC/p160 coactivator protein family members (SRC-1, GRIP-1, and ACTR, respectively) to ERα and ERβ reveal distinctly different patterns for stimulatory and inhibitory ligands. Interestingly, however, compared with estradiol, the novel agonist ligands show some quantitative differences in their ability to recruit SRC-1, -2, and -3 (TABLE 1), implying that these ligands induce receptor conformations that differ somewhat from that induced by estradiol, differences that are thought to be illustrative of the nature of their biological character. These findings highlight the fact that, by changing the shape of the ligand, one generates receptor-ligand complexes of different topology, resulting in differential receptor-coregulator interactions and different pharmacological profiles—namely, changes in profiles of gene expression or other biological responses.

CONCLUSIONS

The research results discussed in this article provide an essential basis for understanding the cell-selective activities of newly developed SERM ligands. The extent to which new generation SERMs act selectively through ERα and ERβ, and the degree to which they provide substantial improvements over estrogens and antiestrogens currently in use for hormone replacement, breast cancer prevention and treatment, osteoporosis prevention, and other biomedical applications, will require careful evaluation. Continued studies with ligands that work as selective agonists or antagonists through the two ER subtypes will be important in developing an improved understanding of the distinct biologies of different SERMs. Because current structural work, and much of the biochemical work as well, derives from studies with just the hormone binding domain alone, it will be important to examine the functional contributions that will be provided by the other domains of the receptors; it is known that the biology of these receptors is critically determined not only by the AF-2, in the ligand binding domain, but also by the AF-1, which is in the N-terminus of these receptors. Elucidating how receptors complexed with different ligands engender distinct receptor-ligand conformations and differentially recruit coregulators from among the diversity of coactivator and corepressor proteins, and characterizing the levels and distributions of these coregulators in different estrogen target cells, should contribute to an understanding of the tissue-selective actions of optimized SERMs and to their further development as medical therapeutic agents.

ACKNOWLEDGMENTS

This research was supported by grants from the National Institutes of Health (Nos. CA18119, DK-15556, 5T32 GM07283, and 5T32 CA09067).

REFERENCES

1. GRESE, T.A. & J.A. DODGE. 1998. Selective estrogen receptor modulators (SERMs). Curr. Pharmacol. Design **4:** 71–92.
2. MCDONNELL, D.P. 1999. The molecular pharmacology of SERMs. Trends Endocrinol. Metab. **10:** 301–311.
3. MCKENNA, N.J. & B.W. O'MALLEY. 2000. An issue of tissues: divining the split personalities of selective estrogen receptor modulators. Nat. Med. **6:** 960–962.
4. KATZENELLENBOGEN, J.A., B.W. O'MALLEY et al. 1996. Tripartite steroid hormone receptor pharmacology: interaction with multiple effector sites as a basis for the cell- and promoter-specific action of these hormones. Mol. Endocrinol. **10:** 119–131.
5. KATZENELLENBOGEN, B.S., M.M. MONTANO et al. 2000. Estrogen receptors: selective ligands, partners, and distinctive pharmacology. Recent Prog. Horm. Res. **55:** 163–195.
6. KATZENELLENBOGEN, B.S. & J.A. KATZENELLENBOGEN. 2000. Estrogen receptor alpha and estrogen receptor beta: regulation by selective estrogen receptor modulators (SERMs) and importance in breast cancer. Breast Cancer Res. **2:** 335–344.
7. CHANG, C., J.D. NORRIS et al. 1999. Dissection of the LXXLL nuclear receptor/coactivator interaction motif using combinatorial peptide libraries: discovery of peptide antagonists of estrogen receptors alpha and beta. Mol. Cell. Biol. **19:** 8226–8239.
8. NORRIS, J.D., L.A. PAIGE et al. 1999. Peptide antagonists of the human estrogen receptor. Science **285:** 744–746.
9. PAIGE, L.A., D.J. CHRISTENSEN et al. 1999. Estrogen receptor (ER) modulators each induce distinct conformational changes in ER alpha and ER beta. Proc. Natl. Acad. Sci. U.S.A. **96:** 3999–4004.
10. BERRY, M., D. METZGER et al. 1990. Role of the two activating domains of the oestrogen receptor in the cell-type and promoter-context dependent agonistic activity of the anti-oestrogen 4-hydroxytamoxifen. EMBO J. **9:** 2811–2818.
11. GRONEMEYER, H. 1991. Transcription activation by estrogen and progesterone receptors. Annu. Rev. Genet. **25:** 89–123.
12. KRAUS, W.L., E.M. MCINERNEY et al. 1995. Ligand-dependent, transcriptionally productive association of the amino- and carboxyl-terminal regions of a steroid hormone nuclear receptor. Proc. Natl. Acad. Sci. U.S.A. **92:** 12314–12318.

13. TZUKERMAN, M.T., A. ESTY et al. 1994. Human estrogen receptor transactivational capacity is determined by both cellular and promoter context and mediated by two functionally distinct intramolecular regions. Mol. Endocrinol. **8:** 21–30.
14. MCINERNEY, E.M., K.E. WEIS et al. 1998. Transcription activation by the human estrogen receptor subtype β (ERβ) studied with ERβ and ERα receptor chimeras. Endocrinology **139:** 4513–4522.
15. MONTANO, M.M. & B.S. KATZENELLENBOGEN. 1997. The quinone reductase gene: a unique estrogen receptor–regulated gene that is activated by antiestrogens. Proc. Natl. Acad. Sci. U.S.A. **94:** 2581–2586.
16. PAECH, K., P. WEBB et al. 1997. Differential ligand activation of estrogen receptors ERα and ERβ at AP1 sites. Science **277:** 1508–1510.
17. WEBB, P., P. NGUYEN et al. 1999. The estrogen receptor enhances AP-1 activity by two distinct mechanisms with different requirements for receptor transactivation functions. Mol. Endocrinol. **13:** 1672–1685.
18. MONTANO, M.M., A.K. JAISWAL et al. 1998. Transcriptional regulation of the human quinone reductase gene by antiestrogen-liganded estrogen receptor-α and estrogen receptor-β. J. Biol. Chem. **273:** 25443–25449.
19. LANGLEY, E., J.A. KEMPPAINEN et al. 1998. Intermolecular NH$_2$-/carboxyl-terminal interactions in androgen receptor dimerization revealed by mutations that cause androgen insensitivity. J. Biol. Chem. **273:** 92–101.
20. TETEL, M.J., P.H. GIANGRANDE et al. 1999. Hormone-dependent interaction between the amino- and carboxyl-terminal domains of progesterone receptor *in vitro* and *in vivo*. Mol. Endocrinol. **13:** 910–924.
21. MCINERNEY, E.M. & B.S. KATZENELLENBOGEN. 1996. Different regions in activation function-1 of the human estrogen receptor required for antiestrogen- and estradiol-dependent transcription activation. J. Biol. Chem. **271:** 24172–24178.
22. MONTANO, M.M., V. MÜLLER et al. 1995. The carboxyl-terminal F domain of the human estrogen receptor: role in the transcriptional activity of the receptor and the effectiveness of antiestrogens as estrogen antagonists. Mol. Endocrinol. **9:** 814–825.
23. HARLOW, K.W., D.N. SMITH et al. 1989. Identification of cysteine-530 as the covalent attachment site of an affinity labeling estrogen (ketononestrol aziridine) and anti-estrogen (tamoxifen aziridine) in the human estrogen receptor. J. Biol. Chem. **264:** 17476–17485.
24. KATZENELLENBOGEN, B.S., B. BHARDWAJ et al. 1993. Hormone binding and transcription activation by estrogen receptors: analyses using mammalian and yeast systems. J. Steroid Biochem. Mol. Biol. **47:** 39–48.
25. PAKDEL, F. & B.S. KATZENELLENBOGEN. 1992. Human estrogen receptor mutants with altered estrogen and antiestrogen ligand discrimination. J. Biol. Chem. **267:** 3429–3437.
26. PAKDEL, F., P. LE GOFF et al. 1993. An assessment of the role of domain F and PEST sequences in estrogen receptor half-life and bioactivity. J. Steroid Biochem. Mol. Biol. **46:** 663–672.
27. REESE, J.C. & B.S. KATZENELLENBOGEN. 1991. Mutagenesis of cysteines in the hormone binding domain of the human estrogen receptor: alterations in binding and transcriptional activation by covalently and reversibly attaching ligands. J. Biol. Chem. **266:** 10880–10887.
28. REESE, J.C., C.H. WOOGE et al. 1992. Identification of two cysteines closely positioned in the ligand binding pocket of the human estrogen receptor: roles in ligand binding and transcriptional activation. Mol. Endocrinol. **6:** 2160–2166.
29. WRENN, C.K. & B.S. KATZENELLENBOGEN. 1993. Structure-function analysis of the hormone binding domain of the human estrogen receptor by region-specific mutagenesis and phenotypic screening in yeast. J. Biol. Chem. **268:** 24089–24098.
30. EKENA, K.E., K.E. WEIS et al. 1996. Identification of amino acids in the hormone binding domain of the human estrogen receptor important in estrogen binding. J. Biol. Chem. **271:** 20053–20059.
31. EKENA, K., K.E. WEIS et al. 1997. Different residues of the human estrogen receptor are involved in the recognition of structurally diverse estrogens and antiestrogens. J. Biol. Chem. **272:** 5069–5075.

32. STAUFFER, S.R., J. SUN et al. 2000. Acyclic amides as estrogen receptor ligands: synthesis, binding, activity, and receptor interaction. Bioorg. Med. Chem. **8:** 1293–1316.
33. SUN, J., M.J. MEYERS et al. 1999. Novel ligands that function as selective estrogens or antiestrogens for estrogen receptor-α or estrogen receptor-β. Endocrinology **140:** 800–804.
34. KRAICHELY, D.M., J. SUN et al. 2000. Conformational changes and coactivator recruitment by novel ligands for estrogen receptor-alpha and estrogen receptor-beta: correlations with biological character and distinct differences among SRC coactivator family members. Endocrinology **141:** 3534–3545.
35. MEYERS, M.J., J. SUN et al. 1999. Estrogen receptor subtype-selective ligands: asymmetric synthesis and biological evaluation of cis- and trans-5,11-dialkyl-5,6,11,12-tetrahydrochrysenes. J. Med. Chem. **42:** 2456–2468.
36. ALLAN, G.F., X. LENG et al. 1992. Hormone and antihormone induce distinct conformational changes which are central to steroid receptor activation. J. Biol. Chem. **267:** 19513–19520.
37. LAZENNEC, G., T.R. EDIGER et al. 1997. Mechanistic aspects of estrogen receptor activation probed with constitutively active estrogen receptors: correlations with DNA and coregulator interactions and receptor conformational changes. Mol. Endocrinol. **11:** 1375–1386.
38. MCDONNELL, D.P., D.L. CLEMM et al. 1995. Analysis of estrogen receptor function in vitro reveals three distinct classes of antiestrogens. Mol. Endocrinol. **9:** 659–669.

Capitalizing on the Complexities of Estrogen Receptor Pharmacology in the Quest for the Perfect SERM

DONALD P. McDONNELL, CHING-YI CHANG, AND JOHN D. NORRIS

Department of Pharmacology and Cancer Biology, Duke University Medical Center, Durham, North Carolina 27710, USA

ABSTRACT: The term Selective Estrogen Receptor Modulators (SERMs) has been used of late to describe a group of pharmaceuticals that manifest estrogen receptor (ER) agonist activity in some tissues, but that oppose estrogen action in others. Whereas the name describing this class of drugs is new, the concept is not. Indeed, compounds exhibiting tissue-selective ER agonist/antagonist properties have been around for nearly 40 years. What is new is the idea that it may be possible to capitalize on the paradoxical activities of these drugs and develop them as treatments for estrogenopathies where it is desirable to direct therapy to a specific estrogen-responsive target organ. This realization has provided the impetus for research in this area and has pushed the development and clinical use of this class of drugs. The objective of this review is to describe how the medical need for SERMs arose and how recent studies of the mechanism of action of the currently available drugs are paving the way for the development of novel drugs with improved selectivity.

KEYWORDS: ERα; ERβ; SERMs; tamoxifen; LXXLL-containing peptides

THERE IS A MEDICAL NEED FOR ESTROGEN RECEPTOR MODULATORS WHOSE ACTIVITIES ARE MANIFEST IN A TISSUE-SELECTIVE MANNER

Initially considered a reproductive hormone, estrogen has been shown to exert regulatory activities in tissues not involved in reproduction.[1] Much of this latter insight has come from a large number of studies performed over the past 50 years on the impact of exogenous estrogen replacement therapy (ERT) on the health and well-being of postmenopausal women.[2,3] First approved for the treatment of climacteric symptoms associated with menopause in women, it is now clear that estrogens have a positive effect in the skeleton, where increases in bone mineral density (BMD) in the spine and hip of 6% and 2%, respectively, have been observed.[4] In the cardiovascular system, a large number of observational studies have shown that ERT is associated with a 50% reduction in cardiovascular disease (CVD) in the primary prevention setting and, in patients with established disease, it reduces by up to 90% the

---

Address for correspondence: Dr. Donald P. McDonnell, Department of Pharmacology and Cancer Biology, Duke University Medical Center, Box 3813, Durham, NC 27710. Voice: 919-684-6035; fax: 919-681-7139.

donald.mcdonnell@duke.edu

chance of a second heart attack.[5–7] Conclusions as to the efficacy of estrogens in the cardiovascular systems have been challenged somewhat by the results of the large placebo-controlled HERS (Heart and Estrogen-progestin Replacement Study) trial, which was unable to demonstrate any overall benefit of estrogen in the cardiovascular systems of women with established heart disease.[8] Given that CVD is the leading cause of death in postmenopausal women, it is very important that these issues be resolved. A proven positive effect of estrogen in the cardiovascular system would set the hurdle for the optimal selective estrogen receptor modulator (SERM). A proven negative effect would suggest that the currently available SERMs are very close to optimal.

Other positive activities ascribed to ERT include the ability to reduce the incidence of macular degeneration, delay the onset of Alzheimer's disease, prevent tooth loss, and reduce the incidence of colon cancer.[9–13] Clearly, ERT has had and will continue to have a large impact on morbidity and mortality in women.[3] Notwithstanding these benefits, only a small percentage of women who could benefit from exogenous estrogens actually take some form of ERT. Indeed, of those who do initiate therapy, the majority discontinue within the first year. Although there are many reasons why therapy may not be started, or is stopped prematurely, it is clear that these decisions are driven in large part by the perception that ERT is associated with a significant increase in the incidence of breast cancer. Repeatedly, studies have shown a moderate increase in risk, about 10% annually, in the incidence of breast cancer in ERT users—an increase similar to what would be expected if menopause were delayed for the same duration.[14] This finding, together with other negative side effects of ERT (i.e., endometrial cancer and deep-vein thrombosis) have raised concern among women in general as to the relative risks and benefits of estrogen-containing medicines.[15,16] The recent findings that the inclusion of a progestin, in the treatment regimens of women with intact uteri, may increase the risk of breast cancer have added more confusion and apprehension.[17,18] Despite these important limitations to ERT, it is apparent that the currently available medicines increase overall survival and improve the quality of life of postmenopausal women.[3] The challenge therefore is to (1) select the women who will benefit most from ERT and (2) develop new ER agonists with improved therapeutic indices. It is out of this environment that the unmet medical need arose for new compounds that act as estrogens in some tissues, but that manifest antagonist or neutral activities in the breast and endometrium.

THE BIRTH OF SERMs

The pharmacological definition of an antagonist is a compound that either competitively or noncompetitively interferes with the action of an activating agonist. Thus, within the confines of the classical models of ER action, the drug tamoxifen was considered to be an antagonist because it could competitively block agonist binding and prevent activation of the receptor.[19,20] It is interesting that, until recently, tamoxifen was classified as an ER antagonist, although as early as 1967, soon after it was first described, it was noted that the agonist/antagonist activities of this compound were tissue- and species-dependent.[21] With respect to pituitary function, it was an antagonist in mice and rats.[21] In the uterus, however, it functioned as a partial agonist in rats and a full agonist in mice. In chickens, it was an antagonist in all tissues examined.[22] (A "partial agonist" in this context is an agent that mimics the activity of estrogen at the ER in a given tissue, but does so to a lesser extent than estrogen.) These findings clearly indicated that tamoxifen was not a pure antagonist and, since its agonist activity was manifest in a tissue-selective manner, it was not appropriate to classify it as a partial agonist either. These initial studies were followed over the next few years by reports that indicated that tamoxifen and a related compound, clomiphene, were bone-protective in rodents and did not cause skeletal deterioration in women as would be expected of an antagonist.[23-25] Regardless of these findings, it was not until a placebo-controlled study demonstrated that tamoxifen could function as an estrogen in the bones of women receiving tamoxifen as adjuvant chemotherapy that the significance of these initial results were realized.[26] This, and similar studies, established the SERM concept and provided the impetus for the pharmaceutical industry to begin the search for other drugs with similar activities.[27] Additionally, the convincing data that indicated that tamoxifen was in fact a tissue-selective estrogen begged a reexamination of the classical models of ER action where such selectivity would not have been predicted.

THE FIRST GENERATION OF SERMs

Tamoxifen was the first drug to be classified as a SERM. However, raloxifene is the only drug of this class currently approved for treatment and prevention of osteoporosis.[28] In the short time that it has been available, raloxifene has established itself as a viable alternative to traditional ERT in some postmenopausal women, although it is still a long way short of being the perfect "estrogen". This drug worsens or has no effect on the climacteric conditions associated with menopause, the primary reason that women begin hormone replacement therapy (HRT).[28] It has been shown to be about half as effective as estrogen or bisphosphonates in increasing BMD in the lumbar spine and, like estrogens, it is not clear whether raloxifene reduces hip fractures.[29] In the cardiovascular system, whereas estrogens and raloxifene lower LDL, the latter drug accomplishes this without a concomitant elevation in triglycerides.[28] The clinical significance of these differences is not known, but suggest that the mechanism or targets of these two drugs are not the same in the cardiovascular system. One of the most important findings, however, with the first generation of SERMs is that they have been shown to significantly reduce or delay the onset of breast cancer in a large number of women.[30] The long-term impact of these drugs on survival is not yet known in women who are disease-free at the initiation of this prophylactic therapy. Although osteoporosis and CVD are much greater killers in postmenopausal women than breast cancer, the ability of SERMs to reduce breast cancer risk may ultimately encourage more women to take some type of HRT.[31] Clearly, the available SERMs are a first step towards the perfect HRT. They dissuade the fears of breast cancer, yet give some of the benefits of estrogen in bone. However, the next generation of SERMs will have to provide additional positive attributes of classical estrogens if they are to have a significant impact on overall mortality and morbidity.

It is worth remembering that the currently available SERMs were not specifically developed as estrogen replacements, but as breast cancer therapeutics. It was the observation that tamoxifen, an antiestrogen, could function as an estrogen in bone and the endometrium that suggested that it was possible for ER-ligand complexes to be recognized differently in different tissues. Raloxifene (formerly called keoxifene) was also developed initially as a breast cancer therapeutic.[32] Like tamoxifen, raloxifene was found to manifest agonist activity in bone, but distinguished itself from tamoxifen in that it functioned as a pure antagonist in the uterus.[33–35] Thus, even within the SERM class, it appears as if there are subclasses of mechanistically distinct compounds.[35,36] These observations have suggested that additional SERMs with unique mechanisms of action remain to be identified. Clearly, the ongoing studies aimed at dissecting the ER-signaling pathway will facilitate the search for the perfect SERM and will help us to understand the molecular basis for the tissue selectivity of the existing members of this class.

THE MOLECULAR MECHANISM OF ACTION OF ER MODULATORS

The biological actions of estrogens, SERMs, and antiestrogens are manifest through high-affinity binding to nuclear receptors located within the target cell nuclei. Until recently, it was considered that all the biological actions of ER modulators were manifest through a single receptor that was biochemically identical in all cells. However, the discovery in 1996 of a second ER significantly increased the biological complexity of estrogen.[37] Unexpectedly, Kuiper and coworkers identified a novel receptor cDNA in the prostate of male rats that encoded a protein that bound 17β-estradiol with an affinity equivalent to that of the previously identified "breast/uterus" estrogen receptors.[37] A human homologue of this novel ER, now called ERβ, was subsequently cloned.[38] With respect to ER pharmacology, the identification of this novel ER is probably one of the most significant discoveries in the past 20 years (FIG. 1). The emergence of a second ER immediately suggested that differential affinity of ligands for each of these receptors, coupled with tissue-specific differences in their expression, could explain how the same compound could exhibit different biological activities in different cells. In support of this hypothesis, it has been shown that genetic disruption of ERα or ERβ in mice does not give rise to the same phenotype, indicating that these two receptors are not functionally equivalent.[1] Consequently, it is inferred from the results of the studies performed thus far that differential activation of these receptors will have different biological consequences. However, as this field has progressed, it has become clear that SERM action is likely to involve more than receptor selectivity since it has been noted that most of the existing drugs of this class do not distinguish between ERα and ERβ.[39,40] In addition, it has been shown that the biological activity of some SERMs can differ among tissues or cells that express the same ER subtype. For instance, using ERα-responsive transcription systems reconstituted in a variety of cells, we have been able to show that tamoxifen can function in some backgrounds as an antagonist, whereas in others it can manifest partial agonist activity.[41,42] Furthermore, in those cells where tamoxifen manifests partial agonist activity, raloxifene, GW5638 (also called DPC 974), droloxifene, and idoxifene function as pure ERα antagonists.[43]

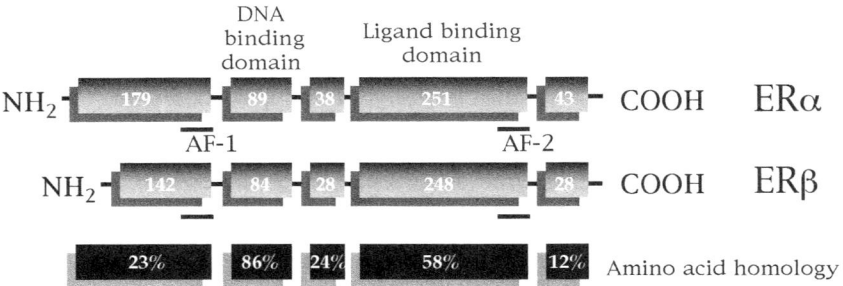

* Numbers in boxes indicate number of amino acids

FIGURE 1. Estrogens and antiestrogens manifest their biological activity through two distinct receptors. Shown is an alignment of the α and β isoforms of the human estrogen receptors. The number of amino acid residues in each functional domain is indicated, as is the percent homology between the two proteins in each domain. Estrogen receptor α contains two distinct activation domains, AF-1 and AF-2.[42,45] ERβ contains an AF-2 domain, but not an AF-1 domain.[40]

This suggests that there are differences in the way that each ER is able to respond to different SERMs. When a similar analysis was done for ERβ, it was determined that all of the known SERMs function as pure antagonists.[40] As yet, no simple explanation has emerged to explain how SERMs can manifest cell-selective agonist activity. It is possible that the cellular backgrounds in which the *in vitro* experiments were performed do not reflect the target cells *in vivo* that are important for SERM agonist activity. It is worth noting that, when tethered to DNA through a promoter-bound AP1 complex, SERM-activated ERβ, but not ERα, can activate transcription.[44] The significance of this observation awaits a demonstration that ER-AP1 interactions occur *in vivo* and are physiologically relevant. As it stands, however, it does not appear that differential activation of ERα or ERβ is sufficient to explain the tissue-selective actions of the known SERMs.

ERα IS A LIGAND-REGULATED TRANSCRIPTION FACTOR

Much of what we know about estrogen action comes from studies of ERα. Although it is acknowledged that ERβ is also likely to be important, the remainder of this review will consider the major advances that have come from the studies of ERα action and the impact of this information on the pharmacology of ER modulators.

The ERα is a ligand-regulated transcription factor that remains inactive when associated with a heat-shock protein complex until an activating ligand binds.[20] This activity promotes the displacement of the receptor from the inhibitory complex, allows receptor dimerization, and facilitates its interaction with specific estrogen response elements located within target gene promoters.[20] Depending on the cellular and promoter context, the DNA-bound promoter can either positively or negatively

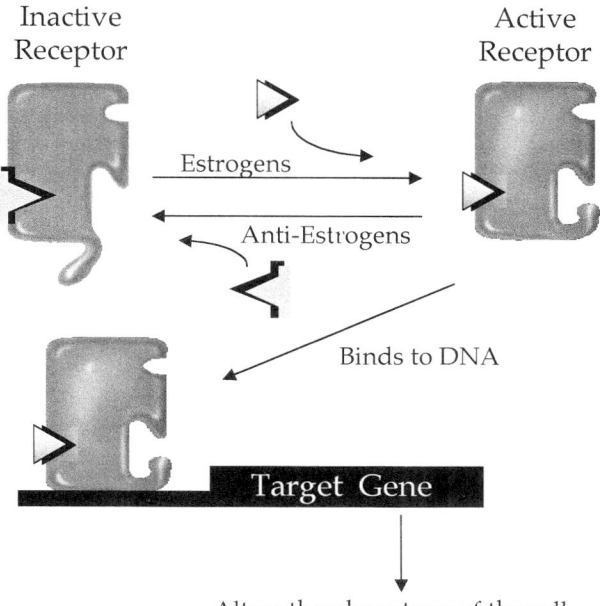

FIGURE 2. Early models of ER action do not explain the complex pharmacology of known ER ligands. The classical models of estrogen action suggested that, in the absence of ligand, the ER existed in the nuclei of target cells in an inactive form.[20] Upon binding an agonist, the ER underwent an activating transformation event that facilitated the interaction of the receptor with specific DNA response elements within target gene promoters. Within the confines of this model, it was hard to explain the molecular pharmacology of tamoxifen and other ligands whose agonist/antagonist activity differed from cell to cell.

regulate target gene transcription.[42,45] In the simplest interpretation of this model, the antiestrogenic activities of SERMs, like tamoxifen, would reflect a displacement of estradiol and the retention of the receptor in an inactive state (FIG. 2). Clearly, this was not the correct interpretation. The first departure from this model describing antagonist action came from the studies of Allan *et al.* that used protease digestion to map the conformational changes in the progesterone receptor (PR) that occur upon ligand binding.[46,47] These important studies demonstrated that agonists and antagonists induce distinct conformational changes in PR upon binding and, importantly, both conformations were distinct from aporeceptor. Thus, antagonists do not merely freeze the receptor in an inactive conformation, but facilitate the formation of a uniquely structured complex. A similar series of studies were later performed with ERα and revealed that the overall conformations of the ERα-tamoxifen and ERα-estradiol complexes were different and distinct from aporeceptor.[41,48] From these studies emerged the concept that cells possess the ability to distinguish between different ERα-ligand complexes and that the same ERα-ligand complex can be recognized in a different manner in different cells.

DEFINING THE MOLECULAR BASIS FOR TAMOXIFEN AGONIST ACTIVITY

The finding that tamoxifen functions as an agonist in the endometrium and bone, whereas a similar SERM, raloxifene, is an agonist in bone and an antagonist in the endometrium indicated that the agonist activities in bone and the endometrium are not occurring in the same manner.[35,49,50] As a first step in understanding SERM pharmacology, we chose to examine the molecular basis of the partial agonist activity of tamoxifen. In large part, this was because we had a model system where estradiol and tamoxifen manifested agonist activity, whereas raloxifene was an antagonist.[41] Specifically, it was observed that estradiol and tamoxifen could activate transcription of a complement 3-luciferase gene transfected into the liver hepatocellular carcinoma cell line, HepG2. We also chose to focus our initial studies on tamoxifen as it had become clear from the work of others that ERα has two distinct activation functions involved in transcriptional activation and that tamoxifen influences the activity of these domains in a differential manner.[41,45] Specifically, it was demonstrated that ERα contains an agonist-dependent activation function within the ligand binding domain (LBD) (AF-2) and a ligand-independent activation function (AF-1) within the amino terminus (see FIG. 1). Using specific mutations that eliminate one or both of these activation domains, it was shown that most cells required both activation domains for maximal transcriptional activity, whereas other cells had preferences for one or the other of the activation domains.[42] As will be discussed below, it is likely that these activation domain preferences are determined by the cell-selective expression of cofactors that interact with ERα and permit it to regulate gene transcription. The importance of the individual activation domains in ERα pharmacology was suggested by the studies of Meyer *et al.*, which demonstrated that tamoxifen is an AF-2 antagonist, an observation confirmed by other groups.[45] Recent crystallographic analysis of the structures of the ERα-LBD in the presence of estradiol or tamoxifen revealed the structural basis of the AF-2 inhibition.[51,52] Cumulatively, these results led to the development of the model depicted in FIGURE 3. This proposes that ERα adopts distinct conformations in the presence of tamoxifen or estradiol. In cells where AF-2 is required (FIG. 3A), the conformation of the ERα-estradiol complex enables AF-2 to interact with a required cofactor and transcription proceeds. The tamoxifen-activated receptor, on the other hand, does not permit this required interaction and ERα transcriptional activity is inhibited. Not surprisingly, therefore, ICI182,780, a compound that inhibits the activity of both activation functions, is an antagonist in this environment. In cells where AF-2 is not required, however, the same ERα-ligand complexes are recognized differently. In this environment (FIG. 3B), the amino-terminal activation function (AF-1) is able to engage a coactivator and, since this activation domain is presented in a ligand-independent manner, both estradiol and tamoxifen can manifest agonist activity. As expected, the pure antagonist ICI182,780 is unable to function as an agonist in this cell and promoter background. The initial interpretation of these data was that tamoxifen is an AF-1 agonist and this activity does not require AF-2. This explanation is likely to be correct, but not complete.

There is a problem with classifying tamoxifen as an ERα–AF-1 agonist. First, in cellular assays where AF-1 is active, we have consistently observed that tamoxifen

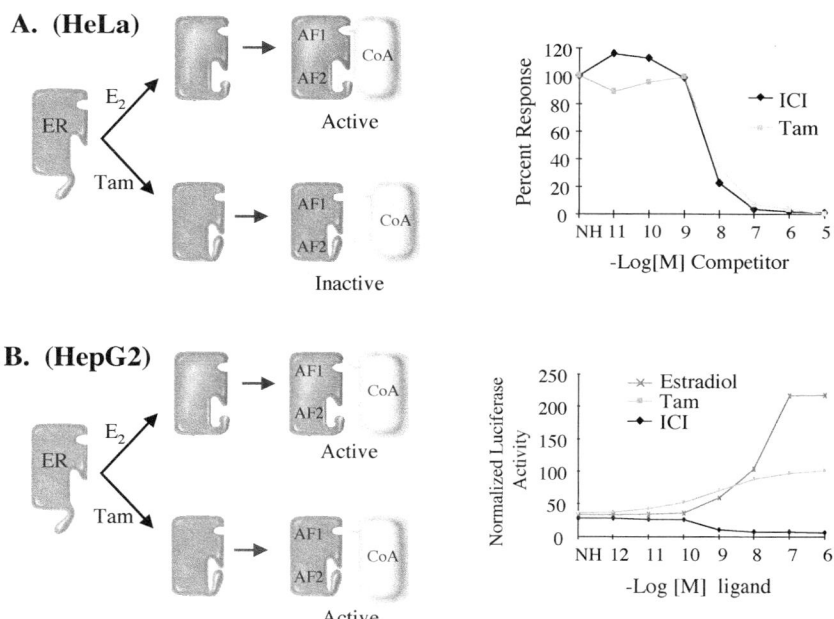

FIGURE 3. Differential coactivator recruitment may explain the tissue-selective agonist/antagonist activities of tamoxifen. The ERα contains two distinct activation functions (AF-1 and AF-2) whose activities are manifest in a cell-selective manner. Upon binding estradiol, the receptor undergoes a conformational change that enables the presentation of both activation domains, whereas tamoxifen binding permits only AF-1 activity to be manifest. **(A)** In some cell contexts, the interaction of both ERα-AFs with a coactivator (CoA) is required for transcriptional activity. In these contexts, estradiol, but not tamoxifen, functions as an agonist. This can be demonstrated pharmacologically by assaying the ability of ERα to regulate the expression of an estrogen-responsive reporter in HeLa cells, a context where both AF-1 and AF-2 are required. In the experiment shown, ERα-dependent transcriptional activity was measured in the presence of estradiol alone (100% response) or in the presence of different concentrations of 4-OH-tamoxifen (Tam) or the pure antagonist ICI182,780 (ICI). These and other published data have led to the conclusion that tamoxifen is an AF-2 antagonist.[41,45] **(B)** In other cell contexts, AF-1 is the primary point of interface between ERα and coactivators required for transcriptional activity. In HepG2 cells, for instance, where AF-2 is not required, both tamoxifen and estrogen function as agonists of ERα-mediated transcription. As discussed in the text, AF-2 is not required for AF-1 activity. However, other sequences within the carboxyl terminus are required for maximal AF-1 transcriptional activity. This observation has led to the conclusion that tamoxifen is an AF-2 antagonist and an AF-1 agonist.

agonist activity never exceeds 50% of that of estradiol.[41,43,53] Second, even in these AF-2-independent cell contexts, we have identified mutations in AF-2 that abolish both AF-1 and tamoxifen activity.[54] Third, deletion of the hormone binding domain yields a totally inactive receptor, which is not what would be expected if AF-1 were a totally independent activation function.[55] Thus, although the AF-2 activation function is dispensable in some contexts, there are domains within the LBD that are required for AF-1 function. These conclusions directed our studies towards the identification of the surfaces on ERα that are presented upon estradiol or tamoxifen binding, as well as an examination of the potential role of these surfaces in facilitating functionally important protein-protein interactions.

IDENTIFICATION OF POTENTIAL PROTEIN-PROTEIN INTERACTION SURFACES ON ERα-LIGAND COMPLEXES USING COMBINATORIAL PHAGE DISPLAY

The identification of the p160 class of the nuclear receptor coactivators SRC-1, SRC-2, and SRC-3 (steroid receptor coactivator-1, -2, -3) and the demonstration that they could interact with ERα–AF-2 in the presence of agonists, but not antagonists, provided a molecular explanation for most of the pharmacological activities of these two classes of compounds.[56,57] Specifically, it was demonstrated that agonist-activated ERα can nucleate the assemblage of large multiprotein complexes at target gene promoters that facilitate transcription by (1) stabilizing the preinitiation complex and (2) acetylating histones H3 and H4 with a subsequent local decondensation of chromatin.[57] Sequence comparisons and mapping studies demonstrated that the p160 coactivators contain a repeated LXXLL motif that is necessary and sufficient for nuclear receptor interaction.[58,59] Crystallization of ERα with a peptide derived from the nuclear interaction domain of SRC-2 (GRIP-1, glucocorticoid receptor interacting protein-1) revealed that the LXXLL motifs fit into a hydrophobic pocket contained within the AF-2 domain and that this pocket is occluded when tamoxifen binds to the receptor.[52] Thus, a mechanistic explanation for the AF-2 antagonist activity of tamoxifen was provided. The crystallographic analysis also appears to indicate that the LXXLL motif is merely required for receptor-coactivator docking, a conclusion that has important pharmacological consequences. If the LXXLL motif is merely a docking module, then access of coactivators to ERα will be regulated by simple competition and thus the relative expression levels of a given coactivator would determine which ERα-coactivator complexes are formed. If, on the other hand, there are different types of LXXLL motifs that are recognized differentially by ERα, then the absolute level of a given coactivator would be the most important determinant of complex composition and resulting transcriptional response. To address this issue, a library of 10^8 different peptides in the format -X_7LXXLLX_7- was created in a vector that enabled the expression and presentation of the peptides on the surface of the M13 bacteriophage.[59] Using estradiol-activated ERα immobilized to plastic, a large number of specific, high-affinity LXXLL-expressing phage were affinity-selected (FIG. 4). Sequencing of the phage revealed three distinct classes of LXXLL motif based on the residues found at the amino terminus of the first fixed leucine. Interestingly, the same three sequence-based classifications were apparent when the LXXLL motifs of the known coactivators were compared in a similar manner (FIG. 5). The significance of these results, however, was not apparent until we studied the impact of AF-2 mutations on the ability of the peptides to interact with the receptor. This was done using a mammalian two-hybrid assay, wherein the peptide to be studied was expressed as a Gal4-peptide fusion and the full-length ERα

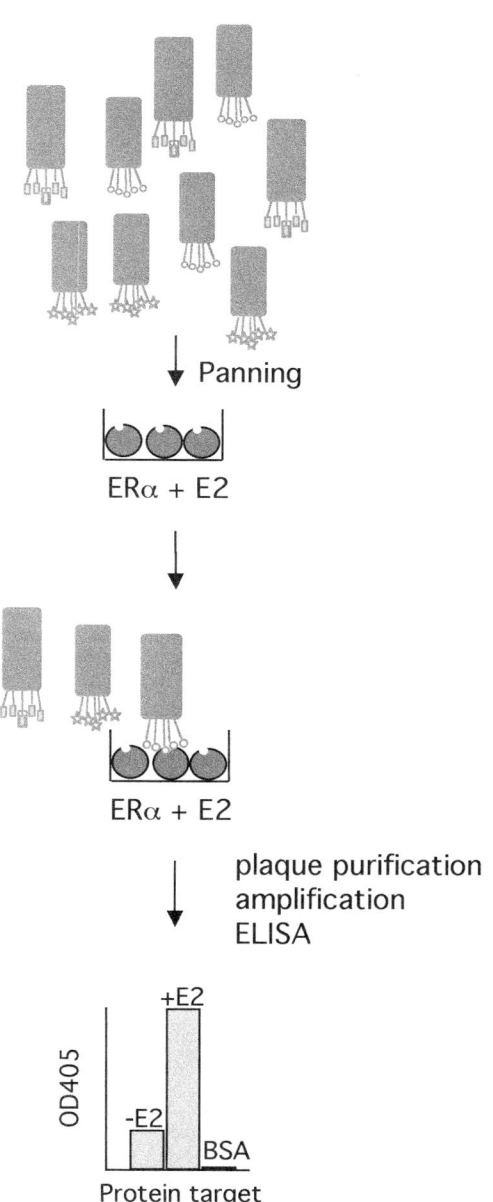

FIGURE 4. Affinity selection of ER binding motifs using phage display technology. Baculovirus-expressed full-length ERα was treated with 10^{-6} M 17β-estradiol and immobilized on 96-well Immulon-4 plates. M13 phage–based random peptide libraries were incubated with target proteins and ERα-binding phage were retained, while the unbound phage were washed away. Bound phage were eluted using a low-pH buffer, amplified in DH5αF′ cells, and subjected to subsequent rounds of selection. The selection process was repeated 2–3 times to enrich for ERα-binding phage. Individual phage were plaque-purified and amplified, and their binding characteristics were examined by ELISA. Phage that interacted specifically with estradiol-activated ERα were selected and the peptide sequences were deduced by DNA sequencing.

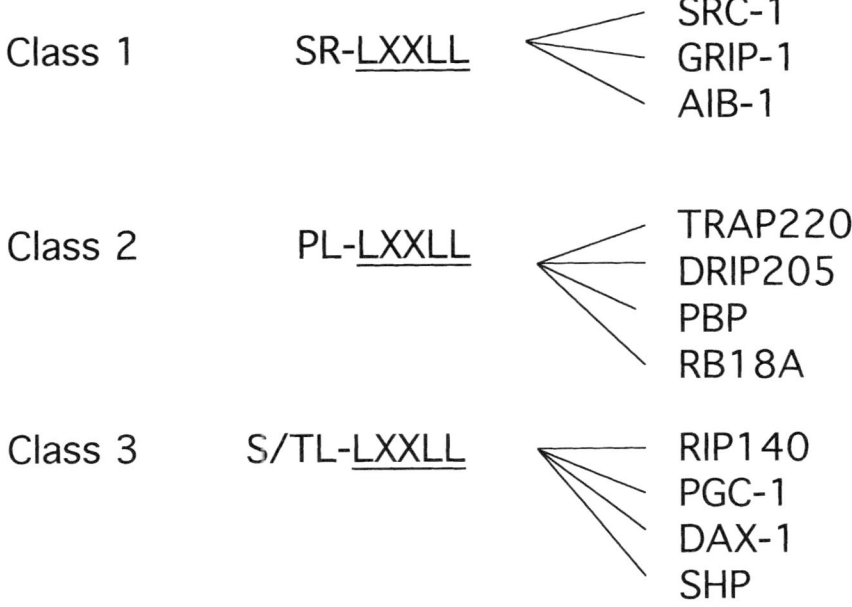

FIGURE 5. Each of the three classes of ERα-interacting LXXLL motifs are found within known coactivators.

was modified so as to contain an acidic activation domain at the amino terminus. The results of a typical experiment are shown in FIGURE 6. The striking conclusion was that the binding of most of the peptides to ERα was sensitive to mutations in the AF-2 pocket. However, the class III peptides were able to interact very well with a receptor mutant (ERα-3X) in which three charged residues, thought to be important for LXXLL binding, were changed to their corresponding amides. The interaction between the class III peptides and ERα was not tolerant of alterations in critical hydrophobic residues in the AF-2 pocket (ERα-LL), confirming the general requirement for the hydrophobic pocket. These results indicate that all of the LXXLL-containing peptides identified interact with the AF-2 domain, although not in an identical manner. More importantly, however, these data provide an explanation for the observation that AF-1 transcriptional activity is dependent on sequences within the LBD. Specifically, it has been shown that the ERα-3X mutant, which is unable to interact with the p160 coactivators, is unresponsive to estrogen activation in most cell backgrounds.[42,58] However, in some cells, the estradiol responsiveness of this mutant receptor is indistinguishable from that of the wild-type receptor. This led to the conclusion that, in these cellular contexts, AF-1 is able to function in an autonomous manner. It now appears that this conclusion is not correct as the mutations chosen to disrupt AF-2 do not prevent the interaction of ERα with all classes of LXXLL motif.[59] Indeed, we have been able to show that coactivators that contain a class III motif, such as PGC-1, can interact with the ERα-3X mutant.[60] Thus, we

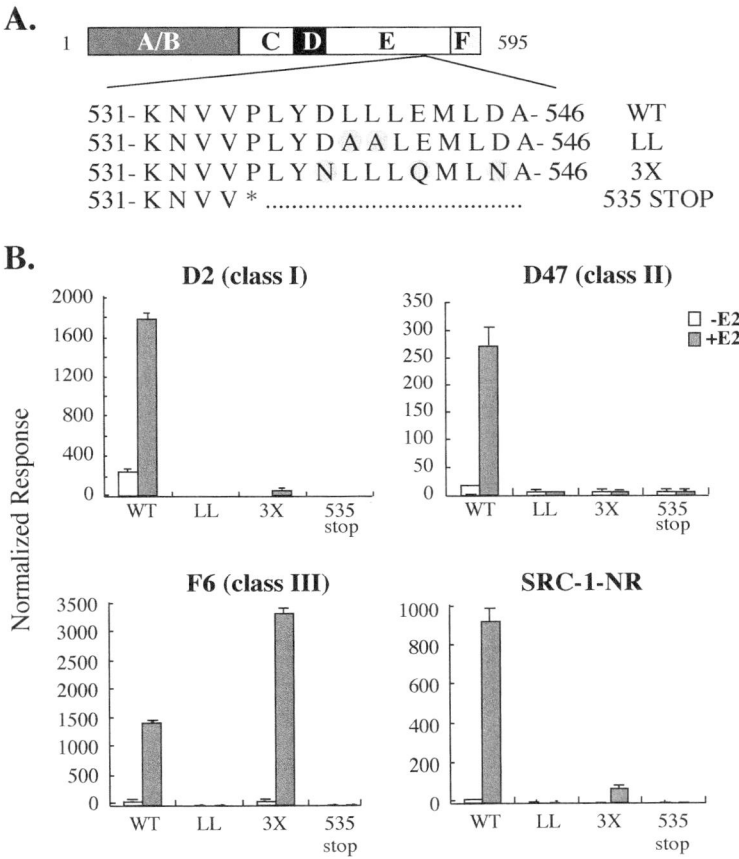

FIGURE 6. Three classes of LXXLL-containing peptides were identified that interact with the ERα–AF-2 domain in different ways. (**A**) Schematic of ERα and corresponding mutants used in this study. (**B**) The three classes of LXXLL-containing peptides (D2, D47, and F6) interact differentially with ERα helix-12 mutants. Selected peptides from each of the three classes and different ERα mutants were expressed as fusion proteins to the Gal4DBD and VP16, respectively. The binding activity of different peptides to ERα mutants was assessed on a 5× Gal4Luc3 reporter construct. The SRC-1-NR construct contains the center three copies of an LXXLL motif (amino acids 621–765) fused to Gal4DBD.

now believe that AF-1 is not an independent activation function and requires AF-2.[59] Rather, AF-1 activity can be enabled by different classes of coactivators that do not interact with ERα in the same manner. This conclusion is supported by the fact that overexpression of peptides corresponding to the class III peptide in cells where ERα-3X is active will block its activation in the presence of estradiol (FIG. 7). These important results suggest that there are different classes of ERα–AF-2–interacting

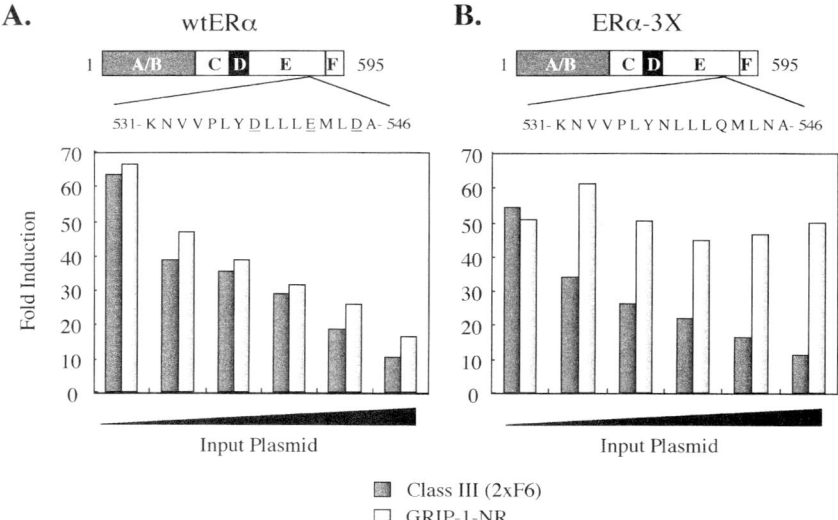

FIGURE 7. LXXLL-containing peptides disrupt ERα transcriptional activity when overexpressed in target cells. HepG2 cells were transfected with plasmids expressing **(A)** wtERα (wild-type ERα) or **(B)** ERα-3X, along with the 3XERE-TATA-Luc reporter and increasing amounts of a construct expressing the peptide-Gal4DBD fusions as indicated. Note that 2× F6 contains two copies of the class III (F6) peptide, with 50 amino acids separating the two LXXLL motifs; and GRIP-1-NR contains the center three NR boxes from the coactivator GRIP-1. All these peptides were expressed as fusion proteins to Gal4DBD. In addition, a pCMVβgal plasmid was cotransfected to normalize for transfection efficiency. After transfection, cells were induced with 10^{-7} M 17β-estradiol for 16 h before assaying. Fold induction represents the ratio of estradiol-induced activity versus no-hormone control for each transfection.

proteins and, consequently, it is likely that the ERα-estradiol complex is not recognized in the same manner in all cells.

The discovery of three distinct classes of LXXLL and the observation that they interact with ERα–AF-2 in different ways suggest that subtle ligand-induced changes in this coactivator binding pocket may favor the binding of one class of coactivator over another. We have done some preliminary studies to test this idea, the results of which are shown in FIGURE 8. Specifically, using a mammalian two-hybrid assay, we were able to show that estradiol-activated ERα interacts equally well with class I and class II peptides, whereas the genistein-activated receptor interacts preferentially with class II peptides. The significance of the observed peptide binding preferences remains to be determined; however, it suggests that, even among classical ERα agonists, there may be functionally distinct subclasses of compounds. These data also highlight the utility of receptor/coactivator-based screens in new drug discovery.

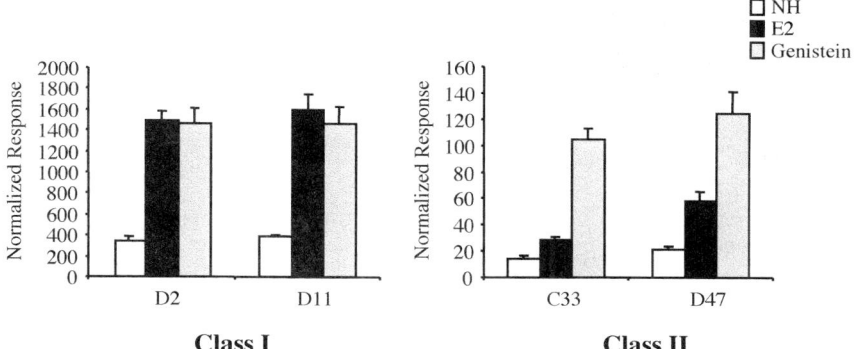

FIGURE 8. Both estradiol- and genistein-activated ERα display LXXLL-binding preferences. The binding preferences of different LXXLL motifs were analyzed using a mammalian two-hybrid assay. LXXLL-containing peptides were made as fusion proteins to the yeast Gal4DBD, and full-length ERα was fused to the VP16 acidic transactivation domain. The interactions between the LXXLL peptides and ERα were determined by a luciferase reporter gene containing Gal4 response elements. HepG2 cells were cotransfected with individual Gal4DBD-peptide fusions, VP16-ERα, the reporter 5×Gal4-luc3, and a normalization plasmid pCMVβgal. After transfection, cells were treated with vehicle control (NH), 100 nM 17β-estradiol (E2), or 1 μM genistein for 16 h. The luciferase activity was normalized to the β-galactosidase activity and expressed as normalized response as indicated.

THE AGONIST ACTIVITIES OF TAMOXIFEN AND ESTRADIOL DO NOT OCCUR IN THE SAME MANNER

The identification of three functionally different classes of LXXLL motifs was enlightening with respect to the cell-specific activities of different ERα agonists. However, since the AF-2 pocket within ERα is occluded in the presence of tamoxifen, it was unclear why tamoxifen could function as an agonist in some circumstances. Predictably, overexpression of any of the three classes of LXXLL motif described above has no effect on ERα-mediated tamoxifen partial agonist activity. We concluded from these results that tamoxifen may present a surface on the receptor that facilitates its interaction with a factor (or factors), the consequence of which is to enable AF-1. Using phage display, we identified peptides that interact with the LBD of ERα in the presence of tamoxifen, but not in the presence of estradiol.[61,62] Initially, these probes were considered to be merely surrogate markers of receptor conformation. However, when expressed in cells capable of supporting tamoxifen partial agonist activity, these peptides were able to block the agonist activity of this compound, while having no effect on estradiol-mediated transcriptional activity.[62] These data indicate that the agonist activities of tamoxifen and estradiol do not occur in the same manner and imply that these two ERα-ligand complexes interact with different coactivators. Since tamoxifen is a synthetic pharmaceutical with no physiologically relevant chemical equivalent (that we know of), this finding implies that this drug facilitates the ectopic interaction of ERα with a coactivator with which it

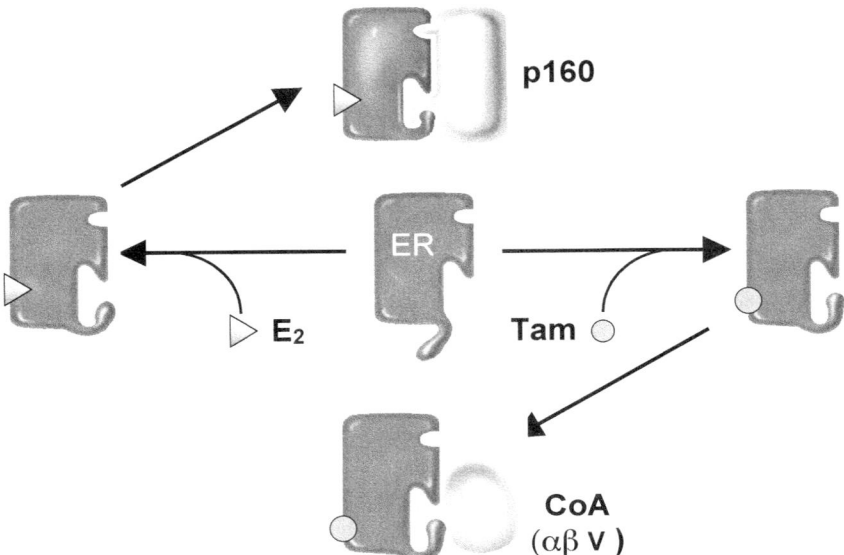

FIGURE 9. The mechanisms by which estradiol and tamoxifen manifest agonist activity are dissimilar. Using peptide antagonists that inhibit specific protein-protein interactions, it has been possible to show that the mechanisms by which estradiol and tamoxifen manifest agonist activity are dissimilar. Estradiol binding enables ERα to adopt a structure that is compatible with the binding of the p160 class of coactivators. Tamoxifen binding, on the other hand, induces a unique alteration in receptor structure that permits an ectopic interaction of the receptor with an as yet unidentified coactivator. The existence of this coactivator is supported by the fact that peptides of the α/β V class (see FIG. 10) will inhibit tamoxifen, but not estradiol-mediated transcriptional activity when expressed in target cells.

would not normally couple. A model depicting how we imagine this occuring is shown in FIGURE 9. Thus, although the hormone binding domain is required for ERα–AF-1 function, it is not used in the same manner and some of the tissue-selective agonist activity of tamoxifen will be regulated by the availability of factors that can interact with the tamoxifen-ERα complex.

IMPORTANT MECHANISTIC DIFFERENCES AMONG SERMs

The observation that tamoxifen-activated ERα adopts a structure that facilitates a specific receptor-coactivator interaction suggested that compounds that do not permit this specific protein-protein interaction would have a different pharmacological profile. We addressed this possibility by dissecting the molecular mechanism of action of additional SERMs. Several years ago, a triphenylethylene-derived antiestrogen, GW5638, which is similar in structure to tamoxifen, was identified and shown to function as an antiresorptive agent in rodent bone, but which did not display the partial agonist activity of tamoxifen in the uterus.[63,64] When assayed in cells capable of supporting tamoxifen agonist activity, this compound exhibited only

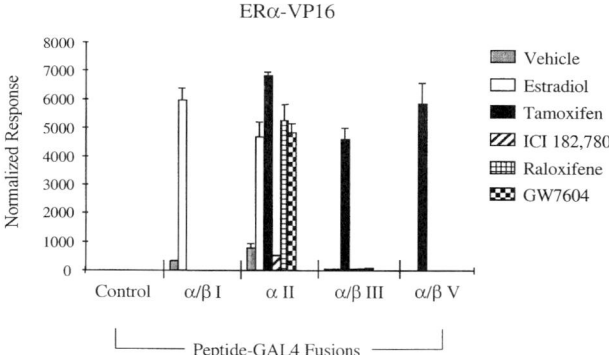

FIGURE 10. The currently available SERMs can be differentiated using peptide probes whose ability to interact with ERα is influenced by receptor structure. HepG2 cells were transiently transfected with expression vectors for ERα-VP16, the peptide-Gal4 fusion proteins, and a luciferase reporter construct under the control of five copies of a Gal4 upstream enhancer element. Transfection of the Gal4DBD alone is included as a control. Cells were then treated with various ligands (100 nM) as indicated in the figure and assayed for luciferase and β-galactosidase activity.

antagonist activity.[43,64] Thus, it appears that the agonist activities of SERMs in bone and the uterus of rodents do not occur in the same manner and that the *in vitro* systems that we have developed to study tamoxifen agonist activity model the activity of this compound in the uterus, but not in bone. Since we have shown that tamoxifen agonist activity in these *in vitro* systems requires the presentation of specific surfaces on ERα, we hypothesized that SERMs that do not exhibit uterotrophic activity, like GW5638 and raloxifene, may not permit these required surfaces to be presented. To test this hypothesis, we again resorted to the two-hybrid assay and surveyed the surfaces presented on ERα following its interaction with several different classes of SERMs.[62] The results of this experiment are shown in FIGURE 10. The peptide α/βI, an LXXLL, interacted only with ERα in the presence of the pure agonist 17β-estradiol. The peptide αII interacted with all ERα-ligand complexes, although not to the same degree.[43,62] However, the most important finding is that the peptides α/βIII and V, whose overexpression was previously shown to inhibit tamoxifen partial agonist activity, interacted with the tamoxifen-activated ERα alone. Thus, a correlation between the presentation of surfaces capable of interacting with the tamoxifen-specific peptides and agonist activity in the uterus (and partial agonist activity in some cells) was established. Identification of the cellular proteins that interact with these surfaces remains a research priority in our laboratory.

One of the most important findings of the peptide binding studies is that the structure of ERα is affected differently upon binding different ligands. In the case of tamoxifen, we have been able to show that one surface presented permits a protein-protein interaction required for partial agonist activity.[62] The relationship between structure and function with respect to agonists and antagonists is well established, having been supported by protease digestion experiments, crystallography, and (more recently) peptide binding studies.[46–48,52,65] However, until the advent of the peptide binding approach, it was difficult to distinguish the conformational changes in ERα induced by raloxifene and tamoxifen, and consequently an explanation as to their different pharmacologies was not forthcoming. The peptide binding studies, however, clearly demonstrate that ERα-tamoxifen and ERα-raloxifene complexes are quite different.[62] The conclusion that different SERMs permit ERα to adopt different conformations has been confirmed by additional studies in our laboratory that have led to the identification of peptides that recognize the GW5638-activated ERα complex, but that do not interact with the receptor when occupied by other ligands.[66] The challenge, though, is to demonstrate that the conformational changes in ERα that occur following ligand binding are functionally relevant and not just microallosteric changes of minimal consequence. The finding that peptides, which interact specifically with the ERα-tamoxifen complex, can inhibit the partial agonist activity of this compound when expressed in target cells argues that conformation is a key determinant of function. However, a complete understanding of the relationship between structure and function will require an evaluation of the functional significance of the surfaces presented on the ERα in the presence of other ligands.

THE FUTURE OF SERMs

It is clear that the main role of ERα in transcription is to facilitate the assembly of large multiprotein complexes at target gene promoters and that the ultimate response to a given ligand is regulated by the composition of the complex.[56,57] The observation that the shape of the ERα-ligand complex has a major impact on which protein-protein interactions occur suggests that it may be possible to develop improved tissue-selective estrogens and SERMs by selecting for compounds that favor one type of protein-protein interaction over another. An efficient way to do this would be to identify the coactivator proteins that are (1) most abundant in the target tissue or (2) most important for a specific biological response, and screen for compounds that facilitate the interaction of ER with these proteins at the expense of others. It is possible, although not likely, that absolute specificity will be achieved in this manner since the known coactivators have a fairly wide tissue distribution. However, in the search for improved ER modulators, it is appropriate to consider that synthetic pharmaceuticals (like tamoxifen) may be found that will enable ER to interact with proteins that it does not interact with under normal physiological circumstances. Indeed, given the opportunities provided by the combined advances in genomics, combinatorial chemistry, and technologies such as phage display, it seems assured that the currently available SERMs will be surpassed in the next 10 years by highly selective designer estrogens. These efforts will be helped and hastened by a continued dissection of the molecular mechanism(s) that can enable cells to distinguish between different ER-ligand complexes.

ACKNOWLEDGMENTS

We would like to thank Trena Martelon for help with the preparation of this manuscript. This work was supported by a grant from the National Institutes of Health (No. DK 48807) (to D. P. McDonnell) and by a postdoctoral fellowship grant

(No. DAMD17-99-1-9173) from the United States Army Medical Research Acquisition Activity (to C-Y. Chang).

REFERENCES

1. COUSE, J.F. & K.S. KORACH. 1999. Estrogen receptor null mice: what have we learned and where will they lead us? Endocr. Rev. **20:** 358–417.
2. HENDERSON, B.E., A. PAGANINI-HILL & R.K. ROSS. 1991. Decreased mortality in users of estrogen replacement therapy. Arch. Intern. Med. **151:** 75–78.
3. PAGANINI-HILL, A. 1995. The risks and benefits of estrogen replacement therapy: leisure world. Int. J. Fertil. **40:** 54–62.
4. THE WRITING GROUP FOR THE PEPI TRIAL. 1996. Effects of hormone therapy on bone mineral density. JAMA **276:** 1389–1396.
5. GRODSTEIN, F., M.J. STAMPFER, J.E. MANSON et al. 1996. Postmenopausal estrogen and progestin use and the risk of cardiovascular disease. N. Engl. J. Med. **335:** 453–461.
6. SULLIVAN, J.M., R.V. ZWAAG & E.F. LEMP. 1988. Postmenopausal estrogen use and coronary atherosclerosis. Ann. Intern. Med. **108:** 358–363.
7. SULLIVAN, J.M., R.V. ZWAAG, J.P. HUGHES et al. 1990. Estrogen replacement and coronary artery disease: effect on survival in postmenopausal women. Arch. Intern. Med. **150:** 2557–2562.
8. HERRINGTON, D.M. 1999. The HERS trial results: paradigms lost? Ann. Intern. Med. **131:** 463–466.
9. GRODSTEIN, F., G.A. COLDITZ & M.J. STAMPFER. 1996. Post-menopausal hormone use and tooth loss: a prospective study. JADA **127:** 370–377.
10. BIRGE, S.J. & K.F. MORTEL. 1997. Estrogen and the treatment of Alzheimer's disease. Am. J. Med. **103:** 36S–45S.
11. CALLE, E.E., H.L. MIRACLE-MCMAHILL, M.J. THUN et al. 1995. Estrogen replacement therapy and risk of fatal colon cancer in a prospective cohort of postmenopausal women. J. Natl. Cancer Inst. **87:** 517–523.
12. CALLE, E.E. 1997. Hormone replacement therapy and colorectal cancer: interpreting the evidence. Cancer Causes Control **8:** 127–129.
13. THE EYE-DISEASE CASE-CONTROL STUDY GROUP. 1992. Risk factors for neovascular age-related macular degeneration. Arch. Ophthalmol. **110:** 1701–1708.
14. COLLABORATIVE GROUP ON HORMONAL FACTORS IN BREAST CANCER. 1997. Breast cancer and hormone replacement therapy: collaborative reanalysis of data from 51 epidemiological studies of 52,705 women with breast cancer and 108,411 women without breast cancer. Lancet **350:** 1047–1059.
15. PERSSON, I., J. YUEN, L. BERGKVIST et al. 1996. Cancer incidence and mortality in women receiving estrogen and estrogen-progestin replacement therapy—long-term follow-up of a Swedish cohort. Int. J. Cancer **67:** 327–332.
16. DALY, E., M.P. VESSEY, M.M. HAWKINS et al. 1996. Risk of venous thromboembolism in users of hormone replacement therapy. Lancet **348:** 977–980.
17. SCHAIRER, C., J. LUBIN, R. TROISI et al. 2000. Menopausal estrogen and estrogen-progestin replacement therapy and breast cancer risk. JAMA **283:** 485–491.
18. ROSS, R.K., A. PAGANINI-HILL, P.C. WAN et al. 2000. Effect of hormone replacement therapy on breast cancer risk: estrogen versus estrogen plus progestin. J. Natl. Cancer Inst. **92:** 328–332.
19. CLARK, J.H. & E.J. PECK. 1979. Female Sex Steroids: Receptors and Function. Springer-Verlag. New York/Berlin.
20. CLARK, J.H. & B.M. MARKAVERICH. 1988. Actions of ovarian steroid hormones. In Actions of Ovarian Steroid Hormones, pp. 675–724. Raven Press. New York.
21. HARPER, M.J.K. & A.L. WALPOLE. 1967. A new derivative of triphenylethylene: effect on implantation and mode of action in rats. J. Reprod. Fertil. **13:** 101–119.
22. SUTHERLAND, R., J. MESTER & E-E. BAULIEU. 1977. Tamoxifen is a potent "pure" anti-oestrogen in chick oviduct. Nature **267:** 434–435.
23. MOON, L.Y., G.K. WAKLEY & R.T. TURNER. 1991. Dose-dependent effects of tamoxifen on long bones in growing rats: influence of ovarian status. Endocrinology **129:** 1568–1574.

24. BEALL, P.T., L.K. MISRA, R.L. YOUNG et al. 1984. Clomiphene protects against osteoporosis in the mature ovariectomized rat. Calcif. Tissue Int. **36:** 123–125.
25. TURNER, R.T., G.K. WAKLEY, K.S. HANNON et al. 1987. Tamoxifen prevents the skeletal effects of ovarian hormone deficiency in rats. J. Bone Miner. Res. **2:** 449–456.
26. LOVE, R.R., R.B. MAZESS, H.S. BARDEN et al. 1992. Effects of tamoxifen on bone mineral density in postmenopausal women with breast cancer. N. Engl. J. Med. **326:** 852–856.
27. NEVEN, P. 2000. Other selective oestrogen receptor modulators (SERMs) in development. Eur. J. Cancer **36:** S65–S67.
28. DELMAS, P.D., N.H. BJARNASON, B.H. MITLAK et al. 1997. Effects of raloxifene on bone mineral density, serum cholesterol concentrations, and uterine endometrium in postmenopausal women. N. Engl. J. Med. **337:** 1641–1647.
29. ETTINGER, B., D.M. BLACK, B.H. MITLAK et al. 1999. Reduction of vertebral risk in postmenopausal women with osteoporosis treated with raloxifene: results from a 3-year randomized clinical trial—Multiple Outcomes of Raloxifene Evaluation (MORE) Investigators. JAMA **282:** 637–645.
30. FISHER, B., J.P. COSTANTINO, D.L. WICKERHAM et al. 1998. Tamoxifen for prevention of breast cancer: report of the National Surgical Adjuvant Breast and Bowel Project P-1 Study. J. Natl. Cancer Inst. **90:** 1371–1388.
31. NATIONAL CENTER FOR HEALTH STATISTICS. 1996. Vital Statistics of the United States, 1992, Vol. II—Mortality, Part A. DHHS Publication 96-1101. U.S. Dept. of Health and Human Services, Public Health Service.
32. AMERICAN HOSPITAL FORMULARY SERVICE (AHFS). 1998. Estrogen agonist-antagonist **68:** 16.12.
33. BAKER, V.L., M. DRAPER, S. PAUL et al. 1998. Reproductive endocrine and endometrial effects of raloxifene hydrochloride, a selective estrogen receptor modulator, in women with regular menstrual cycles. J. Clin. Endocrinol. Metab. **83:** 6–13.
34. BOSS, S.M., W.J. HUSTER, J.A. NEILD et al. 1997. Effects of raloxifene hydrochloride on the endometrium of postmenopausal women. Am. J. Obstet. Gynecol. **177:** 1458–1464.
35. SATO, M., M.K. RIPPY & H.U. BRYANT. 1996. Raloxifene, tamoxifen, nafoxidine, or estrogen effects on reproductive and nonreproductive tissues in ovariectomized rats. FASEB J. **10:** 905–912.
36. MCDONNELL, D.P. 1999. The molecular pharmacology of SERMs. TEM **10:** 301–311.
37. KUIPER, G.G.J.M., E. ENMARK, M. PELTO-HUIKKO et al. 1996. Cloning of a novel estrogen receptor expressed in rat prostate and ovary. Proc. Natl. Acad. Sci. U.S.A. **93:** 5925–5930.
38. MOSSELMAN, S., J. POLMAN & R. DIJKEMA. 1996. ERβ: identification and characterization of a novel human estrogen receptor. FEBS Lett. **392:** 49–53.
39. KUIPER, G.G.J.M., B. CARLSSON, K. GRANDIEN et al. 1997. Comparison of the ligand binding specificity and transcript tissue distribution of estrogen receptors α and β. Endocrinology **138:** 863–870.
40. HALL, J.M. & D.P. MCDONNELL. 1999. The estrogen receptor β-isoform (ERβ) of the human estrogen receptor modulates ERα transcriptional activity and is a key regulator of the cellular response to estrogens and antiestrogens. Endocrinology **140:** 5566–5578.
41. MCDONNELL, D.P., D.L. CLEMM, T. HERMANN et al. 1995. Analysis of estrogen receptor function in vitro reveals three distinct classes of antiestrogens. Mol. Endocrinol. **9:** 659–668.
42. TZUKERMAN, M.T., A. ESTY, D. SANTISO-MERE et al. 1994. Human estrogen receptor transactivational capacity is determined by both cellular and promoter context and mediated by two functionally distinct intramolecular regions. Mol. Endocrinol. **8:** 21–30.
43. WIJAYARATNE, A.L., S.C. NAGEL, L.A. PAIGE et al. 1999. Comparative analyses of the mechanistic differences among antiestrogens. Endocrinology **140:** 5828–5840.
44. PAECH, K., P. WEBB, G.G.J.M. KUIPER et al. 1997. Differential ligand activation of estrogen receptors ERα and ERβ at AP1 sites. Science **277:** 1508–1510.
45. MEYER, M-E., H. GRONEMEYER, B. TURCOTTE et al. 1989. Steroid hormone receptors compete for factors that mediate their enhancer function. Cell **57:** 433–442.
46. ALLAN, G.F., S.Y. TSAI, M-J. TSAI et al. 1992. Ligand-dependent conformational changes in the progesterone receptor are necessary for events that follow DNA binding. Proc. Natl. Acad. Sci. U.S.A. **89:** 11750–11754.

47. ALLAN, G.F., X. LENG, S.Y. TSAI et al. 1992. Hormone and antihormone induce distinct conformational changes which are central to steroid receptor activation. J. Biol. Chem. **267:** 19513–19520.
48. BEEKMAN, J.M., G.F. ALLAN, S.Y. TSAI et al. 1993. Transcriptional activation by the estrogen receptor requires a conformational change in the ligand binding domain. Mol. Endocrinol. **7:** 1266–1274.
49. ASHBY, J., J. ODUM & J.R. FOSTER. 1997. Activity of raloxifene in immature and ovariectomized rat uterotrophic assays. Regul. Toxicol. Pharmacol. **25:** 226–231.
50. BLACK, L.J., M. SATO, E.R. ROWLEY et al. 1994. Raloxifene (LY139481 HCI) prevents bone loss and reduces serum cholesterol without causing uterine hypertrophy in ovariectomized rats. J. Clin. Invest. **93:** 63–69.
51. BRZOZOWSKI, A.M., A.C. PIKE, Z. DAUTER et al. 1997. Molecular basis of agonism and antagonism in the oestrogen receptor. Nature **389:** 753–758.
52. SHIAU, A.K., D. BARSTAD, P.M. LORIA et al. 1998. The structural basis of estrogen receptor/coactivator recognition and the antagonism of this interaction by tamoxifen. Cell **95:** 927–937.
53. NORRIS, J.D., D. FAN & D.P. MCDONNELL. 1996. Identification of the sequences within the human complement 3 promoter required for estrogen responsiveness provides insight into the mechanism of tamoxifen mixed agonist activity. Mol. Endocrinol. **10:** 1605–1616.
54. NORRIS, J.D., D. FAN, M.R. STALLCUP et al. 1998. Enhancement of estrogen receptor transcriptional activity by the coactivator GRIP-1 highlights the role of activation function 2 in determining estrogen receptor pharmacology. J. Biol. Chem. **273:** 6679–6688.
55. NORRIS, J.D., D. FAN, S.A. KERNER et al. 1997. Identification of a third autonomous activation domain within the human estrogen receptor. Mol. Endocrinol. **11:** 747–754.
56. MCKENNA, N.J. & B.W. O'MALLEY. 2000. An issue of tissues: divining the split personalities of selective estrogen receptor modulators. Nat. Med. **6:** 960–962.
57. MCKENNA, N.J., R.B. LANZ & B.W. O'MALLEY. 1999. Nuclear receptor coregulators: cellular and molecular biology. Endocr. Rev. **20:** 321–344.
58. WHITE, R., M. SJÖBERG, E. KALKHOVEN et al. 1997. Ligand-independent activation of the oestrogen receptor by mutation of a conserved tyrosine. EMBO J. **16:** 1427–1435.
59. CHANG, C-Y., J.D. NORRIS, H. GRØN et al. 1999. Dissection of the LXXLL nuclear receptor-coactivator interaction motif using combinatorial peptide libraries: discovery of peptide antagonists of estrogen receptors α and β. Mol. Cell. Biol. **19:** 8226–8239.
60. TCHEREPANOVA, I., P. PUIGSERVER, J.D. NORRIS et al. 2000. Modulation of estrogen receptor-α transcriptional activity by the coactivator PGC-1. J. Biol. Chem. **275:** 16302–16308.
61. PAIGE, L.A., D.J. CHRISTENSEN, H. GRØN et al. 1999. Estrogen receptor (ER) modulators each induce distinct conformational changes in ERα and ERβ. Proc. Natl. Acad. Sci. U.S.A. **96:** 3999–4004.
62. NORRIS, J.D., L.A. PAIGE, D.J. CHRISTENSEN et al. 1999. Peptide antagonists of the human estrogen receptor. Science **285:** 744–746.
63. WILLSON, T.M., B.R. HENKE, T.M. MOMTAHEN et al. 1994. 3-[4-(1,2-Diphenylbut-1-enyl)phenyl]acrylic acid: a non-steroidal estrogen with functional selectivity for bone over uterus in rats. J. Med. Chem. **37:** 1550–1552.
64. WILLSON, T.M., J.D. NORRIS, B.L. WAGNER et al. 1997. Dissection of the molecular mechanism of action of GW5638, a novel estrogen receptor ligand, provides insights into the role of ER in bone. Endocrinology **138:** 3901–3911.
65. GREENE, G., L. CHENG, P.M. LORIS et al. 1998. Mechanistic complexities in endocrine modulation: estrogen receptor structure, modulators, and targets. *In* Mechanistic Complexities in Endocrine Modulation: Estrogen Receptor Structure, Modulators, and Targets. ILSI Press. Washington, D.C.
66. CONNOR, C.E., J.D. NORRIS, G. BROADWATER et al. 2001. Circumventing tamoxifen resistance in breast cancers using antiestrogens that induce unique conformational changes in the estrogen receptor. Cancer Res. **61:** in press.

Developing Animal Models for Analyzing SERM Activity

JUDITH M. A. EMMEN AND KENNETH S. KORACH

Laboratory of Reproductive and Developmental Toxicology, Receptor Biology Section, National Institute of Environmental Health Sciences, National Institutes of Health, Research Triangle Park, North Carolina 27709, USA

> ABSTRACT: Estrogens have effects on many organ systems, beyond the reproductive system, in both females and males. Estrogen effects are exerted through specific receptors, of which there are two types: estrogen receptor (ER) α and estrogen receptor (ER) β. To study the roles of each receptor *in vivo*, a series of mice were generated lacking either a functional ERα or ERβ or both. These mice, labeled αERKO, βERKO, or αβERKO, respectively, have been useful in defining the tissue specificities, localization, and functions of each of the estrogen receptors. These mouse models also show great promise for use in defining the effectiveness of putative SERMs.
>
> KEYWORDS: ERα; ERβ; SERMs

INTRODUCTION

There is a very broad spectrum of organ systems that respond or have been suggested to respond to estrogen hormones, including the female reproductive tract and mammary gland, the skeleton, the cardiovascular system, and the central nervous system. Estrogens exert their effects through specific estrogen receptors. Two types of estrogen receptors, estrogen receptor α (ERα) and estrogen receptor β (ERβ) have been cloned and characterized.[1–4] To study the roles of each of these estrogen receptors *in vivo*, mice were generated lacking either a functional ERα or ERβ, referred to as αERKO and βERKO mice, respectively.[5,6] More recently, mice lacking both estrogen receptors, αβERKO mice, have been generated.[7,8] These mice are viable and quite healthy. This was somewhat surprising since it was thought that estrogens were essential for prenatal survival, suggesting the possibility that another estrogen receptor has yet to be cloned. Studies in rodents showed that the tissue distribution of the two receptors differs: ERα is expressed in many different tissues, including the female and male reproductive tract, skeletal and cardiac muscle, kidney, liver, lung, hypothalamus, and pituitary gland. ERβ expression is more limited and is expressed principally in the ovary, male reproductive tract, lung, and hypothalamus. αERKO mice express ERβ at wild-type levels and, vice versa, βERKO mice express ERα at normal levels. αERKO and βERKO mice have proven

---

Address for correspondence: Dr. K. S. Korach, Receptor Biology Section, LRDT, NIEHS, NIH, MD B3-02, P.O. Box 12233, Research Triangle Park, NC 27709. Voice: 919-541-3521; fax: 919-541-0696.
Korach@niehs.nih.gov

to be highly useful in understanding the distinct roles of both estrogen receptors in various tissues. These knockout models are also suitable for evaluating individual receptor-mediated action of particular ligands or selective estrogen receptor modulators (SERMs) *in vivo* because disruption of a specific receptor form generates mice that will show responsiveness to the other estrogen receptor. In this review, several of the phenotypes seen in specific organ systems of the different estrogen receptor knockout mice will be described.[9]

FEMALE REPRODUCTIVE PHENOTYPE

The Uterus

Estrogens and progesterone, as well as many growth factors, play key roles in female reproductive tract function. Under the influence of these steroids, the uterus is prepared for a possible establishment and maintenance of pregnancy. Estrogen stimulates proliferation of the uterine epithelial cells and induces the progesterone receptor (PR) protein. Progesterone, subsequently, induces stromal cell proliferation and differentiation and opposes the estrogen-induced epithelial proliferation.

The ERα is the predominant estrogen receptor in the adult mouse uterus.[10] ERβ is detectable in the uterus of both wild-type and αERKO mouse uteri, but only at a very low level. Both αERKO and βERKO mice have properly differentiated female reproductive tracts possessing the constituent structures, such as uteri.[5,6] In addition, uteri of adult βERKO mice show no appreciable morphological or histological differences when compared to uteri of wild-type mice, and they demonstrate a proper response to circulating ovarian hormones.[5,8] In contrast, uteri of adult αERKO female mice are hypoplastic and have lost their estrogen responsiveness, as measured by a uterotropic bioassay.[6,11] In this bioassay, ovariectomized mice are treated for three days with vehicle or an estrogen receptor agonist (estradiol, tamoxifen, or diethylstilbestrol). The uteri of wild-type animals respond to the three different types of agonist in a similar way, showing an increase in uterine wet weight. In αERKO mice, however, no uterine stimulation is seen after administration of any of these three agonists. In addition, not only are uterine growth and morphogenesis lacking in αERKO mice, but also hyperemia and water imbibition, classical early estrogen responses, are lacking, linking these responses to a functional ERα. Further analysis revealed that estrogen-treated αERKO uteri did not demonstrate increased DNA synthesis nor increased gene expression of PR, lactoferrin, and glucose-6-phosphate dehydrogenase, all known estrogen-induced genes in the adult uterus, within 24 h.[12] However, basal levels of PR mRNA and protein in αERKO uteri do not differ from those in wild-type uteri. In addition, PR-mediated progesterone actions appeared to be preserved in αERKO uteri.[13]

The uterine phenotype observed in the αβERKO is very similar to the αERKO.[7] However, Dupont *et al.*[8] reported an aggravation of αERKO uterine phenotype in the αβERKO uterus. The uterine diameter and wall thickness were reduced in the αβERKO uterus in comparison with the αERKO uterus. They suggested at least some compensatory role of ERβ in the mouse uterus.

The Ovary

The ovary is involved in two basic endocrine and physiological actions, folliculogenesis and steroidogenesis. Understanding the role of the estrogen receptor in these ovarian functions has been very difficult. This is due to the fact that the action of estrogen had to be studied in the tissue that is making the hormone itself. Interference with ERα or ERβ action through targeted gene disruption in mice provided us with novel genetic models, which may allow an evaluation of the possible role of estrogen and ER-mediated actions in the ovary. Some of the interesting phenotypes that have evolved from the ER knockout mice confirm the importance of estrogen in the ovary.

In contrast to the uterus, in which ERα can be considered the predominant receptor, both ERα and ERβ are clearly present in adult rodent ovaries.[2,10,14] The distribution pattern of both receptors, however, differs among the different ovarian cell types. ERβ is predominantly localized in the granulosa cells of the ovary, whereas ERα expression is limited to the thecal and interstitial cells. In line with these different expression patterns, analysis of αERKO and βERKO females revealed distinct ovarian phenotypes.[5,6,15] Both ERα and ERβ are not essential for perinatal ovarian development. αERKO females are found to be infertile in continuous mating studies, whereas βERKO females are subfertile. Histological analysis of the αERKO ovary showed a polycystic, or PCOS, type morphology, with enlarged hemorrhagic cystic follicles, no corpora lutea, and no indication of ovulation. Further analysis revealed that the anovulation develops and worsens as the αERKO females age.[15,16] Immature αERKO females studied prior to development of the overt ovarian phenotype are responsive to superovulation treatment, but with a reduced response when compared with immature wild-type females.

Disruption of the ERα gene severely affects the negative feedback action of estradiol on the hypothalamic-pituitary axis, resulting in highly elevated estradiol and luteinizing hormone (LH) serum levels. The chronic elevation of LH serum levels is considered to be the major cause of the ovarian phenotype seen in αERKO females. This hypothesis is supported by the finding that, in αERKO females treated with gonadotropin-releasing hormone (GnRH) antagonist, serum LH levels are suppressed to wild-type range and the polycystic ovarian phenotype is prevented.[17] Moreover, the same polycystic ovarian phenotype is seen in transgenic females overexpressing LH.[18]

βERKO female ovaries, in contrast, have a totally different phenotype.[5] In these ovaries, follicles are seen at various stages of development, from primordial up to large antral follicles. Upon superovulation treatment, βERKO females revealed an obvious ovarian phenotype, exhibiting numerous ovulatory, but unruptured follicles. Serum LH, follicle-stimulating hormone (FSH), and estradiol levels are within the normal wild-type range. The observed subfertility in βERKO females appears to be primarily caused by this compromised ovary as there are no indications that the uterus is dysfunctional. Whether this dysfunction is intrinsic to the βERKO ovary or caused by a disturbed hypothalamic-pituitary axis has not been determined. The ovarian phenotype found in mice lacking a functional progesterone receptor[19] or prostaglandin synthase-2[20] is very similar to that observed in βERKO females. Therefore, expression of these genes is being evaluated in βERKO ovaries.

The αβERKO adult ovaries demonstrate a phenotype that is quite distinct from that seen in either αERKO or βERKO ovaries.[7,8] αβERKO ovaries contain follicles that predominantly reach the small antral stage, with only a few follicles possessing a large antrum and no corpora lutea. Remarkably, however, structures were observed within these ovaries that resembled testicular cordlike structures containing Sertoli-like cells. These structures are only observed in the adult αβERKO ovaries and not in the prepubertal ovaries. The granulosa cells of these "sex-reversed" follicles have undergone redifferentiation to a Sertoli cell phenotype, determined by both morphological and biochemical markers. Thus, ERα and ERβ actions appear not to be essential in ovary determination, but are involved in maintaining the proper differentiation state of the granulosa cells.

Mice lacking the capacity to produce estrogen due to targeted deletion of the aromatase gene, ArKO mice, have an ovarian phenotype, which is more similar to that seen in αERKO females.[21] Serum levels of LH, FSH, and testosterone are elevated in ArKO females, but there is no detectable estradiol. This is in contrast to αERKO females, which have highly elevated levels of estradiol and LH, but not FSH. ArKO ovaries contain follicles at different developmental stages, but no corpora lutea, and are infertile. With age, the ArKO ovaries develop into polycystic hemorrhagic ovaries, similar to what is seen in the αERKO ovaries.[22] Obviously, the lack of both ERα and ERβ leads to a different ovarian phenotype from that seen with lack of estrogen alone. Although this difference cannot be explained at the present time, a different hypothesis can be proposed. There is evidence that polypeptide growth factors, including epidermal growth factor and insulin-like growth factor I, can stimulate ER activity in an estrogen-independent manner, although the significance *in vivo* is not known yet.[23,24] Due to the presence of both a functional ERα and ERβ, such nonestradiol estrogen receptor signaling pathways will still be functional in ArKO females. Another hypothesis explaining the difference in ovarian phenotype between ArKO and αβERKO mice is exposure of the developing ovary to maternal estrogens. Although ArKO females have undetectable estrogen serum levels, these animals are still responsive to estrogens. During prenatal development, maternal estrogens can induce changes in the ovary of ArKO female fetuses. This might lead to the observed and different ovarian phenotype in ArKO and αβERKO females at a later stage of ovarian differentiation.

The Mammary Gland

The mammary gland, in addition to the uterus, is one of the organ systems that is appropriate for evaluation of SERM activity. The mammary gland consists of a ductal and lobuloalveolar network, embedded in stromal tissue.[25] At birth, a rudimentary ductal system is present in the nipple area. During puberty, the ductal system expands through proliferation at the terminal end buds of each branch. During pregnancy and lactation, the ductal system undergoes further branching, and formation of lobuloalveolar structures can be observed. Many studies have implied a role for both estrogen and progesterone in mammary gland differentiation and function.

Estrogen stimulates proliferation of the mammary epithelial cells and induces expression of the PR protein. Progesterone, in turn, induces formation of lobuloalveolar structures. Analysis of the mammary glands of both ER and PR knockout mice supports these previous observations.[19,26] Additionally, these mouse models have proven to be very useful in studying the distinct roles of these two hormones in mammary gland function.

ERα mRNA is very highly expressed in the adult mouse mammary gland. ERβ mRNA is undetectable by RNase protection assay, but is detectable by RT-PCR in adult mouse mammary glands.[9] The mammary gland of βERKO females appears to be normally developed and these females are able to lactate following pregnancy. In contrast, the αERKO mammary gland shows normal prenatal and prepubertal development, but remains rudimentary after puberty, lacking epithelial branching and lobuloalveolar development.[26] The αβERKO mammary gland phenotype resembles that of αERKO adult females. Tissue recombinant experiments have shown that the presence of ERα in the stromal compartment is essential for ductal growth and branching.[27]

PR is a very well known estrogen-responsive gene in the uterus and in the mammary gland. In PR knockout mice, ductal development does occur in the mammary gland, but lobuloalveolar development is lacking.[19] In αERKO mammary glands, basal PR expression is significantly reduced and estrogen-stimulated increase in PR gene expression is lost.[26] The lack of PR induction may contribute to the αERKO mammary gland phenotype. In addition, disruption of the ERα gene also affects the positive feedback action of estradiol on the prolactin (PRL)–secreting cells in the pituitary. PRL is essential for full mammary gland development as shown by the presence of abnormal mammary glands in PRL receptor knockout mice.[28] PRL mRNA appeared to be significantly reduced in the αERKO pituitary, and PRL serum levels are lowered in the αERKO.[29] The pituitary transplantation technique was used to determine whether the observed mammary gland phenotype in αERKO was due to the loss of PRL secretion by the pituitary.[30] An elevation of PRL and mammary gland development could be achieved in αERKO female mice when transplanted with a heterozygous pituitary. Mammary gland development, however, was only seen in transplanted animals with intact ovaries and not in ovariectomized recipients, implicating the need for additional ovarian factors.

Additionally, hormonal replacement studies showed that both progesterone and estradiol, but not PRL, were needed. Treatment of αERKO female animals with high-dose estradiol and progesterone did induce branching and alveolar development in the mammary gland, whereas progesterone alone or in combination with PRL did not. Estradiol alone does cause growth in the αERKO mammary gland, but the combined actions of estradiol and progesterone are needed for the fullest response. In conclusion, the phenotype seen in the αERKO female mammary gland occurs not only via a direct action of estrogens on the gland itself, but also via indirect mechanisms involving the hypothalamic-pituitary axis.

MALE REPRODUCTIVE PHENOTYPE

SERMs were developed because of concern about undesired effects of estrogens in women undergoing hormone replacement therapy. The generation of αERKO mice, however, indicated that estrogen is also essential for male fertility. Therefore, SERMs may also exert important effects on male fertility.

Male αERKO mice are infertile with extensive dysmorphogenesis of seminiferous tubules and disruption of spermatogenesis, reflected by a lower sperm count and decreased sperm motility in comparison with the wild-type male.[31] Although the presence of both ERβ mRNA and protein has been demonstrated in the male reproductive tract, βERKO male mice are fertile and show no apparent or obvious morphological phenotypes.[5,32] The αβERKO male mice are infertile and show a clear and overt phenotype with respect to dysmorphogenesis of the seminiferous tubules and impaired spermatogenesis. This phenotype is similar to that of the αERKO male, suggesting that estrogen action in the male tract related to fertility appears to be mainly regulated through ERα.[8,9]

Further studies showed that impaired spermatogenesis is not caused by any defects in the germ cell itself, but is indirect through disruption in the somatic cells of the αERKO male reproductive tract.[33] A role for estrogens in the luminal fluid balance in the head of the epididymis was suggested based on the observation of dilated efferent ducts and a morphologically abnormal epithelium that has lost its ability to reabsorb fluid from the tubules in the ERKO male.[31,34] This leads to the accumulation of fluid in the efferent tubules and testis, eventually producing testicular atrophy. This αERKO phenotype can be at least partially reproduced in wild-type animals through blockage of ER action with the pure antiestrogen, ICI 182,780.[35] Although no alteration in hormone androgen action has been detected, serum testosterone levels are slightly elevated in the αERKO male in comparison with those of wild-type males.[31] These findings suggest that there is a physiological requirement for estrogen in these male tissues.

It was speculated that the phenotype of the male ArKO mice, being estrogen-deficient, might have been very similar to that of the male αβERKO mice. However, ArKO male mice appeared to be much less severely affected than male mice lacking only ERα or both ERα and ERβ. ArKO male mice are fertile and no morphological changes are observed in the testis.[21] Again, this difference might be the result of ligand-independent estrogen receptor activation pathways that are still functional in ArKO male mice and not in the αERKO or αβERKO male.[9]

CONCLUSIONS

Targeted disruption of the different ER genes has resulted in animal models that are very valuable in evaluating the distinct and cooperative roles of ERα and ERβ in reproductive and nonreproductive tissues. These gene knockout mice should represent useful models in the development and search for tissue-specific SERMs, in analyzing and detecting possible side effects of SERMs, and in the understanding of similar as well as different mechanisms of action of the ER and SERMs.

ACKNOWLEDGMENTS

We wish to thank the many contributors in the Korach lab as well as collaborators all over the world who have contributed to the work described herein.

REFERENCES

1. GREEN, S., P. WALTER, V. KUMAR et al. 1986. Human oestrogen receptor cDNA: sequence, expression, and homology to v-erb-A. Nature **320**: 134–139.

2. KUIPER, G.G., E. ENMARK, M. PELTO-HUIKKO *et al.* 1996. Cloning of a novel receptor expressed in rat prostate and ovary. Proc. Natl. Acad. Sci. U.S.A. **93:** 5925–5930.
3. MOSSELMAN, S., J. POLMA & R. DIJKEMA. 1996. ER beta: identification and characterization of a novel human estrogen receptor. FEBS Lett. **392:** 49–53.
4. TREMBLAY, G.B., A. TREMBLAY, N.G. COPELAND *et al.* 1997. Cloning, chromosomal localization, and functional analysis of the murine estrogen receptor beta. Mol. Endocrinol. **11:** 353–365.
5. KREGE, J.H., J.B. HODGIN, J.F. COUSE *et al.* 1998. Generation and reproductive phenotypes of mice lacking estrogen receptor beta. Proc. Natl. Acad. Sci. U.S.A. **95:** 15677–15682.
6. LUBAHN, D.B., J.S. MOYER, T.S. GOLDING *et al.* 1993. Alteration of reproductive function, but not prenatal sexual development after insertional disruption of the mouse estrogen receptor gene. Proc. Natl. Acad. Sci. U.S.A. **90:** 11162–11166.
7. COUSE, J.F., S.C. HEWIT, D.O. BUNCH *et al.* 1999. Postnatal sex reversal of the ovaries in mice lacking estrogen receptors alpha and beta. Science **286:** 2328–2331.
8. DUPONT, S., A. KRUST, A. GANSMULLER *et al.* 2000. Effect of single and compound knockouts of estrogen receptors alpha (ERalpha) and beta (ERbeta) on mouse reproductive phenotypes. Development **127:** 4277–4291.
9. COUSE, J.F. & K.S. KORACH. 1999. Estrogen receptor null mice: what have we learned and where will they lead us? Endocr. Rev. **20:** 358–417. [Erratum. 1999. Endocr. Rev. **20(4):** 459.]
10. COUSE, J.F., J. LINDZEY, K. GRANDIEN *et al.* 1997. Tissue distribution and quantitative analysis of estrogen receptor-alpha (ERalpha) and estrogen receptor-beta (ERbeta) messenger ribonucleic acid in the wild-type and ERalpha-knockout mouse. Endocrinology **138:** 4613–4621.
11. KORACH, K.S. 1994. Insights from the study of animals lacking functional estrogen receptor. Science **266:** 1524–1527.
12. COUSE, J.F., S.W. CURTIS, T.F. WASHBURN *et al.* 1995. Analysis of transcription and estrogen insensitivity in the female mouse after targeted disruption of the estrogen receptor gene. Mol. Endocrinol. **9:** 1441–1454.
13. CURTIS, S.W., J. CLARK, P. MYERS *et al.* 1999. Disruption of estrogen signaling does not prevent progesterone action in the estrogen receptor alpha knockout mouse uterus. Proc. Natl. Acad. Sci. U.S.A. **96:** 3646–3651.
14. SAR, M. & F. WELSCH. 1999. Differential expression of estrogen receptor-beta and estrogen receptor-alpha in the rat ovary. Endocrinology **140:** 963–971.
15. SCHOMBERG, D.W., J.F. COUSE, A. MUKHERJEE *et al.* 1999. Targeted disruption of the estrogen receptor-alpha gene in female mice: characterization of ovarian responses and phenotype in the adult. Endocrinology **140:** 2733–2744.
16. ROSENFELD, C.S., A.A. MURRAY, G. SIMMER *et al.* 2000. Gonadotropin induction of ovulation and corpus luteum formation in young estrogen receptor-alpha knockout mice. Biol. Reprod. **62:** 599–605.
17. COUSE, J.F., D.O. BUNCH, J. LINDZEY *et al.* 1999. Prevention of the polycystic ovarian phenotype and characterization of ovulatory capacity in the estrogen receptor-alpha knockout mouse. Endocrinology **140:** 5855–5865.
18. RISMA, K.A., C.M. CLAY, T.M. NETT *et al.* 1995. Targeted overexpression of luteinizing hormone in transgenic mice leads to infertility, polycystic ovaries, and ovarian tumors. Proc. Natl. Acad. Sci. U.S.A. **92:** 1322–1326.
19. LYDON, J.P., F.J. DEMAYO, C.R. FUNK *et al.* 1995. Mice lacking progesterone receptor exhibit pleiotropic reproductive abnormalities. Genes Dev. **9:** 2266–2278.
20. LIM, H., B.C. PARIA, S.K. DAS *et al.* 1997. Multiple female reproductive failures in cyclooxygenase 2–deficient mice. Cell **91:** 197–208.
21. FISHER, C.R., K.H. GRAVES, A.F. PARLOW *et al.* 1998. Characterization of mice deficient in aromatase (ArKO) because of targeted disruption of the Cyp19 gene. Proc. Natl. Acad. Sci. U.S.A. **95:** 6965–6970.
22. BRITT, K.L., A.E. DRUMMOND, V.A. COX *et al.* 2000. An age-related ovarian phenotype in mice with targeted disruption of the Cyp19 (aromatase) gene. Endocrinology **141:** 2614–2623.

23. CURTIS, S.W., T. WASHBURN, C. SEWALL et al. 1996. Physiological coupling of growth factor and steroid receptor signaling pathways: estrogen receptor knockout mice lack estrogen-like response to epidermal growth factor. Proc. Natl. Acad. Sci. U.S.A. **93:** 12626–12630.
24. SMITH, C.L. 1998. Cross-talk between peptide growth factor and estrogen receptor signaling pathways. Biol. Reprod. **58:** 627–632.
25. IMAGAWA, W., J. YANG, R. GUZMAN et al. 1994. Control of mammary gland development. In The Physiology of Reproduction, pp. 1033–1063. Raven Press. New York.
26. BOCCHINFUSO, W.P. & K.S. KORACH. 1997. Mammary gland development and tumorigenesis in estrogen receptor knockout mice. J. Mammary Gland Biol. Neoplasia **2:** 323–344.
27. CUNHA, G.R., P. YOUNG, Y.K. HOM et al. 1997. Elucidation of a role for stromal steroid hormone receptors in mammary gland growth and development using tissue recombinants. J. Mammary Gland Biol. Neoplasia **2:** 393–402.
28. BRISKEN, C., S. KAUR, T.E. CHAVARRIA et al. 1999. Prolactin controls mammary gland development via direct and indirect mechanisms. Dev. Biol. **210:** 96–106.
29. SCULLY, K.M., A.S. GLEIBERMAN, J. LINDZEY et al. 1997. Role of estrogen receptor-alpha in the anterior pituitary gland. Mol. Endocrinol. **11:** 674–681.
30. BOCCHINFUSO, W.P., J.K. LINDZEY, S.C. HEWITT et al. 2000. Induction of mammary gland development in estrogen receptor-alpha knockout mice. Endocrinology **141:** 2982–2994.
31. EDDY, E.M., T.F. WASHBURN, D.O. BUNCH et al. 1996. Targeted disruption of the estrogen receptor gene in male mice causes alteration of spermatogenesis and infertility. Endocrinology **137:** 4796–4805.
32. KUIPER, G.G., B. CARLSSON, K. GRANDIEN et al. 1997. Comparison of the ligand binding specificity and transcript tissue distribution of estrogen receptors alpha and beta. Endocrinology **138:** 863–870.
33. MAHATO, D., E.H. GOULDING, K.S. KORACH et al. 2000. Spermatogenic cells do not require estrogen receptor-alpha for development or function. Endocrinology **141:** 1273–1276.
34. HESS, R.A., D. BUNICK, K. LEE et al. 1997. A role for oestrogens in the male reproductive system. Nature **390:** 509–512.
35. LEE, K.H., R.A. HESS, J.M. BAHR et al. 2000. Estrogen receptor alpha has a functional role in the mouse rete testis and efferent ductules. Biol. Reprod. **63:** 1873–1880.

Androgen Receptor: Structural Domains and Functional Dynamics after Ligand-Receptor Interaction

ARUN K. ROY,[a] RAKESH K. TYAGI,[a] CHUNG S. SONG,[a,b] YAN LAVROVSKY,[a] SOON C. AHN,[a] TAE-SUNG OH,[a] AND BANDANA CHATTERJEE[a,b]

[a]*Department of Cellular and Structural Biology, University of Texas Health Science Center at San Antonio, San Antonio, Texas 78229, USA*

[b]*South Texas Veterans Health Care System, San Antonio, Texas 78229, USA*

ABSTRACT: Androgens are C-19 steroids secreted primarily from the testes and adrenals that play a critical role in reproduction. Reproductive functions of androgens are mediated through coordination of diverse physiological processes ranging from brain functions to specific cell proliferation and apoptosis. At the molecular level, most of these regulatory influences are exerted by altered expression of appropriate genes by the androgen receptor (AR), a member of the nuclear receptor (NR) superfamily. The unliganded AR is a cytoplasmic protein and, upon ligand binding, it translocates into the nucleus. Thereafter, in conjunction with other transcription factors and coactivators, the AR influences transcription of target genes through a multistep process that includes its clustering in a subnuclear compartment. Here, we describe the genomic organization of the AR, the role of individual structural domains in specific AR function, and the influence of agonistic/antagonistic ligands in the intracellular movement of the receptor. We also show that the AR is capable of undergoing multiple rounds of nucleocytoplasmic recycling after ligand binding and dissociation. Xenobiotic ligands, considered as selective androgen receptor modulators (SARMs), can modulate AR activity by inhibiting either its nuclear translocation or its subnuclear clustering and subsequent transactivation function.

KEYWORDS: androgen receptor; SARM; endocrine disrupters; vinclozolin; procymidone; chlozolinate; receptor recycling; green fluorescent protein

STRUCTURAL DOMAINS OF THE ANDROGEN RECEPTOR AND THEIR SPECIFIC ROLES IN RECEPTOR FUNCTION

The androgen receptor (AR) is a member of the superfamily of nuclear receptors (NRs), produced from a single-copy gene on the X chromosome.[1] The genomic DNA encoding the approximately 110-kDa human AR spans 90-kilobase (kb) pairs of the chromosomal DNA at the Xq11-q12 site.[2–4] The spliced and processed transcript from the AR gene is about 11 kb in size and contains an open reading frame

Address for correspondence: Arun K. Roy, Ph.D., Department of Cellular and Structural Biology, University of Texas Health Science Center at San Antonio, 7703 Floyd Curl Drive, San Antonio, TX 78229. Voice: 210-567-3850; fax: 210-567-3846.

roy@uthscsa.edu

of ~2.8 kb. Additionally, alternate splicing within the 6-kb-long 3′ untranslated region (UTR) generates a minor 8-kb-long mRNA species.[4] The human AR gene is organized as 8 exons, all of which contribute to the protein-coding sequence. The relatively long first exon specifies the N-terminal domain containing the major transactivating function (AF-1) of the receptor protein and all of the 5′ UTR. Exons 2 and 3 encode the DNA-binding domain, while the ligand-binding domain is specified by the coding sequences contributed by exons 4 through 8. A second and less effective transactivation function (AF-2) resides within the ligand-binding domain of the AR. The 6-kb-long 3′ UTR is part of exon 8.[5–8] The three major structural domains, that is, the AF-1-containing N-terminal domain, the centrally positioned DNA-binding domain, and the C-terminally located ligand-binding domain, are the signature motifs for all NRs. In the case of AR, the exon 1–derived N-terminal domain shows structural polymorphism due to the variable numbers of glutamine (Q) and glycine (G) repeats. Although the number of glutamine repeats appears to vary within a range of 11 to 35, on average the normal population contains 21 consecutively positioned glutamine residues. The glycine repeat located further downstream within the N-terminal domain varies in glycine residues from 10 to 31, with the majority of the human population containing 24 residues. Expansion of the glutamine repeat can sequester coactivators such as the CREB-binding protein (CBP), leading to the age-dependent pathology of spinal and bulbar muscular atrophy (Kennedy's disease).[9,10] Shortening of the polyglutamine or the polyglycine stretch may also cause detrimental effects and is suggested to be associated with predisposition to prostatic neoplasia.[11,12] The genomic origin and functional domains of the AR are summarized in FIGURE 1.

In the absence of the agonist, the ligand-binding domain (LBD) at the carboxyl terminus of the AR prevents the transactivation function of the N-terminal domain. Deletion of the LBD makes the receptor constitutively active by allowing its interaction with coactivator proteins. Structure-function analysis of the mutated AR and steroid receptor coactivator-1 (SRC-1) has shown that almost the entire N-terminal domain (residues 1–494) is required for maximum transactivation function. This region of AR interacts with a glutamine-rich region of SRC-1 (residues 949–1240), which is highly conserved among the coactivator proteins of the p160 family[13] that includes SRC-1, the glucocorticoid receptor–interacting protein (GRIP-1)/TIF2 (transcription intermediary factor 2), and AIB-1 (amplified in breast cancer-1). On the other hand, the weakly acting activation function (AF-2) at the carboxyl terminus interacts with the leucine rich LXXLL motif of the coactivator.[14] Since the unliganded AR is transcriptionally inactive and the C-terminally located AF-2 provides only weak activation function, the AR with a deleted LBD is capable of showing transcriptional activity nearly to its full potential. Thus, not only does the LBD in its unliganded form appear to exert an inhibitory effect on the AF-1 function, but the altered three-dimensional structure resulting from its interaction with the cognate ligand also provides an appropriate surface structure that is conducive to coactivator-receptor interaction at the AF-2 site. Structural realignment at the LBD, in turn, creates the desired conformational change at the N-terminal domain, which then interacts with p160 and possibly other coactivator proteins, leading to the functional integration of the two transactivation domains, and generates a transcriptionally competent stable multiprotein complex.

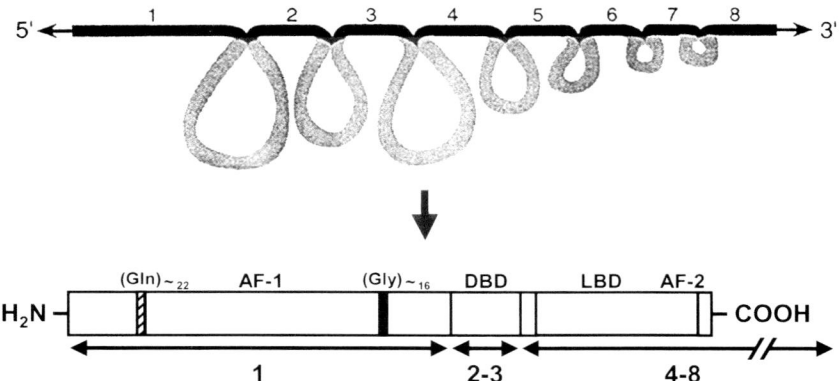

FIGURE 1. Exon-intron organization and domain structure of the androgen receptor (AR) gene and the corresponding protein. **(Top)** The genomic structure of the AR. The natural gene for the AR is organized as 8 exons and 7 introns. **(Bottom)** The domain structure of the AR protein. The three major domains of the AR contributed by exon 1 for the N-terminal domain, exons 2 and 3 for the DNA-binding domain (DBD), and exons 4–8 for the ligand-binding domain (LBD). Part of exon 1 also specifies the 5′ UTR, and a major portion of exon 8 specifies the 3′ UTR. The transactivation functions AF-1 and AF-2 are located within the N-terminal domain and LBD, respectively. Relative positions of glutamine and glycine repeats within the N-terminal domain are shown by the indicated boxes.

SRC-1 can interact with CBP/p300, a global coactivator, that also interacts with the receptor directly, and the two coactivators together show synergy in potentiating the receptor's transactivating function.[15] The histone acetylase (HAT) activity of CBP/p300 and the CBP-associated factor p/CAF ensures that the hormone-bound receptor is able to induce chromatin remodeling that helps open up the surrounding chromatin region, facilitating access of transcription factors to the regulatory site. Ligand binding also enables AF-1/AF-2 to associate with a multisubunit complex of coactivator proteins known as DRIP or TRAP. This coactivating complex is thought to recruit additional regulatory proteins that connect the AR-coactivator complex to RNA polymerase II and the associated transcription factors that are anchored at the core promoter.[16]

The centrally located DNA-binding domain (residues 559–624), specified by exons 2 and 3, contains 9 cysteine residues, of which 8 are involved in forming 2 zinc fingers that are hallmarks of all NRs. These 2 zinc-coordinated stem-loop structures enable the receptor protein to bind to the regulatory region of target genes by interacting with the major groove of the DNA duplex. Studies with hybrid receptors indicate that the first zinc finger (proximal to the N-terminal domain) determines the sequence specificity, while the second finger helps stabilize the DNA-receptor complex.[17,18] Despite their exquisite functional specificity in the physiological context, receptors for androgens, glucocorticoids, progesterone, and mineralocorticoids can recognize the same DNA response element both in *in vitro* binding assay and in functional analysis utilizing transiently transfected cells. This paradox has remained an endocrinological enigma for more than 25 years and may be resolved only when we learn more about the role of chromatin remodeling and chromatin-associated multiprotein complex formation in steroid hormone action.

Although the three-dimensional structure of a holoreceptor has not yet been reported, the crystal structures of the DNA-binding domains as well as of the LBDs of several members of the NR superfamily in the presence and absence of the cognate ligand have been resolved by several groups.[19] Based on these studies, a striking consensus picture has emerged. Despite their difference in the amino acid sequence, the folding patterns of the LBDs among the members of the NR family are remarkably similar. The LBDs are made up of 12 discrete α-helices. In the unliganded receptor, the outermost α-helix (helix 12) is positioned farther away from the ligand-binding pocket. Insertion of an agonist into the ligand-binding pocket changes the LBD conformation in such a way that the helix 12 folds back on top of the ligand-binding site, serving as a lid to retard dissociation of the captured ligand. The agonist-mediated repositioning of the helix 12 also relieves the inhibitory influence of the LBD on AF-1 and, at the same time, creates the appropriate site of interaction between AF-2 and the LXXLL motif of the p160 coactivator proteins. X-ray crystallographic analysis of the LBD of the human AR in the presence and absence of a potent synthetic agonist, R1881, has shown that a total of 18 amino acid residues within the ligand-binding pocket interact with the ligand mostly through hydrophobic interaction involving the steroid scaffold.[20] At least two hydrogen bonds, one with the oxygen at C-3 of the steroid and Arg-752 of the receptor and another with the 17-β hydroxyl group and the Asn-705, add to the stabilization of the androgen-AR complex. These findings are consistent with the structural requirements of the androgenic steroids where the 3-keto and 17-β hydroxyl groups are considered essential for their biological function.[21]

NUCLEOCYTOPLASMIC RECYCLING AND SUBNUCLEAR CLUSTERING OF AR

Most of the unliganded AR is localized in the cytoplasmic compartment of target cells,[22] where it is sequestered as a multiprotein complex with heat-shock proteins and immunophilins.[23] Upon ligand binding, the conformational change of the receptor protein facilitates its dissociation from the multiprotein complex, its homodimerization, and unmasking of the nuclear localization signal (NLS). The exposed NLS is then able to bind to importins, which serve as chaperones for transport of the ligand-activated AR into the nuclear compartment. This aspect of AR function differs from estrogen action since the unliganded estrogen receptor (ER) resides in the nucleus and binding of the estrogenic ligand promotes interaction of the ER with the requisite coactivators in preparation for the subsequent steps of hormonal signaling. The dynamics of receptor movement inside a single living cell can be monitored with AR tagged to the jellyfish green fluorescent protein (GFP-AR). FIGURE 2 shows androgen-mediated nuclear import of GFP-AR from the cytoplasm in transfected COS1 cells. As seen from these fluorescence images, the ligand-dependent nuclear import of the AR is rapid and almost complete within 60 min. A time-lapse movie showing this movement of GFP-AR after dihydrotestosterone (DHT) treatment can be found at the web site, http://www.uthscsa.edu/csb/faculty2/roy.html. This pattern

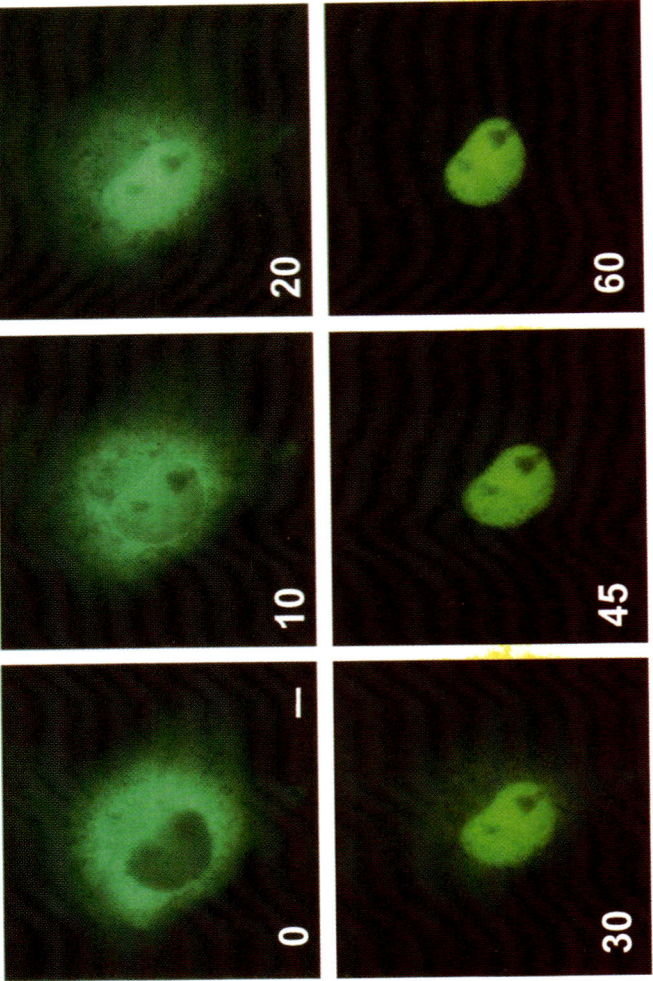

FIGURE 2. Androgen-dependent nuclear translocation of the GFP-AR in transfected cells. The picture shows images of a COS1 cell at various time points (minutes) after DHT treatment. Cells were grown in 5% charcoal-stripped fetal bovine serum, transfected with GFP-AR, and allowed to express the GFP-labeled AR for 30 h before treatment with DHT (10 nM). Images from the same cell were acquired at 0, 10, 20, 30, 45, and 60 min after the hormone treatment. Fluorescence imaging of live cells was performed using an E400 Eclipse epifluorescence microscope and water immersion objectives (Nikon, Melville, NY) connected to a video monitor through a cooled charge-coupled device camera. *Magnification bar* = 10 μm.

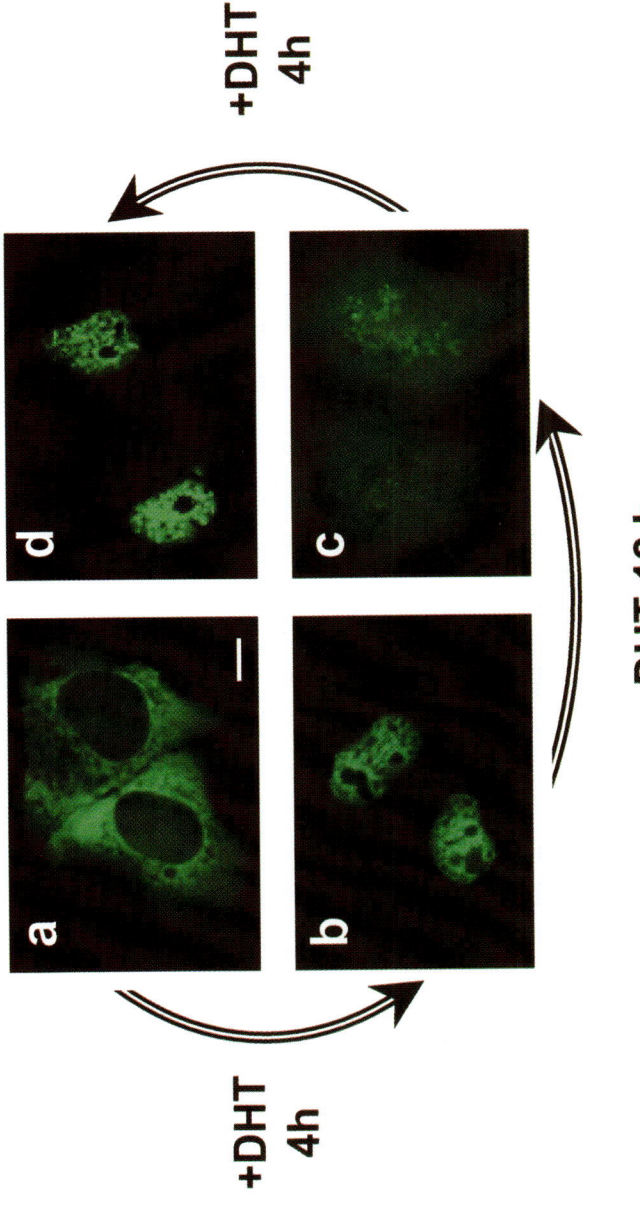

FIGURE 3. Nucleocytoplasmic recycling of the GFP-AR following sequential androgen treatment and androgen withdrawal. Intracellular distribution of the GFP-AR before hormone treatment (**a**), 4 h after treatment with 10 nM DHT (**b**), 12 h after hormone withdrawal in the presence of 50 μg/mL cycloheximide (**c**), and 4 h after DHT treatment (in the presence of cycloheximide) to DHT-withdrawn cells (**d**). *Magnification bar* = 10 μm.

of ligand-mediated nuclear movement of the AR is also observed in other cell types such as PC3 (prostate cancer–derived), HeLa (uterine cancer–derived), CV1 (monkey kidney–derived), and CWR-22 (prostate cancer–derived).

Upon its nuclear entry, the ligand-receptor complex appears to move into a subnuclear compartment, the nature of which has not been clearly defined.[22,24,25] These subnuclear compartments, commonly referred to as nuclear foci, appear to be the congregation sites for the receptor and other associated factors such as the coactivators that are needed for transcriptional activation of target genes. Interestingly, AR bound to only transcriptionally active hormonal ligands and partial agonists (e.g., cyproterone acetate) can support migration of the receptor to the nuclear foci, whereas pure antagonists such as casodex, despite promoting nuclear translocation, fail to deliver the AR to the nuclear foci.[22]

Not only does the AR require ligand activation for its cytoplasmic to nuclear translocation, but ligand association of the receptor appears to be essential for its retention inside the nucleus. This is evident from the finding that, after its androgen-mediated nuclear import, androgen withdrawal (by transferring cells to a DHT-free medium) results in export of the receptor back into the cytoplasmic compartment (FIG. 3). Importantly, the exported receptor is competent to undertake subsequent rounds of hormonal signaling. Under conditions of total inhibition of new receptor synthesis in the presence of cycloheximide, we have recorded four rounds of recycling of the same group of GFP-AR upon sequentially exposing the cells to DHT followed by DHT withdrawal. Since normal cell function is expected to be impaired after prolonged (96 h) inhibition of protein synthesis by cycloheximide, it is likely that, in the absence of this inhibitor, one molecule of AR may be able to undertake more than the observed four rounds of hormonal signaling.

In contrast to the recycling of AR, Nawaz *et al.* have reported that the ER undergoes proteosomal degradation after its participation in the transcriptional activation of target genes, and this process is suggested to serve as the termination signal for estrogen action.[26] The ability of one molecule of the AR to undertake multiple rounds of androgen signaling indicates that, unlike the ER, ligand dissociation and/or inactivation may play a more critical role in the termination of androgen signaling. From the standpoint of cellular efficiency, it makes more sense to keep the receptor functioning for multiple rounds of signal transduction rather than degrading it after every round of hormonal stimulation. It is also interesting that the leptomycin B–sensitive exportins, which are the predominant mediators of the nuclear export, are not involved in exporting the AR from the nucleus to cytoplasm, suggesting the role of an alternative type of export mechanism for the transfer of the unliganded AR from the nuclear to the cytoplasmic compartment.[22]

The calcium-binding protein, calreticulin, inhibits association of the AR with its cognate DNA element due to protein-protein interaction involving a specific peptide sequence of calreticulin and the KXGFFKR (X = G, A, or V) sequence motif present within the DNA-binding domain of a number of NRs including the AR.[26,27] Based on the inhibitory effect of calreticulin on AR function, we have postulated that upregulation of calreticulin may serve to modulate androgen action in target cells, especially in the Leydig cells and in the cells of the adrenal cortex that contain high levels of both the AR and steroidal agonists.[21] In a recent report, calreticulin is shown to function as a chaperone for the nuclear export of the glucocorticoid receptor (GR) by interacting with its DNA-binding domain.[28,29] It appears that, at least for the GR and possibly also for the AR, following ligand dissociation from the receptor, calreticulin may serve as the termination signal for hormone-regulated target gene expression by competing for the ligand-free receptor at the DNA response element and then chaperoning the receptor out of the nucleus in preparation for another round of signaling.

MODULATION OF AR FUNCTION BY ENVIRONMENTAL ENDOCRINE DISRUPTERS AND POTENTIAL SARMs

The suggestion that hydrophobic interactions between the steroid backbone and the side chains of the amino acid residues lining the steroid-binding pocket are primarily responsible for capturing and retaining the androgenic steroids by the AR has been recently authenticated by X-ray crystallographic analysis.[20] Since the hydrophobic interactions are not sufficiently specific, a number of other steroids can potentially enter the ligand-binding pocket of the AR and be retained there for a transient, albeit functionally sufficient, time period through a concentration-dependent dynamic equilibrium. This may explain the limited cross-reactivity of the AR with other hormonal steroids such as estradiol-17β and progesterone. At a 100-fold higher concentration, both of these cross-reactive hormones are about 60–80% as efficient as DHT in promoting nuclear translocation of the GFP-AR and about 8–10% as competent as DHT in driving its transactivation function.[22] Cross-reactivity of the AR at the LBD also accounts for its functional inhibition by a number of structurally unrelated synthetic chemicals. Some of these xenobiotics were designed to serve as pharmacological inhibitors of androgen action, while others were accidentally dis-

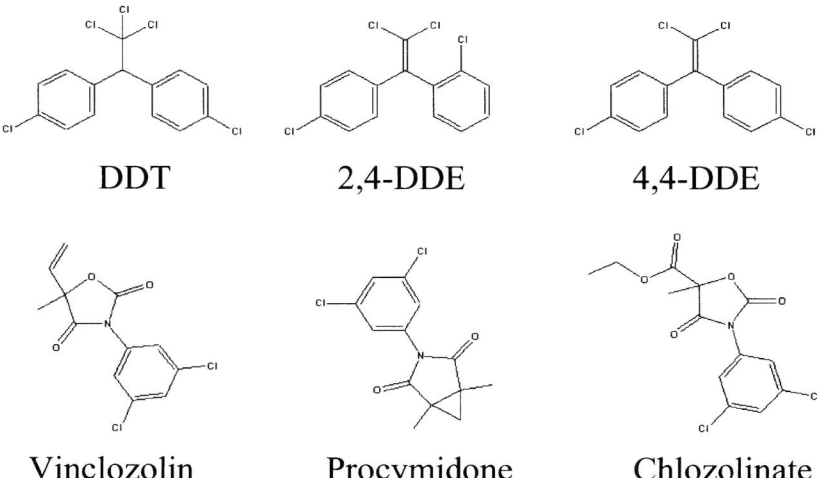

FIGURE 4. Chemical structures of the xenobiotic endocrine disrupters used in this study.

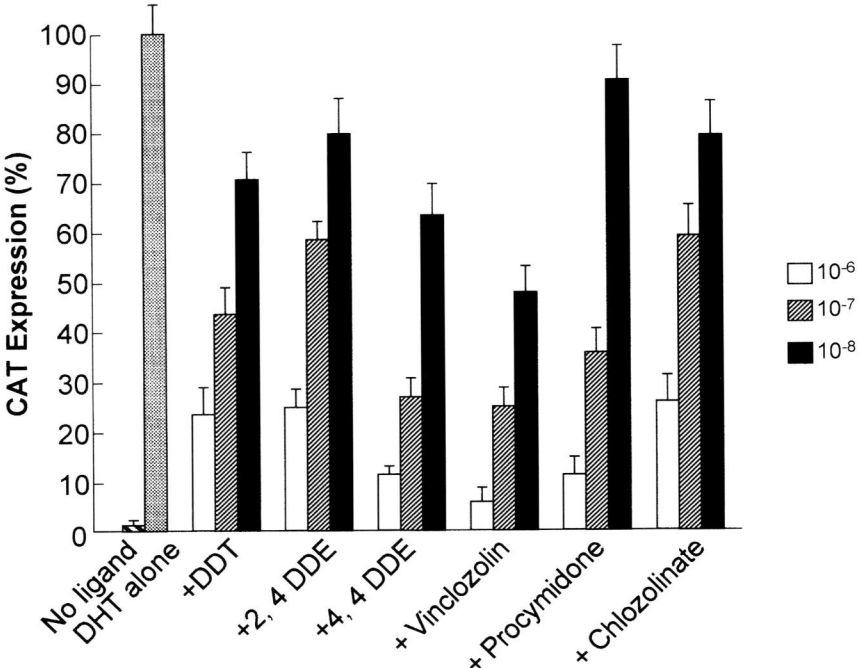

FIGURE 5A. Inhibition of the androgen-dependent transactivation function of AR by endocrine disrupters/SARMs at a subsaturating concentration of DHT. PC3 cells were transfected with the AR expression plasmid (CMV-AR) along with the MMTV-CAT promoter-reporter construct. Cells were treated with 10^{-10} M DHT alone or along with 100-, 1000-, and 10,000-fold molar excesses of each of the endocrine disrupters, as indicated. Values represent means (+ SEM) of four independent experiments conducted in triplicate. None of these SARMs inhibited GR-mediated transactivation of the MMTV-CAT reporter plasmid (not shown in the figure).

covered when they were found to act as environmental endocrine disrupters. Many of these chemicals meet the criteria for their classification as selective androgen receptor modulators (SARMs), deserving further investigation.

Based on their known effects on androgen action and/or male reproductive functions, we selected a number of these xenobiotic chemicals to examine their comparative effects in modifying the cellular dynamics of androgen receptor action in living cells.[30–32] These include the insecticide DDT (dichloro-diphenyl-trichloro-ethane) and its two metabolites (2,4-DDE and 4,4-DDE), as well as three agricultural fungicides, vinclozolin (dichlorophenyl-methyl-vinyloxazolidine-dione), procymidone (dichlorophenyl-methyl-cyclopropane-dicarboxymide), and chlozolinate (ethyl-dichlorophenyl-methyl-dioxo-oxazolidine carboxylate). Chemical structures of these compounds are shown in FIGURE 4. Results presented in FIGURES 5A and 5B show the relative potencies of these chemicals in inhibiting the DHT-mediated transactivation function of the AR (FIG. 5A) and in promoting nuclear translocation of the

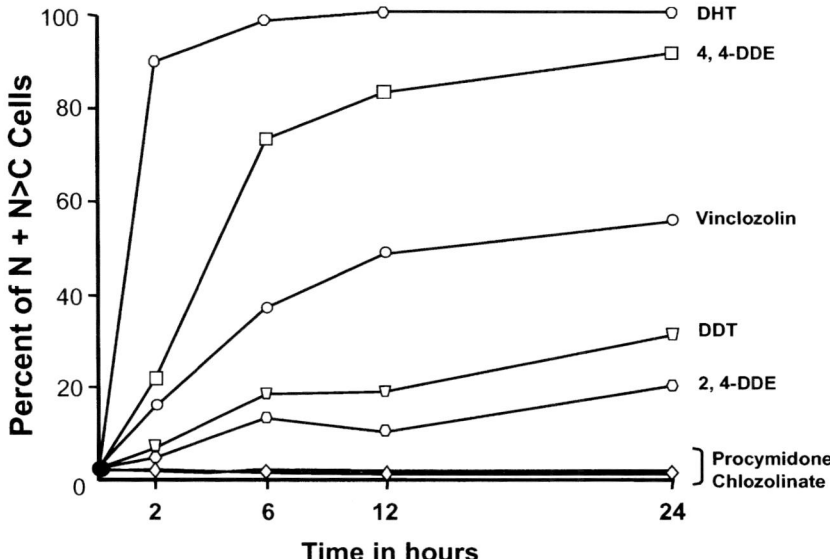

FIGURE 5B. Kinetics of the nuclear translocation of GFP-AR initiated by DHT and selected endocrine disrupters. PC3 cells were transfected with GFP-AR and, after 24 h, cells were treated with DHT (10 nM) or with one of the endocrine disrupters (1 µM) as labeled. Subcellular distribution of the receptor in a field of 100 cells in the same culture dish was determined at various time points after ligand treatment. The vertical coordinate represents the percent of cell showing predominantly nuclear (N + N>C) localization of the GFP-AR. Each point is an average of two independent experiments.

GFP-AR in living cells (FIG. 5B). Although all of these chemicals displayed anti-androgenic activities in transactivation assays, only some of them were effective in translocating the AR into the nuclear compartment. As compared to the natural agonist DHT, 4,4-DDE and vinclozolin were most potent in promoting nuclear import of the GFP-AR. DDT and 2,4-DDE were also able to promote nuclear import to a relatively small extent. However, both procymidone and chlozolinate were totally ineffective. Additionally, despite their effectiveness in promoting nuclear translocation, we observed that 4,4-DDE, vinclozolin, DDT, and 2,4-DDE were unable to induce formation of the nuclear foci. This is consistent with the observation that none of these chemicals by themselves was able to promote transcriptional activation by the AR (data not shown). However, when used in the presence of DHT, procymidone, vinclozolin, and 4,4-DDE were highly effective in preventing the formation of the nuclear foci (FIG. 6). 2,4-DDE, DDT, and chlozolinate were relatively less effective in inhibiting this particular step in AR function. Again, the relative efficiencies of these three xenobiotics in preventing the formation of nuclear foci correlate with their relative potencies in inhibiting the transactivation function of the AR as determined by cell transfection assay. These results also suggest that the conformational transition induced by a certain group of nonhormonal AR ligands such as procymi-

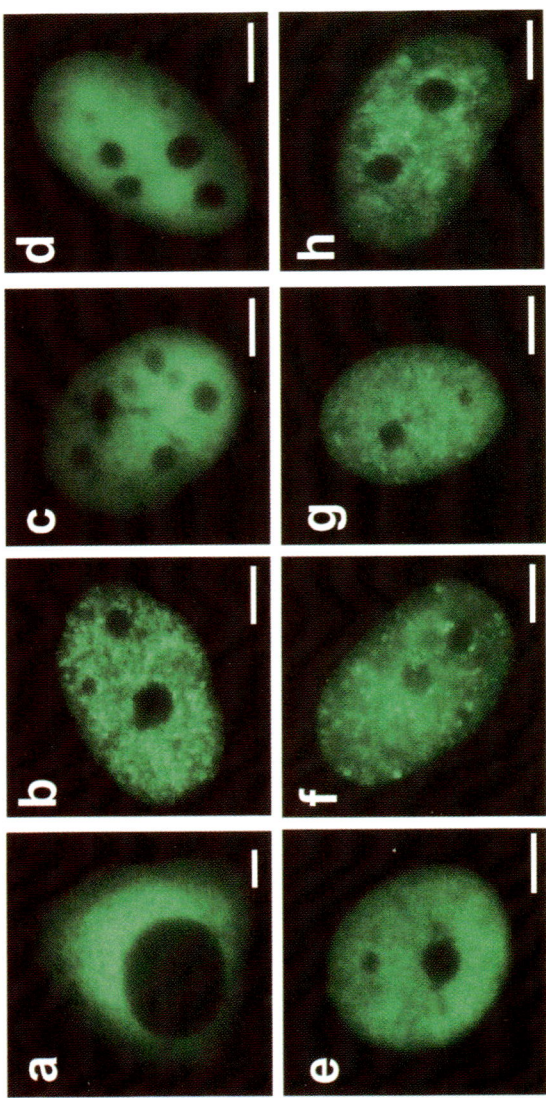

FIGURE 6. Inhibition of DHT-mediated subnuclear clustering of the GFP-AR by xenobiotic endocrine disrupters. PC3 cells transfected with the GFP-AR were treated simultaneously with DHT (10^{-9} M) along with one of the endocrine disrupters (10^{-6} M). After 15 h of treatment, imaging was performed to analyze subnuclear distribution patterns of the AR. Each panel shows the fluorescence distribution pattern in a typical nucleus of the treatment group: **(a)** no hormone; **(b)** DHT alone; **(c)** DHT + procymidone; **(d)** DHT + vinclozolin; **(e)** DHT + 4,4-DDE; **(f)** DHT + 2,4-DDE; **(g)** DHT + DDT; **(h)** DHT + chlozolinate. *Magnification bar* = 10 μm.

done and chlozolinate is inadequate for dissociation of the receptor from other cytoplasmic proteins and/or exposure of the NLS to promote its interaction with importins for its nuclear import. On the other hand, interaction of the AR with the other group of SARMs such as 4,4-DDE, vinclozolin, DDT, and 2,4-DDE removes the first hurdle—namely, its import into the nuclear compartment—but fails to initiate the subsequent nuclear steps that result in transactivation. This mechanism may be similar to the one reported earlier with the pure antagonist, casodex, which also can promote nuclear translocation of the AR, but does not induce formation of the nuclear foci.[22] We speculate that an aberrant folding of the helix 12 at the LBD may be responsible for creating an inappropriate conformational change, which inhibits the attachment of the steroid receptor to coactivators. Additional analyses will be needed to clearly delineate the mechanism of action of these antagonists in inhibiting discrete steps in androgen action.

CONCLUSIONS

Nuclear transmission of the transcription regulatory signal by androgens is initiated in response to binding of the androgenic ligand to the cytoplasmic AR, triggering release of the receptor-associated proteins and unmasking of the nuclear localization signal of the receptor to facilitate its interaction with importins and translocation to the nucleus. Once transported into the nucleus, the transcriptionally active AR accumulates within a subnuclear compartment (nuclear foci) and subsequently regulates target gene expression. Androgen withdrawal results in export of the AR to the cytoplasm in a form that is competent to undertake the next round of nucleocytoplasmic shuttling. Multiple rounds of receptor recycling in live cells can be demonstrated by repeated sequential exposure of the receptor to DHT in hormone-treated cells followed by hormone withdrawal. The AR's ability to undergo repeated nucleocytoplasmic shuttling suggests that, rather than receptor degradation, ligand inactivation and its dissociation from the receptor protein are likely to be the major termination signal of androgen action. Calreticulin may be actively involved in both promoting dissociation of the unliganded AR from the target gene and its subsequent nuclear export.

The nuclear foci are likely to serve as the platforms where the receptor and coactivators form the multiprotein complex before migrating to the target gene promoter. X-ray crystallography of the agonist-bound AR LBD has shown that the ligand is held to the ligand-binding pocket mostly through hydrophobic interactions between the steroid backbone and the side chains of the amino acid residues lining the ligand-binding site. The generally weak nature of the hydrophobic interactions accounts for the limited cross-reactivity of the AR to the nonandrogenic steroids, estrogen and progesterone, and also to a chemically diverse class of xenobiotic agents functioning as AR modulators (SARMs). All of these chemicals can bind to the AR and inhibit DHT-mediated AR transactivation activity. However, they may influence AR function in two distinct manners. One group of inhibitors can promote nuclear translocation of the AR, but fail to deliver the receptor to the subnuclear compartment, a step considered essential for transcriptional function. The other group binds to the AR, but cannot promote its nuclear translocation. We speculate that, in the latter case, binding of the SARM to the receptor leads to an early block in androgen action, possibly due to an impediment in the dissociation of the receptor-associated proteins and/or unmasking of the nuclear localization signal. On the other hand, for the first group of endocrine disrupters/SARMs, it is likely that an aberrant folding of the LBD helix 12 prevents conformational alignment between AF-2 and AF-1, hindering the receptor's ability to bind to the coactivators. A definitive understanding of all of these discrete events would allow further dissection of various steps in androgen action and development of therapeutically relevant SARMs.

ACKNOWLEDGMENTS

Studies in our laboratory on androgen action were supported by grants from the National Institutes of Health (Nos. RO1 DK14744 and R37 AG10486). We also thank Gilbert Torralva for technical assistance.

REFERENCES

1. KOKONTIS, J.M. & S. LIAO. 1999. Molecular action of androgen in the normal and neoplastic prostate. Vitam. Horm. **55:** 219–307.
2. BROWN, C.J., S.J. GOSS, D.B. LUBAHN et al. 1989. Androgen receptor locus on the human X chromosome: regional localization to Xq11-12 and description of a DNA polymorphism. Am. J. Hum. Genet. **44:** 264–269.
3. KUIPER, G.G., P.W. FABER, H.C. VAN ROOIJ et al. 1989. Structural organization of the human androgen receptor gene. J. Mol. Endocrinol. **2:** R1–R4.
4. FABER, P.W., H.C. VAN ROOIJ, J.A. VAN DER KORPUT et al. 1991. Characterization of the human androgen receptor transcription unit. J. Biol. Chem. **266:** 10743–10749.
5. LIAO, S.S., J. KOKONTIS, T. SAI et al. 1989. Androgen receptors: structures, mutations, antibodies, and cellular dynamics. J. Steroid Biochem. **34:** 41–51.
6. RUNDLETT, S.E., X.P. WU & R.L. MIESFELD. 1990. Functional characterizations of the androgen receptor confirm that the molecular basis of androgen action is transcriptional regulation. Mol. Endocrinol. **4:** 708–714.
7. SIMENTAL, J.A., M. SAR & E.M. WILSON. 1992. Domain functions of the androgen receptor. J. Steroid Biochem. Mol. Biol. **43:** 37–41.
8. JENSTER, G., J.A. VAN DER KORPUT, J. TRAPMAN et al. 1992. Functional domains of the human androgen receptor. J. Steroid Biochem. Mol. Biol. **41:** 671–675.
9. NUCIFORA, F.C., M. SASAKI, M.F. PETERS et al. 2001. Interference by huntingtin and atrophin-1 with CBP-mediated transcription leading to cellular toxicity. Science **291:** 2423–2428.
10. GOTTLIEB, B., D.M. VASILIOU, R. LUMBROSO et al. 1999. Analysis of exon 1 mutations in the androgen receptor gene. Hum. Mutat. **14:** 527–539.
11. QUIGLEY, C.A., A. DE BELLIS, K.B. MARSCHKE et al. 1995. Androgen receptor defects: historical, clinical, and molecular perspectives. Endocr. Rev. **16:** 271–321.
12. HAKIMI, J.M., M.P. SCHOENBERG, R.H. RONDINELLI et al. 1997. Androgen receptor variants with short glutamine or glycine repeats may identify unique subpopulations of men with prostate cancer. Clin. Cancer Res. **3:** 1599–1608.
13. ROBYR, D., A.P. WOLFFE & W. WAHLI. 2000. Nuclear hormone receptor coregulators in action: diversity for shared tasks. Mol. Endocrinol. **14:** 329–347.
14. BEVAN, C.L., S. HOARE et al. 1999. The AF1 and AF2 domains of the androgen receptor interact with distinct regions of SRC1. Mol. Cell. Biol. **19:** 8383–8392.
15. MCKENNA, N.J., R.B. LANZ & B.W. O'MALLEY. 1999. Nuclear receptor coregulators: cellular and molecular biology. Endocr. Rev. **20:** 321–344.
16. FREEDMAN, L.P. 1999. Strategies for transcriptional activation by steroid/nuclear receptors. J. Cell. Biochem. Suppl. **32/33:** 103–109.

17. UMESONO, K. & R.M. EVANS. 1989. Determinants of target gene specificity for steroid/thyroid hormone receptors. Cell **57:** 1139–1146.
18. TSAI, M.J. & B.W. O'MALLEY. 1994. Molecular mechanisms of action of steroid/thyroid receptor superfamily members. Annu. Rev. Biochem. **63:** 451–486.
19. MORAS, D. & H. GRONEMEYER. 1998. The nuclear receptor ligand-binding domain: structure and function. Curr. Opin. Cell Biol. **10:** 384–391.
20. MATIAS, P.M., P. DONNER, R. COELHO et al. 2000. Structural evidence for ligand specificity in the binding domain of the human androgen receptor: implications for pathogenic gene mutations. J. Biol. Chem. **275:** 26164–26171.
21. ROY, A.K., Y. LAVROVSKY, C.S. SONG et al. 1999. Regulation of androgen action. Vitam. Horm. **55:** 309–352.
22. TYAGI, R.K., Y. LAVROVSKY, S.C. AHN et al. 2000. Dynamics of intracellular movement and nucleocytoplasmic recycling of the ligand-activated androgen receptor in living cells. Mol. Endocrinol. **14:** 1162–1174.
23. DEFRANCO, D.B. 1999. Regulation of steroid receptor subcellular trafficking. Cell Biochem. Biophys. **30:** 1–24.
24. HTUN, H., L.T. HOLTH, D. WALKER et al. 1999. Direct visualization of the human estrogen receptor alpha reveals a role for ligand in the nuclear distribution of the receptor. Mol. Biol. Cell **10:** 471–486.
25. STENOIEN, D.L., M.G. MANCINI, K. PATEL et al. 2000. Subnuclear trafficking of estrogen receptor-alpha and steroid receptor coactivator-1. Mol. Endocrinol. **14:** 518–534.
26. NAWAZ, Z., D.M. LONARD, C.L. SMITH et al. 1999. The Angelman syndrome–associated protein, E6-AP, is a coactivator for the nuclear hormone receptor superfamily. Mol. Cell. Biol. **19:** 1182–1189.
27. DEDHAR, S., P.S. RENNIE, M. SHAGO et al. 1994. Inhibition of nuclear hormone receptor activity by calreticulin. Nature **367:** 480–483.
28. BRUCHOVSKY, N., R. SNOEK, P.S. RENNIE et al. 1996. Control of tumor progression by maintenance of apoptosis. Prostate Suppl. **6:** 13–21.
29. HOLASKA, J.M., B.E. BLACK, D.C. LOVE et al. 2001. Calreticulin is a receptor for nuclear export. J. Cell. Biol. **152:** 127–140.
30. SONNENSCHEIN, C. & A.M. SOTO. 1998. An updated review of environmental estrogen and androgen mimics and antagonists. J. Steroid Biochem. Mol. Biol. **65:** 143–150.
31. KELCE, W.R., C.R. STONE, S.C. LAWS et al. 1995. Persistent DDT metabolite p,p'-DDE is a potent androgen receptor antagonist. Nature **375:** 581–585.
32. WONG, C., W.R. KELCE, M. SAR et al. 1995. Androgen receptor antagonist versus agonist activities of the fungicide vinclozolin relative to hydroxyflutamide. J. Biol. Chem. **270:** 19998–20003.

Tissue-Specific Estrogen Biosynthesis and Metabolism

EVAN R. SIMPSON,[a,b] COLIN CLYNE,[a] CAROLINE SPEED,[a] GARY RUBIN,[a] AND SERDAR BULUN[c]

[a]*Prince Henry's Institute of Medical Research and* [b]*Department of Biochemistry and Molecular Biology, Monash University, Melbourne, Australia*

[c]*Division of Reproductive Endocrinology, Department of Obstetrics and Gynecology, University of Illinois at Chicago, Chicago, Illinois, USA*

ABSTRACT: While the ovaries are the principal source of systemic estrogen in the premenopausal nonpregnant woman, other sites of estrogen biosynthesis are present throughout the body and these become the major sources of estrogen beyond menopause. These extragonadal sources of estrogen are small, but may play an important, though hitherto largely unrecognized, physiological and pathophysiological role. Aromatase activity in extragonadal sites contributes to this source of estrogen and may contribute to breast tumor development and/or growth. Selective aromatase modulators (SAMs) may have a role to play in the treatment of estrogen-dependent diseases, such as breast cancer.

KEYWORDS: ERα; ERβ; aromatase; SAMs

INTRODUCTION

Models of estrogen insufficiency have revealed new and often unexpected roles for estradiol in both females and males.[1] These models include natural mutations in humans of the aromatase gene, of which there are some 10 cases known, of whom 2 are men, as well as 1 man with a mutation in the estrogen receptor (ER) α. They also include mice with targeted disruptions of the ERα and ERβ, the double ERα and β knockout,[2–4] as well as the aromatase knockout (ArKO) mouse.[5] Some of these roles challenge the definition of the terms estrogen and androgen. For example, the lipid and carbohydrate phenotype of estrogen insufficiency is nonsexually dimorphic and appears to apply equally to males and females,[6,7] as does the bone phenotype of undermineralization and failure of epiphyseal closure. Even more dramatically, the role of estradiol in male germ cell development would indicate that, at least in this local context, estradiol would be more appropriately defined as an androgen.[8] The second important point is that in men and in postmenopausal women, when the ovaries cease to produce estrogens, estradiol does not function as a circulating hormone. It is no longer an endocrine factor; instead, estradiol is produced in a number

---

Address for correspondence: Dr. Evan R. Simpson, Prince Henry's Institute of Medical Research, Monash Medical Center, Level 4–Block E, 246 Clayton Road, Clayton, VIC 3168, Australia. Voice: 61-3-9594-4397; fax: 61-3-9594-6376.

evan.simpson@med.monash.edu.au

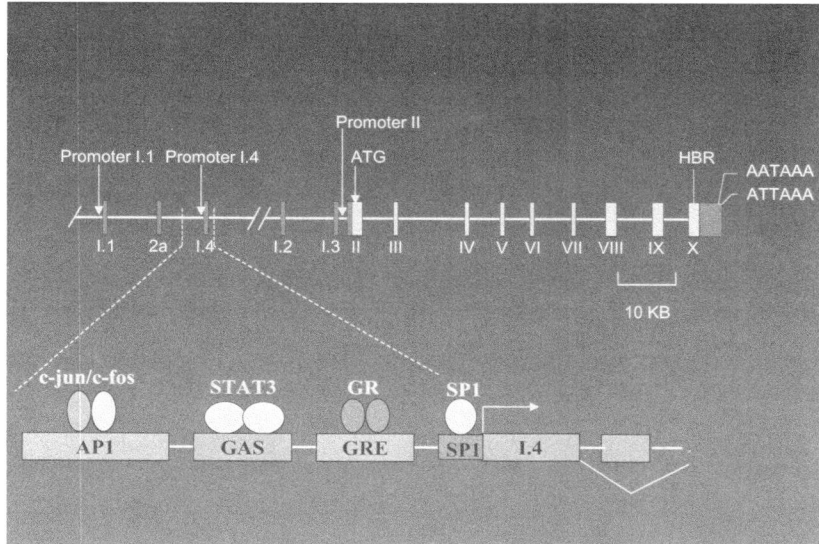

FIGURE 1. Structure of the *CYP19* gene encoding human aromatase cytochrome P450, showing the coding exons (II through X), the heme-binding region (HBR), and the start of translation (ATG). Also shown are the various untranslated exons I and their upstream promoter regions, with an expanded view of promoter I.4 showing the characterized response elements.

of extragonadal sites and acts locally at these sites as a paracrine or even intracrine factor.[9,10] These sites include the mesenchymal cells of adipose tissue, osteoblasts and chondrocytes of bone, numerous sites in the brain, and also the Leydig cells and germ cells of the testes. Thus, circulating levels of estrogens in postmenopausal women and in men do not drive estrogen action. Rather, they are derived from the production of estrogen in extragonadal sites where it has acted locally and which then escapes local metabolism to reenter the circulation. Hence, circulating levels reflect, rather than direct, estrogen action in postmenopausal women and men.

Estrogens are synthesized from androgens and the enzyme responsible for this is called aromatase, which is a member of the superfamily of genes known collectively as cytochrome P450. Aromatase belongs to family 19—hence its designation as *CYP19*. In humans, aromatase is expressed in a number of tissue sites corresponding to the sites of estrogen biosynthesis. An important feature of this expression is that tissue-specific expression of aromatase is regulated by a number of upstream untranslated first exons that are spliced into the mature transcript in a tissue-specific fashion[11] (FIG. 1). Therefore, expression in the gonads as well as in estrogen-synthesizing tumors is driven by a proximal promoter immediately upstream of the start of translation, promoter II. By contrast, expression in placenta is driven by a distal promoter, promoter I.1, whereas expression in mesenchymal cells of adipose tissue is driven by another distal promoter, promoter I.4. However, in adipose tissue proximal to a breast tumor, promoter II is the dominant promoter utilized. Each of these promoters is regulated by a different cohort of signaling pathways and transcription factors. Thus, estrogen biosynthesis is differentially regulated in the various tissue sites of expression. In gonads and in tumors, expression is regulated primarily by cyclic AMP. In the ovary, the factor that drives cyclic AMP formation is FSH (follicle-stimulating hormone). In tumors, it appears to be prostaglandin E2 (PGE2). In normal adipose mesenchymal cells, expression from promoter I.4 is driven primarily by class 1 cytokines such as interleukin 6, interleukin 11, LIF (leukemia inhibitory factor), and oncostatin M via a Jak 1–Stat 3 (Janus kinase-1–signal transducer and activator of transcription 3) pathway. TNFα (tumor necrosis factor-α) also activates expression from promoter I.4 probably via an MAP (mitogen-activated protein) kinase–AP-1 (activator protein-1) pathway. The untranslated first exons downstream of these tissue-specific promoters are all spliced into a common 3′-splice junction upstream of the start of translation. Thus, the coding region in each of the tissue-specific sites of expression is identical and the aromatase protein in each of these sites is the same.[11]

In this presentation, we will discuss the importance of local estrogen biosynthesis in two pathological situations—namely, endometriosis and breast cancer.

AROMATASE EXPRESSION AND ENDOMETRIOSIS

Our previous studies have shown that, using a semiquantitative RT-PCR (reverse transcription–polymerase chain reaction) technique, aromatase expression was undetectable in normal healthy endometrium, but was readily apparent in endometriotic implants.[12] This is particularly true of endometriotic implants in the cul-de-sac of the abdominal wall where aromatase expression is extremely high. This is also evidenced when stromal cells from these implants are placed in culture and aromatase activity determined—it was found that activity on a milligram protein basis was as high as would be found in syncytiotrophoblasts of the placenta. A subsequent study of the mechanism of regulation of aromatase expression in endometriotic stromal cells in culture employing exon-specific RT-PCR found that the predominant promoter utilized in endometriotic stromal cells was the proximal promoter II, the same promoter employed in ovary and in tumor cells. Predictably, then, we found that cyclic AMP was a powerful stimulus of aromatase expression in endometriotic stromal cells, as it is in ovarian granulosa cells. However, whereas in granulosa cells the factor that regulates adenylate cyclase is FSH, in the case of endometriotic stromal cells PGE2 appears to be the principal factor involved in regulating aromatase expression via cyclic AMP.[13] This is produced locally within the endometriotic plaque itself.

Employing promoter II–containing luciferase constructs transfected into these endometriotic stromal cells, it was possible to show that cyclic AMP indeed is a powerful stimulator of reporter gene expression in this system. Using granulosa cells, it has been shown that an orphan member of the nuclear receptor family, namely, steroidogenic factor-1 (SF1), is required for aromatase expression via promoter II.[14] When an SF1 expression plasmid was cotransfected into endometriotic stromal cells together with the promoter II reporter gene construct, there was a dramatic stimulation of the reporter gene activity, indicating that SF1 was also involved in promoter

II regulation in these cells. Another orphan member of the nuclear receptor family that also binds to the site, but in an inhibitory fashion, is chicken ovalbumin upstream promoter–transcription factor (COUP-TF). When a COUP-TF expression plasmid was cotransfected into the endometriotic stromal cells along with the promoter II reporter gene, there was a marked inhibition of reporter gene expression. Consequently, a study was conducted to determine which of these transcription factors might be present in normal healthy endometrium as well as in endometriotic plaques.

Employing the SF1 response element in promoter II as a probe and using recombinant COUP-TF and recombinant SF1 as controls, it was found that both of these transcription factors bound to the probe, but that the position of the retarded band in each case was different.[14] Nuclear extracts from normal endometrium or endometriotic tissue were then utilized to determine if any binding proteins were present in these extracts. It was found that endometriotic tissue contained proteins giving bands corresponding to both SF1 and COUP-TF. However, only COUP-TF was detectable in nuclear extracts from healthy endometrium. This was confirmed by analysis of the transcripts by RT-PCR. It was found that the transcripts for COUP-TF were present in both endometriotic cells and cells derived from healthy endometrium, whereas SF1 transcripts were only detectable in the tissue derived from endometriotic plaques. Hence, from this, it was possible to propose the following mechanism: namely that, in normal healthy endometrium, SF1 is absent. Also, instead, the response element on promoter II is occupied by the repressor COUP-TF. This would provide an explanation as to why there is no detectable aromatase activity in normal healthy endometrium. By contrast, in endometriotic tissue, SF1 is expressed and therefore competes with COUP-TF for the half site. Thus, aromatase expression is initiated because of the presence of the SF1 in endometriotic cells.[15]

The question that arises then is the role that local estrogen biosynthesis plays in endometriotic implants. This was examined in a 57-year-old postmenopausal woman with severe recurrent endometriosis.[15] Her condition was so severe that she already had one kidney removed and appeared resistant to all other forms of treatment. Based on the above studies, it was decided to treat her with anastrozole, which is a phase III inhibitor of aromatase. Because of concern that the aromatase inhibitor might give rise to bone demineralization, she was also placed on calcium and alendronate. Results were dramatic. Within 1 month of treatment her pain had disappeared, and within 9 months most of the endometriotic lesions had essentially disappeared. Thus, treatment with the aromatase inhibitor had a dramatic effect on her disease, whereas other previous forms of treatment had been ineffective. However, there was a negative aspect to this, namely, the patient did suffer considerable bone loss over the period of treatment in spite of being simultaneously treated with alendronate and calcium. The reason for this is that aromatase inhibitors such as anastrozole inhibit aromatase activity in a global fashion regardless of whether it is in the bone, breast, brain, or endometriotic plaque.

Since it is probably impossible to inhibit aromatase catalytic activity in a tissue-specific fashion, ideal therapy would be to inhibit aromatase expression in a tissue-specific fashion. From the previous discussion of the regulation of aromatase in endometriotic cells, it can be seen that in theory this would be possible in the case of endometriosis—namely, if there were a ligand for COUP-TF that enhanced this

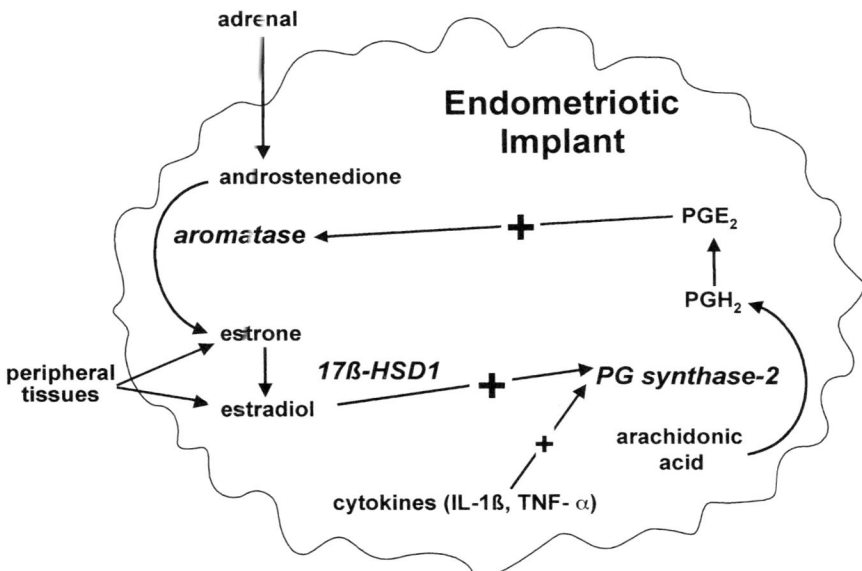

FIGURE 2. Diagram of estrogen biosynthesis in an endometriotic explant. PGE2 appears to be the major factor regulating aromatase expression in this tissue, via cAMP and promoter II. This is made possible by the presence of SF1 (steroidogenic factor-1) in the cells of the endometriotic implant. Since the major substrate for aromatase is androstenedione produced by the adrenal cortex, the initial product is estrone, which is converted to estradiol by the action of 17β-hydroxysteroid dehydrogenase type 1 also present within the implant.

repressive action on aromatase expression, this would be a selective inhibitor for aromatase expression in endometriotic implants. It would have no effect whatsoever on aromatase expression in bone because promoter II does not drive aromatase expression in bone[15] nor should it influence aromatase expression in normal adipose tissue driven by promoter I.4. Thus, it would be selective for endometriosis.

Another aspect of this work relates to the fact that in endometriotic implants, as in other extragonadal sites of estrogen biosynthesis, the substrate for aromatase is circulating androstenedione. This is because extragonadal sites of estrogen biosynthesis are incapable of synthesizing the androgenic substrate from C_{27} precursors. Because androstenedione is the principal circulating C_{19} androgenic steroid, the first product of the aromatase reaction in endometriotic implants is estrone, which has essentially no estrogenic activity. In order to have biological activity, it must first be converted to estradiol. It turns out that the enzyme required to do this, namely, 17β-hydroxysteroid dehydrogenase type 1, is present within endometriotic implants, but is not present in normal healthy endometrium. Instead, the type 2 enzyme is present in normal endometrium, which catalyzes the opposite conversion, namely, estradiol to estrone.[17] Thus, because the type 1 enzyme is present in endometriotic implants together with aromatase, it is possible to form estradiol within endometriotic tissue from circulating androstenedione. Hence, the 17β-HSD type 1 would be another potential target for drug activity to inhibit estrogen biosynthesis in endometriotic tissue. The pathways leading to estrogen biosynthesis in endometriotic plaques are summarized in FIGURE 2.

BREAST CANCER

In studies conducted within the United States in which large numbers of women were given either tamoxifen or raloxifene,[18] there was a substantial decrease in the incidence of invasive breast cancer in women of all ages regardless of whether they were pre- or postmenopausal. This implies that there is a source of estrogen in postmenopausal women that directs breast cancer development, in spite of the fact that the ovaries cease to make estrogens at the time of menopause. This source of estrogen appears to be aromatase expression either within the breast tumor itself or within the mesenchymal cells of the breast surrounding the tumor. It has been shown that the levels of estradiol present in breast tumors are at least an order of magnitude greater than those present in the circulating plasma of postmenopausal women.[19] This can only be due to local estrogen biosynthesis. As an aside, this helps to account for the fact that hormone replacement therapy (HRT) appears to present little increase in the risk of breast cancer, at most 0.30-fold.[20] Even if HRT resulted in an increase in the circulating plasma estrogen levels of severalfold, these levels would still be much lower than those present within the tumor due to local synthesis. This again illustrates the concept that was stated earlier, namely that circulating levels of estrogens in postmenopausal women are not the drivers of estrogen action, but rather reflect local production at extragonadal sites. We conclude, therefore, that local aromatase expression within the breast is the main source of estrogen implicated in breast cancer development in postmenopausal women.

Over the years,[11] we have studied the regulation of aromatase expression in breast and have shown that, in normal breast adipose mesenchymal tissue, aromatase expression is driven primarily by class 1 cytokines and TNFα as described in the INTRODUCTION (FIG. 3). This is because the principal promoter utilized in this tissue is the distal promoter I.4, which responds to signaling pathways stimulated by these factors. However, if a breast tumor is present, there is a switch in promoter utilization such that promoter II, the proximal promoter, is now the major promoter utilized, as was the case in endometriotic tissue. Once again, as in endometriotic tissue, the factor that is driving expression via promoter II appears to be PGE2, produced either by the epithelial cells of the tumor or else by macrophages recruited to the tumor site.[21] This results in a gradient of aromatase expression with highest levels within and proximal to the tumor, and decreasing with increased distance from the tumor.

As mentioned previously, if promoter II reporter gene constructs are transfected into ovarian granulosa cells, then addition of forskolin, which stimulates adenylate cyclase, results in an increase in reporter gene expression. If the SF1 half site on promoter II is mutated, this results in a dramatic loss of reporter activity. When similar experiments were conducted in mouse 3T3L1 cells, which are of adipose mesenchymal origin, a different result was observed. When the SF1 site was mutated, in fact there was an increase in reporter gene activity instead of a loss of reporter gene activity. This suggests that, just as was the case with cells derived from endo-

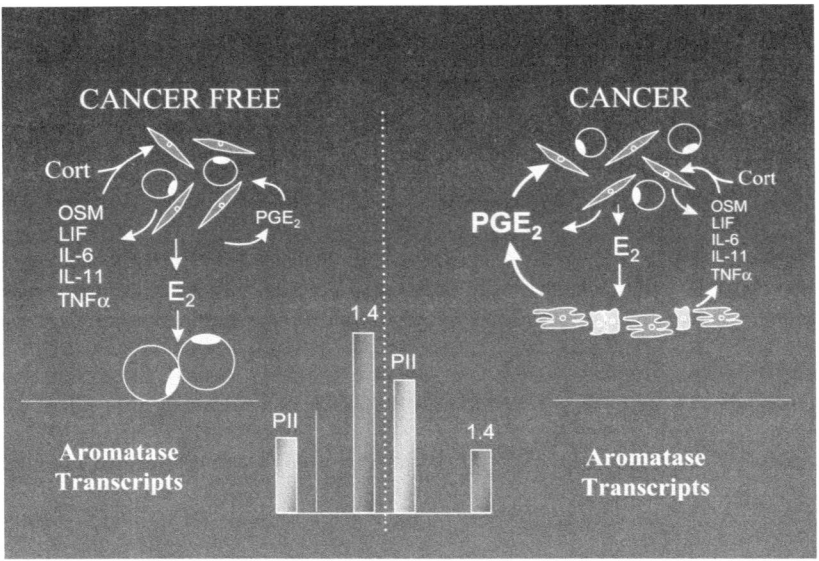

FIGURE 3. Regulation of aromatase expression in breast adipose mesenchymal cells distal and proximal to a tumor. In the cancer-free condition, regulation is regulated primarily by class I cytokines and/or TNFα produced locally within the adipose tissue. Under these conditions, promoter I.4 is the major promoter driving expression. Proximal to a tumor, promoters II and I.3 predominate, indicative of regulation via cAMP. This appears to be because the major factor driving expression is now PGE2, produced in the adipose as well as in tumorous epithelium and macrophages recruited to the tumor site.

metriotic plaques, in these adipose-derived fibroblasts there is a factor that is bound to the SF1 site under normal circumstances and that represses aromatase expression. When the cells were cotransfected with an SF1 expression plasmid, just as was observed with endometriosis-derived cells, there was once again a large increase in reporter gene expression. Current efforts are directed towards cloning and characterizing this putative repressive protein present in adipose fibroblasts of breast. In endometrial tissue, this repressor protein appears to be COUP-TF. Preliminary results, though, indicate that in adipose tissue this is not the case. However, if this repressor protein turns out to be an orphan member of the nuclear receptor family, then in principle it might be possible to discover a ligand for this factor that increases its repressive activity. Since promoter II is not involved in aromatase expression in bone cells, such a ligand would prove to be a highly specific inhibitor of aromatase expression in breast tissue.

Although this putative repressor protein has yet to be characterized, there is another class of compounds that we have found to be potent inhibitors of aromatase expression in breast adipose cells, namely, ligands for peroxisome proliferator–activated receptor γ (PPARγ) and for retinoid X receptor (RXR). PPARγ-RXR heterodimers are critical factors involved in adipocyte differentiation. Our studies have shown that, in adipose tissue, aromatase is expressed primarily in the pre-

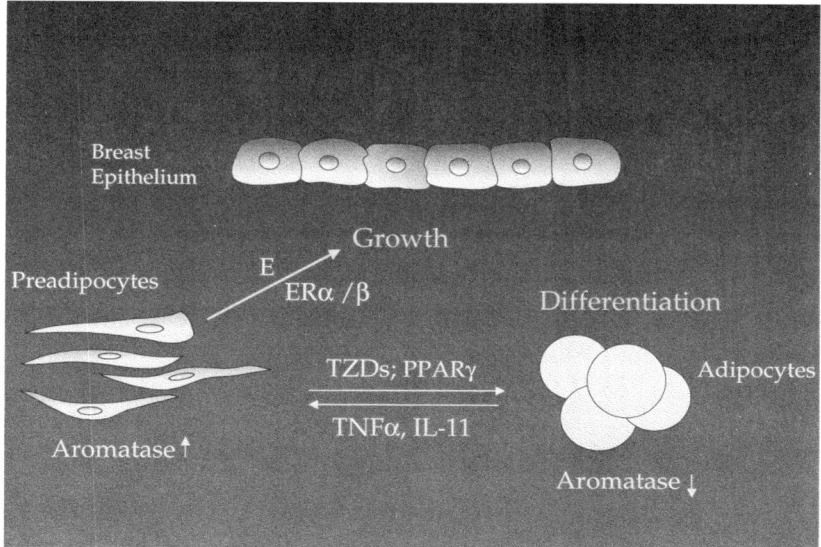

FIGURE 4. Diagram of the regulation of aromatase expression in breast adipose mesenchymal tissue and its role in tumor development.

adipocyte stromal mesenchymal cells rather than in mature adipocytes. Since factors that stimulate aromatase expression in these cells, namely, class 1 cytokines and TNFα, are all inhibitors of adipocyte differentiation, then one might predict that stimulators of adipocyte differentiation would inhibit aromatase expression. Ligands for PPARγ, such as troglitazone and rosiglitazone, and the putative natural ligand 15-deoxy-Δ^{12-14}-prostaglandin J2 are all powerful stimulators of adipocyte differentiation in model systems. We have examined the effect of these compounds on aromatase expression in breast adipose stromal cells and have found that, as predicted, they are powerful inhibitors of aromatase expression in these cells[22] (FIG. 4). The synthetic PPARγ ligands have found utility in the management of type 2 insulin-resistant diabetes. Based on the above results, we suggest that they would also be potentially useful in breast cancer therapy.

SELECTIVE AROMATASE MODULATORS

In conclusion, therefore, we wish to introduce the concept of selective aromatase modulators (SAMs). This concept is critically dependent on the fact that, in postmenopausal women as in men, estradiol does not function as a circulating hormone, but rather functions in a paracrine and intracrine fashion—namely, it is produced locally in a number of extragonadal sites and acts within the same site to effect its biological activity. It is also dependent on the finding that tissue-specific expression of aromatase is dependent on tissue-specific promoters that are differentially regulated by a variety of stimulatory or inhibitory cofactors. Clearly, if estradiol functioned primarily as a circulating hormone in postmenopausal women, these principles would not apply. As we proceed to analyze the specific coactivators and corepressors of aromatase in the various tissue sites of expression, it should be possible to select targets for the development of drugs that will inhibit aromatase in a tissue-specific fashion. The first generation of SAMs might well be ligands of PPARγ and RXR, but we believe that there are other possibilities waiting to be discovered.

As was stated previously, the problem with the phase 3 inhibitors of aromatase activity is that they inhibit this activity globally, not only in the desired site, but also in other sites such as bone and brain. While this may not be so critical in elderly women with advanced breast cancer, it becomes an issue when considering treatment of young women with early disease or even as chemoprevention. Thus, we would anticipate that tissue-specific inhibitors of aromatase expression—that is, SAMs— would find utility in breast cancer treatment, not only as a backup therapy, for example, following tamoxifen breakthrough, but also as first-line therapy in their own right.

ACKNOWLEDGMENTS

This work was supported by USPHS Grant No. R-37 AG 08174 as well as by the Victorian Breast Cancer Research Consortium. Sue Elger provided skilled editorial assistance.

REFERENCES

1. GRUMBACH, M.M. & R.J. AUCHUS. 1999. Estrogen: consequences and implications of human mutations in synthesis and action. J. Clin. Endocrinol. Metab. **85:** 4677–4694.
2. LUBAHN, D.B., J.S. MOYES, T.S. GOLDING et al. 1993. Alteration of function, but not pre-natal sexual development after insertional disruption of the mouse estrogen receptor gene. Proc. Natl. Acad. Sci. U.S.A. **90:** 11162–11166.
3. KREGE, J.H., J.B. HODGIN, J.F. COUSE et al. 1998. Generation and reproductive phenotypes of mice lacking estrogen receptor β. Proc. Natl. Acad. Sci. U.S.A. **95:** 15677–15682.
4. COUSE, J.F., S.C. HEWITT, D.O. BUNCH et al. 1999. Postnatal sex reversal of the ovaries in mice lacking estrogen receptors alpha and beta. Science **286:** 2328–2331.
5. FISHER, C.R., K.H. GRAVES, A.F. PARLOW & E.R. SIMPSON. 1998. Characterization of mice deficient in aromatase (ArKO) because of targeted disruption of the cyp19 gene. Proc. Natl. Acad. Sci. U.S.A. **95:** 6965–6970.
6. JONES, M.E.E., A.W. THORBURN, K.L. BRITT et al. 2000. Aromatase-deficient (ArKO) mice have a phenotype of increased adiposity. Proc. Natl. Acad. Sci. U.S.A. **97:** 12735–12740.
7. HEINE, P.A., J.A. TAYLOR, G.A. IWAMOTO et al. 2000. Increased adipose tissue in male and female estrogen receptor-α knockout mice. Proc. Natl. Acad. Sci. U.S.A. **97:** 12729–12734.
8. ROBERTSON, K.M., L. O'DONNELL, M.E.E. JONES et al. 1999. Impairment of spermatogenesis in mice lacking a functional aromatase (cyp19) gene. Proc. Natl. Acad. Sci. U.S.A. **96:** 7986–7991.
9. LABRIE, F., A. BELANGER, L. CUSAN et al. 1997. Physiological changes in dehydroepiandrosterone are not reflected by serum levels of active androgens and estrogens, but of their metabolites: intracrinology. J. Clin. Endocrinol. Metab. **82:** 2403–2409.

10. SIMPSON, E.R. & S.R. DAVIS. 1998. Why do the clinical sequelae of estrogen deficiency affect women more frequently than men? J. Clin. Endocrinol. Metab. **83:** 2214.
11. SIMPSON, E.R., Y. ZHAO, V.R. AGARWAL et al. 1997. Aromatase expression in health and disease. Recent Prog. Horm. Res. **52:** 185–213.
12. NOBLE, L.S., E.R. SIMPSON, A. JOHNS & S.E. BULUN. 1996. Aromatase expression in endometriosis. J. Clin. Endocrinol. Metab. **81:** 174–179.
13. NOBLE, L.S., K. TAKAYAMA, K.M. ZEITOUN et al. 1997. Prostaglandin E2 stimulates aromatase expression in endometriosis-derived stromal cells. J. Clin. Endocrinol. Metab. **82:** 600–606.
14. ZEITOUN, K., K. TAKAYAMA, M.D. MICHAEL & S.E. BULUN. 1999. Stimulation of aromatase P450 promoter (II) activity in endometriosis and its inhibition in endometrium are regulated by competitive binding of steroidogenic factor-1 and chicken ovalbumin upstream promoter transcription factor to the same cis-acting element. Mol. Endocrinol. **13:** 239–253.
15. BULUN, S.E., K.M. ZEITOUN, K. TAKAYAMA et al. 2000. Aromatase as a therapeutic target in endometriosis. Trends Endocrinol. Metab. **11:** 22–27.
16. SHOZU, M. & E.R. SIMPSON. 1998. Aromatase expression of human osteoblast-like cells. Mol. Cell. Endocrinol. **139:** 117–129.
17. ZEITOUN, K., K. TAKAYAMA, H. SASANO et al. 1998. Deficient 17β-hydroxysteroid dehydrogenase type 2 expression in endometriosis: failure to metabolize 17β-estradiol. J. Clin. Endocrinol. Metab. **83:** 4474–4480.
18. JORDAN, V.C. 1999. Targeted antiestrogens to prevent breast cancer. Trends Endocrinol. Metab. **10:** 312–317.
19. PASQUALINI, J.R., G. CHETRITE, C. BLACKER et al. 1996. Concentrations of estrone, estradiol, and estrone sulfate and evaluation of sulfatose and aromatase activities in pre- and postmenopausal breast cancer patients. J. Clin. Endocrinol. Metab. **81:** 1460–1464.
20. COLLABORATIVE GROUP ON HORMONAL FACTORS IN BREAST CANCER. 1997. Collaborative re-analysis of data from 51 epidemiological studies of 52,705 women with breast cancer and 108,441 women without breast cancer. Lancet **350:** 1047–1059.
21. ZHAO, Y., V.R. AGARWAL, C.R. MENDELSON & E.R. SIMPSON. 1996. Estrogen biosynthesis proximal to a breast tumor is stimulated by PGE2 via cyclic AMP, leading to activation of promoter II of the cyp19 gene. Endocrinology **137:** 5739–5742.
22. RUBIN, G.L., Y. ZHAO, A.M. KALUS & E.R. SIMPSON. 2000. Peroxisome proliferator-activated receptor gamma ligands inhibit estrogen biosynthesis in human breast adipose tissue: possible implications for breast cancer therapy. Cancer Res. **60:** 1604–1608.

Cancer Treatment and Prevention
Introduction

BARBARA K. DUNN[a] AND BARRY KRAMER[b]

[a]*Division of Cancer Prevention, Basic Prevention Science Research Group, National Cancer Institute, Bethesda, Maryland, USA*

[b]*Office of Disease Prevention, National Institutes of Health, Bethesda, Maryland, USA*

The "Basic Biology of SERMs" papers offered insight into the mechanism of action of selective estrogen modulators (SERMs) at the molecular level. Clearly, the best-defined route of SERM action appears to be via interaction with the estrogen receptor(s) (ER). The chief molecular consequence of this interaction is competition with estrogen for the ER, with resulting estrogen agonism or antagonism depending on the nature of this alternative SERM ligand-receptor interaction. While the net impact of the SERM-ER complex on target gene activation and cellular proliferation emerges in part from the molecular characteristics of the SERM in question, the specific cellular environment, that is, the presence of coactivators and corepressors, also contributes to this outcome. Since ERs are observed in multiple tissue types and the cellular environment varies with the target tissue, the clinical consequences of SERM-ER interaction encompass multiple organ systems, each of which is characterized by a distinct proestrogenic or antiestrogenic profile from intervention with a given SERM.

    The best-studied clinical application of SERMs involves the target disease site breast cancer. In fact, the best-studied SERM, tamoxifen, a first-generation triphenylethylene, although initially investigated as a fertility drug, was ultimately developed primarily for its efficacy in breast cancer.[1,2] Following the traditional sequence of clinical testing first in metastatic disease, then in localized disease, and finally in high-risk women for its efficacy as a breast cancer preventive agent,[3-5] tamoxifen has proven to be a major success story among anticancer drugs. Tamoxifen is the most commonly used hormonal agent for ER-positive disease in both the adjuvant and metastatic settings, and it is approved to reduce the risk of breast cancer in women at increased risk for the disease.[6,7]

    Despite its efficacy and widespread use in breast cancer, tamoxifen has two major limitations: limited range of efficacy and toxicity. First, tamoxifen is limited by its lack of 100% efficacy in the various breast cancer settings in which it is currently the standard of care. On the one hand, its predominant mechanism of action restricts its

---

Address for correspondence: Barbara K. Dunn, Ph.D., M.D., Division of Cancer Prevention, Basic Prevention Science Research Group, National Cancer Institute, EPN 2056, Bethesda, MD 20892-7215. Voice: 301-402-1209; fax: 301-480-4110.
    dunnb@mail.nih.gov

applicability to ER-positive breast cancers in metastatic and adjuvant breast cancer. In the preventive setting, only ER-positive cancers are reduced in incidence.[3] Even among the ER-positive cancers, only a subset respond to tamoxifen: in the metastatic setting, only 50% either regress or remain stable with tamoxifen; only a 50% annual reduction in recurrence is seen with adjuvant tamoxifen in localized disease; and 69% of ER-positive breast cancers are prevented by tamoxifen.[3,6] This imperfect record with regard to efficacy is exacerbated by the frequent development of tamoxifen resistance, manifest as progressive growth of distant stable disease and reemergence of disease while on adjuvant tamoxifen.[8,9]

Second, use of tamoxifen is restricted by virtue of its toxic side effects. At least two of these are potentially life-threatening: endometrial cancer and thromboembolic disease. These limitations of tamoxifen, combined with a growing understanding of the molecular basis for SERM action, have motivated an ongoing search for SERMs that lack the undesirable effects of tamoxifen, but retain or enhance its beneficial outcomes. Thus, tamoxifen has paved the way for the application of newer, more potent, and more specifically targeted SERMs to the treatment and prevention of breast cancer.

Another important issue that has emerged from the studies of tamoxifen is that of risk-benefit evaluation of agents with established potential in disease treatment and prevention. In the treatment setting, the toxicities of tamoxifen have been viewed as relatively minor in comparison to those of commonly used chemotherapeutic agents and in comparison to the adverse outcome of the untreated disease itself. However, in the prevention setting, the healthy, although high-risk, recipients of the drug represent an entirely different cohort in which drug-related toxicity plays a larger role in the decision to take tamoxifen. These concerns have spawned a series of publications offering statistically based models for risk/benefit assessment[10,11] and addressing the appropriate approaches to physician-patient decision-making regarding the use of preventive tamoxifen.[12] Despite such misgivings regarding tamoxifen's toxic side effects, evaluations show that the quality of life of women taking tamoxifen as part of ongoing breast cancer prevention trials has not been adversely affected[13,14] and are addressed in this section on "Cancer Treatment and Prevention."

In addition, concerns about tamoxifen-related toxicities have instigated studies of newer SERMs in the high-risk setting. Most prominent of these agents is raloxifene, now in a phase 3 study (National Surgical Adjuvant Breast and Bowel Project's P-2 Study of Tamoxifen and Raloxifene: STAR) of its ability, relative to that of tamoxifen, to reduce the incidence of breast cancer in high-risk women.[15,16] However, smaller phase I and II studies of SERM efficacy focusing on biomarkers as surrogates for clinical end points are also ongoing.[17-20] Finally, the risk/benefit issue with tamoxifen is also being addressed directly by studies examining efficacy of lower, and therefore potentially less toxic, doses, again using surrogate end point biomarkers.[18,19]

The papers in this section span the gamut of breast cancer studies, exploring the application of SERMs to the treatment of metastatic disease through adjuvant therapy in localized disease through prevention in high-risk women. In particular, controversial issues evolving from the definitively positive NSABP BCPT trial,[3] demonstrating the efficacy of tamoxifen versus placebo in reducing the incidence of breast cancer in high-risk women, are discussed and analyzed in light of results from two independent European trials.[4,5,21] Interestingly, more recent data from the Italian group suggest that continued follow-up of the Italian trial is revealing that tamoxifen may, in fact, reduce breast cancer incidence in their average-risk population.[22,23] The hope has been expressed that results from the yet uncompleted International Breast Cancer Intervention Study (IBIS) will help to resolve some of the issues relating to the differences between the European and American trials.[24]

While the papers in this section center mainly on tamoxifen, which is the focus of most clinical cancer studies and by far the SERM most widely used in clinical practice for breast cancer, other SERMs are discussed. These newer SERMs are now under clinical investigation for both the treatment and prevention of breast cancer. Raloxifene, a second-generation SERM that lacked efficacy in limited studies of the treatment of existing breast cancer,[25] was suggested as a preventive agent by secondary findings in a placebo-controlled osteoporosis study.[15] It is now being compared to tamoxifen for its efficacy in the breast cancer preventive setting in the Study of Tamoxifen and Raloxifene, STAR.[16] A recently published phase I study of LY353381 (SERM-3) in pretreated metastatic breast cancer showed that all tested doses (up to 100 mg per day) were well tolerated and no endometrial thickening was observed after 12 weeks of treatment as assessed by transvaginal ultrasound.[26] The only SERM besides tamoxifen that is FDA-approved for clinical use in breast cancer is toremifene, a second-generation triphenylethylene. Touted for less DNA adduct formation relative to tamoxifen in preclinical models, its approved use is limited to treatment of metastatic disease in postmenopausal women.[27] The development of new, more specifically targeted SERMs with more potency at their primary target sites, as well as efforts to explore a range of dosages of existing agents such as tamoxifen, in order to optimize the risk/benefit ratio,[18,19] are the foci of current clinical SERM research in oncology and are addressed in several of the papers in this section. Despite promising early data suggesting greater efficacy or lesser toxicity of specific SERMs in various breast cancer settings, development of most of these second- and third-generation agents has been hampered either by excess toxicity or by the absence of greater efficacy than the standard, tamoxifen.

REFERENCES

1. FURR, B.J. & V.C. JORDAN. 1984. The pharmacology and clinical uses of tamoxifen. Pharmacol. Ther. **25:** 127–205.
2. JORDAN, V.C. 1999. Introduction: foundations. In Tamoxifen for the Treatment and Prevention of Breast Cancer, pp. 23–28. PRR. Melville, NY.
3. FISHER, B., J.P. COSTANTINO, D.L. WICKERHAM et al. 1998. Tamoxifen for prevention of breast cancer: report of the National Surgical Adjuvant Breast and Bowel Project P-1 Study. J. Natl. Cancer Inst. **90:** 1371–1388.
4. POWLES, T., R. EELES, S. ASHLEY et al. 1998. Interim analysis of the incidence of breast cancer in the Royal Marsden Hospital tamoxifen randomised chemoprevention trial. Lancet **352:** 98–101.
5. VERONESI, U., P. MAISONNEUVE, A. COSTA et al. 1998. Prevention of breast cancer with tamoxifen: preliminary findings from the Italian randomised trial among hysterectomised women: Italian Tamoxifen Prevention Study. Lancet **352:** 93–97.
6. OSBORNE, C.K. 1998. Drug therapy: tamoxifen in the treatment of breast cancer. N. Engl. J. Med. **889:** 1609–1618.

7. INGLE, J.N. 2001. Aromatase inhibition and antiestrogen therapy in early breast cancer treatment and chemoprevention. Oncology **15**(suppl.): 28–34.
8. CLARKE, R. & M.E. LIPPMAN. 1993. Acquisition of antiestrogen resistance in breast cancer. *In* Drug Resistance in Oncology, pp. 501–536. Dekker. New York.
9. MAMOUNAS, E. 2001. Adjuvant exemestane therapy after 5 years of tamoxifen: rationale for the NSABP B-33 trial. Oncology **15**(suppl.): 35–39.
10. GAIL, M.H., J.P. COSTANTINO, J. BRYANT *et al.* 1999. Weighing the risks and benefits of tamoxifen treatment for preventing breast cancer. J. Natl. Cancer Inst. **91**: 1829–1846.
11. TAYLOR, A.L., L.L. ADAMS-CAMPBELL & J.T. WRIGHT, JR. 1999. Risk/benefit assessment of tamoxifen to prevent breast cancer—still a work in progress? J. Natl. Cancer Inst. **91**(21): 1792–1793.
12. CHLEBOWSKI, R.T., D.E. COLLYAR, M.R. SOMERFIELD & D.G. PFISTER. 1999. American Society of Clinical Oncology technology assessment on breast cancer risk reduction strategies: tamoxifen and raloxifene. J. Clin. Oncol. **17**: 1939–1955.
13. DAY, R., P.A. GANZ, J.P. COSTANTINO *et al.* 1999. Health-related quality of life and tamoxifen in breast cancer prevention: a report from the National Surgical Adjuvant Breast and Bowel Project P-1 study. J. Clin. Oncol. **17**: 2659–2669.
14. FALLOWFIELD, L., A. FLEISSIG, R. EDWARDS *et al.* 2001. Tamoxifen for the prevention of breast cancer: psychosocial impact on women participating in two randomized controlled trials. J. Clin. Oncol. **19**: 1886–1892.
15. CUMMINGS, S.R., S. ECKERT, K.A. KRUEGER *et al.* 1999. The effect of raloxifene on risk of breast cancer in postmenopausal women: results from the MORE randomized trial—Multiple Outcomes of Raloxifene Evaluation. JAMA **281**: 2189–2197.
16. WOLMARK, N. 1999. The Breast Cancer Prevention Trial, tamoxifen, and the woman at high risk for breast cancer. Primary Care Cancer **19**(suppl. 2): 11–16.
17. FABIAN, C.J., B.F. KIMLER, R.M. ELLEDGE *et al.* 1998. Models for early chemoprevention trials in breast cancer. Hematol. Oncol. Clin. N. Am. **12**: 993–1017.
18. DECENSI, A., B. BONANNI, A. GUERRIERI-GONZAGA *et al.* 1998. Biologic activity of tamoxifen at low doses in healthy women. J. Natl. Cancer Inst. **90**: 1461–1467.
19. DECENSI, A., S. GANDINI, A. GUERRIERI-GONZAGA *et al.* 1999. Effect of blood tamoxifen concentrations on surrogate biomarkers in a trial of dose reduction in healthy women. J. Clin. Oncol. **17**: 2633–2638.
20. DUNN, B.K. & L.G. FORD. 2000. Prevention of breast cancer. Semin. Breast Dis. **3**: 90–99.
21. PRITCHARD, K.I. 1998. Is tamoxifen effective in prevention of breast cancer? Lancet **352**: 80–81.
22. DECENSI, A., B. BONANNI, N. ROTMENSZ *et al.* 2000. Update on tamoxifen to prevent breast cancer: the Italian Tamoxifen Prevention Study. Eur. J. Cancer **36**: S49–S56.
23. DECENSI, A., N. ROTMENSZ, P. MAISONNEUVE *et al.* 2001. Prevention of breast cancer with tamoxifen: update of the Italian trial in hysterectomized women. Abstract 4441, p. 827. Proc. Am. Assoc. Cancer Res. (Ninety-second Meeting, New Orleans).
24. CUZICK, J. 1998. Point of view: continuation of the International Breast Cancer Intervention Study (IBIS). Eur. J. Cancer **34**: 1647–1648.
25. BUZDAR, A.U., M.C. HOLMES, F. HOLMES *et al.* 1988. Phase II evaluation of LY156758 in metastatic breast cancer. Oncology **45**: 344–345.
26. MÜNSTER, P.N., A. BUZDAR, K. DHINGRA *et al.* 2001. Phase I study of a third-generation selective estrogen receptor modulator, LY353381.HCl, in metastatic breast cancer. J. Clin. Oncol. **19**: 2202–2209.
27. BUZDAR, A.U. & G.N. HORTOBAGYI. 1998. Tamoxifen and toremifene in breast cancer: comparison of safety and efficacy. J. Clin. Oncol. **16**: 348–353.

The Past, Present, and Future of Selective Estrogen Receptor Modulation

V. CRAIG JORDAN

Robert H. Lurie Comprehensive Cancer Center, Northwestern University Medical School, Chicago, Illinois 60611, USA

ABSTRACT: The recognition of selective estrogen receptor modulation in the mid-1980s provided a unique opportunity to develop multifunctional drugs. Tamoxifen, the first selective estrogen receptor modulator (SERM), is the first antiestrogen to be tested successfully for the prevention of breast cancer in high-risk women. However, the recognition that SERMs maintain bone density and lower circulating cholesterol suggested that the prevention of osteoporosis and coronary heart disease would be beneficial side effects of tamoxifen treatment. This hypothesis has not been pursued in clinical trial, but an alternate hypothesis, that SERMs could be developed to prevent osteoporosis and potentially reduce the risk of breast cancer, has been pursued with raloxifene. Current molecule modeling of the SERM-ER complex has identified the reason for the promiscuous estrogen-like actions of tamoxifen compared with raloxifene. Future studies of the signal transduction pathways of the ER alpha (α)– and beta (β)–SERM complexes hold the promise of new drug discoveries and a menu of preventive medicine in clinical practice.

KEYWORDS: SERM; tamoxifen; raloxifene; estrogen receptor; breast cancer

INTRODUCTION

In 1936, Professor Antoine Lacassagne presented a paper at the American Association for Cancer Research that provided a vision for the prevention of breast cancer in well women.[1] In the summary of his paper, he stated the following:

> If one accepts the consideration of adenocarcinoma of the breast as the consequence of a special hereditary sensitivity to the proliferative actions of oestrone, one is led to imagine a therapeutic preventive for subjects predisposed by their heredity to this cancer. It would consist—perhaps in the very near future when the knowledge and use of hormones will be better understood—in the suitable use of hormones, antagonistic or excretory, to prevent the stagnation of oestrone in the ducts of the breast.

However, in 1936, the target for hormone action was unknown and there were no antagonists for estrogen action. In 1962, Jensen[2] first described the estrogen receptor (ER) in estrogen target tissues and applied this knowledge to establish a predictive test to identify breast tumors that would respond to endocrine therapy.[3] Lerner and coworkers[4] independently reported the pharmacological properties of MER 25, the first nonsteroidal antiestrogen. MER 25 is a complete antiestrogen with no other

Address for correspondence: V. Craig Jordan, Ph.D., D.Sc., Robert H. Lurie Comprehensive Cancer Center, Northwestern University Medical School, 303 East Chicago Avenue, 8258 Olson Pavilion, Chicago, IL 60611. Voice: 312-908-4148; fax: 312-908-1372.

vcjordan@northwestern.edu

hormonal or antihormonal activities in any species. However, MER 25 was not developed for clinical use because of low potency and unacceptable side effects.[5]

In retrospect, the early clinical development of a pure antiestrogen with no estrogen-like activity would not have advanced the science of selective estrogen receptor modulators (SERMs). It can be argued that, if estrogens are important to maintain bone density and decrease circulating cholesterol, then a complete antiestrogen could prevent breast cancer, but predispose well women to osteoporosis and coronary heart disease in later life. The shift towards the examination of triphenylethylene-based nonsteroidal antiestrogens[6] and the subsequent development of tamoxifen for the treatment of advanced breast cancer[7] provided a unique opportunity to study the laboratory and clinical pharmacology of a partial estrogen agonist with antiestrogenic actions in breast cancer.[8]

TAMOXIFEN FOR THE TREATMENT OF BREAST CANCER

Tamoxifen blocks the binding of estradiol to the human breast cancer ER[9] and is effective in controlling the growth of ER-positive, but not ER-negative, breast tumors in laboratory models *in vivo*.[10,11] However, tamoxifen is not a tumoricidal agent and long-term therapy is more effective in animal models than short-term therapy.[12–14] These laboratory principles have been tested in clinical trials over the past 30 years.

Tamoxifen is more effective in treating ER- or ER/PgR (progesterone receptor)–positive advanced breast cancer[15,16] than receptor-negative disease. Similarly, tamoxifen is more effective as an adjuvant in ER-positive disease, but without advantage for patients with ER-negative disease.[17] However, the duration of adjuvant tamoxifen therapy is critical to enhance survival. Five years of tamoxifen is superior to either 1 or 2 years of adjuvant tamoxifen[17] and the benefit of tamoxifen lasts for at least a decade after tamoxifen is stopped. The reason for this property of tamoxifen is unclear, but it may be related to the observation that tamoxifen-resistant (stimulated) disease becomes supersensitive to physiologic concentrations of estradiol, which kills the cancer cells.[18]

It is now estimated that 400,000 women are alive today because of the widespread use of adjuvant tamoxifen. The safe use of tamoxifen in node-negative breast cancer, coupled with the observations that tamoxifen prevents rat mammary carcinogenesis[19] and reduces the incidence of contralateral breast cancer,[20–22] raised the possibility that tamoxifen could be used as a chemopreventive agent in high-risk women. Trevor Powles, at the Royal Marsden Hospital in England, initiated a pilot study to assess the feasibility of recruiting 2000 women with a first-degree relative with breast cancer to be randomized into placebo or tamoxifen-treated groups.[23] However, in 1986 when these preliminary clinical studies were getting started, it was unclear whether long-term tamoxifen therapy would place well women at risk for osteoporosis and coronary heart disease.

RECOGNITION OF THE SERM PRINCIPLE

In the mid-1980s, an intense laboratory research program was initiated to study the selective pharmacology of tamoxifen in different target sites.

Tamoxifen was found to be estrogen-like in bone in the ovariectomized rat,[24–26] despite having well-defined partial estrogenic/antiestrogenic actions in the uterus[27] and antiestrogenic/antitumor actions in the mammary gland.[14] Similarly, tamoxifen is estrogen-like in the mouse uterus,[28] but is an antiestrogen/antitumor agent in breast or mammary tissue.[29,30] Indeed, the bitransplantation of a breast and an endometrial tumor into athymic mice treated with tamoxifen results in the control of breast cancer growth, but a continuation of endometrial cancer growth.[31] To explain these findings, it was proposed that the tamoxifen-ER complex acts as an estrogen at some sites, but as an inhibitor of estrogen action at other select sites.[29,31]

These laboratory observations translated to women with the findings that tamoxifen maintains bone density in postmenopausal women[32] and lowers circulating cholesterol.[33,34] The selective action of tamoxifen on breast and endometrial cancer growth was observed in clinical trials with a reduction of the incidence of contralateral breast cancer, but an increase in the detection of endometrial cancer.[21]

These data allowed advancement of the strategy for testing the worth of tamoxifen in the prevention of breast cancer in high-risk women. However, it was clear that tamoxifen was not suitable for well women without high-risk factors for breast cancer. A new strategy for the general application of SERMs was proposed in 1989 and subsequently published as a road map for the development of SERMs in the 1990s. The new paradigm shift for the broad application of SERMs was simply stated:

> We have obtained valuable clinical information about this group of drugs that can be applied in other disease states. Research does not travel in straight lines and observations in one field of science often become major discoveries in another. Important clues have been garnered about the effects of tamoxifen on bone and lipids, so it is possible that derivatives could find targeted applications to retard osteoporosis or atherosclerosis. The ubiquitous application of novel compounds to prevent diseases associated with the progressive changes after menopause may, as a side effect, significantly retard the development of breast cancer. The target population would be postmenopausal women in general, thereby avoiding the requirement to select a high-risk group to prevent breast cancer.[6]

TAMOXIFEN AND RALOXIFENE AS PREVENTIVES

Tamoxifen is proven to reduce the incidence of primary breast cancer in high-risk pre- and postmenopausal women.[35] Tamoxifen is the first drug to be approved by the FDA for the reduction of breast cancer risk. Most importantly, tamoxifen demonstrated the properties of a SERM: there was a nonsignificant decrease in fractures, a reduction in breast cancer incidence, and an increase in the incidence of endometrial cancer, but this was confined to postmenopausal women.[35] Coronary heart disease was not affected by tamoxifen treatment,[36,37] but this is not a surprise as the drug has not been tested prospectively in women with high risk for coronary heart disease. The uncertainty of the value of estrogen in preventing coronary heart disease is another complicating factor.[36]

Raloxifene has been evaluated and tested clinically based on the Lerner/Jordan hypothesis stated above. In the early 1980s, raloxifene was known as keoxifene or LY156758.[38] The compound has very little estrogen-like action in the rodent uterus, and compounds of this class can block the estrogen-like action of tamoxifen in the rodent uterus.[39] The drug was destined for development as a breast cancer drug, but poor performance against tamoxifen in laboratory models[40,41] and in tamoxifen-resistant breast cancer patients[42] terminated development. A major concern for the development of raloxifene as a breast cancer drug is the fact that there is only 2% bioavailability because of severe first-pass metabolism in the liver.[43]

In 1992, raloxifene was proposed for development as a preventive for osteoporosis with breast and uterine safety. Raloxifene maintains bone density in postmenopausal women[44] and reduces fractures of the spine.[45] Raloxifene also reduces circulating cholesterol[46] and is currently being evaluated as a preventive for coronary heart disease. To test the veracity of the hypothesis[6] that a SERM for osteoporosis would reduce the incidence of breast cancer, events were monitored during a trial of osteoporosis.[47] By the third year of treatment with raloxifene, there was a significant decrease in breast cancer incidence. In associated studies, no stimulation of the uterus was found.[48] These data provided the rationale for testing tamoxifen and raloxifene for reducing the risk of breast cancer in high-risk postmenopausal women. This is the Study of Tamoxifen and Raloxifene (STAR) trial.

Despite the advances in chemoprevention, it is important to elucidate the mechanism of action of SERMs at the ER so that, in the future, novel therapeutic agents can be developed.

MOLECULAR MECHANISMS

During the 1980s, numerous molecular models of estrogen, partial estrogen, and antiestrogen action were developed based on structure-activity relationships of the ligand bound in the ER.[49–51] In its simplest form, the model stated that the intrinsic activity of the receptor complex is controlled by sealing an estrogen in the ligand-binding domain, but an antiestrogen blocks estrogen action by wedging in the ligand-binding domain. The antiestrogen side chain of the molecule interacts with an "antiestrogen region" to block full activation of the ER complex. The length of the side chain controls antiestrogen action, so partial agonists result from a mixture of different-shaped complexes with different properties. However, the cloning of the ER[52] allowed examination of the structure-function relationships of the ligand with the receptor protein.

The discovery of a mutated surface amino acid D351Y (aspartate residue converted to tyrosine) in a tamoxifen-stimulated tumor,[53] which enhanced the estrogen-like properties of tamoxifen and converted raloxifene from an antiestrogen to a partial estrogen,[54,55] illustrated for the first time how a natural mutation could control the estrogen-like actions of a SERM. The subsequent publication of the X-ray crystallographic data of the ligand-binding domain of ER with tamoxifen and raloxifene[56,57] demonstrated that the antiestrogenic side chain interacts with D351. Indeed, raloxifene has a tight interaction shielding the exposed carboxylic acid of aspartate, whereas tamoxifen is unable to provide neutralization of the charge. To address the hypothesis that D351 controls the promiscuous estrogen-like effects of tamoxifen, a D351G mutant (aspartate residue converted to glycine) has been constructed that allosterically converts tamoxifen from an estrogen to a complete antiestrogen.[58] Conversely, removing the piperidine ring of raloxifene and replacing it with a cyclohexane or replacing aspartate with glutamate or tyrosine at 351 results in an allosteric reactivation of the estrogenic activity in the raloxifene-ER complex in the AF-1 region.[59,60]

The goal of future studies is to amplify or suppress the target tissue–specific actions of novel ligands. New model systems of drug resistance to SERMs can help in this process by identifying the cooperative subcellular signal transduction pathways that can be used to explain SERM action *in vivo*. As the first step in this process, we have developed a new model of drug resistance to tamoxifen using T47D cells grown in athymic mice. The pharmacology of SERMs in the model *in vivo*[61–63] replicates the pharmacology of SERMs in *in vitro* assay systems.[64]

The integration of the SERM with signal transduction pathways through ERα and ERβ, as well as their interaction with coactivators and corepressors, will provide insight not only for advancing breast and endometrial cancer prevention, but also for the prevention of coronary heart disease and osteoporosis.

ACKNOWLEDGMENTS

V. C. Jordan is the Diana, Princess of Wales, Professor of Cancer Research. The studies were supported by SPORE Grant No. CA89018-01, the generosity of the Lynn Sage Breast Cancer Research Foundation of Northwestern Memorial Hospital, and the Avon Products Foundation.

REFERENCES

1. LACASSAGNE, A. 1936. Hormonal pathogenesis of adenocarcinoma of the breast. Am. J. Cancer **27:** 217–225.
2. JENSEN, E.V. & H.I. JACOBSON. 1962. Basic guides to the mechanism of estrogen action. Recent Prog. Horm. Res. **18:** 387–414.
3. JENSEN, E.V., G.E. BLOCK, S. SMITH *et al.* 1971. Estrogen receptors and breast cancer response to adrenalectomy. Natl. Cancer Inst. Monogr. **34:** 55–70.
4. LERNER, L.J., J.F. HOLTHAUS & C.R. THOMPSON. 1958. A non-steroidal estrogen antagonist 1-(*p*-2-diethylaminoethoxyphenyl)-1-phenyl-2-*p*-methoxyphenylethanol. Endocrinology **63:** 295–318.
5. LERNER, L.J. 1981. The first non-steroidal antiestrogen—MER 25. In Nonsteroidal Antioestrogens: Molecular Pharmacology and Antitumour Activity, pp. 1–6. Academic Press. Sydney.
6. LERNER, L.J. & V.C. JORDAN. 1990. Development of antiestrogens and their use in breast cancer: Eighth Cain Memorial Award lecture. Cancer Res. **50:** 4177–4189.
7. JORDAN, V.C. 1988. The development of tamoxifen for breast cancer therapy: a tribute to the late Arthur L. Walpole. Breast Cancer Res. Treat. **11:** 197–209.
8. FURR, B.J. & V.C. JORDAN. 1984. The pharmacology and clinical uses of tamoxifen. Pharmacol. Ther. **25:** 127–205.
9. JORDAN, V.C. & S. KOERNER. 1975. Tamoxifen (ICI 46,474) and the human carcinoma 8S oestrogen receptor. Eur. J. Cancer **11:** 205–206.
10. JORDAN, V.C. & T. JASPAN. 1976. Tamoxifen as an antitumour agent: oestrogen binding as a predictive test for tumour response. J. Endocrinol. **68:** 453–460.
11. OSBORNE, C.K., K. HOBBS & G.M. CLARK. 1985. Effect of estrogens and antiestrogens on growth of human breast cancer cells in athymic nude mice. Cancer Res. **45:** 584–590.
12. JORDAN, V.C., C.J. DIX & K.E. ALLEN. 1979. The effectiveness of long-term tamoxifen treatment in a laboratory model for adjuvant hormone therapy of breast cancer. In Adjuvant Therapy of Cancer, pp. 19–26. Grune & Stratton. New York.

13. JORDAN, V.C., K.E. ALLEN & C.J. DIX. 1980. Pharmacology of tamoxifen in laboratory animals. Cancer Treat. Rep. **64:** 745–759.
14. JORDAN, V.C. & K.E. ALLEN. 1980. Evaluation of the antitumour activity of the nonsteroidal antioestrogen monohydroxytamoxifen in the DMBA-induced rat mammary carcinoma model. Eur. J. Cancer **16:** 239–251.
15. KIANG, D.T. & B.J. KENNEDY. 1977. Tamoxifen (antiestrogen) therapy in advanced breast cancer. Ann. Intern. Med. **87:** 687–690.
16. RAVDIN, P.M., S. GREEN, T.M. DORR et al. 1992. Prognostic significance of progesterone receptor levels in estrogen receptor–positive patients with metastatic breast cancer treated with tamoxifen: results of a prospective Southwest Oncology Group study. J. Clin. Oncol. **10:** 1284–1291.
17. EARLY BREAST CANCER TRIALISTS' COLLABORATIVE GROUP. 1998. Tamoxifen for early breast cancer: an overview of the randomized trials. Lancet **351:** 1451–1467.
18. YAO, K., E.S. LEE, D.J. BENTREM et al. 2000. Antitumor action of physiological estradiol on tamoxifen-stimulated breast tumors grown in athymic mice [in process citation]. Clin. Cancer Res. **6:** 2028–2036.
19. JORDAN, V.C. 1976. Effect of tamoxifen (ICI 46,474) on initiation and growth of DMBA-induced rat mammary carcinomata. Eur. J. Cancer **12:** 419–424.
20. CUZICK, J. & M. BAUM. 1985. Tamoxifen and contralateral breast cancer [letter]. Lancet **2:** 282.
21. FORNANDER, T., L.E. RUTQVIST, B. CEDERMARK et al. 1989. Adjuvant tamoxifen in early breast cancer: occurrence of new primary cancers. Lancet **1:** 117–120.
22. FISHER, B., J. COSTANTINO, C. REDMOND et al. 1989. A randomized clinical trial evaluating tamoxifen in the treatment of patients with node-negative breast cancer who have estrogen-receptor-positive tumors. N. Engl. J. Med. **320:** 479–484.
23. POWLES, T.J., J.R. HARDY, S.E. ASHLEY et al. 1989. A pilot trial to evaluate the acute toxicity and feasibility of tamoxifen for prevention of breast cancer. Br. J. Cancer **60:** 126–131.
24. JORDAN, V.C., E. PHELPS & J.U. LINDGREN. 1987. Effects of anti-estrogens on bone in castrated and intact female rats. Breast Cancer Res. Treat. **10:** 31–35.
25. TURNER, R.T., G.K. WAKLEY, K.S. HANNON et al. 1987. Tamoxifen prevents the skeletal effects of ovarian hormone deficiency in rats. J. Bone Miner. Res. **2:** 449–456.
26. TURNER, R.T., G.K. WAKLEY, K.S. HANNON et al. 1988. Tamoxifen inhibits osteoclast-mediated resorption of trabecular bone in ovarian hormone-deficient rats. Endocrinology **122:** 1146–1150.
27. HARPER, M.J. & A.L. WALPOLE. 1967. A new derivative of triphenylethylene: effect on implantation and mode of action in rats. J. Reprod. Fertil. **13:** 101–119.
28. TERENIUS, L. 1971. Structure-activity relationships of anti-oestrogens with regard to interaction with 17-beta-oestradiol in the mouse uterus and vagina. Acta Endocrinol. (Copenh.) **66:** 431–447.
29. JORDAN, V.C. & S.P. ROBINSON. 1987. Species-specific pharmacology of antiestrogens: role of metabolism. Fed. Proc. **46:** 1870–1874.
30. JORDAN, V.C., M.K. LABABIDI & S. LANGAN-FAHEY. 1991. Suppression of mouse mammary tumorigenesis by long-term tamoxifen therapy. J. Natl. Cancer Inst. **83:** 492–496.
31. GOTTARDIS, M.M., S.P. ROBINSON, P.G. SATYASWAROOP et al. 1988. Contrasting actions of tamoxifen on endometrial and breast tumor growth in the athymic mouse. Cancer Res. **48:** 812–815.
32. LOVE, R.R., R.B. MAZESS, H.S. BARDEN et al. 1992. Effects of tamoxifen on bone mineral density in postmenopausal women with breast cancer. N. Engl. J. Med. **326:** 852–856.
33. LOVE, R.R., D.A. WIEBE, P.A. NEWCOMB et al. 1991. Effects of tamoxifen on cardiovascular risk factors in postmenopausal women. Ann. Intern. Med. **115:** 860–864.
34. POWLES, T.J., T. HICKISH, J.A. KANIS et al. 1996. Effect of tamoxifen on bone mineral density measured by dual-energy X-ray absorptiometry in healthy premenopausal and postmenopausal women. J. Clin. Oncol. **14:** 78–84.
35. FISHER, B., J.P. COSTANTINO, D.L. WICKERHAM et al. 1998. Tamoxifen for prevention of breast cancer: report of the National Surgical Adjuvant Breast and Bowel Project P-1 Study. J. Natl. Cancer Inst. **90:** 1371–1388.

36. JORDAN, V.C. 2001. Estrogen, selective estrogen receptor modulation, and coronary heart disease: something or nothing. J. Natl. Cancer Inst. **93:** 2–4.
37. REIS, S.E., J.P. COSTANTINO, D.L. WICKERHAM *et al.* 2001. Cardiovascular effects of tamoxifen in women with and without heart disease: Breast Cancer Prevention Trial. J. Natl. Cancer Inst. **93:** 16–21.
38. BLACK, L.J., C.D. JONES & J.F. FALCONE. 1983. Antagonism of estrogen action with a new benzothiophene derived antiestrogen. Life Sci. **32:** 1031–1036.
39. JORDAN, V.C. & B. GOSDEN. 1983. Inhibition of the uterotropic activity of estrogens and antiestrogens by the short acting antiestrogen LY117018. Endocrinology **113:** 463–468.
40. CLEMENS, J.A., D.R. BENNETT, L.J. BLACK *et al.* 1983. Effects of a new antiestrogen, keoxifene (LY156758), on growth of carcinogen-induced mammary tumors and on LH and prolactin levels. Life Sci. **32:** 2869–2875.
41. GOTTARDIS, M.M. & V.C. JORDAN. 1987. Antitumor actions of keoxifene and tamoxifen in the *N*-nitrosomethylurea-induced rat mammary carcinoma model. Cancer Res. **47:** 4020–4024.
42. BUZDAR, A.U., C. MARCUS, F. HOLMES *et al.* 1988. Phase II evaluation of LY156758 in metastatic breast cancer. Oncology **45:** 344–345.
43. SNYDER, K.R., N. SPARANO & J.M. MALINOWSKI. 2000. Raloxifene hydrochloride. Am. J. Health Syst. Pharmacol. **57:** 1669–1678 [quiz: 76–78].
44. DELMAS, P.D., N.H. BJARNASON, B.H. MITLAK *et al.* 1997. Effects of raloxifene on bone mineral density, serum cholesterol concentrations, and uterine endometrium in postmenopausal women [see comments]. N. Engl. J. Med. **337:** 1641–1647.
45. ETTINGER, B., D.M. BLACK, B.H. MITLAK *et al.* 1999. Reduction of vertebral fracture risk in postmenopausal women with osteoporosis treated with raloxifene: results from a 3-year randomized clinical trial—Multiple Outcomes of Raloxifene Evaluation (MORE) Investigators [see comments]. JAMA **282:** 637–645.
46. WALSH, B.W., L.H. KULLER, R.A. WILD *et al.* 1998. Effects of raloxifene on serum lipids and coagulation factors in healthy postmenopausal women. JAMA **279:** 1445–1451.
47. CUMMINGS, S.R., S. ECKERT, K.A. KRUEGER *et al.* 1999. The effect of raloxifene on risk of breast cancer in postmenopausal women: results from the MORE randomized trial—Multiple Outcomes of Raloxifene Evaluation. JAMA **281:** 2189–2197.
48. COHEN, F.J., S. WATTS, A. SHAH *et al.* 2000. Uterine effects of 3-year raloxifene therapy in postmenopausal women younger than age 60. Obstet. Gynecol. **95:** 104–110.
49. LIEBERMAN, M.E., J. GORSKI & V.C. JORDAN. 1983. An estrogen receptor model to describe the regulation of prolactin synthesis by antiestrogens *in vitro*. J. Biol. Chem. **258:** 4741–4745.
50. TATE, A.C., G.L. GREENE *et al.* 1984. Differences between estrogen- and antiestrogen-estrogen receptor complexes from human breast tumors identified with an antibody raised against the estrogen receptor. Cancer Res. **44:** 1012–1018.
51. JORDAN, V.C., M.E. LIEBERMAN, E. CORMIER *et al.* 1984. Structural requirements for the pharmacological activity of nonsteroidal antiestrogens *in vitro*. Mol. Pharmacol. **26:** 272–278.
52. GREENE, G.L., P. GILNA, M. WATERFIELD *et al.* 1986. Sequence and expression of human estrogen receptor complementary DNA. Science **231:** 1150–1154.
53. WOLF, D.M. & V.C. JORDAN. 1994. The estrogen receptor from a tamoxifen stimulated MCF-7 tumor variant contains a point mutation in the ligand binding domain. Breast Cancer Res. Treat. **31:** 129–138.
54. CATHERINO, W.H., D.M. WOLF & V.C. JORDAN. 1995. A naturally occurring estrogen receptor mutation results in increased estrogenicity of a tamoxifen analog. Mol. Endocrinol. **9:** 1053–1063.
55. LEVENSON, A.S., W.H. CATHERINO & V.C. JORDAN. 1997. Estrogenic activity is increased for an antiestrogen by a natural mutation of the estrogen receptor. J. Steroid Biochem. Mol. Biol. **60:** 261–268.
56. BRZOZOWSKI, A.M., A.C. PIKE, Z. DAUTER *et al.* 1997. Molecular basis of agonism and antagonism in the oestrogen receptor. Nature **389:** 753–758.
57. SHIAU, A.K., D. BARSTAD, P.M. LORIA *et al.* 1998. The structural basis of estrogen receptor/coactivator recognition and the antagonism of this interaction by tamoxifen. Cell **95:** 927–937.

58. MACGREGOR SCHAFER, J., H. LIU, D.J. BENTREM et al. 2000. Allosteric silencing of activating function 1 in the 4-hydroxytamoxifen estrogen receptor complex is induced by substituting glycine for aspartate at amino acid 351. Cancer Res. **60:** 5097–5105.
59. LIU, H., E.S. LEE, A. DE LOS REYES et al. 2001. Silencing and reactivation of the estrogen receptor modulator (SERM)–ER alpha complex. Cancer Res. **61:** 3632–3639.
60. LIU, H., D.J. BENTREM, R. DARDES et al. 2001. The role of amino acid 351 on the ligand binding domain of estrogen receptor alpha in agonist activity of SERMs Abstract 1447, p. 269. Proc. Am. Assoc. Cancer Res. (Ninety-second Meeting, New Orleans).
61. MACGREGOR SCHAFER, J.I., E.S. LEE, R.M. O'REGAN et al. 2000. Rapid development of tamoxifen stimulated mutant p53 breast tumors (T47D) in athymic mice. Clin. Cancer Res. **6:** 4374–4381.
62. LEE, E.S., J. MACGREGOR SCHAFER, K. YAO et al. 2000. Cross resistance of triphenylethylene-type antiestrogen, but not ICI 182,780 in tamoxifen-stimulated breast tumors grown in athymic mice. Clin. Cancer Res. **6:** 4893–4899.
63. MACGREGOR SCHAFER, J., E.S. LEE, R.C. DARDES et al. 2001. Analysis of cross-resistance of the selective estrogen receptor modulators arzoxifene (LY353381) and LY117018 in tamoxifen-stimulated breast cancer xenografts. Clin. Cancer Res. **7:** 2505–2512.
64. LEVENSON, A.S. & V.C. JORDAN. 1999. Selective oestrogen receptor modulation: molecular pharmacology for the millennium. Eur. J. Cancer **35:** 1628–1639.

Use of SERMs for the Adjuvant Therapy of Early-Stage Breast Cancer

ANTONIO C. WOLFF AND NANCY E. DAVIDSON

The Johns Hopkins Oncology Center, The Johns Hopkins University School of Medicine, Baltimore, Maryland 21231, USA

ABSTRACT: Tamoxifen was the first in a class of drugs now commonly referred to as selective estrogen receptor modulators or SERMs. SERMs exhibit tissue-specific estrogenic agonist/antagonist activity through their ability to bind to the estrogen receptor α (ER) protein and interact with coregulatory proteins, thereby modulating transcription of estrogen target genes. Since its first approval by the United States Food and Drug Administration (FDA) in 1977, tamoxifen has been found to (a) lower the risk of recurrence and death for women with early-stage hormone receptor–positive breast cancer, irrespective of menopausal or node status or use of adjuvant chemotherapy; (b) reduce the risk of invasive breast cancer following breast conservation in women with ductal carcinoma *in situ* (DCIS); and (c) reduce the risk of breast cancer in high-risk women. Toremifene is the only other SERM approved by the FDA for breast cancer treatment. However, it offers no clear clinical advantage over tamoxifen in the adjuvant or metastatic settings. Several other SERMs are in various phases of clinical development. In addition, strategies to combine SERMs with other endocrine therapy like ovarian suppression or aromatase inhibitors are active areas of investigations. At present, SERMs are recognized as the first targeted and relatively nontoxic medical therapy for women with high-risk or steroid hormone receptor–positive breast cancer.

KEYWORDS: selective estrogen receptor modulator (SERM); early-stage breast cancer; adjuvant therapy; metastatic therapy; tamoxifen; raloxifene

INTRODUCTION

It has been long known that breast cancer may be estrogen-dependent and that surgical hormonal manipulation (such as oophorectomy, adrenalectomy, and hypophysectomy) can induce tumor regression.[1] Most of the effects of estrogen are exerted through binding to nuclear estrogen receptor proteins that regulate transcriptional activation of estrogen-responsive genes. Selective estrogen receptor modulators (SERMs) such as tamoxifen exert their modulatory effects through similar mechanisms, but may function as estrogen receptor agonists, antagonists, or mixed agonist-antagonists depending on the target tissue. SERMs are broadly classified in three categories. These include triphenylethylene derivatives (e.g., tamoxifen), nonsteroidal antiestrogens (e.g., the benzothiophene raloxifene), and steroidal anti-

---

Address for correspondence: Antonio C. Wolff, M.D., Division of Medical Oncology, The Johns Hopkins Oncology Center, Cancer Research Building, 1650 Orleans Street, Room 189, Baltimore, MD 21231-1000. Voice: 410-614-4192; fax: 410-955-0125.
  awolff@jhmi.edu

estrogens (e.g., ICI 182,780 or fulvestrant). Presently, our most extensive clinical experience with SERMs in breast cancer is with tamoxifen. In the United States, it is approved for the management of advanced disease, adjuvant treatment of both node-negative and node-positive hormone receptor–positive disease, reduction in the risk of invasive breast cancer following breast conservation in women with ductal carcinoma *in situ* (DCIS), and risk reduction in high-risk women. However, as tamoxifen has undesirable effects in the uterus, vagina, and central nervous system, several other SERMs with different profiles are also under investigation.

TAMOXIFEN IN METASTATIC DISEASE

Endocrine therapy is considered the initial treatment of choice for most women with hormone receptor–positive metastatic breast cancer who are not facing a "visceral crisis". Many of these women, particularly those with few symptoms and indolent disease, are candidates for sequential hormonal manipulation, often with tamoxifen as the first-line option. Postmenopausal status and positive progesterone receptors (PR) are strong positive predictors of response.[2] Tamoxifen offers similar results to ovarian ablation in premenopausal women[3,4] and seems to be superior to progestational agents. Tamoxifen has shown activity in women previously treated with adjuvant tamoxifen.[5] These data support a commonly employed algorithm of ovarian suppression/ablation or tamoxifen, sequentially or in combination in premenopausal women. However, in postmenopausal women, recent data suggest at least equivalent (and possibly superior) activity of aromatase inhibitors (AI) when compared with tamoxifen as first-line endocrine therapy in patients with metastatic[6,7] or locally advanced disease.[8] Thus, an AI followed by tamoxifen or the reverse sequence is now considered appropriate hormone therapy for postmenopausal women with advanced hormone receptor–positive breast cancer. Presently, it is unknown whether the order of hormonal intervention affects survival. In summary, though, tamoxifen remains one of the mainstays in the serial hormone treatment of advanced disease in women with hormone receptor–positive disease.

TAMOXIFEN IN THE ADJUVANT SETTING

The very substantial activity of tamoxifen in advanced breast cancer led to its testing in early-stage breast cancer. Perhaps the largest contribution to our understanding of the use of adjuvant tamoxifen comes from the Early Breast Cancer Trialists' Collaborative Group (EBCTCG) metanalysis.[9] The 1995 update included 37,000 women in 55 trials that began before 1990 comparing adjuvant tamoxifen versus no adjuvant tamoxifen. This represented approximately 87% of the worldwide evidence at the time. Nearly 8000 of these women had low or no ER protein detected in their primary tumor, and there is little or no benefit from adjuvant tamoxifen in this group. In the remaining 30,000 women (18,000 with ER-positive and 12,000 with untested tumors), the proportional reductions in recurrence and mortality produced with approximately 10 years of follow-up were, respectively, 21% and 12% (1 year of tamoxifen use), 29% and 17% (2 years), and 47% and 26% (5 years). One important observation is that the benefits from 5 years of tamoxifen persist at

10 years. The absolute improvement in recurrence was greater during the first 5 years, whereas the improvement in survival grew steadily larger throughout the first 10 years. The proportional mortality reductions were similar for women with node-positive and node-negative disease. This translated into absolute improvements in 10-year survival for tamoxifen versus control of 10.9% for node-positive (61.4% versus 50.5%, $2P < 0.00001$) and 5.6% for node-negative (78.9% versus 73.3%, $2P < 0.00001$) patients, irrespective of age, menopausal status, tamoxifen dose, or use of adjuvant chemotherapy.[9] There was a higher incidence of endometrial cancer, but the absolute decrease in contralateral breast cancer was about twice the absolute increase in endometrial cancer. There was no apparent effect on the incidence of colorectal cancer. Interestingly, no impact on other causes of death such as coronary disease was observed, despite data from individual trials suggesting a cardiovascular benefit from adjuvant tamoxifen.[10,11] The 2000 update of the EBCTCG database, now showing benefits extending to 15 years, was presented at the November 2000 National Institutes of Health (NIH) Consensus Development Conference on Adjuvant Therapy for Breast Cancer (http://consensus.nih.gov).

The largest database from a single trial on the use of adjuvant tamoxifen comes from the National Surgical Adjuvant Breast and Bowel Project (NSABP) B-14, a randomized trial of tamoxifen versus placebo in 2818 women with node-negative, ER-positive breast cancer.[12,13] Through 10 years of follow-up, significant benefits were seen in disease-free survival (69% versus 57%, $P < 0.0001$), distant disease-free survival (76% versus 67%, $P < 0.0001$), and overall survival (80% versus 76%, $P = 0.02$), favoring tamoxifen over placebo. This survival benefit was present in all age groups. There was a small increase in the risk of endometrial cancer (annual hazard rate of 0.2/1000 in the placebo group versus 1.6/1000 in the tamoxifen group), although these tumors were mostly of early stage and good-moderate histologic grade.[14] Another important observation was a 37% reduction in the incidence of contralateral breast cancer ($P = 0.007$) and these data helped to set the stage for several trials assessing tamoxifen as a chemopreventive agent.[15–17]

An issue that remains controversial is the question of duration of adjuvant tamoxifen. NSABP B-14 was the largest trial to address this issue explicitly.[13] Initially, 2818 patients were randomized to 5 years of tamoxifen or placebo. Patients who remained disease-free after 5 years of tamoxifen were then randomized to receive another 5 years of tamoxifen ($n = 322$) or placebo ($n = 321$). After the study began, another group of 1211 patients who met the same protocol eligibility requirements as the randomly assigned patients were registered to receive tamoxifen. Registered patients who were disease-free after 5 years of tamoxifen were also randomly assigned to another 5 years of tamoxifen ($n = 261$) or placebo ($n = 249$).[13] At a median follow-up of 5.6 years after randomization, better disease-free survival (92% versus 86%, $P = 0.003$) and distant disease-free survival (96% versus 90%, $P = 0.01$) were seen favoring the group that discontinued tamoxifen at 5 years, but survival was similar (96% versus 94%, $P = 0.08$). In the Scottish trial of adjuvant tamoxifen in node-negative breast cancer, 236 among the 747 original patients had a second randomization to continue tamoxifen indefinitely or stop tamoxifen after 5 years.[18] There was no additional benefit seen with longer duration of adjuvant tamoxifen,[19] similar to findings from NSABP B-14.[13] Both studies show a trend towards more complications (e.g., endometrial cancer and thromboembolic disease) with longer duration of adjuvant tamoxifen, but further follow-up is needed. A smaller trial in node-positive patients by the Eastern Cooperative Oncology Group (ECOG) looked at 5 years versus indefinite use and detected a nonstatistically significant trend in favor of the longer duration of tamoxifen.[20] Ongoing large studies such as the ATLAS (Adjuvant Tamoxifen Longer Against Shorter) and aTTom (Adjuvant Tamoxifen Treatment, Offer More?) trials plan to randomize 20,000 patients and should help settle the duration issue.

Another unsettled issue is how to define steroid receptor positivity, particularly the choice of ER/PR assay. Most of the data discussed above come from studies that assessed ER status using ligand-binding assays (LBA). This biochemical assay requires fresh tissue and does not permit histologic correlation. Since then, immunohistochemistry (IHC) has become the preferred assay as it is an easier and cheaper technique that allows testing of archival paraffin material and correlation with tissue histology. Unfortunately, IHC assays have been neither properly standardized across different pathology laboratories nor correlated with clinical outcome data. A recent study from Harvey *et al.* compared both techniques in 1982 specimens from the San Antonio Tumor Bank and showed that determination of ER-positive status by IHC (defined as having as few as 1–10% weakly positive cells) was better than LBA in predicting improved disease-free survival and equivalent at predicting overall survival in primary breast cancer.[21] Nonetheless, a rigorous standardization of both technique and interpretation is lacking.

TAMOXIFEN FOLLOWING BREAST CONSERVATION IN DCIS

Most patients with DCIS can be treated with breast conservation techniques and some investigators have argued that many patients will do well with wide excision alone.[22] However, randomized clinical trials conducted by the NSABP[23] and the European Organization for the Research and Treatment of Cancer (EORTC)[24] have shown an additional local control benefit of radiation therapy after local excision for DCIS as compared with local excision alone. Furthermore, NSABP B-24 has now shown that the addition of 5 years of tamoxifen to lumpectomy and radiation therapy further improves local control and also decreases the incidence of contralateral breast cancer.[25] In this study with 1804 women, there was a decrease in the cumulative incidence of breast cancer events at 5 years, such as all-invasive events (7.2% versus 4.1%, $P = 0.004$), ipsilateral invasive events (4.2% versus 2.1%, $P = 0.03$), and contralateral invasive events (2.3% versus 1.8%, $P = 0.22$). Where both noninvasive and invasive breast cancers were evaluated together, a reduction was observed in contralateral ($P = 0.01$) as well as ipsilateral ($P = 0.04$) and total ($P = 0.0009$) events.

OTHER SERMs

Toremifene, another triphenylethylene derivative that differs from tamoxifen by one chlorine atom at the 4-position, is approved by the FDA in metastatic breast cancer. Its theoretical advantage is that it does not induce DNA adduct formation or liver cancer, a documented toxicity of tamoxifen in rats. However, no excess risk of liver cancer has been seen in women receiving tamoxifen and thus tamoxifen hepatocarcinogenicity is not a concern in humans.[26] Due to its estrogenic activity in the uterus,[27] diminished estrogenic effects on bones,[28] and complete cross-resistance with tamoxifen,[29] toremifene offers no clinical advantage over tamoxifen. An overview of randomized trials comparing toremifene with tamoxifen in metastatic breast cancer showed both drugs to be equally effective and well tolerated.[30] An adjuvant randomized trial of toremifene versus tamoxifen is in progress.[31] An initial safety analysis in 889 patients indicates similar toxicity and efficacy. Another member of this class, idoxifene, showed activity in patients with tamoxifen-resistant tumors,[32] but was associated with development of uterine polyps and prolapse. Droloxifene (3-hydroxytamoxifen) has a similar preclinical profile to both toremifene and tamoxifen, but is no longer under development due to its poor performance against tamoxifen.[33]

The nonsteroidal SERM, raloxifene, has been developed as a drug for osteoporosis. A pivotal study showed that it decreases the risk of vertebral fractures in postmenopausal women.[34] This osteoporosis study in a population with a presumably lower baseline breast cancer risk also showed a reduced incidence of breast cancer diagnosis in raloxifene-treated women compared with placebo.[35] However, raloxifene use was not associated with changes in endometrial thickness or increased risk of endometrial cancer. A study of raloxifene for treatment of women with advanced breast cancer who had received tamoxifen showed little activity.[36] Taken together, these limited data do not support raloxifene's use for treatment of breast cancer or for primary risk reduction.[37] However, the findings in aggregate do support the Study of Tamoxifen and Raloxifene (STAR) trial, a randomized comparison of raloxifene and tamoxifen for postmenopausal women at high risk for breast cancer development. Two other raloxifene analogues, LY353381 (SERM-3) and LY357489, appear to be more potent anti–breast cancer drugs *in vitro* and lack intrinsic estrogenic activity.[38] SERM-3 is undergoing clinical evaluation.

The steroidal pure antiestrogen ICI 182,780 (fulvestrant) holds the greatest promise as a new anti–breast cancer drug among existing SERMs. It binds to both the AF-1 and AF-2 transactivating domains of the ER and induces degradation of the ER.[39] It has a 100-fold greater affinity for the ER than tamoxifen and has documented clinical activity in patients with tamoxifen-resistant disease.[40] Although it is considered a pure antiestrogen, little is known about its bone effects in humans and the data in rats are conflicting. It does not appear to cross the blood-brain barrier and, consequently, it may not induce hot flashes.[39] Randomized clinical trials show activity at least comparable to that seen with the aromatase inhibitor, anastrozole, in metastatic disease, and its administration schedule (a monthly 5-mL intramuscular injection) was not a deterrent to patients.[41,42] Data comparing fulvestrant and tamoxifen as first-line therapy in metastatic disease should be available in the near future.

TAMOXIFEN COMBINED WITH NONCYTOTOXIC DRUGS

A number of studies have focused on combination endocrine therapy in order to effect a "total estrogen blockade". Significant interest exists in combining tamoxifen with an aromatase inhibitor in postmenopausal women. Results from the adjuvant ATAC trial (Anastrazole and Tamoxifen Alone or in Combination) in about 9000 women with early breast cancer are expected in the very near future. A recent metanalysis of a combined luteinizing hormone–releasing hormone (LHRH) agonist with or without tamoxifen in premenopausal women with advanced breast cancer showed both a survival and progression-free survival advantage favoring the combination.[43] However, combination therapy is not uniformly beneficial. A recent trial examining the combination of tamoxifen and octreotide in the adjuvant setting (NSABP B-29) was closed early because of unacceptable octreotide-related biliary toxicity. The combination of tamoxifen and fenretinide [*N*-(4-hydroxyphenyl) retinamide] appears to have synergistic antitumor and chemopreventive activity against mammary cancer in preclinical studies, and its safety and tolerability were demonstrated in a pilot trial.[44] However, a North American Intergroup adjuvant trial of fenretinide versus placebo in elderly women receiving tamoxifen was stopped prematurely due to an excessive number of patient withdrawals in the fenretinide and tamoxifen group.[45]

CONCLUSIONS

Tamoxifen is the most well studied of the SERMs. Data from the EBCTCG overview confirm its significant benefit in reducing the odds of death and recurrence in women with ER-positive early-stage breast cancer. This benefit extends beyond the initial 5 years of tamoxifen administration and its adjuvant benefit is seen in all age groups, regardless of menopausal status or chemotherapy administration.

Based on these data (and other findings not reviewed here), a non-Federal panel of experts convened for an NIH Consensus Development Conference in November 2000 considered the adjuvant use of SERMs as part of an evidence-based review of therapy for early breast cancer. The panel recommended 5 years of adjuvant tamoxifen therapy for all women with hormone receptor–positive tumors, regardless of age, menopausal status, axillary lymph node status, tumor size, or use of adjuvant chemotherapy. Possible exceptions would include women with node-negative tumors less than 10 mm in size who wished to avoid the side effects of tamoxifen. Ovarian ablation or suppression could be an alternative for premenopausal women. The decision to recommend adjuvant hormonal therapy should be based on the presence of ERs and/or PRs as assessed by immunohistochemical staining. In the absence of sufficient tumor to determine hormone receptor status, it should be considered positive, especially in postmenopausal women. Tamoxifen administration was not recommended for women with ER- and PR-negative invasive breast cancers. The expression pattern of the *HER-2* gene should not influence the decision to recommend hormonal therapy. The panel emphasized that, for most women, the benefit from adjuvant tamoxifen far outweighs any risk, such as endometrial cancer and venous thromboembolism, and that neither transvaginal ultrasonography nor endometrial biopsies are indicated as screening tests for endometrial cancer in asymptomatic women taking tamoxifen. Finally, the panel acknowledged the lack of data at present to support the use of any other agents such as raloxifene, toremifene, or aromatase inhibitors alone or in combination in the adjuvant setting. However, much remains to be understood about the optimal use of SERMs in the treatment and prevention of breast cancer alone or in combination with other agents.

REFERENCES

1. OSBORNE, C.K. 1998. Tamoxifen in the treatment of breast cancer. N. Engl. J. Med. **339:** 1609–1618.
2. RAVDIN, P.M., S. GREEN, T.M. DORR et al. 1992. Prognostic significance of progesterone receptor levels in estrogen receptor–positive patients with metastatic breast cancer treated with tamoxifen: results of a prospective Southwest Oncology Group study. J. Clin. Oncol. **10:** 1284–1291.
3. BUCHANAN, R.B., R.W. BLAMEY, K.R. DURRANT et al. 1986. A randomized comparison of tamoxifen with surgical oophorectomy in premenopausal patients with advanced breast cancer. J. Clin. Oncol. **4:** 1326–1330.
4. INGLE, J.N., J.E. KROOK, S.J. GREEN et al. 1986. Randomized trial of bilateral oophorectomy versus tamoxifen in premenopausal women with metastatic breast cancer. J. Clin. Oncol. **4:** 178–185.
5. MUSS, H.B., L.R. SMITH & M.R. COOPER. 1987. Tamoxifen rechallenge: response to tamoxifen following relapse after adjuvant chemohormonal therapy for breast cancer. J. Clin. Oncol. **5:** 1556–1558.
6. BONNETERRE, J., B. THURLIMANN, J.F. ROBERTSON et al. 2000. Anastrozole versus tamoxifen as first-line therapy for advanced breast cancer in 668 postmenopausal women: results of the tamoxifen or arimidex randomized group efficacy and tolerability study. J. Clin. Oncol. **18:** 3748–3757.
7. NABHOLTZ, J.M., A. BUZDAR, M. POLLAK et al. 2000. Anastrozole is superior to tamoxifen as first-line therapy for advanced breast cancer in postmenopausal women: results of a North American multicenter randomized trial. J. Clin. Oncol. **18:** 3758–3767.
8. ELLIS, M.J., F. JAENICKE, A. LLOMBART-CUSSAC et al. 2000. A randomized double-blind multicenter study of preoperative tamoxifen versus Femara (letrozole) for postmenopausal women with ER and/or PgR positive breast cancer ineligible for breast-conserving surgery: correlation of clinical response with tumor expression and proliferation [abstract 14]. Breast Cancer Res. Treat. **64:** 29.
9. EARLY BREAST CANCER TRIALISTS' COLLABORATIVE GROUP. 1998. Tamoxifen for early breast cancer: an overview of the randomized trials. Lancet **351:** 1451–1467.
10. COSTANTINO, J.P., L.H. KULLER, D.G. IVES et al. 1997. Coronary heart disease mortality and adjuvant tamoxifen therapy. J. Natl. Cancer Inst. **89:** 776–782.
11. MCDONALD, C.C., F.E. ALEXANDER, B.W. WHYTE et al. 1995. Cardiac and vascular morbidity in women receiving adjuvant tamoxifen for breast cancer in a randomised trial: the Scottish Cancer Trials Breast Group. Br. Med. J. **311:** 977–980.
12. FISHER, B., J. COSTANTINO, C. REDMOND et al. 1989. A randomized clinical trial evaluating tamoxifen in the treatment of patients with node-negative breast cancer who have estrogen-receptor-positive tumors. N. Engl. J. Med. **320:** 479–484.
13. FISHER, B., J. DIGNAM, J. BRYANT et al. 1996. Five versus more than five years of tamoxifen therapy for breast cancer patients with negative lymph nodes and estrogen receptor–positive tumors. J. Natl. Cancer Inst. **88:** 1529–1542.
14. FISHER, B., J.P. COSTANTINO, C.K. REDMOND et al. 1994. Endometrial cancer in tamoxifen-treated breast cancer patients: findings from the National Surgical Adjuvant Breast and Bowel Project (NSABP) B-14. J. Natl. Cancer Inst. **86:** 527–537.
15. FISHER, B., J.P. COSTANTINO, D.L. WICKERHAM et al. 1998. Tamoxifen for prevention of breast cancer: report of the National Surgical Adjuvant Breast and Bowel Project P-1 Study. J. Natl. Cancer Inst. **90:** 1371–1388.
16. POWLES, T., R. EELES, S. ASHLEY et al. 1998. Interim analysis of the incidence of breast cancer in the Royal Marsden Hospital tamoxifen randomised chemoprevention trial. Lancet **352:** 98–101.
17. VERONESI, U., P. MAISONNEUVE, A. COSTA et al. 1998. Prevention of breast cancer with tamoxifen: preliminary findings from the Italian randomised trial among hysterectomised women—Italian Tamoxifen Prevention Study. Lancet **352:** 93–97.
18. STEWART, H.J. 1992. The Scottish trial of adjuvant tamoxifen in node-negative breast cancer: the Scottish Cancer Trials Breast Group. J. Natl. Cancer Inst. Monogr. **311:** 117–120.

19. STEWART, H.J., A.P. FORREST, D. EVERINGTON *et al.* 1996. Randomised comparison of 5 years of adjuvant tamoxifen with continuous therapy for operable breast cancer: the Scottish Cancer Trials Breast Group. Br. J. Cancer **74:** 297–299.
20. TORMEY, D.C., R. GRAY & H.C. FALKSON. 1996. Postchemotherapy adjuvant tamoxifen therapy beyond five years in patients with lymph node–positive breast cancer: Eastern Cooperative Oncology Group [see comments]. J. Natl. Cancer Inst. **88:** 1828–1833.
21. HARVEY, J.M., G.M. CLARK, C.K. OSBORNE *et al.* 1999. Estrogen receptor status by immunohistochemistry is superior to the ligand-binding assay for predicting response to adjuvant endocrine therapy in breast cancer. J. Clin. Oncol. **17:** 1474–1481.
22. SILVERSTEIN, M.J., M.D. LAGIOS, S. GROSHEN *et al.* 1999. The influence of margin width on local control of ductal carcinoma *in situ* of the breast [see comments]. N. Engl. J. Med. **340:** 1455–1461.
23. FISHER, B., J. DIGNAM, N. WOLMARK *et al.* 1998. Lumpectomy and radiation therapy for the treatment of intraductal breast cancer: findings from National Surgical Adjuvant Breast and Bowel Project B-17. J. Clin. Oncol. **16:** 441–452.
24. JULIEN, J.P., N. BIJKER, I.S. FENTIMAN *et al.* 2000. Radiotherapy in breast-conserving treatment for ductal carcinoma *in situ*—first results of the EORTC randomised phase III trial 10853: EORTC Breast Cancer Cooperative Group and EORTC Radiotherapy Group [see comments]. Lancet **355:** 528–533.
25. FISHER, B., J. DIGNAM, N. WOLMARK *et al.* 1999. Tamoxifen in treatment of intraductal breast cancer: National Surgical Adjuvant Breast and Bowel Project B-24 randomised controlled trial [see comments]. Lancet **353:** 1993–2000.
26. HARD, G.C., M.J. IATROPOULOS, K. JORDAN *et al.* 1993. Major difference in the hepatocarcinogenicity and DNA adduct forming ability between toremifene and tamoxifen in female Crl:CD(BR) rats. Cancer Res. **53:** 4534–4541.
27. O'REGAN, R.M., A. CISNEROS, G.M. ENGLAND *et al.* 1998. Effects of the antiestrogens tamoxifen, toremifene, and ICI 182,780 on endometrial cancer growth. J. Natl. Cancer Inst. **90:** 1552–1558.
28. MARTTUNEN, M.B., P. HIETANEN, A. TIITINEN *et al.* 1998. Comparison of effects of tamoxifen and toremifene on bone biochemistry and bone mineral density in postmenopausal breast cancer patients. J. Clin. Endocrinol. Metab. **83:** 1158–1162.
29. VOGEL, C.L., I. SHEMANO, J. SCHOENFELDER *et al.* 1993. Multicenter phase II efficacy trial of toremifene in tamoxifen-refractory patients with advanced breast cancer. J. Clin. Oncol. **11:** 345–350.
30. PYRHONEN, S., J. ELLMEN, J. VUORINEN *et al.* 1999. Meta-analysis of trials comparing toremifene with tamoxifen and factors predicting outcome of antiestrogen therapy in postmenopausal women with breast cancer. Breast Cancer Res. Treat. **56:** 133–143.
31. HOLLI, K., R. VALAVAARA, G. BLANCO *et al.* 2000. Safety and efficacy results of a randomized trial comparing adjuvant toremifene and tamoxifen in postmenopausal patients with node-positive breast cancer. J. Clin. Oncol. **18:** 3487–3494.
32. COOMBES, R.C., B.P. HAYNES, M. DOWSETT *et al.* 1995. Idoxifene: report of a phase I study in patients with metastatic breast cancer. Cancer Res. **55:** 1070–1074.
33. RAUSCHNING, W. & K.I. PRITCHARD. 1994. Droloxifene, a new antiestrogen: its role in metastatic breast cancer. Breast Cancer Res. Treat. **31:** 83–94.
34. ETTINGER, B., D.M. BLACK, B.H. MITLAK *et al.* 1999. Reduction of vertebral fracture risk in postmenopausal women with osteoporosis treated with raloxifene: results from a 3-year randomized clinical trial—Multiple Outcomes of Raloxifene Evaluation (MORE) Investigators [see comments]. JAMA **282:** 637–645. [1999. Erratum. JAMA **282**(22): 2124.]
35. CUMMINGS, S.R., S. ECKERT, K.A. KRUEGER *et al.* 1999. The effect of raloxifene on risk of breast cancer in postmenopausal women: results from the MORE randomized trial—Multiple Outcomes of Raloxifene Evaluation [see comments]. JAMA **281:** 2189–2197. [1999. Erratum. JAMA **282**(22): 2124.]
36. GRADISHAR, W., J. GLUSMAN, Y. LUM *et al.* 2000. Effects of high dose raloxifene in selected patients with advanced breast carcinoma. Cancer **88:** 2047–2053.
37. CHLEBOWSKI, R.T., D.E. COLLYAR, M.R. SOMERFIELD *et al.* 1999. American Society of Clinical Oncology technology assessment on breast cancer risk reduction strategies: tamoxifen and raloxifene—ASCO special article. J. Clin. Oncol. **17:** 1939–1955.

38. DHINGRA, K. 1999. Antiestrogens—tamoxifen, SERMs, and beyond. Invest. New Drugs **17:** 285–311.
39. OSBORNE, C.K., H. ZHAO & S.A. FUQUA. 2000. Selective estrogen receptor modulators: structure, function, and clinical use. J. Clin. Oncol. **18:** 3172–3186.
40. HOWELL, A., D. DEFRIEND, J. ROBERTSON et al. 1995. Response to a specific anti-oestrogen (ICI 182780) in tamoxifen-resistant breast cancer [see comments]. Lancet **345:** 29–30.
41. HOWELL, A., J.F. ROBERTSON, A.J. QUARESMA et al. 2000. Comparison of efficacy and tolerability of fulvestrant (Faslodex) with anastrozole (Arimidex) in postmenopausal (PM) women with advanced breast cancer (ABC)—preliminary results [abstract 6]. Breast Cancer Res. Treat. **64:** 27.
42. OSBORNE, C.K. 2000. On behalf of the North American Faslodex Investigator Group: a double-blind randomized trial of Faslodex (fulvestrant) with Arimidex (anastrozole) in post-menopausal (PM) women with advanced breast cancer (ABC) [abstract 7]. Breast Cancer Res. Treat. **64:** a7.
43. KLIJN, J.G.M., R.W. BLAMEY, F. BOCCARDO et al. 2001. Combined tamoxifen and luteinizing hormone–releasing hormone (LHRH) agonist versus LHRH agonist alone in premenopausal advanced breast: a meta-analysis of four randomized trials. J. Clin. Oncol. **19:** 343–353.
44. CONLEY, B., J. O'SHAUGHNESSY, S. PRINDIVILLE et al. 2000. Pilot trial of the safety, tolerability, and retinoid levels of N-(4-hydroxyphenyl) retinamide in combination with tamoxifen in patients at high risk for developing invasive breast cancer. J. Clin. Oncol. **18:** 275–283.
45. COBLEIGH, M.A., R. GRAY, M. GRAHAM et al. 2000. Fenretinide (FEN) vs. placebo in postmenopausal breast cancer patients receiving adjuvant tamoxifen (TAM), an Eastern Cooperative Oncology Group phase III intergroup trial (EB193, INT-0151) [abstract 328]. Proc. Am. Soc. Clin. Oncol. **19:** 86a.

Breast Cancer Prevention with Selective Estrogen Receptor Modulators

A Perspective

KATHLEEN I. PRITCHARD

Division of Clinical Trials and Epidemiology, Toronto-Sunnybrook Regional Cancer Centre, Toronto, Ontario M4N 3M5, Canada

ABSTRACT: Chemoprevention for breast cancer is both old and new. It has long been appreciated that early ovarian ablation dramatically reduces the incidence of breast cancer in premenopausal women. It was subsequently demonstrated, in the Early Breast Cancer Trialists' Collaborative Group (EBCTCG) overview, that tamoxifen results in a 40% or greater reduction in the incidence of contralateral breast cancer. Now, the National Surgical Adjuvant Breast and Bowel Project (NSABP) has shown a similar reduction in a randomized trial [Breast Cancer Prevention Trial (BCPT)] comparing tamoxifen and placebo in women aged 35 years or over at increased risk of developing breast cancer because of age, family history, or other factors. In this trial, the incidences of both ductal carcinoma *in situ* (DCIS) and invasive cancer were reduced. Reduction in incidence was similar over all years of the study and in all subgroups of high-risk women. However, all of the reduction was confined to estrogen receptor (ER)–positive tumors. Raloxifene, a newer selective estrogen receptor modulator (SERM) originally developed for osteoporosis, also appears to have a major preventive effect on breast cancer incidence. Limitations in the design and patient population of raloxifene trials, however, have made it difficult to as yet recommend raloxifene for risk reduction of breast cancer. The randomized Study of Tamoxifen and Raloxifene (STAR) study, which will compare raloxifene to tamoxifen in over 20,000 postmenopausal women at increased risk of breast cancer, as well as ongoing and proposed placebo-controlled studies of tamoxifen, the aromatase inhibitor anastrozole, and other antiestrogens in high- or average-risk postmenopausal women, will provide further results on optimal prevention strategies.

KEYWORDS: breast cancer; invasive breast cancer; ductal carcinoma *in situ*; prevention; risk reduction; selective estrogen receptor modulators (SERMs); tamoxifen; raloxifene

INTRODUCTION

It has long been appreciated that early menarche and late menopause increase the risk of breast cancer,[1] while early oophorectomy without hormone replacement

---

Address for correspondence: Kathleen I. Pritchard, M.D., F.R.C.P.C., Professor, University of Toronto, Head, Division of Clinical Trials and Epidemiology, Toronto-Sunnybrook Regional Cancer Centre, 2075 Bayview Avenue, Toronto, Ontario M4N 3M5, Canada. Voice: 416-480-4616; fax: 416-480-6002.

kathy.pritchard@tsrcc.on.ca

therapy can reduce the risk of developing breast cancer by as much as 60%.[2] More recently, tamoxifen has been shown in the Oxford Overview[3] and in other studies[4] to reduce the incidence of breast cancer by more than 40%. Even more recently, raloxifene, a new selective estrogen receptor modulator (SERM), has also been discovered, somewhat serendipitously, to be associated with a reduced incidence of breast cancer.[5] Now, one must examine these results in order to compare the risks and benefits of the various approaches for the chemoprevention of breast cancer. The purpose of this manuscript is to summarize the results of the published trials of SERMs as breast cancer "preventives" or "risk reducers" and to put in perspective the results of these studies.

In discussing the colloquially labeled Breast Cancer "Prevention" Trials, it seems important to first clarify what we mean by prevention:

- Prevent: Keep from; to keep from happening; to hinder. To prevent is to keep a person or thing from doing something or making progress by acting to set up an obstacle to stop him/her or it. Synonyms are hinder and impede.
- Hinder: Hold back so that making, starting, going ahead, or finishing is late, difficult, or impossible.
- Impede: Slow up movement and progress by putting something binding, falling, etc., on or in the way.[6]

The dictionary definition of prevention certainly has the connotation of "preventing permanently", but some definitions do not necessarily include the permanence. Because of uncertainty about the meaning of this word, the term "risk reduction" has come to be applied to the results achieved in Breast Cancer "Prevention" Trials. This terminology carries with it the concept that it is not clear whether the incidence of cancer in the tamoxifen-treated women will eventually "catch up" to that in the placebo-treated women. The substantial and lengthy proportional risk reductions achieved with tamoxifen, however, seem to consign the discussion of "prevention" versus "risk reduction" to somewhat that of a semantic quibble.

OVARIAN ABLATION/ESTROGEN WITHDRAWAL

Although this approach to breast cancer risk reduction fits perhaps only loosely under the title "chemoprevention", it actually represents the earliest and best-known hormonal approach to the prevention of breast cancer.

Many observational studies have shown that early menarche and late menopause increase the risk of breast cancer[1] and that early surgical menopause without hormone replacement is associated with as much as a 60% reduction in the risk of developing breast cancer.[2] In addition, the Oxford Overview of ovarian ablation as adjuvant therapy given to premenopausal women with breast cancer also shows a risk reduction of over 40% in the incidence of new primary contralateral breast cancers.[7] Ovarian ablation, which presumably carries out its effect either by reducing estrogen levels or by eliminating estrogenic and progestational cycling, is therefore a form of chemoprevention for breast cancer and may serve as a model for other approaches. Like the more "modern" chemopreventive approaches, however, ovarian ablation is associated with short- and long-term side effects including vasomotor symptoms and urogenital atrophy as well as exacerbation of osteoporosis and cardiovascular disease. Thus, like the newer chemopreventive approaches, risk and benefit must be weighed. The development of luteinizing hormone–releasing hormone (LHRH) agonists raises the possibility that chemical approaches to ovarian ablation might be tested for their role in risk reduction.

TAMOXIFEN

Tamoxifen is a selective estrogen receptor modulator (SERM) that competes with estrogen for binding to the estrogen receptor. In different tissues and in different animal species, tamoxifen, like other SERMs, may act as an agonist or antagonist of estrogen. In humans, tamoxifen acts as an estrogen antagonist in breast tissue, inhibiting the growth of estrogen-dependent breast tumors. In other tissues such as endometrium or bone, and in the serum lipoprotein fractions, tamoxifen acts as an estrogen agonist in that it induces endometrial proliferation, preserves bone mass in postmenopausal women, and lowers LDL cholesterol.[8–11]

Tamoxifen was first appreciated as a breast cancer preventive from the results of the Oxford Overview, which showed a reduction in contralateral breast cancer that has persisted up until the most recent follow-up.[3] With the support of these data, the National Surgical Adjuvant Breast and Bowel Project (NSABP) began their Breast Cancer Prevention Trial (BCPT, P-1) to evaluate the role of tamoxifen in reducing the risk of primary invasive breast cancer in women at increased risk of the disease. Between 1 June 1991 and 30 September 1997, 13,388 women were randomly assigned to receive tamoxifen at 20 mg daily or placebo. These women aged 35 years or greater were at increased risk of breast cancer because they (1) were 60 years of age or older, (2) were 35–59 years of age, with a 5-year predicted risk of breast cancer of at least 1.66%, or (3) had a history of lobular carcinoma *in situ* (LCIS). As of 31 July 1998, a total of 368 invasive and noninvasive breast cancers had occurred among these women. There were 175 cases of invasive breast cancer in the placebo group compared with 89 in the tamoxifen group [relative risk (RR) = 0.51; 95% confidence intervals (CI) = 0.39–0.66; $P \le 0.0001$]. The annual event rate for invasive breast cancer in women taking tamoxifen was 3.4/1000 women compared with 6.8/1000 women taking placebo. There was a similar reduction in the risk of noninvasive breast cancer [1.4/1000 vs. 2.7/1000 (RR = 0.50; 95% CI = 0.33–0.77; $P = 0.002$)] (TABLE 1).

There was a reduced risk of developing invasive breast cancer among all age groups in this study. Risk ratios were 0.56 for women less than 49 years of age, 0.49 for women 50 to 59 years of age, and 0.45 for women 60 years of age or older. Benefit was also seen in a variety of other subgroups of women including those with LCIS [RR = 0.44; 95% CI = 0.16–1.06] and women with a history of atypical hyperplasia [RR = 0.14; 95% CI = 0.03–0.47]. Reduced risk ratios were also seen at all projected levels of risk and among women with any number of first-degree relatives with a history of invasive breast cancer.

The reduction in risk of invasive breast cancer was seen within the first year of the trial. Lower breast cancer incidence rates were seen for each subsequent year of the trial throughout 6 years of maximum follow-up (FIG. 1). The distribution of primary tumor size and pathologic involvement of the axillary lymph nodes was not

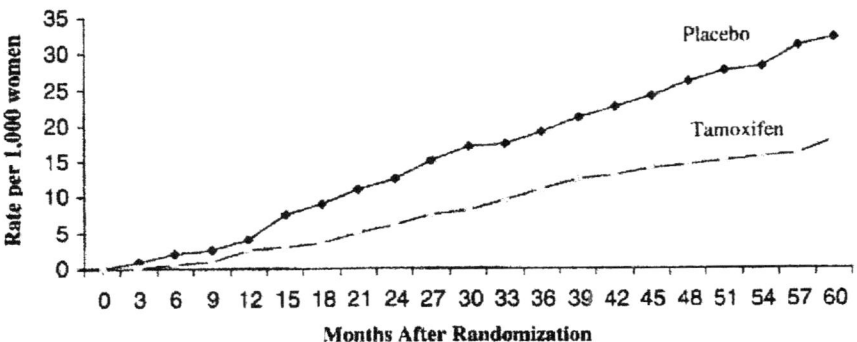

FIGURE 1. Incidence of invasive breast cancer in the NSABP Breast Cancer Prevention Trial among women taking placebo (*upper line*; $n = 6707$) versus tamoxifen (*lower line*; $n = 6681$). Data from Ref. 4.

markedly different between women taking tamoxifen and placebo. Virtually all of the reduction in breast cancer incidence associated with tamoxifen, however, was accounted for by a reduced incidence rate of ER-positive breast cancer. The rate of ER-positive breast cancers was 5/1000 women in the placebo group compared with 1.6/1000 women in the tamoxifen group, a 69% reduction. Rates of ER-negative tumors were not significantly different between the two treatment groups.

Women who received tamoxifen in the Breast Cancer Prevention Trial had a 2.5 times greater risk of developing invasive endometrial cancer. The average annual rates of endometrial cancer were 0.9/1000 women in the placebo group and 2.3/1000 women in the tamoxifen group. All of the 36 invasive endometrial cancers that occurred among women who received tamoxifen were Federation of Gynecology and Obstetrics (FIGO) stage I (TABLE 1).

A total of 955 women experienced bone fractures in the BCPT. The incidence of osteoporotic fracture events involving the spine, hip, or lower radius was reduced from 137 events in the placebo group to 111 events in the tamoxifen group. The most striking reduction was in fractures of the hip (see TABLE 1). There was also an increase in the number of thromboembolic vascular events among women taking tamoxifen in the BCPT (TABLE 1). Only the event rate for pulmonary embolism reached statistical significance, but there may be increases in event rates for stroke, transient ischemic attack (TIA), and deep vein thrombosis (DVT), particularly among women 50 years of age and older who took tamoxifen.

There was also an increase in the rate of cataract development among women who took tamoxifen in the BCPT. The number of cataract operations was also increased in the tamoxifen-treated women. Hot flashes and vaginal discharge were more common in women receiving tamoxifen (46% vs. 29%, and 29% vs. 13%, respectively).[4]

In addition to the NSABP P-1 trial, two other large studies of tamoxifen as a preventive have been published[12,13] (TABLE 2).

The Italian tamoxifen prevention study randomized 5408 hysterectomized women, aged 35 to 70, to 20 mg tamoxifen daily for 5 years or placebo. The women in this study had low to normal risk of developing breast cancer. At a median follow-

TABLE 1. Average annual rates for outcomes in the Breast Cancer Prevention Trial

Cancer outcome	Rate per 1000 women		Risk ratio (95% CI)
	Tamoxifen	Placebo	
Invasive breast cancer	3.4	6.8	0.51 (0.39–0.66)
Noninvasive breast cancer	1.4	2.7	0.50 (0.33–0.77)
Invasive BrCa by patient characteristic			
Age, years			
≤49	3.8	6.7	0.56 (0.37–0.85)
50–59	3.1	6.3	0.49 (0.29–0.81)
≥60	3.3	7.2	0.45 (0.27–0.74)
History of LCIS			
Yes	5.7	13.0	0.44 (0.16–1.06)
No	3.3	6.4	0.51 (0.39–0.68)
History of atypical hyperplasia			
Yes	1.4	10.1	0.14 (0.03–0.47)
No	3.6	6.4	0.56 (0.42–0.73)
Number of first-degree relatives with BrCa			
0	3.0	6.4	0.46 (0.24–0.84)
1	3.0	6.0	0.51 (0.35–0.73)
2	4.8	8.7	0.55 (0.30–0.97)
≥3	7.0	13.7	0.51 (0.15–1.55)
Risk of breast cancer within 5 years (%)			
≤2	2.1	5.5	0.37 (0.18–0.72)
2.01–3.0	3.5	5.2	0.68 (0.41–1.11)
3.01–5.0	3.9	5.9	0.66 (0.39–1.09)
≥5.01	4.5	13.3	0.34 (0.19–0.58)
Invasive endometrial cancer			
Age, years			
≤49	1.3	1.1	1.21 (0.41–3.60)
≥50	3.0	0.8	4.01 (1.70–10.90)
Fractures			
Hip	0.5	0.8	0.55 (0.25–1.15)
Hip, spine, lower radius combined	4.3	5.3	0.81 (0.63–1.05)
Thromboembolic events			
Stroke	1.4	0.9	1.59 (0.93–2.77)
Transient ischemic attack	0.7	1.0	0.76 (0.40–1.44)
Pulmonary embolism	0.7	0.2	3.01 (1.15–9.27)
Deep vein thrombosis	1.3	0.8	1.60 (0.91–2.86)

NOTE: From Ref. 4.

up of 46 months, the Italian trial found no significant difference in the incidence of breast cancer between the treatment groups, except in women on hormone replacement therapy (HRT). A total of 22 breast cancers were diagnosed in the placebo

TABLE 2. Summary of tamoxifen prevention trials

Trial	Sample size	Risk of breast cancer	Women-years of follow-up	Breast cancers/1000 women-years	
				Placebo	Tamoxifen
NSABP P-1	13,388	high (modified Gail model)	52,401	6.8	3.4
Royal Marsden	2471	based on family history	12,355	5.0	4.7
Italian	5408	low to normal	20,731	2.3	2.1

group compared to 19 in the tamoxifen-treated group. Of the women who were taking HRT, 8 breast cancers were found in the placebo group ($n = 390$) compared to 1 in the tamoxifen group ($n = 362$) [hazard ratio = 0.13; 95% CI = 0.02–1.02]. Accrual to this trial was halted by an independent data monitoring committee due to problems with compliance. Twenty-six percent of the women discontinued their study drug in the first year. This study does not confirm the BCPT results, but the low-risk study population, the relatively low power of the trial, and compliance issues make interpretation of this study difficult.[14]

The Royal Marsden Hospital Tamoxifen Prevention Pilot Trial enrolled 2471 women with a family history of breast cancer. In this study, family history was the only risk criterion. Postmenopausal women taking HRT were eligible to participate without having to stop such therapy and women in the trial were allowed to start HRT if symptoms developed. The study population in this British trial were younger (61% under age 50) than the BCPT population (40% under age 50). With a median follow-up of 17 months, this trial found no advantage to tamoxifen over placebo. Thirty-four cases of breast cancer were found in the tamoxifen group and 36 in the placebo group. The investigators found no interaction between HRT and tamoxifen. Powles calculated that the Royal Marsden trial had a 90% power to detect a 50% reduction in breast cancer incidence. While it is less clear why this study does not confirm the NSABP BCPT results, a lower risk population, the use of family history as the only risk criterion, and the younger population may have played a role. There was an estimated 30% noncompliance at 5 years.[14]

Another large international study, the International Breast Cancer Intervention Study (IBIS), is continuing to randomize women at high risk of breast cancer to receive tamoxifen or placebo for 5 years. This study aims to accrue over 7000 patients and is well on its way to achieving those goals.[14]

It is important to note that even the NSABP BCPT has, as yet, shown no difference in overall survival between tamoxifen- and placebo-treated women. Clearly, much longer follow-up would be required to show any such results. Because of the design of the NSABP study, which planned for disclosure of results and unblinding to patients and investigators once a highly significant decrease in incidence was seen, the possibility of following patients receiving their original therapy long enough to detect a survival benefit is extremely low. In the Italian study, most women have also discontinued their original therapy. Women in the Royal Marsden study and in the IBIS study, however, may continue their randomized therapy longer; and it is possible that long-term follow-up of these women, plus the women from the NSABP P-1—even though many changed therapy following treatment unblinding—may provide worthwhile data concerning possible survival benefit.

RALOXIFENE

Raloxifene (keoxifene, LY156758) is a benzothiophene SERM that has been shown to increase bone density in postmenopausal women and is currently indicated for the prevention and treatment of osteoporosis in this population.[15] This drug is of particular interest because it appears, in preclinical and early clinical testing, to be less likely to cause endometrial stimulation and/or to result in endometrial cancer.

The Multiple Outcomes of Raloxifene Evaluation (MORE) trial is a randomized placebo-controlled double-blind trial that was originally designed to determine whether raloxifene reduced the risk of fracture in postmenopausal women with osteoporosis.[5] In this trial, 7704 women with a mean age of 66.5 years were randomized to receive 60 mg daily of raloxifene, 120 mg daily of raloxifene, or placebo. Osteoporosis was a primary end point of this trial. The development of breast cancer was a secondary end point, so the women selected were not necessarily at high risk of developing breast cancer. In fact, breast cancer risk factors were not routinely ascertained at baseline.[16]

When data from both raloxifene dosage groups were pooled, with 40 months median follow-up, 13 cases of breast cancer were found among women assigned to raloxifene versus 27 among women assigned to placebo [RR = 0.24; 95% CI = 0.13–0.44; $P < 0.001$]. Raloxifene decreased the risk of ER-positive breast cancer by 90% [RR = 0.10; 95% CI = 0.04–0.24]. The incidence of ER-negative breast cancers was not reduced. Raloxifene was associated with an increased risk of venous thromboembolic disease [RR = 3.1; 95% CI = 1.5–6.2]. The risk of endometrial cancer was not increased [RR = 0.8; 95% CI = 0.2–2.7].[5,17]

In a recent metanalysis, data were combined from the MORE trial and other randomized placebo-controlled trials of raloxifene. In a total of 10,553 postmenopausal women with no personal history of breast cancer, the relative risk for all breast cancers (invasive and noninvasive) was 0.46 with raloxifene. In the placebo group, there were 3.7 cases of breast cancer per 1000 women compared with 1.7 cases per 1000 women in the raloxifene-treated groups[18] (TABLE 3). The ongoing RUTH trial (Raloxifene Use for the Heart), which is testing raloxifene versus placebo in 10,000

TABLE 3. Metanalysis of raloxifene placebo-controlled clinical trials

Time to diagnosis	Cases ($n = 10,553$)	Rate per 1000 patient-years		RR (95% CI)
		Placebo	Raloxifene	
All	58	3.7	1.7	0.46 (0.28–0.75)
0–6 months	11	1.8	2.4	1.30 (0.35–4.88)
6–18 months	12	2.1	1.0	0.49 (0.16–1.50)
>18 months	35	5.9	1.9	0.32 (0.17–0.62)

women at high risk for coronary disease, will collect additional data on cardiac and breast events related to tamoxifen as well.

A number of new trials are under way to examine SERM therapy in reduction of breast cancer risk. There is an NSABP Study of Tamoxifen and Raloxifene (STAR, or P-2 Trial) and a proposed IBIS II trial that will randomize women at increased risk of developing breast cancer to receive one of (1) placebo, (2) tamoxifen 20 mg daily, or (3) Arimidex 1 mg daily for 5 years. The results of these trials will not be known for many years. The STAR trial opened in July 1999 and has already randomized over 7000 of a projected 22,000 women to receive 20 mg daily of tamoxifen or 60 mg daily of raloxifene for 5 years.

It has been postulated by investigators from the NSABP that, in the United States, based on the women who showed benefit in their P-1 study, over 30 million women could be candidates for tamoxifen prevention. Three million of these women would be premenopausal and, if at high risk by virtue of LCIS, atypical hyperplasia, or family history, could get the best balance of risk and benefit, in that they have little or no increased risk of the serious side effects seen mainly in older women such as endometrial cancer or deep vein thromboses and pulmonary emboli. It is interesting to ask, however, whether these women, or indeed even a small proportion of them, are actually taking tamoxifen or even considering it. It seems that nowhere near this number are taking tamoxifen for prevention or are even approached by their physicians to consider it, for reasons that are not altogether clear.

Certainly, many of the women who are eligible in terms of the women treated in the P-1 trial are also eligible to receive HRT. HRT clearly has its own short-term benefits and may have additional long-term benefits including osteoporosis prevention and cardiovascular protection, although perhaps this latter issue is coming into increasing question. Thus, a woman who might consider tamoxifen prevention may have to consider whether this means discontinuing or not starting HRT. Are these two strategies for peri- and postmenopausal "wellness" in competition? It seems so and the issue of which is more beneficial on balance or of whether they could be combined is far from being clarified.

Furthermore, many women are taking other medication for osteoporosis. Drugs such as Didronel (etidronate) and Fosamax (alendronate) or indeed raloxifene are used widely for this purpose and are seen by many women as of more importance and with fewer side effects than either HRT or tamoxifen.

Exercise and a diet high in calcium, vegetables, fruit, and fiber and low in fat seem like motherhood. Such lifestyle alterations are clearly beneficial for a variety of symptoms and may be seen by many women as replacing the need for any type of medication to prevent osteoporosis, heart disease, or breast cancer. Indeed, here the phenomenon of well women wishing to avoid pills including birth control pills, HRT, and perhaps tamoxifen or raloxifene for breast cancer risk reduction comes into play. It is intuitive for many healthy individuals to see medication as a last resort for "wellness."

SUMMARY

It has been clear for many years that early ovarian ablation would reduce the incidence of breast cancer. Because of its side effects, though, this maneuver has not been considered an acceptable preventive treatment. Now, the NSABP BCPT has found a highly significant reduction in the incidence of breast cancer with the use of 5 years of tamoxifen. While the Italian and British tamoxifen trials did not confirm these results, the differences between these studies are most likely due to differences in study populations, treatment intervention, and design.[14] In Canada and the United States, regulatory agencies have approved tamoxifen for use in the reduction of breast cancer risk in healthy women at high risk for the disease. Women may not be using this drug to nearly the degree they could, however, for reasons that are not totally clear. Results from raloxifene remain more preliminary. While the results of the MORE trial and of the metanalysis are exciting, statistical and design limitations have prevented any recommendation for the use of raloxifene in either treatment or prevention of breast cancer outside of clinical trials.

A 1999 ASCO technology assessment[19] stressed the importance of assessing risks and benefits in giving tamoxifen to women as a breast cancer preventive and encouraged physicians to discuss and outline these risks with their patients as clearly as possible so that an informed choice can be made by each patient together with her physician. This paper also stressed that there is currently no role for the use of raloxifene in treatment or prevention of breast cancer, except in the setting of clinical trials such as the ongoing STAR study. The results of currently ongoing and proposed clinical trials in these areas will be awaited with great interest.

REFERENCES

1. HENDERSON, B.E. 1989. The cancer question: an overview of recent epidemiologic and retrospective data. Am. J. Obstet. Gynecol. **161:** 1859–1864.
2. HENDERSON, B.E., R.K. ROSS & M.C. PIKE. 1997. The prevention of hormone-related cancer in women. Adv. Oncol. **13:** 10–14.
3. EARLY BREAST CANCER TRIALISTS' COLLABORATIVE GROUP. 1998. Tamoxifen for early breast cancer: an overview of the randomized trials. Lancet **351:** 1451–1467.
4. FISHER, B., J.P. COSTANTINO, D.L. WICKERHAM et al. 1998. Tamoxifen for prevention of breast cancer: report of the National Surgical Adjuvant Breast and Bowel Project P-1 Study. J. Natl. Cancer Inst. **90:** 1371–1388.
5. CUMMINGS, S.R., S. ECKERT, K.A. KRUEGER et al. 1999. The effect of raloxifene on risk of breast cancer in postmenopausal women: results from the MORE randomized trial—Multiple Outcomes of Raloxifene Evaluation. JAMA **281:** 2189–2197.
6. COLLINS GEM ENGLISH DICTIONARY (Canadian Edition). 1998. Collins–Clear Type Press. Toronto.
7. EARLY BREAST CANCER TRIALISTS' COLLABORATIVE GROUP. 1996. Ovarian ablation in early breast cancer: an overview of the randomized trials. Lancet **348:** 1189–1196.
8. FISHER, B., J.P. COSTANTINO, C. REDMOND et al. 1994. Endometrial cancer in tamoxifen-treated breast cancer patients: findings from the National Surgical Adjuvant Breast and Bowel Project (NSABP) B-14. J. Natl. Cancer Inst. **86:** 527–537.
9. KRISTENSEN, B., B. EJLERSTEN, P. DALGAARD et al. 1994. Tamoxifen and bone metabolism in postmenopausal low-risk breast cancer patients: a randomized study. J. Clin. Oncol. **12:** 992–997.
10. LOVE, R.R., R.B. MAZESS, H.S. BARDEN et al. 1992. Effects of tamoxifen on bone mineral density in postmenopausal women with breast cancer. N. Engl. J. Med. **326:** 852–856.
11. LOVE, R.R., D.A. WIEBE, P.A. NEWCOMB et al. 1991. Effects of tamoxifen on cardiovascular risk factors in postmenopausal women. Ann. Intern. Med. **115:** 860–864.
12. VERONESI, U., P. MAISONNEUVE, A. COSTA et al. 1998. Prevention of breast cancer with tamoxifen: preliminary findings from the Italian randomized trial among hysterectomized women. Lancet **352:** 93–97.

13. POWLES, T.J., R. EELES, S. ASHLEY *et al.* 1998. Interim analysis of the incidence of breast cancer in the Royal Marsden Hospital tamoxifen randomized chemoprevention trial. Lancet **352:** 98–101.
14. PRITCHARD, K.I. 1998. Is tamoxifen effective in prevention of breast cancer? Lancet **352:** 80–81.
15. DELMAS, P.D., N.H. BJARNASON, B.H. MITLAK *et al.* 1997. Effects of raloxifene on bone mineral density, serum cholesterol concentrations, and uterine endometrium in postmenopausal women. N. Engl. J. Med. **337:** 1641–1647.
16. FRANKS, A.L. & K.K. STEINBERG. 1999. Encouraging news from the SERM frontier. JAMA **281:** 2243–2244.
17. CUMMINGS, S.R., L. NORTON, S. ECKERT & J. GRADY. 1998. Raloxifene reduces the risk of breast cancer and may decrease the risk of endometrial cancer in postmenopausal women: two-year findings from the multiple outcomes of raloxifene evaluation (MORE) trial [abstract 3]. Proc. Am. Soc. Clin. Oncol. **17:** 2a.
18. JORDAN, V.C., J.E. GLUSMAN, S. ECKERT *et al.* 1998. Raloxifene reduces incident primary breast cancer: integrated data from multicenter double-blind placebo-controlled randomized trials in postmenopausal women [abstract 2]. Breast Cancer Res. Treat. **50:** 227.
19. CHLEBOWSKI, R.T., D.E. COLLYAR, M.R. SOMERFIELD *et al.* 1999. American Society of Clinical Oncology technology assessment on breast cancer risk reduction strategies: tamoxifen and raloxifene—ASCO special article. J. Clin. Oncol. **17:** 1939–1955.

The Role of Tamoxifen in Breast Cancer Prevention

Issues Sparked by the NSABP Breast Cancer Prevention Trial (P-1)

NORMAN WOLMARK[a] AND BARBARA K. DUNN[b]

[a]*Department of Human Oncology, Allegheny General Hospital, Pittsburgh, Pennsylvania 15212, USA*

[b]*Division of Cancer Prevention, National Cancer Institute, Bethesda, Maryland 20892, USA*

ABSTRACT: The Breast Cancer Prevention Trial (P-1: BCPT) of the National Surgical Adjuvant Breast and Bowel Project (NSABP) randomized 13,388 women, ≥35 years of age, at increased risk for breast cancer [≥1.66% by Gail model criteria or with a history of lobular carcinoma *in situ* (LCIS)] to 5 years of tamoxifen or placebo. A 49% reduction ($P < 0.00001$) in invasive breast cancers occurred, 175 with placebo versus 89 with tamoxifen, mainly among estrogen receptor (ER)–positive tumors (130 with placebo vs. 41 with tamoxifen). The major toxicities of tamoxifen were endometrial cancer (15 with placebo vs. 36 with tamoxifen) and thromboembolic disease, both predominantly in women who were ≥50 years old. Ramifications emerging from the P-1 results regarding the efficacy and toxicities of preventive tamoxifen include the following: (1) Does tamoxifen induce more virulent breast cancers? (2) Does tamoxifen induce more virulent endometrial cancers? (3) Tamoxifen is especially efficacious in reducing breast cancer risk in LCIS (18 invasive breast cancers with placebo vs. 8 with tamoxifen group) and atypical ductal hyperplasia (AH) (23 invasive breast cancers with placebo vs. 3 with tamoxifen). (4) Does tamoxifen reduce breast cancer risk in women at increased risk due to genetic mutations? (5) How can we prevent tamoxifen-resistant breast cancers? (6) What do the BCPT results tell us about who should take preventive tamoxifen? In its ongoing effort to lower the incidence of breast cancer, the NSABP is now implementing its second breast cancer prevention trial, the Study of Tamoxifen and Raloxifene (STAR), which is comparing the two agents with regard to efficacy and toxicity.

KEYWORDS: breast cancer; NSABP (National Surgical Adjuvant Breast and Bowel Project); BCPT (Breast Cancer Prevention Trial) P-1; STAR (Study of Tamoxifen and Raloxifene); tamoxifen; raloxifene

---

Address for correspondence: Norman Wolmark, M.D., Department of Human Oncology, Allegheny General Hospital, 320 East North Avenue, Pittsburgh, PA 15212. Voice: 412-359-3336; fax: 412-359-3096.

nwolmark@wpahs.org

INTRODUCTION: SYNOPSIS OF THE NSABP BREAST CANCER PREVENTION TRIAL (BCPT P-1)

The NSABP chemoprevention trial was initiated in June 1992 and followed the typical NSABP format in that it was randomized and double-blind.[1] Between June 1992 and September 1997, 13,388 women, 35 years of age or older, who were at increased risk for the development of breast cancer were randomized to either 5 years of tamoxifen or to placebo. Increased risk was defined as a 5-year predicted incidence of breast cancer of at least 1.66% (that of an average 60-year-old woman) according to modified Gail model criteria[2] or a personal history of lobular carcinoma *in situ* (LCIS). The mean follow-up time was 47 months, whereas the median time on study was 54 months. Through 69 months of follow-up, there were 175 events of invasive breast cancer in the placebo group compared to 89 in the tamoxifen-treated group (TABLE 1), a 49% reduction ($P < 0.00001$), equivalent to a cumulative incidence of 43.4 per 1000 women and 22.0 per 1000 women in the two groups, respectively. There was a concomitant reduction in the incidence of noninvasive breast cancer: 69 events in the placebo arm and 35 in the tamoxifen-treated group. The benefits from tamoxifen were not dependent on the age of the patient and were evident to the same degree in all the age groups that were analyzed: a comparable decrease in risk for invasive breast cancer occurring in women 35–49 years of age as well as those ≥50 years of age.

Of the 834 women who entered the study with a history of LCIS, there were 18 invasive breast cancers in the placebo group compared with 8 in the group receiving tamoxifen; of the 1026 women who entered the trial with a history of atypical hyperplasia (AH), there were 23 invasive breast cancers in the placebo group compared with 3 in the tamoxifen arm. When examined during each of the first 6 yearly intervals of follow-up, a reduction in the annual hazard rate of similar magnitude is noted in the first year and for each year of follow-up. This indicates that the effect of tamoxifen does not end with the last pill and continues beyond the cessation of the treatment. The major influence of tamoxifen appeared to be in the reduction of estrogen receptor (ER)–positive breast cancers, in that there were 130 ER-positive breast cancers arising in women treated with placebo compared to 41 in those who were treated with tamoxifen.

The benefits of tamoxifen came at a price and that is an increased incidence of endometrial cancer and vascular events. There were 15 endometrial cancers in the placebo arm compared with 36 in the tamoxifen group (TABLE 1); this increased risk occurred predominantly in women ≥ 50 years of age. With regard to vascular events, there were 52 events in the placebo arm compared to 91 in the tamoxifen arm: an increase in the rate of deep vein thrombosis (0.84 vs. 1.34 per 1000 women per year), pulmonary emboli (0.23 vs. 0.69 per 1000 women per year), and stroke (0.92 vs. 1.45 per 1000 women per year). These adverse vascular events also occurred more frequently in women ≥ 50 years of age. Of note, in no previous trial was tamoxifen associated with an increased risk of stroke. Therefore, although this increase was not statistically significant in P-1 [RR = 1.59; 95% CI = 0.93–2.77], we wanted to make certain that it was included in the risks associated with tamoxifen. Whether or not this is real will require further analyses and information from other corroborating trials.

A number of issues and novel findings, some controversial, have emerged from the BCPT and merit special attention.

TABLE 1. Numbers of events among participants in the NSABP's P-1 Breast Cancer Prevention Trial

	Events (n)	
	Placebo (6131)	Tamoxifen (6101)
Invasive breast cancer	175	89
Noninvasive breast cancer	69	35
Endometrial cancer	15	36
Deep vein thrombosis	22	35
Pulmonary emboli	6	18
Stroke	24	38
Deaths	71	57
ER-positive breast cancers	130	41
ER-negative breast cancers	31	38
Unknown	14	10
LCIS	18	8
AH	23	3

RAMIFICATIONS OF THE NSABP P-1: BCPT

Does Tamoxifen Induce More Virulent Breast Cancers?

The contention has been made that tamoxifen, in displaying efficacy limited to the better prognosis ER-positive breast cancers, in essence was simply eliminating favorable breast cancers and culling out the more virulent variety, which was left unattenuated. In point of fact, when one analyzes characteristics such as tumor size and nodal status, features classically associated with tumor aggressiveness, that contention is not corroborated in that there is no excess in the unfavorable tumor size or nodal status groups among tumors that arose in the tamoxifen-treated cohort. The only category of aggressive tumor that was not reduced in incidence by tamoxifen was that of ER-negative breast cancers. In contrast to ER-positive tumors, which were reduced by 49%, the ER-negative tumors had the same frequency in the tamoxifen as in the placebo arm. The importance of this finding is that, although ER-negative breast cancer was not prevented by tamoxifen, it also was not stimulated or selected for by this agent. The suppression of the better prognosis ER-positive cancers therefore did not create a tissue milieu that supported emergence of the more aggressive ER-negative cancers.

Does Tamoxifen Induce More Virulent Endometrial Cancers?

Another contentious area involves the increased risk of endometrial cancer in BCPT participants taking tamoxifen. While this elevation of risk is generally accepted as an unfortunate, but tolerable outcome in women being treated with tamoxifen for existing breast cancer, endometrial cancer clearly presents a potential obstacle to the use of tamoxifen in the prevention setting where women are essentially healthy, but are at high risk. Nevertheless, concern over this toxicity is tempered somewhat by several factors. First, the RR of 2.53 observed with tamoxifen in the BCPT is the same as that observed in the adjuvant trials of this agent[3–10] and thus offered no surprises when the P-1 data were analyzed. Second, the increase in risk was confined to women over 50, leaving the younger, very high risk women far less vulnerable to this adverse outcome. Third, among the 37% of BCPT participants who had a hysterectomy, the toxic outcome of endometrial cancer did not apply. This hysterectomized status is even more common among the women over 50, with 43% having had a hysterectomy prior to randomization and an additional 4% undergoing this procedure during the course of follow-up. Fourth, at one time, the suggestion was made that endometrial cancers resulting from tamoxifen therapy were more aggressive than those in the general population.[11] Not only has this concern not been borne out by subsequent studies of tamoxifen-induced endometrial cancers,[7,12] but those endometrial cancers that developed in women on the BCPT also failed to demonstrate increased virulence in association with tamoxifen use. All 36 endometrial cancers that arose on tamoxifen were Federation of Gynecology and Obstetrics (FIGO) stage 1, with the only carcinoma higher than stage 1 (a stage 4) being seen in a placebo-treated participant (the only patient who died from an endometrial cancer). Finally, the risk of endometrial cancer due to tamoxifen is similar to that seen in women taking estrogen replacement therapy,[13–15] a widely employed therapy among healthy postmenopausal women. In summary, without trivializing the significance of endometrial carcinoma, it can be concluded that the level of excess risk for endometrial cancer appears to have been exaggerated when viewed in the larger context of tamoxifen trials as well as in the setting of the BCPT.[1]

Efficacy of Tamoxifen in Reducing Breast Cancer Risk in Lobular Carcinoma in Situ (LCIS) and Atypical Ductal Hyperplasia (AH)

The BCPT yielded novel insights into the efficacy of tamoxifen in preventing invasive breast cancer in women who were at high risk due to documented lobular carcinoma *in situ* (LCIS) or atypical ductal hyperplasia (AH). P-1 was the largest trial _assessing tamoxifen in the setting of LCIS, with 814 women deemed eligible for P-1 as a result of a personal history of LCIS. Similarly, over 1100 women entered into P-1 based on a pathologic diagnosis of AH. Both eligibility criteria offered risk cohorts with high relative risks of breast cancer. LCIS confers a risk that is 7 to 10 times that of the general population,[16] while AH is associated with a relative risk of 4.0 to 5.0.[16,17] The P-1 results demonstrated that both risk cohorts benefited from preventive tamoxifen. Thus, tamoxifen reduced the incidence of invasive breast cancer by 56% in women with LCIS and, even more dramatically, by 86% in women with AH.

Does Tamoxifen Reduce Breast Cancer Risk in Women at Increased Risk due to Genetic Mutations?

An important issue that remains unanswered by the BCPT results is whether high-risk groups defined by their genetic predisposition to breast cancer, such as

BRCA-1 or BRCA-2 mutation-positive women or other genetically disposed risk groups, are appropriate candidates for preventive tamoxifen. Technically, the data at this time do not exist to either support or reject the use of tamoxifen in such genetic risk groups. The BCPT eligibility criteria did not include mutation positivity because the BRCA-1 and BRCA-2 breast cancer susceptibility genes had not yet been cloned and sequenced at the time the BCPT was initiated.[18,19] Yet, as part of the design of the NSABP P-1 study, peripheral white blood cells were stored from study participants in anticipation of the imminent identification of heritable risk genes for breast cancer.[20] The NSABP P-1G study, "A Study of the Association between Inherited Mutations and the Effect of Tamoxifen on Breast Cancer Incidence", which involves sequencing of the BRCA-1 and BRCA-2 genes in DNA samples from a subset of BCPT participants, was begun in 1999 in the laboratory of Mary-Claire King and is well on its way to completion. The primary aim of this study is to determine if any differences exist in the preventive efficacy of tamoxifen in mutation carriers versus high-risk noncarriers, a question that will hopefully be answered in the near future.

A second genetic substudy of P-1 is the NSABP P-1G2, "A Study of the Association between Inherited Mutations in Specific Clotting Factors and the Incidence of Blood Clots in Women Taking Tamoxifen", directed by Judy Garber. P-1G2 addresses the interaction between tamoxifen and the genetic polymorphisms, Factor V Leiden and Prothrombin 20210A, whose main gene effects are increased thrombotic risk.[21–23] The primary objective of this study is to see if this thrombotic propensity is exacerbated by interaction with tamoxifen. Finally, in the near future, we plan to examine a subset of the BCPT DNA samples to assess the interaction of tamoxifen with genetic polymorphisms demonstrated in epidemiologic studies to affect breast cancer or endometrial cancer risk. Selected polymorphisms occur in genes whose protein products metabolize estrogen and tamoxifen or affect estrogen function, for example, the estrogen receptor.

How Can We Prevent Tamoxifen-Resistant Breast Cancers?

The distinctly positive results of the BCPT still fall short of showing 100% efficacy for tamoxifen in reducing breast cancer risk in high-risk women. The following question then arises: how can the tamoxifen-resistant breast cancers be prevented? These breast cancers fall into two groups: the ER-negative breast cancers and the residual 31% of ER-positive breast cancers that were not suppressed by tamoxifen. The ER-negative tumors are not expected to be affected by tamoxifen or any other SERM since, by their very nature, these agents act through the ER. In the near future, drugs that bypass the ER, acting further downstream in the carcinogenic pathway, will be tested for their ability to prevent breast cancer. Similarly, tamoxifen resistance among ER-positive breast cancers may well result from constitutive activity of mutated molecules downstream of the ER, rendering these cancers resistant to tamoxifen despite the presence of an immunologically detectable ER. Here, as well, future drug development will need to target downstream molecules involved in key cell functions such as signal transduction or the cell cycle.

What Do the BCPT Results Tell Us about Who Should Take Preventive Tamoxifen?

Arguably, the most critical question arising from the BCPT results is who is a good candidate for preventive tamoxifen therapy. The BCPT was developed as a phase III, large-scale, long-term, prospective, randomized, double-blinded trial, a design that yields the highest level of evidence for efficacy of an intervention (in this case, tamoxifen) in humans.[24,25] In other words, this was an optimally designed trial that yielded a highly significant positive result for the efficacy of tamoxifen in achieving the primary end point of decreased breast cancer incidence in high-risk women.[26] From this perspective, the data are incontrovertible, as far as demonstrating that tamoxifen can reduce the subsequent incidence of invasive breast cancer. In fact, the FDA approved reduction in breast cancer incidence in high-risk women as an indication for tamoxifen.[27] Had this added indication for tamoxifen applied to the treatment of breast cancer, its introduction into standard clinical practice might well have been a routine matter. However, a number of concerns have impacted the implementation of preventive tamoxifen use.

The hesitancy with regard to universal acceptance of the scientifically confirmed and FDA-approved preventive indication for tamoxifen has been influenced to some extent by the failure of parallel tamoxifen prevention trials in Europe to confirm the NSABP P-1's results on the preventive efficacy of this agent.[28,29] Although multiple reasons have been explored to explain the discrepancies between the British and Italian tamoxifen prevention trial outcomes and that of the BCPT[30,31] (see also Pritchard and Cuzick in these proceedings), the most obvious explanations for the differences in outcomes are the much smaller sizes of the two European trials, which together had fewer than half the number of events of the BCPT (111 breast cancer cases in the Royal Marsden plus Italian studies versus 264 invasive breast cancer events in the BCPT), and differences in study design relating mainly to differing risk levels of the respective cohorts.

An even greater impact on clinical acceptance has come from the nature of the population to which preventive tamoxifen would be applied. On the one hand, the potential users are "healthy" women and, on the other, tamoxifen has toxicities that, although infrequent, can be serious or life-threatening. As a result, the decision regarding who should be considered for preventive tamoxifen must address two issues: first, who is expected to benefit from the drug based on her membership in the tested target population; second, to what extent do the observed risks of tamoxifen, its toxicities, compete with its potential benefits in a given individual. Thus, appropriate patient targeting is a key element in deciding which women will benefit from tamoxifen in a preventive mode. As a starting point, women with the risk factors used as eligibility criteria for the BCPT[2] may be considered appropriate candidates for preventive tamoxifen. The BCPT risk factors centered around age and menopausal status, which contribute to both risk reduction for breast cancer as well as toxicity due to drug. Additional factors that fed into BCPT eligibility include the number of first-degree relatives with breast cancer, a personal history of breast disease, and a history of LCIS, and these should also be considered before instituting preventive therapy. Since the risk of invasive breast cancer in women with a history of localized ductal carcinoma *in situ* (DCIS) is as high (if not higher) as that for women with

LCIS and since tamoxifen has reduced the incidence of contralateral breast cancer in women with DCIS,[32] tamoxifen should also be considered as a preventive agent in the DCIS group. Finally, the role of genetic predisposition to breast cancer (exemplified by mutations in the BRCA-1 and BRCA-2 genes) as a risk factor justifying consideration of preventive tamoxifen therapy must be clarified. A chemopreventive alternative to the only existing modalities of prophylaxis, mastectomy[33] and oophorectomy,[34] would be extremely desirable for this group of high-risk women.

A formal method for assessing breast cancer risk that incorporates Gail model features was developed by the NCI in conjunction with the NSABP. This method is included in a "Risk Disk" available from the NCI (NCI Cancer Information Service: 1-800-4-CANCER—call for "Risk Disk" information; NCI website: http://www.nci.nih.gov—access for sign-up form for "Risk Disk").[35] However, the Risk Disk is only a starting point in evaluating the appropriateness of preventive tamoxifen for a given individual since a woman's susceptibility to the toxic side effects of tamoxifen must be taken into consideration as well, leading to elaboration of an individualized risk-benefit ratio.

In order to synthesize the multiple effects of tamoxifen into a unified risk-benefit model, Gail et al.[36] subjected the risks (primarily endometrial cancer, stroke, pulmonary embolism, and deep vein thrombosis, with some lesser toxic side effects) and benefits (breast cancer and fracture reduction) of tamoxifen as observed in the BCPT to a quantitative analysis that yielded an estimate of the relative risks of this drug for specific clinical end points. Among the considerations that these authors incorporated into their calculations of relative risk were the absolute risk of breast cancer as well as the background rates for the risks and benefits of tamoxifen, which are age-dependent (the adverse effects generally rising with age) and race-dependent, though less data are available in the latter case. A general conclusion that can be drawn from these calculations is that younger women at higher risk will tend to benefit more from preventive tamoxifen. Despite concerns over this attempt to quantify risks and benefits by placing numerical values on essentially human values for clinical outcomes, the model offers interested parties a standardized starting point for clinical decision-making. The emphasis here is on "starting point" since the core of the decision-making process lies in the psychosocial factors that color a woman's perception of her disease. This quantitative risk-benefit model is thus, like the Risk Disk, merely a tool in the decision-making process for an interested woman. In the final analysis, the propriety and utility of using tamoxifen in the prevention setting should remain a choice left to the individual after a consideration of the risks and benefits.[37]

In summary, the BCPT results, in conjunction with the extensive clinical data derived from breast cancer treatment trials, support consideration of tamoxifen as a preventive agent for up to 5 years in women who are at increased risk for breast cancer, especially those considered at increased risk based on eligibility criteria for the P-1 trial. The risk-benefit model described above then offers a method for individualizing estimated outcomes for a particular woman. There are subsets where the benefits clearly outweigh the risks, including women who are <50 years of age; women who are >50 years of age, but have had a hysterectomy; women with a personal history of LCIS; and probably women with a personal history of atypical lobular hyperplasia or ductal hyperplasia. In the end, however, decisions such as these are necessarily both complex and personal.[38,39]

THE NEXT SERM TRIAL—THE NSABP'S P-2: STUDY OF TAMOXIFEN AND RALOXIFENE (STAR)

It would be unfortunate to view the data from the P-1: BCPT chemoprevention trial as an end unto itself. It is simply one point in a continuum. Tamoxifen is not the ideal intervention and we would like to move beyond it. That is the basis and the rationale for the NSABP's current prevention trial, P-2: the Study of Tamoxifen and Raloxifene (STAR), which basically simulates the schema that was used for P-1, namely, tamoxifen being compared to raloxifene in a double-blind fashion.

The selection of raloxifene was based on its demonstrated ability to reduce breast cancer incidence as a secondary end point in the Multiple Outcomes of Raloxifene Evaluation (MORE). In the MORE study, 7704 postmenopausal women with osteoporosis were randomized in double-blinded fashion to receive raloxifene (60 mg or 120 mg per day) or placebo.[40,41] Regarding its primary end point, the MORE trial showed that raloxifene reduced the risk of osteoporosis progressing, as reflected in the preservation of bone mineral density, the reduction of bone turnover, and the decreased incidence of vertebral fractures, thereby contributing to the database that led to the FDA's approval of the drug for this purpose in November 1997.[41,42] As a secondary observation, raloxifene decreased the incidence of invasive breast cancers. Of the total of 54 cases of breast cancer that were confirmed during 40.0 months of follow-up, 22 (0.41%) occurred in women assigned to raloxifene and 32 (0.59%) in women assigned to placebo, yielding a relative risk of 0.35. For the 40 invasive breast cancers, the RR was 0.24 with raloxifene. The risk reduction, which was similar for both doses of raloxifene, was confined to ER-positive tumors (RR = 0.10), with no reduction in risk for ER-negative tumors (RR = 0.88).

These data led to the hypothesis that raloxifene is a chemopreventive agent for breast cancer and, given its potentially nontoxic profile, a prime candidate for testing for preventive efficacy against the recently documented standard, tamoxifen. Therefore, in July 1999, the NSABP began its second breast cancer prevention trial, NSABP P-2: Study of Tamoxifen and Raloxifene (STAR). The entry criteria are similar to those of P-1, with the exception that this trial is restricted to postmenopausal women. In STAR, 22,000 risk-eligible postmenopausal women volunteers will be randomized in double-blinded fashion to receive either tamoxifen (20 mg per day) or raloxifene (60 mg per day) for a duration of 5 years in order to ascertain whether the benefits noted with tamoxifen in P-1 can be achieved with a diminished incidence of adverse events with raloxifene. Participants will be stratified according to age, breast cancer risk, race, and history of LCIS, as was done in the BCPT, as well as by hysterectomy status. If the assumptions that entered into the design of STAR are correct, the anticipated time of the final analysis will be approximately 6.5 years from the time that randomization was initiated in July 1999. This trial was initiated in July 1999 and, as of April 2001, 9688 women have been randomized into this trial.

ACKNOWLEDGMENTS

We wish to pay special tribute to those 13,388 women who, because of their courage and selflessness, entered into the NSABP P-1 and made possible the next logical step, the STAR trial.

REFERENCES

1. FISHER, B., J.P. COSTANTINO, D.L. WICKERHAM et al. 1998. Tamoxifen for prevention of breast cancer: report of the National Surgical Adjuvant Breast and Bowel Project P-1 Study. J. Natl. Cancer Inst. **90:** 1371–1388.
2. GAIL, M.H., L.A. BRINTON, D.P. BYAR et al. 1989. Projecting individualized probabilities of developing breast cancer for white females who are being examined annually. J. Natl. Cancer Inst. **81:** 1879–1886.
3. FORNANDER, T., L.E. RUTQVIST, B. CEDERMARK et al. 1989. Adjuvant tamoxifen in early breast cancer: occurrence of new primary cancers. Lancet **1:** 117–120.
4. FORNANDER, T., L.E. RUTQVIST, B. CEDERMARK et al. 1991. Adjuvant tamoxifen in early-stage breast cancer: effects on intercurrent morbidity and mortality. J. Clin. Oncol. **10:** 1740–1748.
5. FISHER, B., J.P. COSTANTINO, C.K. REDMOND et al. 1994. Endometrial cancer in tamoxifen-treated breast cancer patients: findings from the National Surgical Adjuvant Breast and Bowel Project (NSABP) B-14. J. Natl. Cancer Inst. **86:** 527–537.
6. VAN LEEUWEN, F.E., J. BENRAADT, J.W. COEBERGH & L.A. KIEMENEY. 1994. Risk of endometrial cancer after tamoxifen treatment of breast cancer. Lancet **343:** 448–452.
7. BARAKAT, R.R., G. WONG, J.P. CURTIN et al. 1994. Tamoxifen use in breast cancer patients who subsequently develop corpus cancer is not associated with a higher incidence of adverse histologic features. Gynecol. Oncol. **55:** 164–168.
8. BARAKAT, R.R. 1999. Endometrial cancer and tamoxifen. Primary Care Cancer **19**(suppl. 1): 27–30.
9. RUTQVIST, L.E., H. JOHANSSON, T. SIGNOMKLAO et al. 1995. Adjuvant tamoxifen therapy for early stage breast cancer and second primary malignancies: Stockholm Breast Cancer Study Group. J. Natl. Cancer Inst. **87:** 645–651.
10. BERLIERE, M., A. CHARLES, C. GALANT & J. DONNEZ. 1998. Uterine side effects of tamoxifen: a need for systematic pretreatment screening. Obstet. Gynecol. **91:** 40–44.
11. MARGRIPLES, U., F. NAFTOLIN, P.E. SCHWARTZ & M.L. CARCANGIU. 1993. High-grade endometrial carcinoma in tamoxifen-treated breast cancer patients. J. Clin. Oncol. **11:** 485–490.
12. FORNANDER, T., A-C. HELLSTROM & B. MOBERGER. 1993. Descriptive clinicopathologic study of 17 patients with endometrial cancer during or after adjuvant tamoxifen in early breast cancer. J. Natl. Cancer Inst. **85:** 1850–1855.
13. COLDITZ, G.A., S.E. HANKINSON, D.J. HUNTER et al. 1995. The use of estrogens and progestins and the risk of breast cancer in postmenopausal women. N. Engl. J. Med. **332:** 1589–1593.
14. GRADY, D., T. GEBRETSADIK, K. KERLIKOWSKE et al. 1995. Hormone replacement therapy and endometrial cancer risk: a meta-analysis. Obstet. Gynecol. **85:** 304–313.
15. SUH-BURGMANN, E.J. & A. GOODMAN. 1999. Surveillance for endometrial cancer in women receiving tamoxifen. Ann. Intern. Med. **131:** 127–135.
16. WINER, E.P., M. MORROW, C.K. OSBORNE & J.R. HARRIS. 2001. Malignant tumors of the breast. *In* Cancer: Principles and Practice of Oncology. Sixth edition, pp. 1651–1717. Lippincott/Williams & Williams. Philadelphia.
17. DUPONT, W. & D. PAGE. 1985. Risk factors for breast cancer in women with proliferative breast disease. N. Engl. J. Med. **312:** 146–151.
18. MIKI, Y., J. SWENSEN, D. SHATTUCK-EIDENS et al. 1994. A strong candidate for the breast and ovarian cancer susceptibility gene BRCA1. Science **266:** 66–71.
19. WOOSTER, R., G. BIGNELL, J. LANCASTER et al. 1995. Identification of the breast cancer susceptibility gene BRCA2. Nature **378:** 789–792.
20. HALL, J.M., M.K. LEE, B. NEWMAN et al. 1990. Linkage of early-onset familial breast cancer to chromosome 17q21. Science **250:** 1684–1689.
21. ROSENDAAL, F.R., T. KOSTER, J.P. VANDENBROUCKE et al. 1995. High risk of thrombosis in patients homozygous for Factor V Leiden (activated protein C resistance). Blood **85:** 1504–1508.
22. ROSENDAAL, F.R., C.J.M. DOGGEN, A. ZIVELIN et al. 1998. Geographic distribution of the 20210 G to A Prothrombin variant. Thromb. Haemostasis **79:** 706–708.

23. POORT, S.R., R.R. ROSENDAAL, P.H. REITSMA *et al.* 1996. A common genetic variation in the 3′-untranslated region of the Prothrombin gene is associated with elevated plasma Prothrombin levels and an increase in venous thrombosis. Blood **88:** 3698–3703.
24. PRENTICE, R. 1995. Experimental methods in cancer prevention research. *In* Cancer Prevention and Control, pp. 80–81. Dekker. New York.
25. CHEMOPREVENTION WORKING GROUP. 1999. Prevention of cancer in the next millennium: report of the Chemoprevention Working Group to the American Association for Cancer Research. Cancer Res. **59:** 4743–4758.
26. FISHER, B. 1999. National Surgical Adjuvant Breast and Bowel Project breast cancer prevention trial: a reflective commentary. J. Clin. Oncol. **17:** 1632–1639.
27. ZENECA. 1998. Tamoxifen prescribing information [package insert]. Zeneca. Wilmington, DE.
28. POWLES, T.J., R. EELES, S. ASHLEY *et al.* 1998. Interim analysis of the incidence of breast cancer in the Royal Marsden Hospital tamoxifen randomised chemoprevention trial. Lancet **352:** 98–101.
29. VERONESI, U., P. MAISONNEUVE, A. COSTA *et al.* 1998. Prevention of breast cancer with tamoxifen: preliminary findings from the Italian randomised trial among hysterectomised women. Lancet **352:** 93–97.
30. PRITCHARD, K.I. 1998. Is tamoxifen effective in prevention of breast cancer? Lancet **352:** 80–81.
31. POWLES, T.J. 1999. Re: Tamoxifen for prevention of breast cancer—report of the National Surgical Adjuvant Breast and Bowel Project P-1 study. J. Natl. Cancer Inst. **91:** 730.
32. FISHER, B., J. DIGNAM, N. WOLMARK *et al.* 1999. Tamoxifen in treatment of intraductal breast cancer: National Surgical Adjuvant Breast and Bowel Project B-24 randomised controlled trial. Lancet **353:** 1993–2000.
33. HARTMANN, L.C., D.J. SCHAID, J.E. WOODS *et al.* 1999. Efficacy of bilateral prophylactic mastectomy in women with a family history of breast cancer. N. Engl. J. Med. **340:** 77–84.
34. REBBECK, T.R., A.M. LEVIN, A. EISEN *et al.* 1999. Breast cancer risk after bilateral prophylactic oophorectomy in BRCA1 mutation carriers. J. Natl. Cancer Inst. **91:** 1475–1479.
35. WOLMARK, N. 1999. The Breast Cancer Prevention Trial, tamoxifen, and the woman at high risk for breast cancer. Primary Care Cancer **19**(suppl. 2)**:** 11–16.
36. GAIL, M.H., J.P. COSTANTINO, J. BRYANT *et al.* 1999. Weighing the risks and benefits of tamoxifen treatment for preventing breast cancer. J. Natl. Cancer Inst. **91:** 1829–1846.
37. CHLEBOWSKI, R.T., D.E. COLLYAR, M.R. SOMERFIELD & D.G. PFISTER. 1999. American Society of Clinical Oncology technology assessment on breast cancer risk reduction strategies: tamoxifen and raloxifene. J. Clin. Oncol. **17:** 1939–1955.
38. GOODMAN, S.N. 1999. Probability at the bedside: the knowing of chances or the chances of knowing? Ann. Intern. Med. **130:** 604–606.
39. PHILLIPS, K-A., G. GLENDON & J.A. KNIGHT. 1999. Putting the risk of breast cancer in perspective. N. Engl. J. Med. **340:** 141–144.
40. CUMMINGS, S.R., S. ECKERT, K.A. KRUEGER *et al.* 1999. The effect of raloxifene on risk of breast cancer in postmenopausal women: results from the MORE randomized trial—Multiple Outcomes of Raloxifene Evaluation. JAMA **281:** 2189–2197.
41. ETTINGER, B., D.M. BLACK, B.H. MITLAK *et al.* 1999. Reduction of vertebral fracture risk in postmenopausal women with osteoporosis treated with raloxifene: results from a 3-year randomized clinical trial. JAMA **282:** 637–645.
42. DELMAS, P.D., N.H. BJARNASON, B.H. MITLAK *et al.* 1997. Effects of raloxifene on bone mineral density, serum cholesterol concentrations, and uterine endometrium in postmenopausal women. N. Engl. J. Med. **337:** 1641–1647.

The Royal Marsden Hospital (RMH) Trial
Key Points and Remaining Questions

TREVOR J. POWLES

Royal Marsden Hospital, Sutton Surrey SM2 5PT, United Kingdom

ABSTRACT: The reported interim analysis of the Royal Marsden chemoprevention trial, giving tamoxifen (20 mg/day) for up to 8 years to healthy women at increased risk of breast cancer because of a family history, has failed to confirm the 49% reduction in overall early incidence of breast cancer reported from the National Surgical Adjuvant Breast and Bowel Project (NSABP) P-1 trial. Although statistically compatible, this discrepancy in results raises the possibility that the sensitivity to tamoxifen chemoprevention may depend on the population characteristics of the participants in the two trials. Younger women who do not have lobular carcinoma *in situ* or atypical ductal hyperplasia, or who may be at high risk of carrying a breast cancer predisposing gene, may be relatively resistant to tamoxifen chemoprevention. Furthermore, the clinical benefit of a reduction in the early incidence of breast cancer by using tamoxifen in healthy women has not been clearly established by the P-1 trial because of the lack of mortality data. Use of tamoxifen for risk reduction in healthy women needs to take into account these factors, and more information needs to be gained from the continuing placebo-controlled trials that are under way.

KEYWORDS: tamoxifen; breast cancer; chemoprevention; hormone replacement therapy (HRT)

INTRODUCTION

Based on experimental data showing that tamoxifen reduces the incidence of experimental endocrine-dependent rat mammary cancers[1] and on the reported reduction in the incidence of contralateral breast cancer in patients who were given adjuvant tamoxifen,[2] we started a pilot trial in 1986 to evaluate the use of tamoxifen for chemoprevention of breast cancer in healthy women.[3]

A total of 2494 women were randomized between October 1986 and April 1996 to receive tamoxifen (20 mg/day) or placebo. The median age of participants was 47 years (range: 30–70 years) and 66% of these women were pre- or perimenopausal. Use of hormone replacement therapy (HRT) was not contraindicated in this trial because it was considered that censure and exclusion of women who required HRT while on the trial could introduce a potential bias. Furthermore, we considered it unlikely that tamoxifen would interact negatively with HRT as it has similar efficacy as adjuvant therapy in pre- and postmenopausal women not receiving chemotherapy. Sixteen percent of women were on HRT at the time of randomization and a further

---

Address for correspondence: Dr. Trevor J. Powles, Royal Marsden Hospital, Downs Road, Sutton Surrey SM2 5PT, United Kingdom. Voice: 44-(0)20-8661 3361; fax: 44-(0)20-8770 7313.

trevor.powles@rmh.nthames.nhs.uk

26% of participants required HRT at some time after randomization. Throughout the whole trial, concomitant use of HRT at the same time as tamoxifen occurred during only 13% of the tamoxifen medication period.

Women who were eligible for the trial were aged between 30 and 70 years with no clinical or screening evidence of breast cancer, but with an increased risk of breast cancer because of a family history. Each participant had at least one first-degree relative under the age of 50 with breast cancer, one first-degree relative with bilateral breast cancer, or one affected first-degree relative of any age plus another affected first- or second-degree relative. Twenty-two percent of women had a previous benign breast surgical biopsy. There were no significant differences in distribution of any prognostic factors between treatment groups.

At the time of the interim analysis in 1998,[4] there was a median follow-up of 70 months; compliance was good, with 63% of women taking tamoxifen at 5 years compared to 73% of women taking placebo. Toxicity was low, with an increased incidence of hot flashes ($P < 0.0005$), gynecological problems ($P < 0.005$), and menstrual abnormalities ($P = 0.01$). Noncompliance because of toxicity occurred in 320 women on tamoxifen compared to 176 women on placebo ($P < 0.0005$).

At the time of this analysis, there was no difference in the incidence of breast cancer for women randomized to receive tamoxifen (34) or placebo (36) ($P = 0.8$).[4] Eight patients, four from each group, had ductal carcinoma *in situ*. After adjustment for all pretreatment prognostic factors, the randomized treatment of tamoxifen or placebo was not predictive of breast cancer. Furthermore, there was no identified interaction between the use of HRT and any effect of tamoxifen on breast cancer incidence. Twelve of 523 women who received HRT developed breast cancer compared with 13 of 507 on placebo ($P = 0.6$). Correction for possible confounding factors in multivariate analysis confirmed the result. Compliance was assessed by direct questioning and confirmed by measurement of tamoxifen and its metabolites in participants who developed breast cancer in the trial.

DISCUSSION

It was surprising that the Royal Marsden pilot trial failed to show any effect of tamoxifen with this duration of follow-up and number of events. The NSABP P-1 trial[5] was substantially more powerful than the Royal Marsden trial; however, although the results of both trials are statistically compatible, our negative result would indicate that the overall effect is likely to be less than the reported 49% reduction in early incidence reported in the P-1 trial.[5] This could be compounded by differences in the risk characteristics of the populations of women in the two trials, which could account for a differential response to tamoxifen. There are indications from the NSABP P-1 trial that different risk groups of women may respond differently to the effect of tamoxifen on early incidence. There was a relatively large reduction in breast cancer incidence in women on tamoxifen who had atypical ductal hyperplasia (ADH) (RR = 0.14) or lobular carcinoma *in situ* (LCIS) (RR = 0.44), presumably for the most part in younger women. The remainder of P-1 participants under 50, who were at a risk as defined by the Gail model,[6] were therefore likely to have gained less benefit from tamoxifen. It is possible that the participants in the Royal Marsden trial, who were generally younger than in the P-1 trial and who did not have LCIS or ADH as an entry criterion, were relatively more resistant to the effects of tamoxifen. In these circumstances, our trial would lack the power to show any small reduction in incidence. In the Royal Marsden trial, it was estimated, using the Claus model,[7] that approximately 36% of participants and more than 60% of those who developed breast cancer were likely to have inherited a breast cancer predisposition gene. The estrogen promotion of breast cancer may not be the same for these younger women who have inherited a high-risk breast cancer predisposing gene compared to those who develop sporadic cancers.

REMAINING QUESTIONS

There is no doubt that the NSABP P-1 trial overall has shown a significant reduction in the early incidence of invasive and noninvasive breast cancers. However, uncertainty remains about the long-term benefit of these observed reductions in early incidence of breast cancer because the NSABP P-1 trial was stopped before the mortality data had matured sufficiently to show any survival benefit. It is thus not possible at this time to say whether it was better to have treated 6647 healthy women with tamoxifen rather than having 86 extra patients with breast cancers, as seen in the placebo arm, all of which were estrogen receptor–positive and highly curable.

Furthermore, it is difficult to evaluate any overall clinical benefit without mortality data. Besides the 86 fewer invasive breast cancers, there were 34 fewer noninvasive breast cancers and 26 fewer osteoporotic fractures, which needs to be balanced against 21 additional endometrial cancers together with 14 extra strokes, 12 extra pulmonary emboli, 13 extra deep vein thromboses, and 67 extra cataracts.

CONCLUSIONS

The results of the P-1 trial have clearly shown the possibility that breast cancer can be prevented by giving tamoxifen to healthy women. However, at this time, there is uncertainty whether this observed reduction in early incidence is more effective and less toxic than treatment of cancers as they arise and which groups of women at risk gain benefit. The continued follow-up of the placebo-controlled trials in Europe is essential in order to establish overall, long-term clinical benefit from any observed reduction in incidence and to identify which women are likely to gain this benefit.

REFERENCES

1. JORDAN, V. 1976. Effect of tamoxifen (ICI 46,474) on initiation and growth of DMBA-induced rat mammary carcinomata. Eur. J. Cancer **12:** 419–425.
2. CUZICK, J. & M. BAUM. 1985. Tamoxifen and contralateral breast cancer [letter]. Lancet **ii:** 282.
3. POWLES, T., J. HARDY, S. ASHLEY et al. 1989. A pilot trial to evaluate the acute toxicity and feasibility of tamoxifen for prevention of breast cancer. Br. J. Cancer **60:** 126–131.
4. POWLES, T., R. EELES, S. ASHLEY et al. 1998. Interim analysis of the incidence of breast cancer in the Royal Marsden Hospital tamoxifen randomised chemoprevention trial. Lancet **352:** 98–101.

5. FISHER, B., J. COSTANTINO, D.L. WICKERHAM *et al.* 1998. Tamoxifen for prevention of breast cancer: report of the National Surgical Adjuvant Breast and Bowel Project P-1 Study. J. Natl. Cancer Inst. **90:** 1371–1388.
6. GAIL, M., L. BRINTON, D. BYAR *et al.* 1989. Projecting individualised probabilities of developing breast cancer for white females who are examined annually. J. Natl. Cancer Inst. **81:** 1879–1886.
7. CLAUS, E., N. RISCH & W. THOMPSON. 1990. Age at onset as an indicator of familial risk of breast cancer. Am. J. Epidemiol. **131:** 961–972.

The Italian Breast Cancer Prevention Trial with Tamoxifen

Findings and New Perspectives

ALIANA GUERRIERI-GONZAGA,[a] ARIANNA GALLI,[a] NICOLE ROTMENSZ,[b] AND ANDREA DECENSI[a]

[a]*Division of Chemoprevention and* [b]*Division of Epidemiology and Biostatistics, European Institute of Oncology, Milan, Italy*

ABSTRACT: The Italian Tamoxifen Prevention Study includes 5408 healthy hysterectomized women aged 35–70 years who have been randomized to 20 mg/day of tamoxifen or placebo for 5 years. After 46 months median follow-up, an increased risk of venous vascular events (38 women on tamoxifen vs. 18 women on placebo, $P = 0.0053$), mainly consisting of superficial phlebitis, has been observed and 41 breast cancers have occurred (19 on tamoxifen vs. 22 on placebo, $P = 0.64$). However, subgroup analyses indicated a borderline significant reduction of breast cancer among women continuously on estrogen replacement therapy (ERT, mostly transdermal) and receiving tamoxifen, with 8 cases of breast cancer among 390 ERT users on placebo versus 1 case among 362 ERT users on tamoxifen (RR = 0.13, 95% CI = 0.02–1.02). Withdrawal rate (mainly due to menopausal symptoms) differed according to ERT use, with compliance being 78% and 75% at 3 and 5 years, respectively, for women who never took ERT, and 92% and 88% at 3 and 5 years, respectively, for women not on ERT at baseline, but who took ERT at some time during the trial. Pharmacokinetic and pharmacodynamic (surrogate end point biomarkers) studies showed that a lower dose of tamoxifen (such as 5 mg/day) does not affect the drug's activity on several biomarkers of both cardiovascular and breast cancer risk. We are therefore planning a multicenter placebo-controlled phase III trial in postmenopausal healthy women on hormone replacement therapy (HRT) to test whether the combination of HRT and low-dose tamoxifen retains the benefits while reducing the risks of either agent maintaining a high compliance rate.

KEYWORDS: selective estrogen receptor modulator (SERM); breast cancer prevention; estrogen replacement therapy (ERT); tamoxifen

Tamoxifen is a nonsteroidal triphenylethylene derivative that can be classified as a first-generation selective estrogen receptor modulator (SERM).[1,2] It is widely used for palliative endocrine treatment of advanced breast cancer and as adjuvant therapy to control micrometastatic relapse and new primaries in women treated surgically for

Address for correspondence: Andrea Decensi, M.D., Director, Division of Chemoprevention, European Institute of Oncology, Via Ripamonti, 435, 20141 Milan, Italy. Voice: +39-0257489861; fax: +39-0257489809.
andrea.decensi@ieo.it

early breast cancer.[2] Tamoxifen has also been investigated in three large cooperative phase III trials for breast cancer prevention in at-risk women. While the preliminary results of two European studies, conducted in Italy (Italian Tamoxifen Prevention Study) and in the United Kingdom (Royal Marsden Tamoxifen Chemoprevention Trial), have shown no significant difference so far,[3,4] the American (National Surgical Adjuvant Breast and Bowel Project, NSABP P-1) trial has shown a 50% reduction of the risk of both invasive and noninvasive breast cancer and a 69% reduction of the occurrence of estrogen receptor–positive tumors.[5]

The Italian Tamoxifen Prevention Study is a multicenter, double-blind, placebo-controlled, chemoprevention trial, started in October 1992, to evaluate the effect of a daily dose of 20 mg/day of tamoxifen for five years in reducing breast cancer incidence. Eligible subjects are healthy women, 35–70 years old, who have had prior hysterectomy for nonmalignant conditions. Recruitment was closed on December 1997 with a total of 5408 women randomized. Overall, after a median follow-up of 46 months for adverse events, there was an increased risk of venous vascular events (38 women on tamoxifen vs. 18 women on placebo, $P = 0.0053$), mainly consisting of superficial phlebitis.[4] Seventeen cases of hypertriglyceridemia (15 on tamoxifen vs. 2 on placebo, $P = 0.0013$) were also observed, although abnormal triglyceride levels were based on patient self-reports in addition to laboratory-confirmed findings. Therefore, this information probably underestimates the occurrence of these events in the study. As regards major end points such as death and cancer, a total of 41 breast cancers occurred (19 on tamoxifen and 22 on placebo, $P = 0.64$). Among the 15 deaths from all causes, none was due to breast cancer. However, unplanned subgroup analyses gave more interesting clues. A borderline significant reduction of breast cancer was observed among women who were continuously on estrogen replacement therapy (ERT, mostly by transdermal route) and received tamoxifen. Compared to the 8 cases of breast cancer that occurred among the 390 ERT users on placebo, there was 1 case of breast cancer among the 362 ERT users who were on tamoxifen (RR = 0.13, 95% CI = 0.02–1.02).[4] This beneficial trend has been confirmed in a recent updated analysis.[6] These results are based on subgroup analysis and should therefore be taken cautiously. However, they generate an interesting hypothesis that will be tested in a future randomized trial.

Although our study was regarded as being affected by a high dropout rate,[7] a comparison of the three primary prevention trials of tamoxifen indicated that, in fact, the number of discontinuations for reasons other than major events was 20.7%, 28.8%, and 35.5% in the Italian, American, and English trials, respectively.[8] In our trial, the dropout rate was higher during the first year of recruitment and plateaued thereafter (2% per month in the first year vs. 1% in years 2–5). Since most women who left the study voluntarily did so mainly because of menopausal symptoms, the combination of tamoxifen and ERT might reduce tamoxifen side effects. Indeed, the rate of voluntary withdrawals was different according to ERT use: compliance with treatment was 78% at 3 years and 75% at 5 years for women who never took ERT (FIG. 1, curve A); in contrast, for women who were not on ERT at baseline, but who took ERT at some time during the trial, the compliance was 92% at 3 years and 88% at 5 years (FIG. 1, curve B). The figures for 3 years are based upon 2204, 385, and 433 women, respectively, while those at 5 years are based upon 500, 111, and 151 women for "never on ERT," "no ERT at baseline, then on," and "always on ERT,"

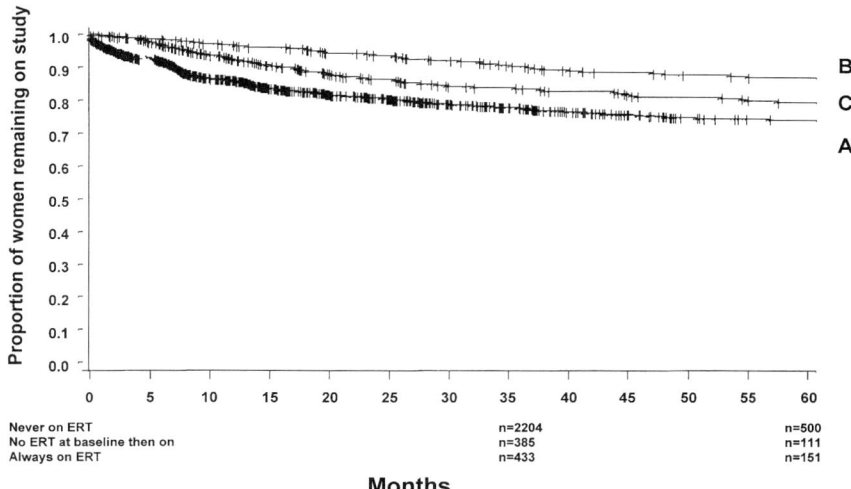

FIGURE 1. Voluntary withdrawal from the Italian tamoxifen prevention trial. The figures for 3 years are based upon 2204, 385, and 433 women, while those at 5 years are based upon 500, 111, and 151 women who were (A) never on ERT, (B) not on ERT at baseline, but then on ERT during the study, and (C) always on ERT, respectively.

respectively (FIG. 1). These data suggest that compliance may be increased by concomitant use of ERT and tamoxifen.

The use of progestins in the hormone replacement therapy (HRT) regimen might reduce the risk of endometrial cancer associated with tamoxifen treatment. Indeed, the NSABP P-1 trial showed that women aged 50 or younger had no increased incidence of adverse events, including endometrial cancer and venous thromboembolic events.[5] This suggests that the concomitant presence of adequate circulating hormone levels might prevent tamoxifen from acting as an estrogen agonist at these target tissues. In addition, previous studies have shown that the combination of HRT and tamoxifen does not adversely influence their biological effects, including bone density and clotting factors,[9] and our group has recently shown that the beneficial effects of tamoxifen on cardiovascular risk factors are unchanged in current HRT users.[10] Altogether, these considerations provide a strong rationale for further investigations of the combination of tamoxifen and HRT in an attempt to reduce the risk while retaining the benefits of both agents.

As regards breast cancer risk associated with HRT use, the metanalysis of 51 epidemiological studies including 52,705 individuals with breast cancer and 108,411 control women, accounting for 90% of the worldwide evidence, has shown that use of oral HRT is associated with an overall increased risk of breast cancer (RR = 1.14, SE = 0.03, $P = 0.00001$).[11] The risk increased with duration of HRT (RR = 1.35, 95% CI = 1.21–1.49 after an average of 11 years) and progressively decreased after HRT discontinuation, with no excess risk after 5 years from cessation. Interestingly, the magnitude of the increased risk (2.3% per year, 95% CI = 1.1%–3.6%) is comparable to that associated with each year of delayed menopause (i.e., 2.8% per year, 95% CI = 2.1%–3.4%), strongly upholding the hypothesis that maintenance of a premenopausal hormonal milieu may account for the reported increased risk in HRT users. Importantly, the increased risk observed in current and recent HRT users was greater for women with lower body mass index (i.e., BMI < 25 kg/m^2).

Although little information was available regarding hormonal type and dose and 80% of these women had used oral estrogen alone, the addition of progestins was associated with a higher RR of breast cancer than estrogen alone. The RR values were 1.15 (SE, 0.19) and 1.53 (SE, 0.33) in current or recent users of estro-progestins for ≤5 years and >5 years, respectively, compared with RR of 0.99 (SE, 0.08) and 1.34 (SE, 0.09) for current or recent users of estrogens alone. Finally, cancers in women who had ever used HRT tended to be less advanced clinically than those in never users. In this regard, a prospective cohort study of 37,105 HRT users in the Iowa Women's Health Study has shown that exposure to HRT was associated with an increased risk of invasive breast cancer with a favorable histologic type, while there was little evidence of association with other invasive ductal or lobular cancers or ductal carcinoma *in situ*.[12] These findings have not been confirmed in other studies.[13] Also, a trend to longer survival in HRT users who developed breast cancer compared to never users has been observed in some studies.[14] A previous analysis from the Nurses' Health Study[15] showed a moderately elevated risk of breast cancer death among postmenopausal women who were taking oral estrogen or had previously used this therapy for 10 or more years. Notably, a recent update of the cohort shows that the addition of progestins was associated with a 9% (SE, 2.5) increased risk per year as compared to 3.3% (SE, 0.84) with estrogen alone.[16] Likewise, a recent analysis from the Breast Cancer Detection Demonstration Project (BCDDP) based on 2082 incident breast cancer cases found that the estrogen-progestin regimens were associated with greater increases in breast cancer risk than estrogen alone (8% per year, 95% CI = 2%–16%, vs. 1% per year, 95% CI = 0.2%–3%, for each year of estrogen alone).[13] Importantly, the increased risk is largely limited to current or recent users and is directly related to duration of use. An updated analysis in a Swedish cohort also found greater risks with combined therapy: for 6 or more years of current or recent use, the risk of breast cancer was increased by 70% for combined therapy, but no increase was seen for estrogen alone.[17] A case-control study recently performed in California among 1897 postmenopausal case subjects and 1637 postmenopausal control subjects also showed that combined estro-progestin therapy was associated with a higher risk of breast cancer compared to unopposed ERT.[18] The OR for 5 years of HRT use was 1.10 (95% CI = 1.02–1.18). Risk was higher for continuous HRT (estro-progestin) users (OR = 1.24, 95% CI = 1.07–1.45) than for ERT users (OR = 1.06, 95% CI = 0.97–1.15). There was a trend for sequential HRT (i.e., with progestins given for 10 or more days per month) being associated with a higher risk (OR = 1.38, 95% CI = 1.13–1.68) than combined continuous HRT (i.e., with progestins given continuously), where the OR was 1.09 (95% CI = 0.88–1.35), but this was not statistically significant. These results were not confirmed in the Swedish cohort, where continuous combined HRT was associated with a higher risk than sequential HRT.[19] Differences between progesterone- and testosterone-derived progestin use may partly account for these discrepancies. Overall, these studies provide firm evidence that addition of progestin to estrogen does not reduce the risk of breast cancer and suggest that the risk is actually increased.[20]

It must be emphasized that all of the above data are based solely on studies making use of orally administered estrogens. Since the extensive use of transdermal HRT is relatively recent, no epidemiological data are available yet on its association with breast cancer risk. However, the parenteral route of administration, in contrast to the oral route, is associated with the following endocrine effects: a trend to an increase in circulating insulin-like growth factor-I (IGF-I) levels, one of the most potent breast mitogens;[21,22] a lower conversion to the weak estrogen, estrone;[23,24] and a higher availability of free estrogen levels due to unchanged sex hormone binding globulin (SHBG) levels.[21,23,25] These effects might be associated with an increased risk of breast cancer. While further studies are needed to clarify this issue, new strategies to minimize the risk of breast cancer are demanded.

From the biological point of view, the increased risk of breast cancer associated with HRT use is linked to an increased expression of estrogen receptors in the breast tissue,[26] thus leading to an enhanced sensitivity to the mitogenic effect of estrogen. The addition of a SERM, such as tamoxifen, capable of reducing this growth-promoting effect on the breast could thus be useful for women's health maintenance. On the other hand, one of the major concerns about this drug is the increased risk of endometrial cancer. In the NSABP P-1 prevention study, the rate of endometrial cancer was increased in the tamoxifen group (RR = 2.53, 95% CI = 1.35–4.97), with the increased risk occurring predominantly in women aged 50 years or older. In women aged 49 or younger, RR was 1.21 with 95% CI = 0.41–3.60; in women aged ≥50, RR was 4.01 with 95% CI = 1.70–10.90. This suggests that the woman's endocrine milieu can influence the pharmacodynamics of tamoxifen at the endometrial level. Specifically, progesterone could neutralize tamoxifen's agonistic activity on the endometrium in much the same manner as progesterone countered the proliferative effect of estrogen in this organ. Moreover, all endometrial cancers observed in the NSABP P-1 trial were stage I and no endometrial cancer deaths were reported in the tamoxifen group.[5]

There is also indirect evidence that the risk of endometrial cancer induced by tamoxifen is both time- and dose-dependent, with the higher relative risk being observed with daily doses of 30 or 40 mg/day of adjuvant tamoxifen.[27] Thus, one plausible way to lower this risk is a reduction of the dose.[28] We therefore studied the biological activity of tamoxifen with a view to establishing a dosing schedule with a better risk-benefit ratio.[29,30] The blood concentrations of tamoxifen and its main metabolites were measured in a dose titration study in 105 healthy women (placebo, tamoxifen 10 mg on alternate days, 10 mg/day, and 20 mg/day). Drug levels measured after 2 months of treatment were correlated with the changes in several biomarkers, such as total cholesterol, HDL cholesterol, LDL cholesterol, triglycerides, lipoprotein (a), blood cell count, fibrinogen, antithrombin III, osteocalcin, and IGF-I. Mean (± SD) tamoxifen and N-desmethyltamoxifen (metabolite X) concentrations were dose-related, being, respectively, 0 and 0 ng/mL with placebo, 26.8 ± 15.1 and 43.7 ± 22.5 ng/mL with 10 mg every other day, 51.2 ± 24.1 and 90.7 ± 48 ng/mL with 10 mg/day, and 136 ± 52.7 and 230.6 ± 75.0 ng/mL with 20 mg/day of tamoxifen. In contrast, the biomarker levels were of comparable magnitudes at all drug concentrations, with the exception of platelet counts and triglyceride levels, both of which showed a trend toward increasing with increasing tamoxifen concentrations. Thus, a 75% reduction of the conventional dose, which resulted in an 80% decrease in serum drug concentration, did not affect tamoxifen activity on several biomarkers of cardiovascular and breast cancer risk and may in fact have a more favorable safety profile.[30]

We have subsequently set up an experiment that is reciprocal and complementary to our previous trial, namely, a study of the correlation of tamoxifen elimination with biomarker recovery in healthy subjects completing the 5-year intervention period.[31] Tamoxifen, N-desmethyltamoxifen, and biomarker levels were measured at 0 (baseline), 2, 4, and 6 weeks after completion of treatment in 23 healthy postmenopausal women allocated to tamoxifen (20 mg/day) and in 6 women allocated to placebo. Mean ($\pm$ SD) serum tamoxifen and N-desmethyltamoxifen concentrations were, respectively, 141 ± 50 and 226 ± 77 ng/mL at baseline, 36 ± 19 and 99 ± 46 ng/mL at 2 weeks, 20 ± 15 and 61 ± 37 ng/mL at 4 weeks, and 12 ± 9 and 36 ± 26 ng/mL at 6 weeks. Compared to baseline values, the percent increase in total cholesterol, LDL cholesterol, and IGF-I at 4 weeks after treatment completion was 5%, 9%, and 14%, respectively. No change during the 6-week period was observed in the placebo arm. After 1 month of treatment discontinuation, the biomarkers' recovery was far from complete, despite tamoxifen concentrations in the range of 10 ng/mL, that is, approximately 15 times lower than the steady state concentrations attained with 20 mg/day.[31] Consistent with observations in breast cancer patients treated for a short term[32] or for longer periods,[33] tamoxifen and N-desmethyltamoxifen serum concentrations were halved after 9 and 13 days, respectively. These findings underscore the importance of assessing the most appropriate schedule for preventive agents based on their pharmacokinetic characteristics. Although the limited observation time and the specific drug pharmacokinetics prevented us from inferring the minimal active concentration, our data suggest that biomarker recovery is slower than tamoxifen elimination from blood. This is in agreement with the observation that tamoxifen is retained in tissues for a long time[34] and indicates that tamoxifen may exert biological effects for several weeks after treatment interruption.

Since tamoxifen has a very high tissue/serum concentration ratio,[34,35] the tissue level attainable with 10 mg every other day exceeds the growth inhibitory concentration of tamoxifen and N-desmethyltamoxifen in breast cancer cell lines, which is approximately 35 ng/mL.[36–38] In addition, the concomitant activity of metabolite X, which has a significant growth inhibitory activity in breast cancer cell lines, may further contribute to the total drug inhibitory activity. Moreover, *in vivo* studies in a spontaneous rat mammary tumor model showed that a dose equivalent to 1 mg/day in humans leads to a 94% inhibition of mammary tumor formation compared to control animals.[39] Interestingly, a recent cross-sectional study conducted in older nursing home residents in New York State long-term facilities has shown a significant reduction of bone fracture rate among women with breast cancer taking 10 mg/day of tamoxifen. During the first 1.5-year period for which bone fractures were documented, the fracture rates were 7.6% in 5196 untreated control women, 3.2% in the 125 women receiving 10 mg/day of tamoxifen, and 6.7% in the 1248 women receiving 20 mg/day of tamoxifen. The OR for 20 mg/day compared to controls is 0.92 (0.72–1.16), while the OR for 10 mg/day versus controls is 0.31 (0.11–0.87, $P = 0.025$).[40] Altogether, these findings provide a strong rationale to assess a lower dose of tamoxifen in a preventive context, as reported in TABLE 1.

Taking into account all the above-mentioned considerations, it seems reasonable to test whether the combination of HRT and low doses of tamoxifen may retain the benefits while reducing the risks of either agent. A summary of the potential benefits

TABLE 1. Tamoxifen: rationale for a dose reduction

- The minimal active dose is unknown
- Tamoxifen's antitumor activity reaches a plateau above the concentration that saturates the ER
- 20 mg/day of tamoxifen is as effective as 30–40 mg/day
- The endometrial effect is dose dependent
- A dose reduction might minimize toxicity while retaining activity

TABLE 2. Potential benefit of the combination of tamoxifen and HRT

- ⇓ Breast cancer risk associated with HRT
- ⇓ Dropout rate in tamoxifen studies[a]
- ⇓ Endometrial cancer associated with tamoxifen
- ⇓ Tamoxifen side effects? (vasomotor and urogenital symptoms)[a]

[a]Reduction in tamoxifen side effects is a major contributor to decreased dropout rates in tamoxifen studies.

of the combination of these two agents is reported in TABLE 2. We are therefore setting up a multicenter placebo-controlled phase III trial in postmenopausal healthy women currently on HRT (no more than 3 years are allowed) or in *de novo* users. Women will be randomized to 5 mg/day of tamoxifen or placebo for 5 years. The study design is shown in FIGURE 2. The study is powered to detect a 40% reduction in the incidence of invasive breast cancer and ductal carcinoma *in situ* in the tamoxifen arm. Secondary end points will be the incidence of other noninvasive breast disorders, endometrial cancer, bone fractures, cardiovascular events, venous thromboembolic events, cataracts, all other cancers (in particular, colorectal and ovary), and overall mortality. An ancillary study is being conducted to assess the minimal active dose and the best treatment schedule of tamoxifen, through the modulation of a set of surrogate end point biomarkers (SEBs) of breast carcinogenesis in 200 postmenopausal healthy women undergoing HRT. Women will be randomized to one of the following arms:

- tamoxifen 5 mg/day + placebo/week,
- tamoxifen 1 mg/day + placebo/week,
- placebo/day + tamoxifen 10 mg/week, *or*
- placebo/day + placebo/week.

Treatment duration will be 1 year. The primary end point is the change in IGF-I at 12 months. Secondary end points will be the changes of endometrial thickness and the occurrence of histological abnormalities of the endometrium; changes of hemogram, lipid profile (total cholesterol, LDL, HDL, triglycerides), fibrinogen, antithrombin III, osteocalcin, homocysteine, and C-reactive protein (CRP); and changes of plasma IGF-I ratio [IGF-I/IGF binding protein-3 (IGFBP-3)]. All of these changes

The study is a randomized, double-blind, placebo-controlled phase III trial with the following design:

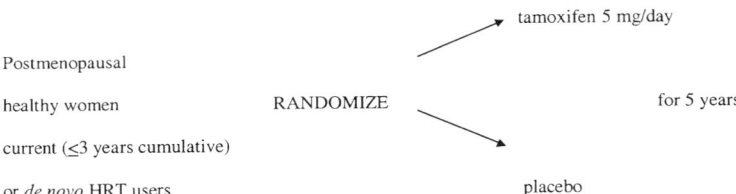

Postmenopausal healthy women current (≤3 years cumulative) or *de novo* HRT users → RANDOMIZE → tamoxifen 5 mg/day / placebo, for 5 years

It will be a multicenter trial, and a total of 8500 subjects is required, 4250 per arm.

Primary endpoint

Incidence of invasive and intraductal breast cancer

Secondary endpoints

Incidence of: other non-invasive breast disorders
endometrial cancer
bone fractures
cardiovascular events
venous thromboembolic events
cataract
all other cancers
overall mortality

Sample size

4250 subjects per arm
Hazard ratio = 0.6
Annual rate of events = 4/1000
Compliance = 80%
Recruitment = 5 years
Follow-up = 5 years
Power = 80%

FIGURE 2. HOT (hormone replacement therapy and tamoxifen) study: design and end points.

will be correlated with tamoxifen and metabolite concentrations. The HOT study is expected to start recruitment by the beginning of the year 2002 and could potentially yield important information regarding breast cancer risk reduction.

REFERENCES

1. PLOWMAN, P.N. 1993. Tamoxifen as adjuvant therapy in breast cancer: current status. Drugs **46:** 819–833.
2. JAIYESIMI, I.A. et al. 1995. Use of tamoxifen for breast cancer: twenty-eight years later. J. Clin. Oncol. **13:** 513–529.
3. POWLES, T. et al. 1998. Interim analysis of the incidence of breast cancer in the Royal Marsden Hospital tamoxifen randomised chemoprevention trial. Lancet **352:** 98–101.
4. VERONESI, U. et al. 1998. Prevention of breast cancer with tamoxifen: preliminary findings from the Italian randomised trial among hysterectomised women—Italian Tamoxifen Prevention Study. Lancet **352:** 93–97.
5. FISHER, B. et al. 1998. Tamoxifen for prevention of breast cancer: report of the National Surgical Adjuvant Breast and Bowel Project P-1 Study. J. Natl. Cancer Inst. **90:** 1371–1388.
6. DECENSI, A. et al. 2001. Prevention of breast cancer with tamoxifen: update of the Italian trial in hysterectomized women [abstract 4441]. Proc. Am. Assoc. Cancer Res. **42:** 827
7. PRITCHARD, K.I. 1998. Is tamoxifen effective in prevention of breast cancer? Lancet **352:** 80–81.
8. VERONESI, U. et al. 1999. Drop-outs in tamoxifen prevention trials. Lancet **353:** 244.
9. CHANG, J. et al. 1996. The effect of tamoxifen and hormone replacement therapy on serum cholesterol, bone mineral density, and coagulation factors in healthy postmenopausal women participating in a randomised, controlled tamoxifen prevention study. Ann. Oncol. **7:** 671–675.
10. DECENSI, A. et al. 1998. Effect of tamoxifen and transdermal hormone replacement therapy on cardiovascular risk factors in a prevention trial: Italian Chemoprevention Group. Br. J. Cancer **78:** 572–578.
11. COLLABORATIVE GROUP ON HORMONAL FACTORS IN BREAST CANCER. 1997. Breast cancer and hormone replacement therapy: collaborative reanalysis of data from 51 epidemiological studies of 52,705 women with breast cancer and 108,411 women without breast cancer. Lancet **350:** 1047–1059.
12. GAPSTUR, S.M., M. MORROW & T.A. SELLERS. 1999. Hormone replacement therapy and risk of breast cancer with a favorable histology: results of the Iowa Women's Health Study. JAMA **281:** 2091–2097.
13. SCHAIRER, C. et al. 2000. Menopausal estrogen and estrogen-progestin replacement therapy and breast cancer risk. JAMA **283:** 485–491.
14. SCHAIRER, C. et al. 1999. Estrogen replacement therapy and breast cancer survival in a large screening study. J. Natl. Cancer Inst. **91:** 264–270.
15. COLDITZ, G.A. et al. 1995. The use of estrogens and progestins and the risk of breast cancer in postmenopausal women. N. Engl. J. Med. **332:** 1589–1593.
16. COLDITZ, G.A. & B. ROSNER. 1998. Use of estrogen plus progestin is associated with greater increase in breast cancer risk than estrogen alone. Am. J. Epidemiol. **147**(suppl.): 64S.
17. PERSSON, I. et al. 1999. Risks of breast and endometrial cancer after estrogen and estrogen-progestin replacement. Cancer Causes Control **10:** 253–260.
18. ROSS, R.K. et al. 2000. Effect of hormone replacement therapy on breast cancer risk: estrogen versus estrogen plus progestin. J. Natl. Cancer Inst. **92:** 328–332.
19. MAGNUSSON, D., I. PERSSON & O. ADAMI. 2000. More about: effect of hormone replacement therapy on breast cancer risk—estrogen versus estrogen plus progestin. J. Natl. Cancer Inst. **92:** 1183–1184.
20. WILLETT, W.C., G. COLDITZ & M. STAMPFER. 2000. Postmenopausal estrogens—opposed, unopposed, or none of the above. JAMA **283:** 534–535.
21. SLOWINSKA-SRZEDNICKA, J. et al. 1992. Transdermal 17-beta-estradiol combined with oral progestogen increases plasma levels of insulin-like growth factor-I in postmenopausal women. J. Endocrinol. Invest. **15:** 533–538.
22. WEISSBERGER, A.J., K.K. HOL & L. LAZARUS. 1991. Contrasting effects of oral and transdermal routes of estrogen replacement therapy on 24-hour growth hormone

(GH) secretion, insulin-like growth factor I, and GH-binding protein in postmenopausal women. J. Clin. Endocrinol. Metab. **72:** 374–381.
23. VAN ERPECUM, K.J. *et al.* 1991. Different hepatobiliary effects of oral and transdermal estradiol in postmenopausal women. Gastroenterology **100:** 482–488.
24. WALSH, B.W., H. LI & F.M. SACKS. 1994. Effects of postmenopausal hormone replacement with oral and transdermal estrogen on high density lipoprotein metabolism. J. Lipid Res. **35:** 2083–2093.
25. CHETKOWSKI, R.J. *et al.* 1986. Biologic effects of transdermal estradiol. N. Engl. J. Med. **314:** 1615–1620.
26. KHAN, S.A. *et al.* 1998. Estrogen receptor expression in benign breast epithelium and breast cancer risk. J. Natl. Cancer Inst. **90:** 37–42.
27. RUTQVIST, L.E. *et al.* 1995. Adjuvant tamoxifen therapy for early stage breast cancer and second primary malignancies: Stockholm Breast Cancer Study Group. J. Natl Cancer Inst. **87:** 645–651.
28. JORDAN, V.C. 1999. Tamoxifen: too much for a good thing? J. Clin. Oncol. **17:** 2629–2630.
29. DECENSI, A. *et al.* 1998. Biologic activity of tamoxifen at low doses in healthy women. J. Natl. Cancer Inst. **90:** 1461–1467.
30. DECENSI, A. *et al.* 1999. Effect of blood tamoxifen concentrations on surrogate biomarkers in a trial of dose reduction. J. Clin. Oncol. **17:** 2633–2638.
31. GUERRIERI-GONZAGA, A. *et al.* 2001. Correlation between tamoxifen elimination and biomarker recovery in a primary prevention trial. Cancer Epidemiol. Biomarker Prev. **10:** 967–970.
32. FABIAN, C. *et al.* 1981. Clinical pharmacology of tamoxifen in patients with breast cancer: correlation with clinical data. Cancer **48:** 876–882.
33. LANGAN-FAHEY, S.M., D.C. TORMEY & V.C. JORDAN. 1990. Tamoxifen metabolites in patients on long-term adjuvant therapy for breast cancer. Eur. J. Cancer **26:** 883–888.
34. LIEN, E.A., E. SOLHEIM & P.M. UELAND. 1991. Distribution of tamoxifen and its metabolites in rat and human tissues during steady-state treatment. Cancer Res. **51:** 4837–4844.
35. ROBINSON, S.P. *et al.* 1991. Metabolites, pharmacodynamics, and pharmacokinetics of tamoxifen in rats and mice compared to the breast cancer patient. Drug Metab. Dispos. **19:** 36–43.
36. SUTHERLAND, R.L. *et al.* 1987. Mechanisms of growth inhibition by nonsteroidal antioestrogens in human breast cancer cells. J. Steroid Biochem. **27:** 891–897.
37. LIPPMAN, M., G. BOLAN & K. HUFF. 1976. The effects of estrogens and antiestrogens on hormone-responsive human breast cancer in long-term tissue culture. Cancer Res. **36:** 4595–4601.
38. WAKELING, A.E. 1989. Comparative studies on the effects of steroidal and nonsteroidal oestrogen antagonists on the proliferation of human breast cancer cells. J. Steroid Biochem. **34:** 183–188.
39. MALTONI, C. *et al.* 1996. Experimental results on the chemopreventive and side effects of tamoxifen using a human-equivalent animal model. *In* The Scientific Bases of Cancer Chemoprevention, pp. 197–217.
40. BREUER, B., S. WALLENSTEIN & R. ANDERSON. 1998. Effect of tamoxifen on bone fractures in older nursing home residents. J. Am. Geriatr. Soc. **46:** 968–972.

A Brief Review of the International Breast Cancer Intervention Study (IBIS), the Other Current Breast Cancer Prevention Trials, and Proposals for Future Trials[a]

J. CUZICK

Department of Mathematics, Statistics, and Epidemiology, Imperial Cancer Research Fund, London WC2A 3PX, United Kingdom

ABSTRACT: The available results from breast cancer chemoprevention trials are reviewed. Four trials using tamoxifen have been performed, of which three have reported efficacy results. A fifth trial using raloxifene has also been published. The largest tamoxifen trial shows approximately a 50% reduction in breast cancer incidence in the short term, but the two smaller trials have not found any incidence reduction. Greater agreement exists for side effects: thromboembolic disease and endometrial cancers are raised about 2- to 3-fold when tamoxifen is used for 5 years. The possible reasons for the discrepancy in breast cancer reduction are explored. A review of trial parameters does not clearly explain this difference, and a metanalysis indicates that all results are compatible with a 42% reduction in short-term incidence. Several important questions remain about the clinical implication of this result, including the effect on mortality, the appropriate risk groups for chemoprevention, and the long-term effects on incidence. Continued follow-up of these trials is crucial for resolving these issues.

KEYWORDS: breast cancer; tamoxifen; raloxifene; metanalysis

INTRODUCTION

Following the observation that tamoxifen reduced the incidence of contralateral breast cancer when used in the adjuvant setting, it was suggested that prevention of breast cancer in high-risk women might also be possible with this drug.[1,2] A pilot study was initiated under the auspices of the United Kingdom Coordinating Committee for Cancer Research (UKCCCR) at the Royal Marsden Hospital (RMH). As a result of the favorable compliance data and lack of unexpected toxicities in the RMH trial, the UKCCCR launched its main trial, the International Breast Cancer

---

Address for correspondence: J. Cuzick, Ph.D., Department of Mathematics, Statistics, and Epidemiology, Imperial Cancer Research Fund, 61 Lincoln's Inn Fields, London WC2A 3PX, United Kingdom. Voice: +44 (0)20-7269-3006; fax: +44 (0)20-7269-3429.
j.cuzick@icrf.icnet.uk

[a]This paper is reproduced from the *European Journal of Cancer* (2000. Vol. 36: 1298–1302) with permission of the publisher and the author. The ADDENDUM is reproduced from an abstract submitted by Dr. Cuzick to the NIH Workshop on Selective Estrogen Receptor Modulators (SERMs), April 26–28, 2000.

Intervention Study (IBIS), in 1992. Subjects were first entered in Australia because the United Kingdom Medical Research Council (MRC) was concerned about hepatic toxicity of tamoxifen in some strains of rats, and their concerns delayed the onset of the study in the United Kingdom until November 1993. A similar trial was initiated in the United States in 1992 under the auspices of the National Surgical Adjuvant Breast and Bowel Project (NSABP). All trials were placebo-controlled studies of 5 years of tamoxifen administration. Three of the studies have published early results on breast cancer reduction. In the largest study, the NSABP P-1 trial, an almost 50% reduction in new tumors was found.[3] This result is very similar to that which was expected from the adjuvant studies[4] and led to the early stopping, unblinding, and curtailment of the American trial. However, the preliminary results of the RMH trial[5] and the Italian trial[6] did not indicate any reduction in breast cancer incidence. These trials remain blinded at the individual level and further follow-up is continuing. In this review, we examine the differences between these trials and look for factors that might explain the difference in results. The IBIS trial is not scheduled to complete recruitment until the end of 2000 and results on the reduction of breast cancer incidence are not available. However, some demographic data are available from this trial and, thus, we can make some comparisons between the four tamoxifen prevention trials. (Details of the IBIS trial are presented as an ADDENDUM to this article.) A fifth trial (MORE: Multiple Outcomes of Raloxifene Evaluation) designed primarily to look at the value of 3 years of the new selective estrogen receptor modulator (SERM), raloxifene, in preventing osteoporosis has also recently reported on breast cancer prevention[7] and is also reviewed.

DEMOGRAPHY

The entry criteria and basic characteristics of the five trials are summarized in TABLES 1 and 2. The number of subjects entered into the P-1 trial is about the same as all the other tamoxifen trials combined. Since P-1 recruited quickly, there is already a median follow-up of 55 months compared with 36 months for the Italian study and (currently) 30 months for IBIS. The smaller RMH study has the longest median follow-up (70 months).

TABLE 1. Breast cancer prevention trials

Trial	Population	Agents (vs. placebo)	Intended duration of treatment (years)
Royal Marsden	high-risk family history	tamoxifen 20 mg	5–8
NSABP P-1	1.6% 5-year risk	tamoxifen 20 mg	5
Italian	normal-risk hysterectomy	tamoxifen 20 mg	5
IBIS	>2-fold risk	tamoxifen 20 mg	5
MORE	normal-risk osteoporotic postmenopausal	raloxifene 60 mg or 120 mg	3

The age ranges for entry were similar among the tamoxifen trials, although a few women below 35 years of age were entered into the RMH trial and a few over 70 years of age entered into P-1. The median age of entry was lower for the RMH and IBIS trials, and more women were below the age of 50 years at entry. The MORE trial entered only postmenopausal women and had a much older median age at entry.

The differences in age of entry are related to different entry criteria for the four trials. The RMH and IBIS trials entered mainly subjects with a family history (96% and 91%, respectively, had at least one first-degree relative with breast cancer). Indeed, the RMH trial had 36% of patients at risk sufficient to be potential carriers of BRCA-1 or BRCA-2. IBIS had 20% of subjects with two or more first-degree relatives with breast cancer and the P-1 trial had 19%.

Because of concerns about tamoxifen-associated endometrial cancer, the Italian trial admitted subjects only if they previously had a hysterectomy. Approximately half of the women also had an oophorectomy, some at a relatively young age, so that many of the women entered into this trial were at a lower than average risk of breast cancer. The entry criteria for P-1 were calculated according to the Gail model, which took into account family history (but not the age of the affected relative), number of breast biopsies, and hormonal risk factors. All women aged 60 years or more were eligible and women less than 60 years had to have a 5-year risk of breast cancer equivalent to that of a woman of 60 years of age. The entry criteria for the IBIS trial are based on family history, benign breast disease, and nulliparity. A range of options for entry was used to approximate a 2-fold risk at age 45–70 years, a 4-fold risk at age 40–44 years, and a 10-fold risk at age 35–39 years. Details are given in reference 8. Although pathological and endocrine risk factors were allowed, in practice, the large majority of subjects were entered because of a history of a young close relative with breast cancer. This was also true of the RMH trial, but was less true for the P-1 study where hormonal risk factors and breast biopsies were more important entry criteria.

The MORE trial was designed primarily to examine osteoporosis and no risk factors for breast cancer were required for entry. Raloxifene was given daily at two doses (60 mg and 120 mg) and these groups were combined for analysis, so there were about twice as many patients in the treated group (5129 vs. 2576).

BREAST CANCER REDUCTION

The early results of three tamoxifen studies have been reported[3,5,6] and are summarized in TABLE 2 and FIGURE 1. The IBIS trial is due to recruit until the end of 2000 and will report 1 or 2 years later. The P-1 trial shows a clear dramatic reduction [OR = 0.51; 95% CI = 0.39–0.66] in the incidence of invasive cancers in the tamoxifen arm. This result is very similar to the reduction in contralateral tumors reported in the overview of tamoxifen adjuvant trials.[4] The RMH and Italian trials do not show appreciable treatment effects. In the RMH trial, the incidence curves for invasive cancers for the two arms are superimposable.[5] When the Italian trial was analyzed according to whether subjects took medication for longer than 1 year, there were indications of an effect (19 cases in the placebo arm vs. 11 in the tamoxifen arm; OR = 0.58), although the numbers are small and this was an unplanned

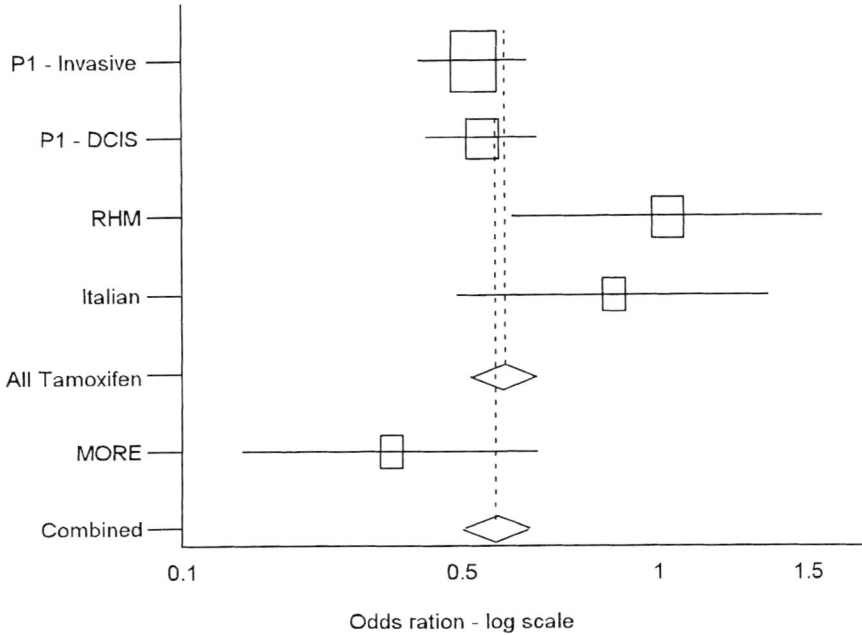

FIGURE 1. Hazard ratios and 95% confidence intervals for the different cancer prevention trials. DCIS = ductal carcinoma *in situ*.

TABLE 2. Numbers of women randomized, follow-up times, and breast cancers detected (including *in situ* lesions)

Trial	Total randomized	Median follow-up (months)	Cancers Total	Tamoxifen/ raloxifene	Placebo	Odds ratio (95% CI)
Royal Marsden	2471	70	70	34	36	0.94
NSABP P-1	13,388	57	368	124	244	0.51 (0.39–0.66)
Italian	5408	46	41	19 (11)[b]	22 (19)[b]	0.91
IBIS[a]	6176	36	96[a]	—[a]	—[a]	—[a]
MORE	7705	40	54	22/2[c]	32	0.35 (0.21–0.58)

[a]As of January 1, 2000 (ongoing and still blinded).
[b]Tamoxifen > 1 year.
[c]2:1 ratio of SERM:placebo in MORE study.

subgroup comparison (FIG. 1). Also, there was 1 case of breast cancer in the tamoxifen + HRT (hormone replacement therapy) group compared with 8 in the placebo + HRT group ($P = 0.02$), suggesting that tamoxifen is particularly effective in preventing cancers associated with exogenous estrogen use.

The MORE trial showed the greatest reduction in breast cancer incidence [RR = 0.35; 95% CI = 0.21–0.58] based on 22 cancers in 5129 women assigned to raloxifene (at 60 mg or 120 mg) and 32 cancers in 2576 women assigned to placebo. The reduction of invasive breast tumors was even greater, giving an odds ratio of 0.24 [95% CI = 0.13–0.44] based on 13 versus 27 cancers.

Very few patients have died in any of these trials and, even for the P-1 trial, there is no direct evidence of a reduction in breast cancer mortality (6 placebo versus 3 tamoxifen).

Estrogen Receptor–Negative Tumors

The incidence reduction in the P-1 and MORE trials is restricted to estrogen receptor (ER)–positive tumors. In the P-1 trial, the reduction was 67% for this group [OR = 0.33; 95% CI = 0.22–0.45], whereas there was a slight increase in ER-negative tumors [OR = 1.22; 95% CI = 0.74–2.03]. Similarly, in the MORE trial, ER-positive tumors were reduced by 90% [OR = 0.10; 95% CI = 0.04–0.24], but there was little effect on ER-negative tumors [OR = 0.88; 95% CI = 0.26–3.0].

SIDE EFFECTS

Endometrial Cancer

Endometrial cancer is the most clearly recognized, if rare, side effect of tamoxifen. Several case reports and case-control studies have found an effect,[9] albeit of highly variable size. The overview of adjuvant trials found 92 endometrial cancers in users of tamoxifen compared with 32 cancers in controls, giving an OR of 2.58 [95% CI = 1.9–3.3]. In the P-1 study, the excess was 36 cases versus 13, leading to a very similar OR of 2.53 [95% CI = 1.35–4.97]. All of the cases identified were FIGO (Federation of Gynecology and Obstetrics) stage 1, except 1 of the control patients who was stage 4, and that is the only patient reported to have died from endometrial cancer. No increase in endometrial cancer was found for women aged less than 50 years and the OR for older women was 4.01. In the RMH study, there were 4 cases of endometrial cancer in the tamoxifen arm versus 1 in the controls, and, of course, there were none in the Italian study because they all had a hysterectomy. No data are available for the IBIS study. In the MORE study, there was no effect on endometrial cancer based on 6 cases in the combined raloxifene groups versus 4 in the control group.

Other Cancers

No cancers other than endometrial are elevated in the adjuvant overview[4] or the P-1 study[3] and it seems increasingly likely that tamoxifen has a minimal effect on the development of other tumors, in contrast to early concerns about liver and colorectal tumors.[10–12]

Vascular Events

Reports from women taking tamoxifen for breast cancer suggested an increase in vascular events, but the relationship to tamoxifen by itself was in question because of the potential confounding effect of chemotherapy and surgery. The P-1 trial has clearly demonstrated that the tamoxifen alone can increase the risk of these events, with a 58% increase in strokes (1.45 vs. 0.92 events per 1000 women-years), a 3-fold increase in pulmonary emboli (0.69 vs. 0.23 cases per 1000 women-years), and a 60% increase in deep vein thromboses (DVT) (1.34 vs. 0.84 cases per 1000 women-years). Three of the 9 pulmonary emboli in the tamoxifen group were fatal. All of these excess risks were again confined to women aged 50 years or older.

Similar results were reported in the Italian trial with 38 vascular events on tamoxifen and 18 on placebo ($P = 0.005$), although most of these were superficial phlebitis and there were only 9 DVTs (6 vs. 3) and 2 pulmonary emboli (1 vs. 1).

Thromboembolic disease was also elevated with raloxifene in the MORE study. The magnitude was approximately 3-fold [OR = 3.1; 95% CI = 1.5–6.2], based on a rate of 3/1000 in the placebo arm and combined raloxifene arms.

Menopausal Symptoms

Both the RMH and P-1 studies have shown a clear increase in menopausal symptoms. The most common of these were hot flushes, which rose from 17% to 33% in the RMH study[13] and from 65% to 78% in the P-1 study.[14] Vaginal discharge and menstrual irregularities were also more common in both trials. Less specific factors such as weight gain, headaches, or depression, which have been suggested as being related to tamoxifen, were not elevated in the tamoxifen groups in either trial.

Other Negative Effects

A few other effects, both positive and negative, appear to be related in a small degree to tamoxifen exposure. The P-1 trial has reported a 14% increase in cataracts, which was of marginal significance, and the RMH trial has suggested a possible loss of bone density in premenopausal women.[15]

OTHER BENEFICIAL EFFECTS

Bone

Several studies have shown that tamoxifen has beneficial effects on bone tumor markers and bone mineral density in postmenopausal women (reviewed in reference 8). It may take some time for this to be fully translated into clinical benefit because of the relatively young age of the women in these trials. However, a nonsignificant 9% reduction in fractures at sites associated with osteoporosis (hip, Colles radius, spine) has already been seen in the P-1 trial, although no reduction in the much larger number of other fractures has been observed.[3]

Raloxifene has been shown to improve bone biomarkers,[16] and recent data show a reduction in vertebral fractures.[17]

Cardiovascular

There is little doubt that tamoxifen reduces low-density lipoprotein (LDL) cholesterol by approximately 20% (reviewed in reference 8). However, the early reports of reductions in cardiovascular disease in adjuvant trials[18,19] have yet to be seen in the prevention trials. This again may relate to the younger age distribution.

CONCLUSIONS

Uncertainty about the interpretation of the apparently disparate results makes it difficult to plan future trials. Much energy has gone into trying to explain the difference between the breast cancer outcomes of the trials. However, a test for heterogeneity between the trials is not significant ($P = 0.06$) if the P-1 *in situ* lesions are taken as a separate stratum and only marginally significant ($P = 0.04$) if they are excluded. Chance must still be considered as a serious explanation for the differences. The results are all consistent with a 42% reduction in breast cancer incidence, but the pooled estimate for the tamoxifen trials still has a 95% confidence interval spanning anywhere from a 30% to a 55% reduction.

The results of the IBIS trial (see ADDENDUM) and continued follow-up of the other trials will be important for evaluating the utility of tamoxifen in chemoprevention.

Two approaches to chemoprevention are being considered in future trials. One is to look for better SERMs that have high protection against breast cancer, but have fewer side effects than tamoxifen. In the United States, the NSABP P-2 is comparing tamoxifen versus raloxifene in this regard. Another approach is to block estrogen production. In premenopausal women, the luteinizing hormone–releasing hormone (LHRH) agonists are the obvious candidates and pilot studies are about to begin to evaluate the acceptability of goserelin in combination with raloxifene, a bisphosphonate, or tibolone in very high risk premenopausal women (e.g., BRCA-1/2 carriers or women with very striking family histories).

In postmenopausal women, the aromatase inhibitors are natural candidates. The IBIS group is currently planning a three-arm study of women at high risk or with newly diagnosed ductal carcinoma *in situ* (DCIS), comparing (1) placebo, (2) tamoxifen alone, and (3) anastrozole alone. This is similar to the ATAC (arimidex, tamoxifen alone, and in combination) adjuvant trial of over 9000 women, but also retains a control arm. The final design of this trial will depend on the results from IBIS and ATAC and on the early results for new SERMs.

Other SERMs are also under development, as well as a range of aromatase inhibitors and LHRH agonists. Validated biomarkers would be very useful in assessing their value and this is a priority area for research in breast cancer chemoprevention.

ADDENDUM

IBIS

Background

Tamoxifen is clearly established as an effective treatment for women with breast cancer. It reduces mortality by about 25% and recurrence rates by about 30%.

TABLE 3. Eligibility criteria for entry[20,21]

For women aged 45–70
(1) First-degree relative who developed breast cancer at age 50 or less
(2) First-degree relative who developed bilateral breast cancer
(3) Two or more first- or second-degree relatives who developed breast cancer
(4) Nulliparous and first-degree relative who developed breast cancer
(5) Benign biopsy and first-degree relative who developed breast cancer
(6) Lobular carcinoma *in situ*
(7) Atypical hyperplasia in a benign lesion

For women aged 40–44
(8) Two or more first- or second-degree relatives who developed breast cancer at age 50 or less
(9) First-degree relative with bilateral breast cancer who developed breast cancer at age 50 or less
(10) Nulliparous and first-degree relative who developed breast cancer at age 40 or less
(11) Benign biopsy and first-degree relative who developed breast cancer at age 40 or less
(12) Lobular carcinoma *in situ*
(13) Atypical hyperplasia in a benign lesion

For women aged 35–39
(14) Two or more first-degree relatives who developed breast cancer at age 50 or less
(15) First-degree relative with bilateral breast cancer who developed first breast cancer at age 40 or less
(16) Lobular carcinoma *in situ*

Adjuvant trials have shown that it is more effective to give tamoxifen as an adjuvant rather than wait until recurrence. These findings and a low incidence of side effects and toxicity prompted interest in the use of tamoxifen to prevent breast cancer. As discussed above, this possibility was further strengthened by the observation in adjuvant trials that tamoxifen reduces the incidence of contralateral tumors by about 50% when given for about 5 years. These studies also showed reductions in LDL cholesterol and increases in bone density in postmenopausal women, suggesting beneficial effects on cardiovascular disease and osteoporosis.

Aims and Design

This placebo-controlled trial has been designed to see if 5 years of tamoxifen at 20 mg/day will have an effect on the incidence of breast cancer in women aged 35 to 70 years with an increased risk of the disease. Entry criteria differ by age and require a higher risk of developing breast cancer for women less than 45. Details are given in TABLE 3. As previously discussed, conflicting preliminary data have been published from trials of a similar design based at the Royal Marsden Hospital and in Italy and North America. The two European trials show no significant chemo-

TABLE 4. IBIS population demographics for the United Kingdom and Europe ($n = 3928$)

Mean age (years)	49
Mean height (cm)	163
Mean weight (kg)	71
Mean BMI	27
Hysterectomy	30%
Hysterectomy with both ovaries retained	13.2%
Hysterectomy with one ovary removed	12.4%
Hysterectomy with both ovaries removed	4.4%
Benign disease	9%
Atypia hyperplasia	3%
Lobular carcinoma *in situ*	1.2%
Postmenopausal	52%
Family history	
Any relative	93%
First-degree relative	83%
Second-degree relative	56%
HRT	
Prior to IBIS	38%
During IBIS	34%

preventive effect of tamoxifen, whereas the North American trial has demonstrated an effect comparable to that found in adjuvant trials. It is very important for IBIS to recruit sufficient women to provide the data required to solve this conflict of evidence.[20,21] It is hoped that the investigators in all the trials will be able to collaborate to provide better information on the longer-term profile of tamoxifen prophylaxis. Additional end points will be breast cancer mortality, cardiovascular disease, other cancers, and fracture rates. Tolerability and toxicity are also being closely monitored. Demographic characteristics of the current European population are shown in TABLE 4 and the age distribution is shown in FIGURE 2.

Numbers and Logistics

The required trial size is 7000 participants and the trial was closed to new entry on February 1, 2001, with a total of 7151 women enrolled. The recruitment rate was about 100 women/month. As of April 1, 2001, a total of 142 breast cancers had been observed. There are 22 United Kingdom centers located in Aberdeen, Belfast, Birmingham, Bristol, Cambridge, Cardiff, Chelmsford, Dundee, Edinburgh, Glasgow, Huddersfield, Kettering, Leeds, Leicester, Liverpool, Guy's Hospital (London), University College Hospital (London), Manchester, Newcastle, Nottingham, Oxford, and Southampton. There are also 10 Australian centers, as well as additional centers in New Zealand, Switzerland, Belgium, Ireland, Spain, and Finland.

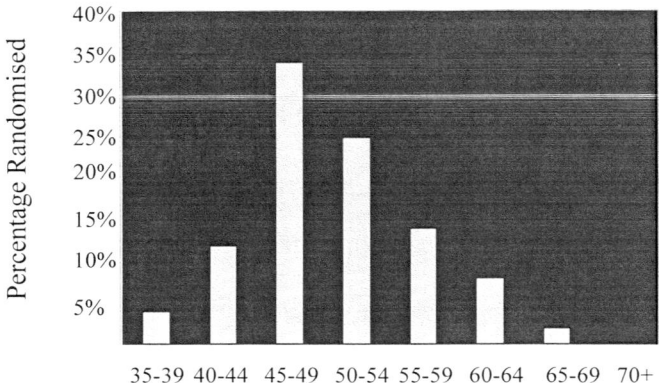

Age Distribution

FIGURE 2. IBIS: Age distribution 1992 to December 1999. Mean age = 50 years. Median age = 49 years.

ACKNOWLEDGMENTS

This study was supported by the Cancer Research Campaign, the Imperial Cancer Research Fund, and the Department of Health under the auspices of the UKCCCR.

REFERENCES

1. CUZICK, J. & N.I. BAUM. 1985. Tamoxifen and contralateral breast cancer. Lancet **ii:** 282.
2. CUZICK, I., D.Y. WANG & R.D. BULBROOK. 1956. The prevention of breast cancer. Lancet **i:** 83–86.
3. FISHER, B., J.P. COSTANTINO, D.L. WICKERHAM *et al.* 1998. Tamoxifen for prevention of breast cancer: report of the National Surgical Adjuvant Breast and Bowel Project P-1 Study. J. Natl. Cancer Inst. **90:** 1371–1388.
4. EARLY BREAST CANCER TRIALISTS' COLLABORATIVE GROUP (EBCTCG). 1998. Tamoxifen for early breast cancer: an overview of the randomised trials. Lancet **351:** 1451–1467.
5. POWLES, T., R. EELES, S. ASHLEY *et al.* 1998. Interim analysis of the incidence of breast cancer in the Royal Marsden Hospital tamoxifen randomised chemoprevention trial. Lancet **352:** 98–101.
6. VERONESI, U., P. MAISONNEUVE, A. COSTA *et al.* 1998. Prevention of breast cancer with tamoxifen: preliminary findings from the Italian randomised trial among hysterectomised women. Lancet **352:** 93–97.
7. CUMMINGS, S.R., S. ECKERT, K.A. KRUEGER *et al.* 1999. The effect of raloxifene on risk of breast cancer in postmenopausal women: results from the MORE randomized trial. JAMA **281:** 2189–2197.
8. CUZICK, J. 1996. Chemoprevention of breast cancer with tamoxifen. *In* Chemoprevention in Cancer Control. IARC Scientific Publication No. 16, pp. 95–109. IARC. Lyon.
9. IARC. 1996. Some pharmaceutical drugs. *In* IARC Monographs on the Evaluation of Carcinogenic Risks to Humans. Vol. 66, pp. 253–365. IARC. Lyon.

10. HAN, X. & J. LIEHR. 1992. Induction of covalent DNA adducts in rodents by tamoxifen. Cancer Res. **52:** 1360–1363.
11. GREAVES, P. 1993. Ten-year carcinogenicity study of tamoxifen in Alderlev Park Wistar–derived rats. Cancer Res. **53:** 3919–3924.
12. RUTQVIST, L.B., H. JOHANSSON, T. SIGNOMKLAO et al. 1995. Adjuvant tamoxifen therapy for early stage breast cancer and second primary malignancies. J. Natl. Cancer Inst. **87:** 645–651.
13. POWLES, T., C.R. TILLYER & A.L. JONES. 1996. Prevention of breast cancer with tamoxifen—an update on the Royal Marsden Hospital pilot programme. Eur. J. Cancer **26:** 680–684.
14. DAY, R., P.A. GANZ, J. COSTANTINO et al. 1999. Health-related quality of life and tamoxifen in breast cancer prevention: a report from the National Surgical Adjuvant Breast and Bowel Project P-1 Study. J. Clin. Oncol. **17:** 2659–2669.
15. POWLES, T., T. HICKISH, A. KANIS et al. 1996. Effect of tamoxifen on bone mineral density measured by dual-energy X-ray absorptiometry in healthy premenopausal and postmenopausal women. J. Clin. Oncol. **14:** 78–84.
16. DELMAS, P.D., N.H. BJARNASON, B.H. MITLAK et al. 1997. Effects of raloxifene on bone mineral density, serum cholesterol concentrations, and uterine endometrium in postmenopausal women. N. Engl. J. Med. **337:** 1641–1647.
17. ETTINGER, B., D.M. BLACK, B.H. MITLAK et al. 1999. Reduction of vertebral fracture risk in postmenopausal women with osteoporosis treated with raloxifene. JAMA **282:** 637–645.
18. MCDONALD, C.C. & H.J. STEWART FOR THE SCOTTISH BREAST CANCER COMMITTEE. 1991. Fatal myocardial infarction in the Scottish adjuvant tamoxifen trial. Br. Med. J. **303:** 435–437.
19. RUTQVIST, L.E. & A. MATTSON. 1993. Cardiac and thromboembolic morbidity among postmenopausal women with early stage breast cancer in a randomised trial of adjuvant tamoxifen. J. Natl. Cancer Inst. **85:** 1398–1406.
20. CUZICK, J. 1998. Point of view: continuation of the International Breast Cancer Intervention Study (IBIS). Eur. J. Cancer **34:** 1647–1648.
21. HUTCHINGS, O., G. EVANS, L. FALLOWFIELD et al. 1998. Effect of early American results on patients in a tamoxifen prevention trial (IBIS) [correspondence]. Lancet **352**: 1222.

The MORE Trial: Multiple Outcomes for Raloxifene Evaluation

Breast Cancer as a Secondary End Point: Implications for Prevention

MAURA N. DICKLER[a] AND LARRY NORTON[b]

[a]*Breast Cancer Medicine Service and* [b]*Division of Solid Tumor Oncology, Department of Medicine, Memorial Sloan-Kettering Cancer Center, New York, New York 10021, USA*

> ABSTRACT: Breast cancer is a common disease in the United States and Europe and is therefore a major target for prevention strategies. Estrogen plays a central role in its pathogenesis, and treatment with estrogen deprivation has long been recognized to be an effective therapy. Tamoxifen is the first selective estrogen receptor modulator (SERM) to be widely used for the treatment of breast cancer and has been demonstrated to reduce the risk of breast cancer in high-risk women. Raloxifene is a second-generation SERM that has estrogenic effects on bone and lipid metabolism, and antiestrogenic effects on breast tissue. Unlike tamoxifen, raloxifene displays antiestrogenic effects on the endometrium and may serve as a safer alternative to tamoxifen in the prevention setting. The MORE trial is a multicenter randomized placebo-controlled trial designed to determine whether 3 years of raloxifene reduces the risk of fracture in postmenopausal women with osteoporosis. As a secondary end point of the trial, raloxifene was shown to reduce the risk of both *in situ* and invasive breast cancer by 65% (RR = 0.35; 95% CI = 0.21–0.58; $P < 0.001$). The benefits were most significant in women who developed estrogen receptor (ER)–positive cancers, with a relative risk of 0.10 (95% CI = 0.04–0.24). This reduced incidence of breast cancer may be due to an anticarcinogenic effect or to a slowing of growth of occult ER-positive cancer, with a shift to the right in the time-to-cancer curve. A second large-scale prevention trial in breast cancer comparing tamoxifen to raloxifene is presently enrolling cancer-free, but high-risk postmenopausal women (the STAR trial). Future directions include combined estrogen blockade of the breast by the addition of an aromatase inhibitor to a SERM. New trial designs, including those based on biochemical changes at the tissue level, will be required to allow future progress in this field with adequate rapidity.
>
> KEYWORDS: raloxifene; breast cancer prevention; MORE trial; aromatase inhibitors

Breast cancer is such a common disease in the United States and Europe that it is a major target for prevention strategies. It is not only the most common malignancy

---

Address for correspondence: Larry Norton, M.D., Head, Division of Solid Tumor Oncology, Department of Medicine, Memorial Sloan-Kettering Cancer Center, 1275 York Avenue, New York, NY 10021. Voice: 212-639-6425; fax: 212-717-3743.
nortonl@mskcc.org

among women in the United States, but is second only to lung cancer as the most common cause of cancer-related mortality.[1] It is estimated that 182,800 new cases of invasive breast cancer will be diagnosed in 2000, and 40,800 women are expected to die of their disease.

Along with prostate cancer in men, one of the distinguishing features of breast cancer etiology is its dependence on normal endocrine function—that is, estrogen plays a central role in the pathogenesis of breast cancer. Several risk factors for breast cancer, including early age of menarche, late age of menopause, and high serum concentrations of estradiol, are linked to an increased cumulative lifetime exposure to estrogen.[2] In addition, treatment of breast cancer with estrogen deprivation has long been recognized to be an effective therapy.[3] We will here consider some recent data concerning the impact of estrogen receptor modulation on the appearance of cancer in the breast and end with speculation concerning future directions in this regard.

Tamoxifen is the first selective estrogen receptor modulator (SERM) to be widely used for the treatment of breast cancer in pre- and postmenopausal women with both early-stage and metastatic disease. Like estrogen, tamoxifen acts as a growth-promoting influence on bone and endometrium, and lowers serum lipids. Its biological effects are mediated through its binding to the estrogen receptor (ER). This leads to inhibition of the normal actions of estrogen on breast tissue plus the initiation of abnormal intracellular signaling with biologic consequences in this tissue that are opposite to that associated with estrogen. Hence, tamoxifen exposure often produces growth arrest or actual apoptosis of the same breast epithelial cells that would respond to estrogen with mitosis. It should therefore not be entirely surprising to find that tamoxifen exposure could reduce the incidence of breast cancer in circumstances in which physiological concentrations of estrogen are associated with high baseline risks.

The National Surgical Adjuvant Breast and Bowel Project (NSABP) has previously reported results from such a study, the Breast Cancer Prevention Trial (P-1). This was a randomized double-blind, placebo-controlled trial of tamoxifen involving 13,388 high-risk women.[1] After a median follow-up of 4.5 years, a 49% reduction in the annual odds of developing invasive breast cancer was observed among the participants randomized to tamoxifen (RR = 0.51; 95% CI = 0.39–0.66). On the negative side, however, tamoxifen was associated with a small, but significant increased incidence of endometrial carcinoma, almost entirely in women greater than 50 years of age (RR = 4.01; 95% CI = 1.70-10.9). There were also slightly increased risks of phlebothromboses, also in older women, similar to those seen with the use of any estrogen-like hormone.

Raloxifene is a second-generation SERM that is FDA-approved for the prevention and treatment of osteoporosis.[2] Like tamoxifen, raloxifene binds to the ER, imparting estrogenic effects on bone and lipid metabolism, and antiestrogenic effects on the breast. Unlike estrogen, however, raloxifene displays antiestrogenic effects on the endometrium. For this reason, it has been theorized that raloxifene could possibly serve as a safer alternative to tamoxifen in the prevention setting.

The MORE trial is a multicenter, randomized, double-blind trial designed to determine whether 3 years of raloxifene use reduces the risk of fracture in postmenopausal women with osteoporosis. This trial has so far demonstrated that raloxifene increases bone mineral density in the spine and femoral neck, and reduces the risk of vertebral fractures. The trial was also designed to prospectively evaluate whether raloxifene reduces the risk of breast cancer, and this end point is the focus of this review.[4]

The MORE trial was conducted at 180 clinical centers in 25 countries, mainly at sites in the United States and Europe, between 1994 and 1998. The trial enrolled 7705 postmenopausal women with a history of osteoporosis. This was defined as having a bone mineral density at least 2.5 standard deviations below the mean for normal young women at the lumbar spine or femoral neck, or having had a least one moderate or two mild vertebral fractures that were detected on radiographs of the spine. Since osteoporosis was required for eligibility, participants were probably at lower risk of breast cancer than the general population, as decreased bone density may serve as a marker of lower cumulative lifetime exposure to estrogen.[5] In addition, only 12.3% of participants reported a family history of breast cancer and, therefore, this cohort was not at high risk based on family history of the disease.

All participants were younger than age 81, with a median age of 66.5 years. Almost all of these women were of European ancestry. Women with a history of breast or endometrial cancer were excluded. In addition, women with estrogen use during the previous 6 months were excluded, and estrogen use during the trial was not permitted.

Subjects were randomized in a double-blind fashion to three treatment arms: raloxifene at 120 mg per day, raloxifene at 60 mg per day, or placebo. Therefore, twice as many women received raloxifene as placebo. All participants also received calcium and vitamin D. Mammography screening was optional after the first year, but was required after 2 and 3 years of treatment. Women who refused mammography were offered a breast ultrasound. The diagnosis of breast cancer was confirmed by review of histopathology, and an oncology adjudication review board, blinded to the assigned treatment, reviewed all the pertinent records. In addition, annual transvaginal ultrasonography was performed in 17 designated centers for all women with an intact uterus, and there also were subsets of patients who received this exam at other centers. Endometrial biopsies were recommended for women with the symptom of vaginal bleeding, with endometrial thickness greater than 8 mm on ultrasound examination, or with an increase in endometrial thickness of at least 5 mm.

After a median follow-up of 40 months, 54 cases of breast cancer were confirmed in the study cohort, including 40 cases of invasive breast cancer. In the 5129 women assigned to raloxifene (recall the 2:1 randomization), 13 cases of invasive breast cancer were noted, as compared to 27 cases in the 2576 women assigned to placebo (RR = 0.24; 95% CI = 0.13-0.44; $P < 0.001$; FIG. 1). The results were similar when all cases of breast cancer were considered (both *in situ* and invasive breast cancer), with a relative risk of 0.35 for women randomized to raloxifene (95% CI = 0.21–0.58; $P < 0.001$; TABLE 1). The reduction in risk of breast cancer was similar for both doses of raloxifene. The benefits were most significant in women who developed ER-positive cancers, with a relative risk of 0.10 (95% CI = 0.04-0.24). Raloxifene did not change the risk of ER-negative breast cancers (RR = 0.88), which is consistent with the results of the NSABP tamoxifen chemoprevention study.

It can therefore be stated with confidence that, in cancer-free women with osteoporosis, the use of raloxifene reduces the incidence of breast cancer, at least over the short term. There is every reason to anticipate that raloxifene should exert a similar effect in women with lesser degrees of bone loss. However, it is not clear if this

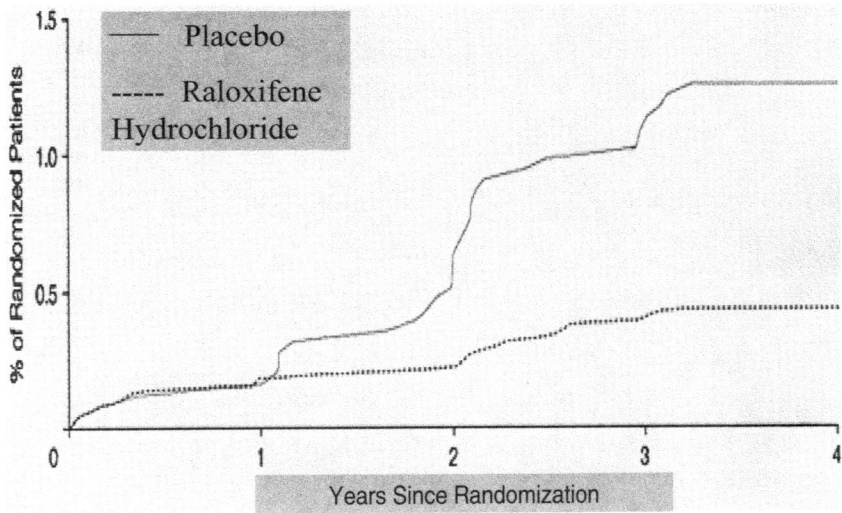

FIGURE 1. Cumulative incidence of breast cancer in study participants, represented as a percentage of all patients randomized to either group ($P < 0.001$). Reproduced with permission from Ref. 4.

TABLE 1. Number, rate, and relative risk of breast cancer by treatment group and ER status

	No. of events		Rate/1000		
	Plac	Tam	Plac	Tam	RR (95% CI)
All breast cancer	32	22	4.3	1.5	0.35 (0.21–0.58)
Invasive breast cancer	27	13	3.6	0.9	0.24 (0.13–0.44)
ER-positive tumors	20	4			0.10 (0.04–0.24)
ER-negative tumors	4	7			0.88 (0.26–3.00)

NOTE: Plac = placebo; Tam = tamoxifen; rate/1000 = rate per 1000 women-years.

reduced incidence of breast cancer is due to an actual anticarcinogenic effect (*chemoprevention*) or to a slowing of the growth of occult ER-positive cancers that happen to arise during or immediately before the study period. A slowing of growth would mean that, at any time point, fewer cancers would have grown to a clinically apparent size, so the time-to-cancer curve would be shifted to the right. We would see this same phenomenon should raloxifene use be associated with a cytoreduction of occult collections of cancer cells. Fewer cells left after therapy means that it would take more time for these residual cells to expand to a clinically meaningful size. Hence, at any time point, fewer patients would have breast cancer. The mathematics of time-to-event curves would indicate that this shift could appear durable, so

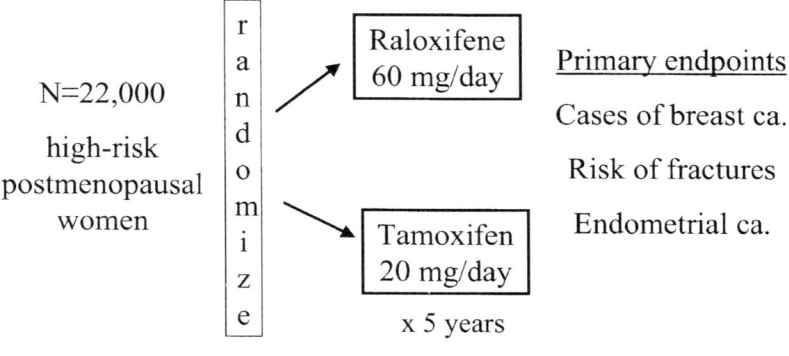

FIGURE 2. The STAR trial (NSABP P-2).

that a treated arm may never fully rejoin a control arm, even though no cancers are actually prevented or eradicated by the therapy. In fact, there are no actual or model-based ways to distinguish real prevention from growth rate reduction or cytoreduction. This is because the result of any mechanism would be fewer clinical cancers at any point in time, which for some patients—those never presenting with disease because their cancers never had time to grow to a noticeable volume—is tantamount to true prevention. (Parenthetically, the above observations are as applicable to the use of anticancer drugs in the postoperative adjuvant setting: No cancer would need to be eradicated to result in a shift of the time-to-recurrence or time-to-death curves to the right. All that is needed is a reduction in the starting number of cancer cells or an inhibition of their growth rates.)

In general, in spite of some predictable side effects, raloxifene was well tolerated in this trial when compared to placebo. Raloxifene-treated patients experienced more hot flashes, leg cramps, and peripheral edema. On the other hand, raloxifene appeared to lower both serum cholesterol and blood pressure. Of great importance, neither vaginal bleeding nor endometrial cancers were increased in women assigned to raloxifene. This observation is, of course, consistent with preclinical data that have established that raloxifene acts like an estrogen antagonist in the endometrium (RR of endometrial cancer = 0.80; 95% CI = 0.2–2.7). Raloxifene, however, like tamoxifen, increased the risk of thromboembolic events such as deep venous thromboses and pulmonary emboli (RR = 3.1; 95% CI = 1.5–6.2).

The results of the Breast Cancer Prevention Trial (NSABP P-1) and the MORE trial have lead to a second large-scale prevention trial in breast cancer, called the STAR trial. The acronym stands for Study of Tamoxifen and Raloxifene. This trial, as the name implies, is comparing tamoxifen to raloxifene in a voluntary group of cancer-free, but high-risk postmenopausal women (FIG. 2). end points of this trial include cases of both breast and endometrial cancer.

It is unfortunate that the lack of reliable surrogate end point biomarkers has made it imperative that we must design chemoprevention trials with such gross end points as the appearance of the actual disease. Two obvious consequences of this failing are that chemoprevention trials now require huge numbers of patients and long follow-up durations. New trial designs, especially those based on biochemical changes at the tissue level, will be required to allow us to make progress with adequate rapidity. This is especially so as many new SERMs are now in preclinical development. Were it necessary to test each one against a standard in a large prospective trial with pure clinical outcomes, it could take us centuries to make substantial progress.

This latter comment is especially germane when we consider that some of the ideas for improvement in hormonal prevention of breast cancer are based on combinations of agents rather than single drugs. For example, there is strong theoretical reason to suspect that combined estrogen blockade of the breast by the addition of an aromatase inhibitor to a SERM may be more effective than an antiestrogen alone for breast cancer chemoprevention. In postmenopausal women, the majority of circulating estrogen is synthesized from the peripheral conversion of androgens to estrogens. The rate-limiting enzyme responsible for the conversion is aromatase. This process of aromatization occurs at peripheral sites, including the adipose tissue, muscle, and liver.[6] Aromatase activity has also been detected in the breasts of women with both benign and malignant disease.[7]

Estrogen levels in the breast are increased in the majority of cancers, with breast tissue estrogen concentrations significantly higher in malignant breast tissue than in nonmalignant tissue. In addition, the concentrations of estrogens in breast tumor tissue in postmenopausal patients are much higher than expected and are similar to those in premenopausal patients, despite the lower circulating estrogens in the postmenopausal population.[8] Therefore, a breast tumor tissue–plasma gradient exists in postmenopausal women, with an estimated tissue:plasma ratio of 10:1 to 50:1.

In theory, this greater-than-expected tissue estrogen concentration in postmenopausal breast cancer may be secondary to increased uptake of estrogen from plasma or from *in situ* estrogen production within the tumor. Yet, Yue *et al.*[9] found that, in preclinical models, *in situ* aromatization could be more important than uptake of peripheral estrogens as a mechanism for the high tumor estrogen concentration. In an ovariectomized athymic nude mouse model, MCF-7 cells transfected with the aromatase gene were able to grow in the presence of androstenedione alone. Sham-transfected MCF-7 cells were not able to grow under these conditions, requiring exogenous estrogen for growth. The highest tumor growth rates and tissue estrogen levels were seen in androstenedione-treated mice rather than mice supplemented with exogenous estrogen, which is evidence that the *in situ* synthesis mechanism may be more important than uptake of peripheral estrogens. The aromatase inhibitor, formestane, was able to reduce the tumor estrogen levels and decrease tumor growth in these mice.

De Jong and colleagues demonstrated the ability of aromatase inhibitors to suppress human breast tumor aromatase activity and thereby reduce estrogen concentrations in a cohort of postmenopausal women with early-stage breast cancer. These investigators treated 11 postmenopausal women with vorozole, a third-generation nonsteroidal aromatase inhibitor, for 7 days prior to definitive surgery.[10] Of 8 evaluable patients, median tissue aromatase activity was 89% lower than that in untreated controls, with a similar reduction in median tissue estrone and estradiol concentrations (64% and 80% lower, respectively). This suggests that not only was the aromatase inhibitor able to inhibit peripheral aromatase activity, but it was also able

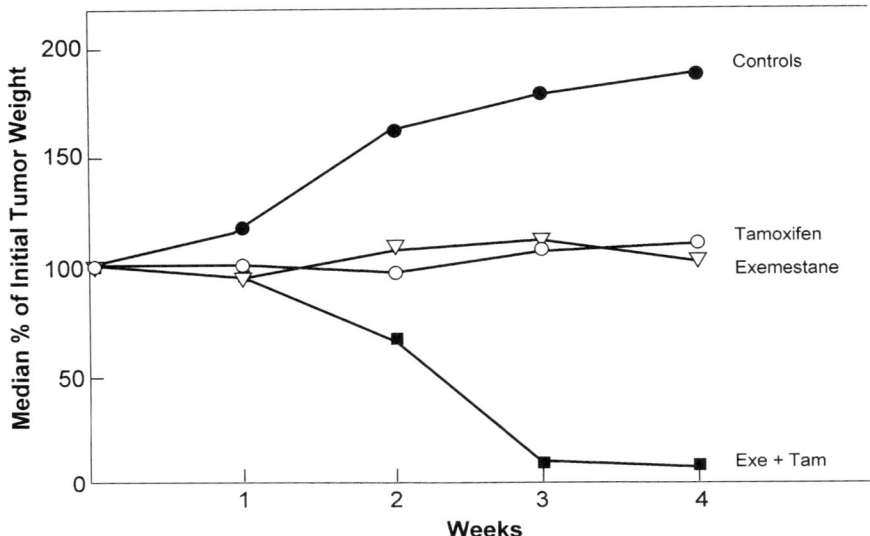

FIGURE 3. Effect of exemestane (20 mg/kg/day sc) and tamoxifen (1 mg/kg/day po), given alone or in combination for 4 weeks, on the growth of DMBA-induced mammary tumors in rats (31–34 tumors per group). Reproduced with permission from Ref. 11.

to inhibit intratumoral aromatase activity and reduce concentrations of breast tissue estrogens. The fact that we can successfully reduce breast tumor estrogens with an aromatase inhibitor, coupled with the known causative role of estrogen in breast carcinogenesis, allows for the investigation of these agents for the prevention of breast cancer.

Preclinical data to support the combination of an antiestrogen with an aromatase inhibitor have been generated in the DMBA-induced rat mammary tumor model.[11] Exemestane, an irreversible steroidal aromatase inhibitor, was administered alone or in combination with tamoxifen. A higher objective response rate of 57% was observed with the combination, as compared with exemestane or tamoxifen alone, with response rates of 44% and 29%, respectively (TABLE 2 and FIG. 3). While the

TABLE 2. Exemestane + tamoxifen on DMBA-induced mammary tumors in rats

	Rats (n)	Tumors (n)	CR (%)	PR (%)	RR (%)	New tumors/rat
Control	21	31	0	6	6	0.9
Exem	22	34	26	18	44	0.4
Tam	21	31	16	13	29	0.5
Exem + tam	21	32	41	16	57	0.1

NOTE: From Ref. 11.

appearance of new tumors was reduced by each treatment alone, the combination of agents was most effective in the prevention of new tumors.

Based on these preclinical models, the combination of an antiestrogen and an aromatase inhibitor may prove to be a more effective strategy for the chemoprevention of breast cancer than the use of an antiestrogen alone. A pilot trial evaluating the combination of raloxifene and exemestane is presently ongoing at our institution to evaluate the safety and tolerability of this approach. end points of the trial include markers of bone turnover, serum lipoproteins, quality of life (in particular, symptoms of estrogen deficiency), and breast density by mammography and MRI. As part of a correlative laboratory study, serial breast biopsy material will be examined to determine whether this combination affects breast tissue aromatase levels, breast tissue estrogens, and potential surrogate end point biological markers of proliferation and apoptosis that may serve as potential intermediate markers for future prevention trials. The use of genomic and expression arrays for examining estrogen-responsive genes for this purpose is in early development.

The importance of this discussion is not the specific combination of a SERM with an agent that reduces breast estrogen levels, even though we believe there is some excitement regarding that particular approach. The point of this discussion is that we must develop better ways of predicting and monitoring anticarcinogenic (or cytoreducing or growth inhibitory) effects or we will not be able to evaluate clinically the many new agents and combinations that both the laboratory and theory will offer us. To some extent, we will have to start believing data in stage IV breast cancer as we have started to do for adjuvant therapy. If something kills cancer cells in the metastatic setting, it will prolong disease-free and likely overall survival as adjuvant treatment. Similarly, if a treatment slows the growth of or kills cancer cells in the metastatic or adjuvant setting, it will probably push the time-to-diagnosis curve to the right in the prevention setting. Of course, to establish this principle, we must have data on both cancer biology and clinical outcomes in enough prospective trials that we can establish the ability of one set of measurements to predict the other. Only when the day arrives that we have total confidence in this correlation can we start to use surrogate end points to accelerate our progress toward the primary prevention of breast cancer. However, it is very important that we make that day arrive as soon as possible.

REFERENCES

1. GREENLEE, R.T., T. MURRAY, S. BOLDEN, *et al.* 2000. Cancer Statistics, 2000. CA Cancer J. Clin. **48:** 7–33.
2. CAULEY, J.A., F.L. LUCAS, L.H. KULLER, *et al.* 1999. Elevated serum estradiol and testosterone concentrations are associated with a high risk for breast cancer. Ann. Intern. Med. **130:** 270–277.
3. BEATSON, A.T. 1896. On the treatment of inoperable cases of carcinoma mamma: suggestions for a new method of treatment with illustrative cases. Lancet **2:** 104–117.
4. FISHER, B., J.P. COSTANTINO, D.L. WICKERHAM *et al.* 1998. Tamoxifen for the prevention of breast cancer: report of the National Surgical Adjuvant Breast and Bowel Project P-1 study. J. Natl. Cancer Inst. **90:** 1371–1388.
5. DELMAS, P.D., N.H. BJARNASON, B.H. MITLAK *et al.* 1997. Effects of raloxifene on bone mineral density, serum cholesterol concentrations, and uterine endometrium in postmenopausal women. N. Engl. J. Med. **337:** 1641–1647.

6. ETTINGER, B., D.M. BLACK, B.H. MITLAK et al. 1999. Reduction of vertebral fracture risk in postmenopausal women with osteoporosis treated with raloxifene: results from a 3-year randomized clinical trial. JAMA **282:** 637–645.
7. CUMMINGS, S.R., S. ECKERT, K.A. KRUEGER et al. 1999. The effect of raloxifene on risk of breast cancer in postmenopausal women: results from the MORE randomized trial. JAMA **281:** 2189–2197.
8. ZHANG, Y., D.P. KIEL, B.E. KREGER et al. 1997. Bone mass and the risk of breast cancer among postmenopausal women. N. Engl. J. Med. **336:** 611–617.
9. HARVEY, H.A. 1998. Emerging role of aromatase inhibitors in the treatment of breast cancer. Oncology **12:** 32–35.
10. O'NEILL, J.S. & W.R. MILLER. 1987. Aromatase activity in breast adipose tissue from women with benign and malignant breast diseases. Br. J. Cancer **56:** 601–604.
11. VAN LANDEGHEM, A.A.J., J. POORTMAN, M. NABUURS et al. 1985. Endogenous concentration and subcellular distribution of estrogens in normal and malignant human breast tissue. Cancer Res. **45:** 2900–2906.

Quality of Life and Tamoxifen in a Breast Cancer Prevention Trial

A Summary of Findings from the NSABP P-1 Study

RICHARD DAY

Department of Biostatistics, Graduate School of Public Health, University of Pittsburgh, Pittsburgh, Pennsylvania 15213, USA

ABSTRACT: This report contains a brief summary of the health-related quality of life findings for 11,064 women taking part in the National Surgical Adjuvant Breast and Bowel Project's P-1 trial. Women taking part in this trial of tamoxifen versus placebo for breast cancer prevention were ≥35 years old and predominantly white, well educated, and middle class, with a strong professional and technical orientation. Key findings included a lack of difference between the tamoxifen and placebo arms with regard to depression, overall physical or mental quality of life, and weight gain. The tamoxifen arm did show consistent increases in vasomotor (hot flashes) and gynecological (vaginal discharge) symptoms, as well as difficulties in certain domains of sexual functioning. It is concluded that an informed discussion with a woman considering tamoxifen therapy should include these points in the risk-benefit discussion.

KEYWORDS: quality of life; tamoxifen; breast cancer; prevention

INTRODUCTION

This is a brief summary of the findings from the health-related quality of life (HRQL) component of the National Surgical Adjuvant Breast and Bowel Project's (NSABP) P-1 trial, a multicenter, double-blinded, placebo-controlled clinical trial designed to evaluate whether 5 years of tamoxifen therapy would reduce the incidence of invasive breast cancer in women at an increased risk for the disease. Detailed descriptions of the rationale, planning, and design of the P-1 study and its HRQL component, as well as specific instruments, are available in separate reports.[1-5]

SUBJECTS AND INSTRUMENTS

This summary focuses on the baseline HRQL examination and the first 36 months of follow-up data on 11,064 women recruited over the first 24 months of the study. The P-1 HRQL questionnaire was composed of the Center for Epidemiological

---

Address for correspondence: Richard Day, Ph.D., Department of Biostatistics, Graduate School of Public Health, University of Pittsburgh, 201 North Craig Street, Suite 350, Pittsburgh, PA 15213. Voice: 412-624-4077; fax: 412-624-9969.

day@nsabp.pitt.edu

Studies–Depression Scale (CES-D), the Medical Outcomes Study (MOS) Short Form (SF-36), the MOS sexual functioning scale, and a symptom checklist (SCL). The questionnaire was to be administered to all participants prior to randomization (baseline), at 3 months, and at each succeeding 6-month examination.

RESULTS

The participants in the P-1 study were predominantly white (96%), well educated (≥65% had some college), married (70%), and professional and technically trained (68.2%) women, who were currently employed (64.9%) and reported a middle to upper-middle class family income (median, $35,000–$49,999).

FIGURE 1 shows the overall proportion and total numbers of women completing the HRQL questionnaire at each examination. It provides a measure of comparative participant adherence with regard to the HRQL questionnaire in the two trial groups. Analysis of sociodemographic and medical variables indicated that participants failing to complete the HRQL questionnaire in each group were similar cohorts of women.

FIGURE 2 shows the proportion of P-1 participants, by group and examination, scoring above the most frequently used clinical cutoff (≥16, i.e., the score above

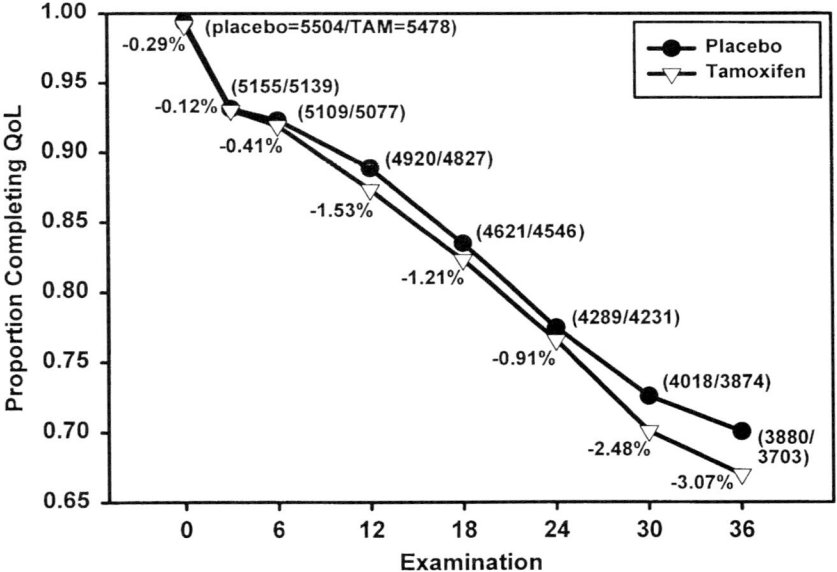

FIGURE 1. Proportion of participants in the tamoxifen ($n = 5527$) and placebo ($n = 5537$) groups completing the QoL questionnaire by examination. *Figures in parentheses* are the number of women in the placebo and tamoxifen groups completing the QoL questionnaire. The difference between the tamoxifen and placebo groups is expressed in terms of percent missing QoL data. QoL, quality of life; TAM, tamoxifen.

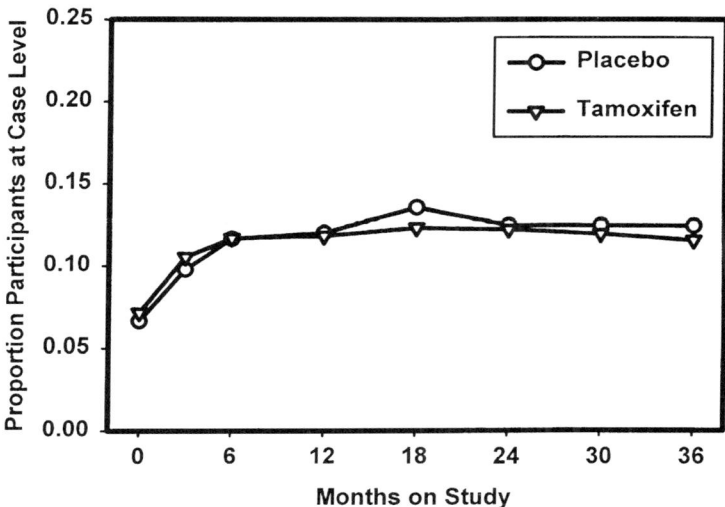

FIGURE 2. Proportion of P-1 participants with CES-D scores at the level of a potential case (≥16) by arm and examination. A CES-D score of ≥16 is the clinical cutoff—that is, it is the score above which depression is considered to be present.

which depression is considered to be present) on the CES-D.[6,7] The youngest age group (35–49 years old) in both trial groups consistently had the highest proportion of members scoring above the clinical cutoff, followed by the 50- to 59-year-old age group. Similar findings with regard to the relationship between the two trial groups emerged from the analysis of the 5-item mental health subscale on the MOS SF-36 (not shown).

The SF-36 results are summarized in FIGURE 3 using the physical and mental component scores (PCS, MCS).[8] Mean PCS declines across the age groups. On follow-up examinations, the tamoxifen group was consistently lower on the PCS only in the 50- to 59-year-old age group (one-sided sign test, $P = 0.065$); however, absolute differences were very small, approximating 1/10th of a standard deviation. No consistent differences emerged on the MCS between the two trial groups.

TABLE 1 provides information on the proportion of women in the tamoxifen and placebo groups reporting symptoms on the SCL at least once during the period that the participants were on treatment—that is, the period excluding baseline, but including the seven follow-up examinations. The five symptoms with the greatest relative difference between the two trial groups are given for each age group and the 10 symptoms with the greatest relative difference are presented for all participants combined.

FIGURE 4 summarizes the information from the five items on the MOS sexual functioning scale. Plate A on FIGURE 4 shows that a greater proportion of participants in the tamoxifen as compared to the placebo group reported being sexually active during the 6 months prior to each follow-up examination. Although apparently consistent, the absolute difference was small (mean = 0.78%) and the findings may have been due

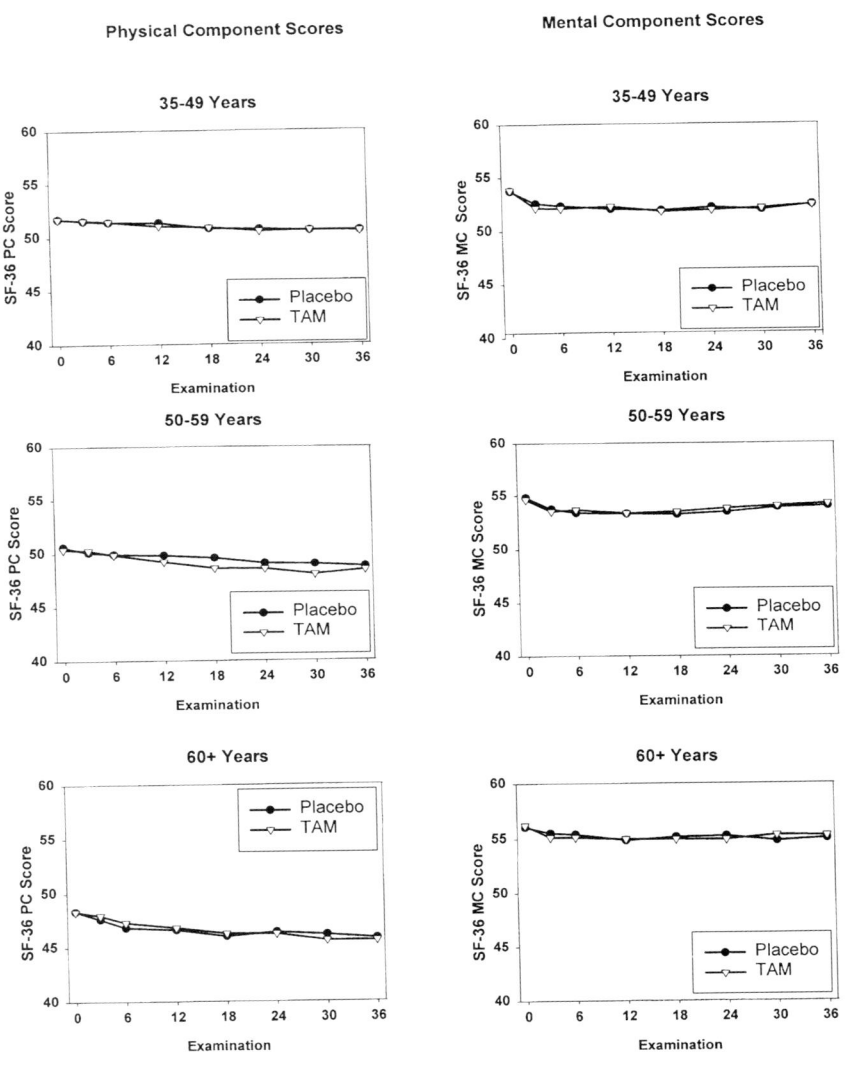

FIGURE 3. Mean scores by age group and examination on SF-36 physical and mental component scores. A higher score represents a better quality of life. TAM, tamoxifen.

TABLE 1. Symptoms reported at least once between 3 and 36 months with the largest relative difference between trial arms

Age group and symptom	Placebo arm proportion (%)	Tamoxifen arm proportion (%)	Relative risk (TAM/placebo)
35–49 Years			
Cold sweats	15.90	22.90	1.44
Vaginal discharge	46.29	62.55	1.35
Pain in intercourse	23.88	31.57	1.32
Night sweats	59.58	74.16	1.24
Hot flashes	65.54	81.28	1.24
50–59 Years			
Cold sweats	16.11	27.00	1.68
Vaginal discharge	32.51	53.47	1.64
Genital itching	36.93	45.24	1.23
Night sweats	62.77	75.88	1.21
Bladder control (laugh)	47.67	56.94	1.19
≥60 Years			
Vaginal bleeding	4.64	10.92	2.35
Vaginal discharge	19.82	45.81	2.31
Genital itching	32.05	40.96	1.28
Hot flashes	51.51	63.59	1.23
Bladder control (laugh)	49.88	56.49	1.13
Overall			
Vaginal discharge	34.13	54.77	1.60
Cold sweats	14.77	21.40	1.45
Genital itching	38.29	47.13	1.23
Night sweats	54.92	66.80	1.22
Hot flashes	65.04	77.66	1.19
Pain in intercourse	24.13	28.19	1.17
Bladder control (laugh)	46.65	52.51	1.13
Bladder control (other)	47.79	52.83	1.11
Weight loss	41.97	44.94	1.07
Vaginal bleeding	21.26	21.96	1.03

to chance. Plates B–E show that a small, but consistently larger percentage of participants in the tamoxifen group reported a definite or serious problem in three of the four specific domains of sexual functioning during the follow-up period.

DISCUSSION

The cohort of women taking part in the P-1 study were not representative of the general population. They were predominantly white, well educated, and middle class, with a strong professional and technical orientation. The initial HRQL findings presented in this report must be assessed within the context of the socioeconomic and cultural characteristics of the P-1 study cohort.

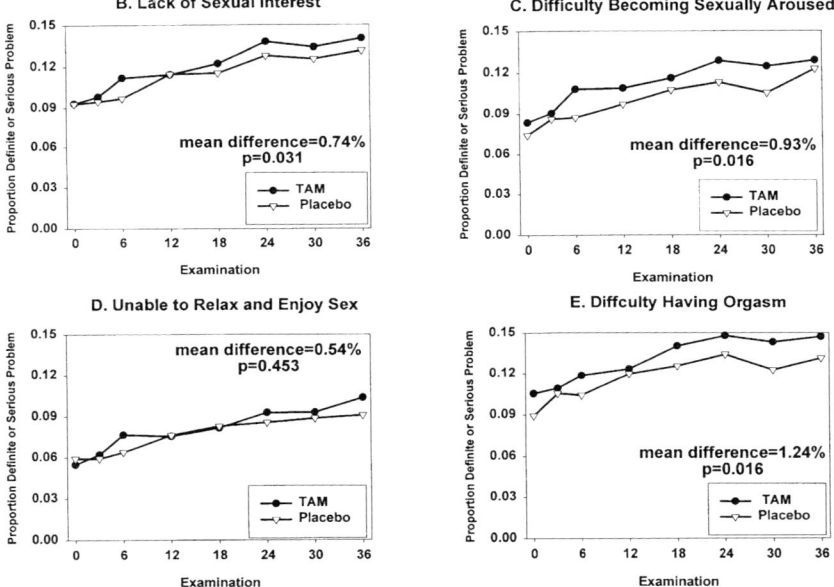

FIGURE 4. Proportion of women in the tamoxifen (TAM) and placebo arms reporting a definite or serious problem in the past 4 weeks on the MOS sexual functioning scale. Plates **B to E** refer only to women who reported being sexually active in the last 6 months.

Although 31.5% of our participants did not complete the 36-month HRQL follow-up examination, we have shown that there is only a small difference in the proportion of nonadherent participants in the tamoxifen and placebo groups and that the nonadherent women in both trial groups are generally similar on key demographic, clinical, and HRQL variables. Given these considerations, it seems unlikely that a maximum difference of 3% in the HRQL follow-up rates between the two groups was sufficient to create a significant bias in our between-group comparisons.

Concern has been expressed regarding the possible relationship between tamoxifen use and the onset of depression.[9–13] Women reporting a history of depressive episodes or of treatment for nervous or mental disorders were not excluded from the trial. If tamoxifen use were associated with the onset of clinically diagnosable depression, we would have expected to see a consistent excess of individuals scoring ≥16 on the CES-D in the tamoxifen group. No such consistent excess was observed.

The MOS SF-36 served in this study as a measure of overall health-related quality of life. We presented data from this instrument in terms of two high-level component scores (PCS and MCS), neither one of which demonstrated any clinically significant differences between the tamoxifen and placebo groups.

The first signs of consistent differences between the tamoxifen and placebo groups were observed in the symptom checklist (SCL). The differences between the trial groups tended to be associated with the types of vasomotor, gynecological, and sexual functioning symptoms previously reported for tamoxifen.[10,14,15]

The data from the MOS sexual functioning scale indicate that relatively small (<4.0%), but consistent differences exist between the two groups with regard to the proportion of women reporting definite or serious problems in at least three specific domains of sexual functioning—sexual interest, arousal, and orgasm. These problems do not appear to be age group–specific. Despite these findings for specific domains of functioning, there is no evidence that these problems result in a reduction in the overall proportion of women in the tamoxifen group who are sexually active.

Based on these data, we would conclude that tamoxifen use is associated with an increase in specific vasomotor, gynecological, and sexual functioning symptoms. At the same time, we did not observe any evidence that overall physical or emotional well-being was significantly affected by these differences in the frequency of symptoms. We also found no evidence on the CES-D or the SF-36 mental health scale for an association in any age group between tamoxifen use and an increase in the proportion of women reporting clinically significant levels of depression.

How should clinicians integrate these research results into decision-making and recommendations to women considering the use of tamoxifen in the setting of prevention? Many symptoms experienced by women who participated in this study are age- and menopause-related and exist independent of the use of tamoxifen. However, several symptoms are substantially more frequent in women using tamoxifen and these include vasomotor symptoms (cold sweats, night sweats, hot flashes), vaginal discharge, and genital itching. Women need to be informed of these possible symptoms. Weight gain and depression, two clinical problems anecdotally associated with tamoxifen treatment in women with breast cancer, were not increased in frequency in this large placebo-controlled trial in healthy women. This is good news that must also be communicated to women.

An informed discussion with a woman considering tamoxifen therapy should include these points in the risk-benefit discussion. Disclosure of likely and unlikely symptoms should prepare a woman for what she might experience and reduce her anxiety or concerns should she embark on preventive therapy. Should a woman experience untoward symptoms after starting tamoxifen treatment, the medication can be discontinued if the symptoms cannot be controlled or her personal assessment of the risks and benefits changes.

REFERENCES

1. FISHER, B., J.P. COSTANTINO, D.L. WICKERHAM et al. 1998. Tamoxifen for the prevention of breast cancer: a report from the NSABP P-1 study. J. Natl. Cancer Inst. **90:** 1371–1388.
2. FISHER, B. & J.P. COSTANTINO. 1997. Highlights of the NSABP Breast Cancer Prevention Trial. Cancer Control **4:** 78–86.
3. GANZ, P.A., R. DAY, J.E. WARE et al. 1995. Baseline quality-of-life assessment in the National Surgical Adjuvant Breast and Bowel Project Breast Cancer Prevention Trial. J. Natl. Cancer Inst. **87:** 1372–1382.
4. GANZ, P.A., R. DAY & J.P. COSTANTINO. 1998. Compliance with quality of life data collection in the NSABP Breast Cancer Prevention Trial. Stat. Med. **17:** 613–622.
5. DAY, R., P.A. GANZ, J.P. COSTANTINO et al. 1999. Health-related quality of life and tamoxifen in breast cancer prevention: a report from the NSABP P-1 study. J. Clin. Oncol. **17:** 2659–2669.
6. RADLOFF, L.S. 1977. The CES-D scale: a self-report depression scale for research in the general population. Appl. Psychol. Meas. **1:** 385–401.
7. ROBERTS, R.E. & S.W. VERNON. 1983. The Center for Epidemiologic Studies Depression Scale: its use in a community sample. Am. J. Psychiatry **140:** 41–46.
8. WARE, J.E., M. KOSINSKI & S.D. KELLER. 1994. SF-36 Physical and Mental Summary Scales: A User's Manual. Third printing revised. The Health Institute, New England Medical Center. Boston.
9. CATHACART, C.K., S.E. JONES, C.S. PUMROY et al. 1993. Clinical recognition and management of depression in node negative breast cancer patients treated with tamoxifen. Breast Cancer Res. Treat. **27:** 277–281.
10. LOVE, R.L., L. CAMERON, B.L. CONNELL et al. 1991. Symptoms associated with tamoxifen treatment in postmenopausal women. Arch. Intern. Med. **151:** 1842–1847.
11. SHARIFF, S., C.E. CUMMING, A. LEES et al. 1995. Mood disorder in women with early breast cancer taking tamoxifen, an estradiol receptor antagonist: an unexpected effect? Ann. N.Y. Acad. Sci. **761:** 365–368.
12. MOREDO ANELLI, T., A. ANELLI, K.N. TRAN et al. 1994. Tamoxifen administration is associated with a high rate of treatment-limiting symptoms in male breast cancer patients. Cancer **74:** 74–77.
13. PLUSS, J.L. & N.J. DIBELLA. 1984. Reversible central nervous system dysfunction due to tamoxifen in a patient with breast cancer. Ann. Intern. Med. **101:** 652.
14. FISHER, B., J. DIGNAM, J. BRYANT et al. 1996. Five versus more than five years of tamoxifen therapy for breast cancer patients with negative lymph nodes and estrogen receptor–positive tumors. J. Natl. Cancer Inst. **88:** 1529–1542.
15. FISHER, B., J.P. COSTANTINO, C. REDMOND et al. 1989. A randomized clinical trial evaluating tamoxifen in the treatment of patients with node-negative breast cancer who have estrogen receptor–positive tumors. N. Engl. J. Med. **320:** 479–484.

Selective Estrogen Receptor Modulators and Cardiovascular Disease

Introduction

DAVID J. GORDON

Division of Heart and Vascular Diseases, National Heart, Lung, and Blood Institute, National Institutes of Health, Bethesda, Maryland 20892, USA

The five papers presented in this section review the evidence for favorable cardiovascular effects of estrogen and compare these effects with those of the new selective estrogen receptor modulators (SERMs).[1–5]

Dr. Herrington has reviewed the many lines of evidence suggesting that oral administration of estrogen may be beneficial in the prevention and treatment of coronary heart disease (CHD) in postmenopausal women.[1] Estrogen has favorable effects on cardiovascular risk factors, including high-density (HDL) and low-density (LDL) lipoprotein cholesterol and fibrinogen, and on measures of vascular endothelial function. Coadministration of medroxyprogesterone acetate (MPA) to protect against endometrial proliferation and neoplasia only partially offsets these putative benefits. CHD incidence and mortality in women generally lag 15 years behind men and are relatively uncommon before menopause. Prospective observational epidemiologic studies in postmenopausal women have shown an association of hormone replacement therapy (HRT), usually combined equine estrogens (CEE) with or without MPA, with marked reduction in risk of CHD and in mortality. However, randomized clinical trials of HRT completed to date have failed to show significant benefit of HRT on clinical CHD events or on the progression of the underlying coronary atherosclerotic lesions and suggest adverse effects on the early incidence of myocardial infarction (MI) and on the incidence of venous thromboembolism (VTE).[1]

The recent advent of the SERMs, which mimic some of the effects of estrogen while antagonizing others, offers the possibility to attain the potential cardiovascular benefits of estrogen therapy without its potential adverse cardiovascular effects or its attendant increased risk of carcinoma of the uterus and breast. In fact, raloxifene, one of the most widely used SERMs, acts as an antiestrogen in the uterus and breast, and does not require coadministration of a progestin in gynecologically intact women.

The articles by Dr. Walsh,[2] Drs. Blum and Cannon,[3] and Dr. Cushman[4] compare the effects of raloxifene and other SERMs with conventional HRT on lipoproteins and on measures of vascular endothelial function, inflammation, and hemostasis.

Address for correspondence: David J. Gordon, M.D., Ph.D., M.P.H., National Heart, Lung, and Blood Institute, Division of Heart and Vascular Diseases, 2 Rockledge Center, Suite 9044, 6701 Rockledge Drive, Bethesda, MD 20892-7540. Voice: 301-435-0564; fax: 301-480-1335.
gordond@nhlbi.nih.gov

While the SERMs are similar to conventional HRT in many ways, there are also differences with potentially important cardiovascular implications. For example, raloxifene lacks the pro-inflammatory effect of estrogen on C-reactive protein (CRP), an important marker of CHD risk. However, unlike estrogen, raloxifene does not raise HDL cholesterol, an important inverse CHD risk factor. The net impact of these differences on CHD risk is uncertain.

Finally, Dr. Mosca describes the design of the Raloxifene Use for the Heart (RUTH) trial, an industry-sponsored randomized trial addressing the effect of raloxifene on the incidence of CHD events and breast cancer in 10,101 women.[5] This is the first randomized trial designed with sufficient power to assess the effects of a SERM on clinical cardiovascular events. Its results, along with those of ongoing large HRT trials like the Women's Health Initiative (WHI), will go a long way toward clarifying the viability of estrogen and SERMs as treatment options for cardiovascular disease.

REFERENCES

1. HERRINGTON, D.M. & K.P. KLEIN. 2001. Cardiovascular trials of estrogen replacement therapy. This volume.
2. WALSH, B.W. 2001. The effects of estrogen and selective estrogen receptor modulators on cardiovascular risk factors. This volume.
3. BLUM, A. & R.O. CANNON III. 2001. Selective estrogen receptor modulator (SERM) effects on serum lipoproteins and vascular function in postmenopausal women and in hypercholesterolemic men. This volume.
4. CUSHMAN, M. 2001. Effects of estrogen and selective estrogen receptor modulators on hemostasis and inflammation: potential differences among drugs. This volume.
5. MOSCA, L. 2001. Rationale and overview of the Raloxifene Use for the Heart (RUTH) trial. This volume.

Cardiovascular Trials of Estrogen Replacement Therapy

DAVID M. HERRINGTON AND KAREN POTVIN KLEIN

Department of Internal Medicine/Cardiology, Wake Forest University School of Medicine, Winston-Salem, North Carolina 27157, USA

ABSTRACT: An impressive body of evidence has suggested that estrogen therapy should be helpful to slow the pathogenesis or progression of atherosclerosis. Estrogen's favorable effects on lipids and endothelial function, coupled with extensive observational epidemiology and data from animal models of atherosclerosis, persuaded many that hormone replacement therapy (HRT) would be helpful for both primary and secondary prevention of coronary disease. Recently, several randomized clinical trials of HRT have been completed, and several more are currently under way. These trials include both primary and secondary prevention cohorts and use clinical as well as anatomic manifestations of atherosclerosis as outcomes. These trials are producing surprising and controversial results that will radically alter contemporary understanding of the role of HRT for cardiovascular disease prevention. This review briefly describes the findings of the Heart and Estrogen/Progestin Replacement Study, the Estrogen Replacement and Atherosclerosis Trial, and other recently completed clinical trials. Trials that are under way are also described and discussed.

KEYWORDS: hormone replacement therapy; cardiovascular disease; women; thrombosis; myocardial infarction; risk factors; menopause

INTRODUCTION

There is an impressive body of evidence suggesting that estrogen therapy should be helpful to slow the pathogenesis or progression of atherosclerosis. The favorable effects of estrogen on lipids and endothelial function, coupled with extensive observational epidemiology and data from animal models of atherosclerosis, have produced a deeply rooted impression that hormone replacement therapy (HRT) would be helpful for both primary and secondary prevention of coronary disease. Nevertheless, without randomized clinical trials, it is impossible to know whether the extensive evidence supporting estrogen use will translate into real clinical benefits and that unanticipated adverse effects do not offset these benefits. During the last 2 years, several trials of HRT have been completed, and several more are currently under way. These trials, including both primary and secondary prevention cohorts using both clinical and anatomic manifestations of atherosclerosis as outcomes, are

---

Address for correspondence: David M. Herrington, M.D., M.H.S., Department of Internal Medicine/Cardiology, Wake Forest University School of Medicine, Medical Center Boulevard, Winston-Salem, NC 27157-1045. Fax: 336-716-9188.
dherring@wfubmc.edu

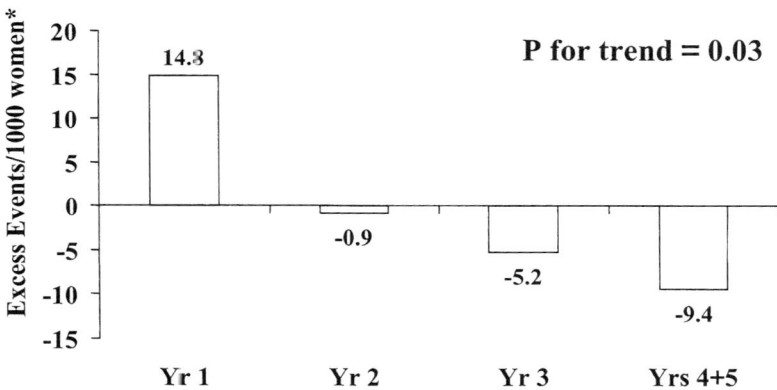

* compared to placebo

FIGURE 1. Excess coronary heart disease events by year in HERS among women taking estrogen plus progestin therapy. *$P = 0.05$ compared to placebo.

producing surprising and controversial results that will radically alter contemporary understanding of the role of HRT for cardiovascular disease prevention.

THE HEART AND ESTROGEN/PROGESTIN STUDY (HERS)

HERS was a multicenter, randomized, double-blind, placebo-controlled trial testing the efficacy of 0.625 mg of conjugated equine estrogens and 2.5 mg of medroxyprogesterone acetate (MPA) for prevention of cardiovascular disease among 2763 women with established CHD. Surprisingly, after 4.1 years of follow-up, the overall rates of myocardial infarction (MI) and CHD death were no different among women in the active treatment group compared to the placebo group.[1] There were also no significant differences among several other secondary cardiovascular end points. Within the overall null effect, there was a pattern of increased risk in the first year among women on active therapy, and decreased risk in the latter years of the trial. The test for trend in the final analysis was nominally significant ($P = 0.03$). However, only the 50% increase in risk in year 1 was significant in the year-specific analyses (FIG. 1). The point estimates for the relative hazards in years 3–5 were less than 1, but not statistically significant.

More questions have been raised than answered by the HERS results. First, is it possible that the HERS results were simply a chance occurrence? This is a tenable question in view of the large amount of previous data suggesting that HRT should have been effective. Second, was the HRT regimen used less effective in terms of cardiovascular protection than other regimens, such as unopposed conjugated equine estrogen or transdermal estradiol? A third issue is whether the pattern of increased risk is real; if so, what is its cause and is it limited to a unique subgroup of women? Finally, is estrogen more effective in primary prevention than it apparently was for secondary prevention? Some of these questions have been addressed with data from newer randomized clinical trials and clinical studies of HRT, which are reviewed below.

CORROBORATING DATA CONCERNING THE PATTERN OF EARLY RISK OBSERVED IN HERS

Recent reports from the Puget Sound Group Health Cooperative[2] and the Nurses' Health Study[3] suggest the presence of an increased risk of MI among new HRT users (TABLE 1). Within the Puget Sound cohort, among healthy women who were new HRT users, the odds ratio for an MI was over twice that of women who had used HRT for 1 to 2 years (<0.5 year, odds ratio [OR] = 1.39, 95% confidence intervals [CI] = 0.52–3.72; 1–2 years, OR = 0.61, 95% CI = 0.23–1.61).[2] A similar pattern was seen in the Nurses' Health Study; of the women with a prior MI (N = 2245), the age-adjusted relative risk for MI recurrence among new HRT users was twice that of women who had used HRT for 1 to 2 years (<1 year, OR = 2.10, 95% CI = 0.88–4.99; 1–2 years, OR = 1.01, 95% CI = 0.31–3.27).[3] Nonetheless, these observations were based on small numbers of women and the confidence intervals were wide and included unity. More recently, the Women's Health Initiative (WHI) investigators announced a similar pattern of early increased risk for cardiovascular events that seemed to decline over time, but specific details are not yet publicly available (see http://www.nhlbi.gov/whi/hrt-en.htm). A reanalysis of the Coronary Drug Project, which examined estrogen in men, also revealed an increased risk of MI within the first 4 months of therapy in men with CHD. For all-cause mortality, the relative hazard was 1.06 (95% CI = 0.91–

TABLE 1. Recent reports of myocardial infarction (MI) risk among new users of HRT in large cohorts or clinical trials

	N	Relative risk for MI	95% confidence intervals
Cohort studies			
Puget Sound[2]	1882		
HRT < 6 months		1.39	0.52–3.72
HRT 1–2 years		0.61	0.23–1.61
Nurses' Health Study[3]	2245		
HRT < 1 year		2.10	0.88–4.99
HRT 1–2 years		1.01	0.31–3.27
Clinical trials			
Coronary Drug Project[4]	5009		
Estrogen < 4 months		1.58	1.04–2.40
Estrogen 1–5 years		0.90	0.80–1.05
HERS[1]	2763		
HRT < 4 months		2.29	0.94–5.56
HRT 1–5 years		0.85	0.67–1.08

1.25).[4] In the aggregate, these data seem to corroborate the pattern of early risk seen in HERS. It is important to note that the data from the Nurses' Health Study and the Coronary Drug Project were from individuals with established coronary artery disease; however, the data from the Puget Sound Group Health Cooperative and the WHI were from women who were largely free of initial evidence of coronary disease. If verified, this could have important implications for the large number of healthy women who use estrogen replacement for prevention of hot flashes or to treat osteoporosis.

POTENTIAL MECHANISMS TO ACCOUNT FOR EARLY RISK WITH HRT

There are several postulated mechanisms for the pattern of early risk observed in HERS. One leading possibility is that the early increase in coronary events was related to a prothrombotic effect of estrogen. It is well established that both postmenopausal HRT and oral contraceptives increase risk for venous thrombosis.[5-7] The new data from women with established coronary disease in HERS complement previous studies of oral contraceptive use in women with coronary risk factors that have also indicated an increased risk for coronary thrombosis.[8,9] Some evidence suggests that women with polymorphisms in one or more genes that regulate thrombosis might be especially at high risk for either an arterial or a venous thrombotic complication of estrogen.[10,11]

One possible explanation for the pattern of early risk is that HRT produced a proinflammatory state. Two large observational studies[12,13] and two clinical trials[14,15] have shown that HRT users have 48% to 260% higher levels of C-reactive protein (CRP), an acute-phase reactant whose hepatic production is primarily regulated by the proinflammatory cytokine, interleukin-6.[16] Furthermore, changes were seen after as little as 4 weeks of treatment.[15] Studies have shown a prospective association between increased CRP levels and cardiovascular events, both in healthy people[17-21] and in patients with established vascular disease.[18,20,22,23] In vitro studies further bolster the idea that CRP and other inflammatory markers are integral in the development of atherosclerosis.[24] More data are needed concerning the effects of estrogen on thrombosis and inflammation and the potential impact on risk for CHD events.

THE ESTROGEN REPLACEMENT AND ATHEROSCLEROSIS (ERA) TRIAL

The ERA trial (funded by the National Heart, Lung, and Blood Institute), like HERS, was a secondary prevention trial. The study examined whether unopposed conjugated equine estrogen or estrogen plus MPA would affect progression of coronary artery atherosclerosis in 309 women with angiographically verified coronary disease. After baseline angiography, women were randomized to receive unopposed conjugated equine estrogen (0.625 mg/day), estrogen plus MPA (2.5 mg/day), or placebo and were followed for a mean of 3.2 years. Follow-up angiography revealed

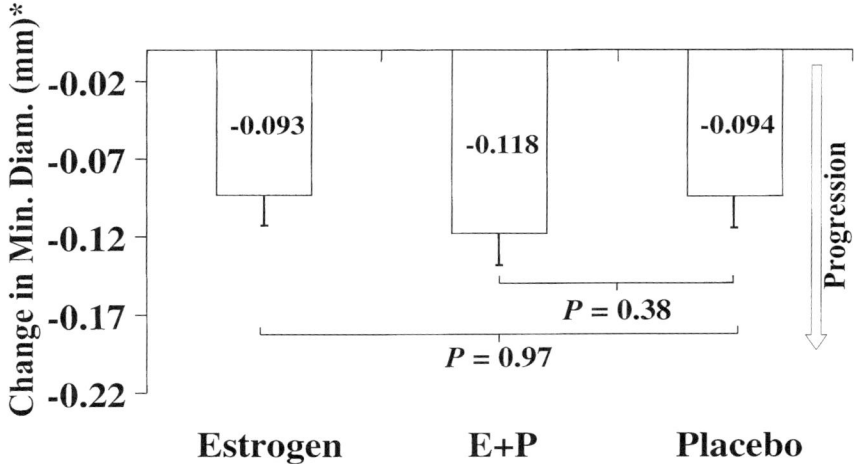

FIGURE 2. Change in mean minimum coronary diameter (adjusted for prespecified covariates) by treatment arm among 248 women in the ERA trial. E + P = estrogen plus progestin.

that women in the two hormone treatment groups had essentially the same rate of progression of coronary disease as the placebo group (FIG. 2).[25] There were also no differences among numerous secondary angiographic outcomes. Since similar results were seen in both the unopposed estrogen and the estrogen plus MPA groups, these data suggest that the null effect in HERS was not a function of the use of MPA.

THE POSTMENOPAUSAL HORMONE REPLACEMENT AGAINST ATHEROSCLEROSIS (PHOREA) TRIAL

The PHOREA trial sought to determine whether hormone replacement would affect the progression of carotid artery atherosclerosis in a population of German postmenopausal women ($N = 321$) at risk for, but who did not yet have, heart disease.[26] Carotid intima-media thickness (IMT) was the primary end point of this 48-week study. After being allocated to two risk strata (≤ 2 risk factors for CHD or >2 risk factors for CHD), participants were randomized to receive no treatment, 1 mg/day oral 17β-estradiol plus 0.025 mg oral gestodene for 12 days/month, or 1 mg/day oral 17β-estradiol plus 0.025 mg oral gestodene for 12 days/every third month. The investigators found that neither hormone regimen slowed the progression of carotid IMT, although both treatments decreased fibrinogen and LDL levels compared to the no-treatment group. The authors speculate that positive effects of HRT may require a longer period of treatment to emerge (as suggested by the HERS results) and that estrogen's protective effects on CHD may be mediated by mechanisms other than inhibition of atherosclerosis.

THE PAPWORTH HRT ATHEROSCLEROSIS STUDY ENQUIRY (PHASE)

The PHASE trial was a United Kingdom–based angiographic trial of HRT among women with angiographically documented coronary disease. Subjects were randomized to receive transdermal 17β-estradiol at 2 mg/day (plus cyclic norethindrone acetate at 4 mg/day in those with an intact uterus) or placebo and were followed for 4 years.[27] The trial was stopped after 3 years of follow-up in only 255 women because of the lack of apparent benefit and the possibility of harm. In the intention-to-treat analysis, the primary end point event rate was 15.6 per 100 person-years in the HRT group compared with 12.6 in the placebo group (OR = 1.23, 95% CI = 0.82–1.86, $P = 0.3$). Of note, the relative risk of CHD events with HRT was greater than 1 for each year of follow-up.

THE ESTROGEN AND PREVENTION OF ATHEROSCLEROSIS TRIAL (EPAT)

EPAT was a randomized clinical trial of estrogen intervention for atherosclerotic disease to include postmenopausal women with elevated LDL cholesterol, but no evidence of coronary disease ($N = 199$).[28] Women were also ineligible if they had diabetes mellitus or a history of smoking. In this study, women were randomized to receive oral 17β-estradiol (1 mg/day) or placebo; all women also received lipid-lowering medication if their baseline LDL cholesterol level exceeded 160 mg/dL. Women were followed for 2 years. The investigators found increased carotid wall thickness in the placebo group, but a small decrease in the estrogen group ($P = 0.045$); however, the difference between the treatment arms was limited to women who were not on lipid-lowering medication. Among this subgroup, there was an even greater increase in carotid wall thickness in the placebo group compared with slight regression in the estrogen group ($P = 0.002$).

ONGOING TRIALS OF HRT FOR CARDIOVASCULAR DISEASE

Secondary Prevention

Three NHLBI-funded angiographic end point trials of HRT in women with established CHD are currently under way (TABLE 2). Among these is the Women's Estrogen-Progestin Lipid Lowering Hormone Atherosclerosis Regression Trial (WELL-HART), a study of 17β-estradiol (plus cyclic MPA in women with a uterus) where all women ($N = 226$) also receive a lipid-lowering agent if their LDL is above 130 mg/dL. Results of WELL-HART should be available sometime in 2001. The Women's Angiographic Vitamin and Estrogen (WAVE) trial, in which women ($N = 400$) receive conjugated equine estrogen (plus 2.5 mg MPA daily for women with a uterus), vitamins C and E, or placebo, will finish in 2002. The Estrogen and Graft Atherosclerosis Research (EAGAR) study (N to date = 99) will examine the effect of 3.5 years of 17β-estradiol plus 2.5 mg MPA daily to prevent graft occlusion in postmenopausal women who have recently undergone coronary artery bypass surgery. This study will be concluded by 2004.

TABLE 2. Summary of completed and ongoing trials of HRT for cardiovascular disease prevention

Study	n	Treatment(s) and results (outcome)[a]	Duration of follow-up	Primary end points
Primary prevention				
PHOREA[26,b]	321	17β-E_2; 17β-E_2 + 0.025 mg gestodene 12 days/month; 17β-E_2 + 0.025 mg gestodene 12 days/every 3 months; no difference in rate of progression	48 weeks	carotid IMT
EPAT[28]	222	17β-E_2; significantly less progression with E_2	2 years	carotid IMT
WHI[30]	27,348	CEE (+ continuous MPA in women with a uterus); N/A	8.5 years	coronary events
WISDOM	34,000	CEE (+ continuous MPA in women with a uterus); N/A	10 years	coronary events
Secondary prevention				
HERS[1]	2763	CEE + MPA; no difference in risk; improvements in lipids	4.1 years	CHD death and nonfatal MI
ERA[25]	309	CEE ± MPA; no difference; improvements in lipids	3.2 years	mean minimum coronary artery diameter
PHASE[27]	255	17β-E_2 ± cyclic norethisterone; no difference	4 years[c]	unstable angina or MI
WEST[29]	652	17β-E_2; no difference	2.7 years	combined nonfatal stroke and death
WELL-HART	144	17β-E_2 + lipid lowering; 5 mg MPA 12 days/year in women with a uterus; N/A	3 years	progression of coronary stenosis
WAVE	400	CEE ± MPA, ± vitamins C and E; N/A	3 years	progression of coronary stenosis
EAGAR	99	17β-E_2 (+ continuous MPA in women with a uterus); N/A	3 years	progression of stenosis (graft)

ABBREVIATIONS: 17β-E_2 = 17β-estradiol; CEE = conjugated equine estrogen; IMT = intima-media thickness; MI = myocardial infarction; MPA = medroxyprogesterone acetate; N/A = not available (study still under way). For explanations of study acronyms, see text.
[a]In these studies, a placebo arm is included. Results are in comparison to placebo.
[b]In PHOREA, results are in comparison to the no-treatment arm.
[c]Trial stopped early at 3 years of follow-up due to lack of apparent benefit and possibility of harm.

The Women's Estrogen for Stroke Trial (WEST) ($N = 652$), funded by NINDS, examined the effect of 1 mg/day oral 17β-estradiol in postmenopausal women with documented transient ischemic attacks or stroke. Women with a uterus received 5 mg

MPA for 12 days, once per year. The primary outcome was a combined outcome of nonfatal stroke or death. After a mean of 2.7 years of follow-up, estradiol did not prevent recurrent stroke or reduce all-cause mortality (combined rate: estradiol group, 27.6%; placebo group, 27.7%; $P = 0.80$).[29]

Primary Prevention

Two large primary prevention trials of HRT are currently under way. The HRT component of the NIH-sponsored Women's Health Initiative ($N = 27,348$) will study risk of heart disease over a mean of 8.5 years of follow-up in women taking conjugated equine estrogen (with or without MPA, depending on uterine status) versus placebo.[30] The Medical Research Council–sponsored Women's International Study of Long Duration Oestrogen after the Menopause (WISDOM) (anticipated $N = 34,000$) will similarly examine its multinational cohort using the same treatments for 10 years. WISDOM is still in the recruitment phase. The WHI results will be reported in 2005. These studies will provide much-needed long-term data on the effects of estrogen (plus MPA in women with a uterus) in mostly healthy postmenopausal women.

In summary, the best available evidence from clinical trials does not support a role of HRT for secondary prevention of coronary disease. The lack of benefit and the possible early increase in risk may be related to previously unrecognized or underemphasized proinflammatory or prothrombotic effects of HRT. Preliminary data in women without evidence of coronary disease are still inconclusive. Results from several newer primary and secondary prevention trials are expected to define further what role, if any, HRT may play for prevention of heart disease. In the meantime, the emphasis should remain on using proven forms of therapy, including lipid lowering when indicated, to reduce the burden of heart disease in women.

ACKNOWLEDGMENT

This work was supported in part by Grant U01HL45488 (D.M. Herrington, PI), National Heart, Lung and Blood Institute, Bethesda, Maryland.

REFERENCES

1. HULLEY, S., D. GRADY, T. BUSH et al. 1998. Randomized trial of estrogen plus progestin for secondary prevention of coronary heart disease in postmenopausal women. J. Am. Med. Assoc. **280:** 605–613.
2. HECKBERT, S.R., N.S. WEISS & B.M. PSATY. 1999. Hormone replacement therapy for secondary prevention of coronary heart disease [letter]. J. Am. Med. Assoc. **281:** 795–796.
3. GRODSTEIN, F., J.E. MANSON & M.J. STAMPFER. 1999. Postmenopausal hormones and recurrence of coronary events in the Nurses' Health Study [abstract]. Circulation **100:** I-871.
4. WENGER, N.K., G.L. KNATTERUD & P.L. CANNER. 2000. Early risks of hormone therapy in patients with coronary heart disease [letter]. J. Am. Med. Assoc. **284:** 41–43.
5. DALY, E., M.P. VESSEY, M.M. HAWKINS et al. 1996. Risk of venous thromboembolism in users of hormone replacement therapy. Lancet **348:** 977–980.

6. JICK, H., L.E. DERBY, M.W. MYERS et al. 1996. Risk of hospital admission for idiopathic venous thromboembolism among users of postmenopausal oestrogens. Lancet **348:** 981–983.
7. GRADY, D., N.K. WENGER, D. HERRINGTON et al. 2000. Postmenopausal hormone therapy increases risk for venous thromboembolic disease: the Heart and Estrogen/Progestin Replacement Study. Ann. Intern. Med. **132:** 689–696.
8. WHO COLLABORATORS. 1999. Acute myocardial infarction and combined oral contraceptives: results of an international multicentre case-control study—WHO Collaborative Study of Cardiovascular Disease and Steroid Hormone Contraception. Lancet **349:** 1202–1209.
9. MANT, J., R. PAINTER & M. VESSEY. 1998. Risk of myocardial infarction, angina, and stroke in users of oral contraceptives: an updated analysis of a cohort study. Br. J. Obstet. Gynaecol. **105:** 890–896.
10. DOGGEN, C.J.M., V. MANGER CATS, R.M. BERTINA et al. 1998. Interaction of coagulation defects and cardiovascular risk factors: increased risk of myocardial infarction associated with factor V Leiden or prothrombin 20210A. Circulation **97:** 1037–1041.
11. GLUECK, C.J., P. WANG, R.N. FONTAINE et al. 2000. The effect of exogenous estrogen on atherothrombotic vascular disease risk relates to the presence or absence of the 20210 G/A prothrombin gene mutation: a cross-sectional study of 230 hyperlipidemic women. Circulation **102**(suppl. II): II-278–II-279.
12. CUSHMAN, M., E.N. MEILAHN, B.M. PSATY et al. 1999. Hormone replacement therapy, inflammation, and hemostasis in elderly women. Arterioscler. Thromb. Vasc. Biol. **19:** 893–899.
13. RIDKER, P.M., C.H. HENNEKENS, N. RIFAI et al. 1999. Hormone replacement therapy and increased plasma concentration of C-reactive protein. Circulation **100:** 713–716.
14. CUSHMAN, M., C. LEGAULT, E. BARRETT-CONNOR et al. 1999. Effect of postmenopausal hormones on inflammation-sensitive proteins: the Postmenopausal Estrogen/Progestin Interventions (PEPI) study. Circulation **100:** 717–722.
15. VAN BAAL, W.M., P. KENEMANS, M.J. VAN DER MOOREN et al. 1999. Increased C-reactive protein levels during short-term hormone replacement therapy in healthy postmenopausal women. Thromb. Haemostasis **81:** 925–928.
16. KUSHNER, I. 1993. Regulation of the acute phase response by cytokines. Perspect. Biol. Med. **36:** 611–622.
17. RIDKER, P.M., M. CUSHMAN, M.J. STAMPFER et al. 1997. Inflammation, aspirin, and the risk of cardiovascular disease in apparently healthy men. N. Engl. J. Med. **336:** 973–979.
18. TRACY, R.P., R.N. LEMAITRE, B.M. PSATY et al. 1997. Relationship of C-reactive protein to risk of cardiovascular disease in the elderly: results from the Cardiovascular Health Study and the Rural Health Promotion Project. Arterioscler. Thromb. Vasc. Biol. **6:** 1121–1127.
19. TOSS, H., B. LINDAHL, A. SIEGBAHN et al. 1997. Prognostic influence of increased fibrinogen and C-reactive protein levels in unstable coronary disease: FRISC (Fragmin during Instability in Coronary Artery Disease). Circulation **96:** 4204–4210.
20. RIDKER, P.M., N. RIFAI, M.A. PFEFFER et al. 1998. Inflammation, pravastatin, and the risk of coronary events after myocardial infarction in patients with average cholesterol levels: Cholesterol and Recurrent Events (CARE) Investigators. Circulation **98:** 839–844.
21. KOENIG, W., M. SUND, M. FROHLICH et al. 1999. C-reactive protein, a sensitive marker of inflammation, predicts future risk of coronary heart disease in initially healthy middle-aged men: results from the MONICA (Monitoring Trends and Determinants in Cardiovascular Disease) Augsburg Cohort Study, 1984 to 1992. Circulation **99:** 237–242.
22. LIUZZO, G., L.M. BIASUCCI, J.R. GALLIMORE et al. 1994. The prognostic value of C-reactive protein and serum amyloid A protein in severe unstable angina. N. Engl. J. Med. **331:** 417–424.
23. ZIMMERMANN, J., S. HERRLINGER, A. PRUY et al. 1999. Inflammation enhances cardiovascular risk and mortality in hemodialysis patients. Kidney Int. **55:** 648–658.
24. LIBBY, P. 1998. The interface of atherosclerosis and thrombosis: basic mechanisms. Vasc. Med. **3:** 225–229.

25. HERRINGTON, D.M., D.M. REBOUSSIN, K.B. BROSNIHAN *et al.* 2000. Effects of estrogen replacement on the progression of coronary-artery atherosclerosis. N. Engl. J. Med. **343:** 522–529.
26. ANGERER, P., S. STORK, W. KOTHNY *et al.* 2001. Effect of oral postmenopausal estrogen replacement on progression of atherosclerosis: a randomized, controlled trial. Arterioscler. Thromb. Vasc. Biol. **21:** 262–268.
27. CLARKE, S., J. KELLEHER, H. LLOYD-JONES *et al.* 2000. Transdermal hormone replacement therapy for secondary prevention of coronary artery disease in postmenopausal women [abstract]. Eur. Heart J. **21**(suppl.)**:** 212.
28. HODIS, H.N., W.J. MACK, R.A. LOBO *et al.* 2000. Estrogen in the prevention of atherosclerosis trial [abstract]. Circulation **102**(suppl. II)**:** II-837.
29. VISCOLI, C.M., L.M. BRASS, W.N. KERNAN *et al.* 2001. Effect of estrogen replacement on risk of recurrent stroke and death in the Women's Estrogen for Stroke Trial (WEST) [abstract]. Stroke **32:** 329.
30. WOMEN'S HEALTH INITIATIVE STUDY GROUP. 1998. Design of the Women's Health Initiative clinical trial and observational study. Control. Clin. Trials **19:** 61–109.

The Effects of Estrogen and Selective Estrogen Receptor Modulators on Cardiovascular Risk Factors

BRIAN W. WALSH

Department of Obstetrics and Gynecology, Brigham and Women's Hospital, Boston, Massachusetts 02115, USA

ABSTRACT: Raloxifene, a selective estrogen receptor modulator, favorably alters several markers of cardiovascular risk in healthy postmenopausal women. While many of its effects are similar to those of conventional hormone replacement therapy (HRT), there are also important differences. Raloxifene lowered low-density lipoprotein cholesterol levels similarly to estrogen. However, raloxifene lacked the potentially beneficial effects of HRT on high-density lipoprotein cholesterol levels and plasminogen activation inhibitor-1, as well as the potentially adverse effects of HRT on triglycerides and C-reactive protein. Raloxifene also had a potentially beneficial fibrinogen-lowering effect not seen with conventional HRT. The net effect of these differences is unclear. Proof that raloxifene or HRT reduces the risk of heart disease must await the results of ongoing clinical trials with cardiovascular event end points.

KEYWORDS: hormone replacement therapy (HRT); selective estrogen receptor modulator; cardiovascular disease; women; risk factors; menopause

Raloxifene, a selective estrogen receptor modulator (SERM), favorably alters several markers of cardiovascular risk in healthy postmenopausal women. This was found in a study of 390 postmenopausal women enrolled in a randomized, placebo-controlled clinical trial.[1] These women were randomly assigned to treatment with raloxifene (60 mg or 120 mg), HRT (equine estrogen 0.625 mg and medroxyprogesterone 2.5 mg), or placebo. Lipids and coagulation factors were measured after daily treatment for 6 months.

Results are displayed in FIGURES 1 and 2 and TABLE 1. Compared with placebo, raloxifene lowered serum levels of low-density lipoprotein (LDL) cholesterol by 12% (similar to the 14% reduction seen with HRT) and lipoprotein(a) by 7% (less than the 19% decrease seen with HRT). This reduction in LDL appears to be sustained over time, as shown in a 2-year study.[2] The decrease in LDL cholesterol by raloxifene would be expected to reduce the risk of coronary artery disease. Epidemiological studies have found that the levels of LDL cholesterol are related to the risk

---

Address for correspondence: Brian W. Walsh, M.D., Department of Obstetrics and Gynecology, Brigham and Women's Hospital, 75 Francis Street, Boston, MA 02115. Voice: 617-732-4285; fax: 617-566-7752.

bwwalsh@bics.bwh.harvard.edu

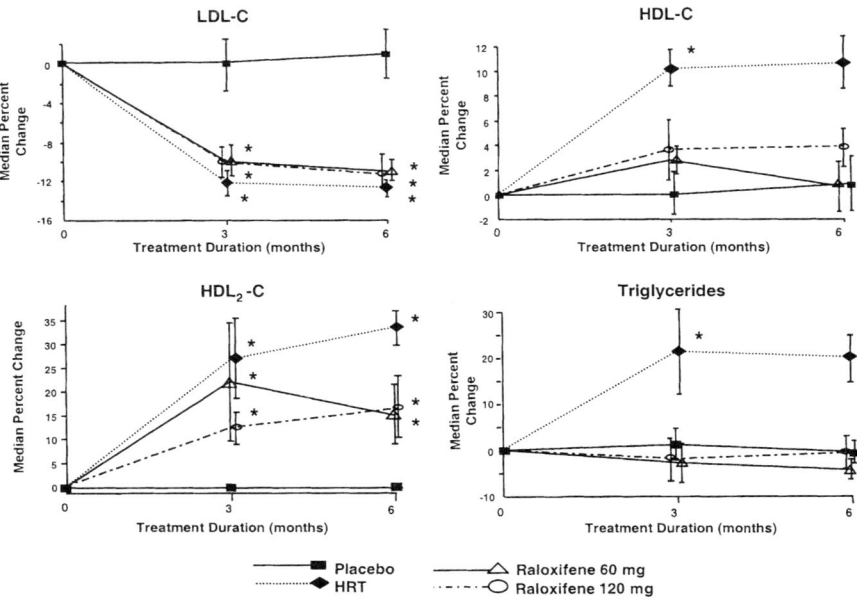

FIGURE 1. Effects of raloxifene and HRT versus placebo on LDL, HDL, and HDL_2 cholesterol and on triglyceride levels.

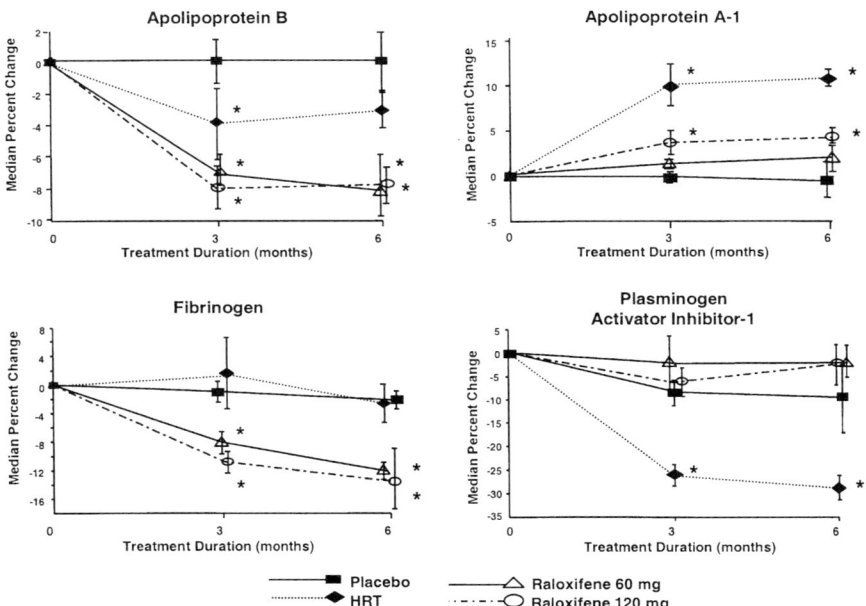

FIGURE 2. Effects of raloxifene and HRT versus placebo on apolipoproteins B and A1, fibrinogen, and PAI-1 levels.

TABLE 1. Comparison of the effects of raloxifene, tamoxifen, and HRT on markers of cardiovascular risk in healthy postmenopausal women: percentage change compared to placebo treatment

Cardiovascular risk marker	Tamoxifen (20 mg/day)	Raloxifene (60 mg/day)	HRT
LDL cholesterol	**−16***	**−12**	**−14**
HDL cholesterol	**+2***	0	**+10**
HDL_2 cholesterol	**+2***	**+15**	**+33**
Triglycerides	0*	−4	**+20**
Apolipoprotein A1	**+7***	+3	**+12**
Apolipoprotein B	**−7**†	**−9**	−3
Lipoprotein(a)	**−32**†	**−7**	**−19**
Fibrinogen	**−24***	**−10**	−1
Plasminogen activator inhibitor-1	**−15**‡	+8	**−19**
Prothrombin fragment 1 and 2	+1‡	+5	**+19**
Fibrinopeptide A	**+11**‡	−4	+3

NOTE: Data on raloxifene and HRT (hormone replacement therapy with conjugated equine estrogen [0.625 mg/day] and medroxyprogesterone acetate [2.5 mg/day]) are from the current study. Data on tamoxifen are from Refs. 13 (*), 14 (†), and 15 (‡), which reported the effect of 3–6 months of treatment. Statistically significant changes are shown in **boldface** type.

of cardiovascular disease (CVD) among both men and women. Moreover, clinical trials that lowered LDL-C levels in women have been found to reduce the incidence of a second cardiac event. One such trial of a lipid-lowering agent found that a 30% reduction in LDL-C levels in women was associated with a 46% reduction in cardiovascular events.[3] This suggests that the 12% reduction in LDL by raloxifene might lower the incidence of heart disease by as much as 18%. The 7% reduction in lipoprotein(a) levels could further decrease this risk.

Raloxifene did not change levels of high-density lipoprotein (HDL) cholesterol, triglycerides, and plasminogen activation inhibitor-1 (PAI-1). In contrast, HRT increased HDL-C by 10% and triglycerides by 20%, and decreased PAI-1 by 19%. Raloxifene did increase the HDL_2 cholesterol subfraction by 15%, but this was less than the 33% elevation with HRT.[1]

Raloxifene lowered fibrinogen by 10%–12%, whereas HRT had no effect.[1] This decline in fibrinogen may be cardioprotective. Fibrinogen levels are an independent risk factor for heart disease, with a reduction of 0.5% for every 0.01-g/L decrease in fibrinogen levels.[4] The 0.42-g/L reduction in fibrinogen induced by raloxifene could reduce cardiovascular events by 21%. For all these effects, there were no differences between the two raloxifene doses.

Raloxifene produces a small, but not statistically significant decrease in serum C-reactive protein (CRP) levels (not shown) after 6 months of treatment.[5] CRP is an independent marker for the risk of cardiovascular disease in men with[6] and without[7] clinically evident coronary artery disease and in postmenopausal women without clinically evident coronary artery disease.[8] This finding suggests a neutral effect of raloxifene on any cardiovascular risk predicted by CRP. In contrast, HRT for 6 months significantly increased serum CRP levels by 84%. This effect was unrelated to effects on the uterus and was observed even when women with concomitant infection or other inflammatory conditions were excluded from the analyses. It remains to be determined whether CRP may be involved in early coronary artery disease events associated with the initiation of HRT in women with existing coronary artery disease.

Raloxifene lowered serum levels of homocysteine by 8% and 6% (not shown), respectively, similar to the 7% reduction with HRT.[5] This is comparable to the 7% reduction observed with tamoxifen in a randomized, placebo-controlled trial in healthy postmenopausal women.[9] The impact of this degree of homocysteine lowering on the incidence of cardiovascular disease events is unknown. The risk of myocardial infarction and death from ischemic heart disease in men with no history of cardiovascular disease was estimated to increase by 84% and 41%, respectively, for each 5-µmol/L increase in the serum homocysteine level.[10] Accordingly, independent of other factors and if sustained over time, the median 0.6- to 1.0-µmol/L decrease in homocysteine levels observed in the present study might be expected to lower the incidence of coronary heart disease by as much as 6% to 17%.

The effect of raloxifene on cardiovascular risk markers resembles that of tamoxifen more than it does HRT (see TABLE 1). This similarity is noteworthy since the changes induced by tamoxifen on cardiovascular risk markers could be responsible for tamoxifen's apparent cardioprotective effect. In some—but not all—randomized, controlled clinical trials, tamoxifen treatment reduced the incidence of fatal myocardial infarction (odds ratio: 0.37; 95% CI: 0.18–0.77)[11] and hospital admissions due to cardiac disease (relative risk: 0.68; 95% CI: 0.48–0.97).[12] Proof that raloxifene reduces the risk of heart disease would require a clinical trial with cardiovascular event end points. Such a study is currently under way.

REFERENCES

1. WALSH, B.W., L.H. KULLER, R.A. WILD et al. 1998. Effects of raloxifene on serum lipids and coagulation factors in healthy postmenopausal women. JAMA **279:** 1445–1451.
2. DELMAS, P.D., N.H. BJARNASON, B.H. MITLAK et al. 1997. The effects of raloxifene on bone mineral density, serum cholesterol, and uterine endometrium. N. Engl. J. Med. **337:** 1641–1647.
3. SACKS, F.M., M.A. PFEFFER, L.A. MOYE et al. 1996. The effect of pravastatin on coronary events after myocardial infarction in patients with average cholesterol levels: Cholesterol and Recurrent Events Trial investigators. N. Engl. J. Med. **335:** 1001–1009.
4. KANNEL, W.B., P.A. WOLF, W.P. CASTELLI et al. 1987. Fibrinogen and risk of cardiovascular disease. JAMA **258:** 1183–1186.
5. WALSH, B.W., S. PAUL, R.A. WILD et al. 2000. The effects of hormone replacement therapy and raloxifene on C-reactive protein and homocysteine in healthy postmenopausal women: a randomized, controlled trial. J. Clin. Endocrinol. Metab. **85:** 214–218.
6. TOSS, H., B. LINDAHL, A. SIEGBAHN et al. 1997. Prognostic influence of increased fibrinogen and C-reactive protein levels in unstable coronary artery disease—FRISC Study Group: Fragmin during Instability in Coronary Artery Disease. Circulation **96:** 4204–4210.
7. TRACY, R.P., R.N. LEMAITRE, B.M. PSATY et al. 1997. Relationship of C-reactive protein to risk of cardiovascular disease in the elderly: results from the Cardiovascular Health Study and the Rural Health Promotion Project. Arterioscler. Thromb. Vasc. Biol. **17:** 1121–1127.

8. RIDKER, P.M., J.E. BURING, J. SHIH et al. 1998. Prospective study of C-reactive protein and the risk of future cardiovascular events among apparently healthy women. Circulation **98:** 731–733.
9. CATTANEO, M.L., M.L. BAGLIETTO, D. ZIGHETTI et al. 1998. Tamoxifen reduces plasma homocysteine levels in healthy women. Br. J. Cancer **77:** 2264–2266.
10. WALD, N.J., H.C. WATT, M.R. LAW et al. 1998. Homocysteine and ischemic heart disease: results of a prospective study with implications regarding prevention. Arch. Intern. Med. **158:** 862–867.
11. MCDONALD, C.C. & H.J. STEWART FOR THE SCOTTISH BREAST CANCER COMMITTEE. 1991. Fatal myocardial infarction in the Scottish adjuvant tamoxifen trial. BMJ **303:** 435–437.
12. RUTQVIST, L.E. & A. MATTSSON FOR THE STOCKHOLM BREAST CANCER STUDY GROUP. 1993. Cardiac and thomboembolic morbidity among postmenopausal women with early stage breast cancer in a randomized trial of adjuvant tamoxifen. J. Natl. Cancer Inst. **85:** 1398–1406.
13. GREY, A.B., J.P. STAPLETON, M.C. EVANS et al. 1995. The effect of the anti-estrogen tamoxifen on cardiovascular risk factors in normal postmenopausal women. J. Clin. Endocrinol. Metab. **80:** 3191–3195.
14. MANNUCCI, P.M., D. BETTEGA, V. CHANTARANGKUL et al. 1996. Effect of tamoxifen on measurements of hemostasis in healthy postmenopausal women. Arch. Intern. Med. **156:** 1806–1810.
15. SHEWMON, D.A., J.L. STOCK, C.J. ROSEN et al. 1994. Tamoxifen and estrogen lower circulating lipoprotein(a) concentrations in healthy postmenopausal women. Arterioscler. Thromb. **14:** 1586–1593.

Selective Estrogen Receptor Modulator Effects on Serum Lipoproteins and Vascular Function in Postmenopausal Women and in Hypercholesterolemic Men

ARNON BLUM[a] AND RICHARD O. CANNON III[b]

[a]*Department of Internal Medicine, Poriya Hospital, Lower Galilee, Israel*

[b]*Cardiology Branch, National Heart, Lung, and Blood Institute, National Institutes of Health, Bethesda, Maryland 20892, USA*

ABSTRACT: Epidemiological observations, clinical mechanistic studies, and basic laboratory research suggest that estrogen therapy is associated with beneficial cardiovascular effects in postmenopausal women. Estrogen has a multitude of biological effects that may account for this apparent benefit (which remains to be proved in randomized clinical trials), including favorable effects on the lipid profile, increased endothelial nitric oxide bioactivity, and enhanced fibrinolysis. However, long-term estrogen therapy increases the risk of breast and endometrial cancers. Raloxifene, a benzothiophene derivative that binds to the estrogen receptor, is a selective estrogen receptor modulator, producing estrogen-agonist effects in some tissues (liver, bone) and estrogen-antagonistic effects in others (breast, uterus), and may prove to be an option for women with atherosclerosis or its risk factors. This review updates the current knowledge of the biological effects of selective estrogen receptor modulators of potential cardiovascular importance in postmenopausal women.

KEYWORDS: estrogen; tamoxifen; raloxifene; atherosclerosis; lipoproteins; nitric oxide; inflammation; hemostasis

INTRODUCTION

Cardiovascular disease is the leading cause of death among women in the United States and other developed societies, as it is among men. However, myocardial infarction and stroke are uncommon in women until their sixth decade and beyond. Clinicians have long suspected that the delay of a decade or more in cardiovascular disease expression in women relative to men is due to protective effects of estrogen before menopause. Thus, women in the Nurses' Health Study who underwent surgical menopause by bilateral oophorectomy without estrogen replacement had more than twice the risk of subsequent coronary heart disease events compared with postoperative women who received estrogen therapy.[1] Reports from population-based

---

Address for correspondence: Richard O. Cannon III, M.D., National Institutes of Health, Building 10, Room 7B15, 10 Center Drive MSC-1650, Bethesda, MD 20892-1650. Voice: 301-496-9895; fax: 301-402-0888.

cannonr@nih.gov

observational studies of the favorable effects of estrogen therapy on cardiovascular morbidity and mortality have led to enthusiasm for widespread use of estrogen by postmenopausal women for prevention of cardiovascular disease events.[2] However, any potential cardiovascular benefit of estrogen, in addition to other benefits such as preservation of bone mass, must be weighed against uterine and breast cancer risks[3] and side effects (breast tenderness, fluid retention, resumption of bleeding, cholelithiasis, deep venous thrombosis) with prolonged use. Thus, intense research has been conducted to find estrogen-like compounds that have the beneficial effects of estrogen without unwanted cancer risks and side effects.

SELECTIVE ESTROGEN RECEPTOR MODULATORS

The first clues to the possibility of an estrogen-like agent that might be devoid of cancer risk were provided by compounds with estrogen antagonist activity for breast cancer and thus were categorized as *antiestrogens*. These agents, exemplified by tamoxifen and raloxifene, were shown to exhibit either full or partial estrogen agonist effects at various tissue sites.[4] Because both the estrogen agonist and antagonist activities of these compounds involve high-affinity interaction with the estrogen receptor,[5] agents displaying this tissue-selective profile were later classified as selective estrogen receptor modulators (SERMs). SERMs exhibit pharmacological profiles distinct from conventional estrogen preparations.[6] Tamoxifen blocks the action of estrogens in several tissues, most notably the breast. However, the same compound exhibits an estrogen-like effect in other tissues, particularly the uterus. Like estrogen, tamoxifen lowers low-density lipoprotein (LDL) cholesterol levels and protects LDL from oxidation; but unlike estrogen, it does not increase levels of the antiatherogenic high-density lipoprotein (HDL).[7] Raloxifene is a nonsteroidal benzothiophene that inhibits the growth of estrogen receptor–dependent mammary tumors and reduces the occurrence of nitrosomethylurea-induced mammary tumors in rats. It has been classified as a SERM on the basis of studies in which it prevented bone loss and lowered serum cholesterol levels without stimulating the endometrium.[8]

LIPOPROTEIN EFFECTS OF RALOXIFENE

Delmas *et al.*[9] studied the effect of raloxifene on serum lipids (among other end points) in 601 postmenopausal women who were randomly assigned to receive 30, 60, or 150 mg of raloxifene or placebo daily for 24 months. Serum concentrations of total cholesterol and LDL cholesterol decreased in all raloxifene treatment groups, whereas serum concentrations of HDL cholesterol and triglycerides did not change. Walsh *et al.*[10] randomized 390 healthy postmenopausal women to receive one of four treatments daily: raloxifene 60 mg, raloxifene 120 mg, conjugated equine estrogens (CEE) 0.625 mg combined with medroxyprogesterone acetate 2.5 mg, or placebo. Both doses of raloxifene lowered LDL cholesterol by 12%, similar to the 14% reduction with CEE. Both doses of raloxifene lowered lipoprotein(a), an atherogenic derivative of LDL, by approximately 8%, but less than the 19% decrease with CEE. Raloxifene did not significantly change levels of HDL cholesterol, triglycerides, or plasminogen activator inhibitor type 1 (PAI-1), an inhibitor of fibrinolysis. In contrast, CEE increased HDL cholesterol levels by 11%, increased triglycerides by 20%, and decreased PAI-1 by 29%. Raloxifene significantly lowered fibrinogen by 12–14%, unlike CEE, which had no effect on this hemostatic protein, increased levels of which are associated with increased risk of myocardial infarction.

RALOXIFENE EFFECTS ON ATHEROSCLEROSIS IN ANIMAL MODELS

Bjarnason et al.[11] ovariectomized 75 female rabbits and treated them with either raloxifene, 17β-estradiol, or placebo; 25 rabbits were sham-operated and treated with placebo. After 45 weeks, the raloxifene-treated animals had two-thirds of the extent of aortic atherosclerosis—as evaluated by the cholesterol content of the aorta—compared with the placebo group. The estrogen-treated group had one-third of the aortic atherosclerosis compared with the placebo-treated animals. The sham-operated group was not significantly different from placebo-treated rabbits. These effects were only partly explained by the changes in serum lipids and lipoproteins. However, another study performed in primates did not find an antiatherogenic effect of raloxifene. Thus, Clarkson et al.[12] treated ovariectomized cynomolgus monkeys fed a moderately atherogenic diet with raloxifene (1 mg/kg/day), raloxifene (5 mg/kg/day), or CEE at a dose estimated to mimic 0.625 mg/day CEE in women, or placebo. Treatment with CEE resulted in an approximately 70% reduction in coronary artery plaque size relative to that in the placebo group, whereas neither the low nor the high dose of raloxifene had an effect on coronary artery plaque size that differed from placebo-treated animals.

SERMS AND ENDOTHELIAL NITRIC OXIDE BIOACTIVITY IN ANIMALS AND IN HUMANS

Figtree et al.[13] suspended rings of coronary artery from adult male and nonpregnant female rabbits, with measurements of isometric tension. Raloxifene added to the organ bath dose dependently induced relaxation in arterial rings from both sexes with the endothelium present. This vasorelaxant effect of raloxifene was partially inhibited by removal of the endothelium, by pharmacologic blockade of nitric oxide synthesis, or by addition of an estrogen receptor antagonist to the organ bath. Herrington and coworkers[14] compared the lipoprotein, hemostatic, and vascular effects of the investigational SERM droloxifene 60 mg daily to those of CEE 0.625 mg daily, each for six weeks in 24 healthy postmenopausal women. Droloxifene and CEE caused similar reductions in LDL cholesterol (16.6% and 12.0%, respectively) and lipoprotein(a) (13.2% and 9.5%, respectively). CEE, but not droloxifene, increased levels of HDL cholesterol. Droloxifene reduced fibrinogen levels to a greater degree than CEE, but had no effect on PAI-1. Thus, the lipoprotein and hemostatic effects of droloxifene appear to be similar to those of raloxifene. Droloxifene improved the brachial artery dilator response to hyeremia following forearm ischemia similar to the effect of CEE, consistent with increased nitric oxide synthesis or bioactivity by vascular endothelium.

EFFECTS OF ESTROGEN AND RALOXIFENE ON MARKERS OF INFLAMMATION IN POSTMENOPAUSAL WOMEN

Enhanced bioavailability of nitric oxide may have additional vascular effects that are atheroprotective. In this regard, nitric oxide donors prevent activation of proinflammatory genes of the endothelium by inhibition of an important nuclear transcriptional factor, kappa B, thus preventing the transcription, synthesis, and expression of adhesion molecules on the endothelial cell surface that attract inflammatory cells to the vessel surface and facilitate their entry into the vessel wall.[15] Cell adhesion molecules, once expressed on the surfaces of endothelial or mononuclear cells in culture following cytokine stimulation, are shed into the supernatant within 24 hours, and are measurable in the sera of humans. The pathophysiologic relevance of soluble cell adhesion molecules measured in human sera has been suggested by their localization in atherosclerotic plaques,[16] higher levels in patients with atherosclerosis relative to control subjects,[17] and association with increased risk of myocardial infarction in apparently healthy (male) subjects.[18] Serum concentrations of E-selectin, ICAM-1, and VCAM-1 were reported to be higher in postmenopausal women with coronary artery disease who were not taking hormone therapy than postmenopausal women with coronary artery disease who were taking hormone therapy at the time of cardiac catheterization.[19] Koh et al.[20] reported that CEE significantly reduced levels of the cell adhesion molecule E-selectin, ICAM-1, and VCAM-1 relative to respective pretreatment values, with the greatest effect noted with E-selectin, the cell adhesion molecule specific to the activated endothelium.

Because SERMs reduce levels of atherogenic lipoproteins and may enhance endothelial synthesis and releasse of nitric oxide, we conducted a study that examined whether raloxifene reduces serum levels of markers of inflammation in postmenopausal women, with comparison to CEE therapy in 23 postmenopausal women.[21] None was diabetic, hypertensive, or a current cigarette smoker. No subject had taken any cholesterol-lowering agent, estrogen therapy, or antioxidant vitamin supplements during the preceding two months. Aspirin and nonsteroidal antiinflammatory agents were stopped 10 days before this randomized, double-blind, three-period crossover treatment trial. Study participants were randomly assigned to raloxifene 60 mg, CEE 0.625 mg, or placebo daily, each for one month, with one month between treatment periods. Compared with placebo, total cholesterol was reduced by approximately 10% both with CEE and with raloxifene therapies. Likewise, LDL cholesterol and apolipoprotein B were reduced by approximately 10% with both therapies. HDL cholesterol and apolipoprotein A-1 were unaffected by raloxifene; however, CEE significantly increased HDL cholesterol and apolipoprotein A-1 levels compared with placebo. Triglyceride levels were not affected by CEE or by raloxifene compared with placebo. Levels of C-reactive protein (CRP), a marker of increased cardiovascular risk in women[22] (and in men), were increased by 50% with CEE, but were unchanged with raloxifene versus placebo values. Levels of interleukin-6 (IL-6), a cytokine implicated in atherosclerosis that also conveys increased risk, were nonsignificantly increased with CEE and with raloxifene relative to placebo. Levels of matrix metalloproteinase–9 (MMP-9) (an enzyme secreted by macrophages and activated smooth muscle cells implicated in plaque rupture by digesting the fibrous cap) were increased by 30% with CEE relative to placebo, but not with raloxifene. E-selectin levels were reduced by 12% with CEE and by 6%

with raloxifene compared with placebo, with CEE having a greater effect on this cell adhesion molecule than raloxifene. Both therapies reduced ICAM-1 levels from placebo, and to a similar degree. VCAM-1 was reduced by 10% with CEE, but raloxifene did not have an effect on VCAM-1 when compared with placebo. Thus, raloxifene lowers levels of cell adhesion molecules to a lesser extent than CEE in otherwise healthy postmenopausal women, but does not increase other markers of inflammation that are raised during CEE therapy (CRP, interleuken-6, and MMP-9). The biologic relevance of these differences in effects on markers of inflammation remains to be determined in clinical trials.

HORMONAL, LIPOPROTEIN, AND VASCULAR EFFECTS OF RALOXIFENE IN HYPERCHOLESTEROLEMIC MEN

Studies of vascular effects of estrogen in men have yielded conflicting results, with one group finding no effect of intracoronary infusion of 17β-estradiol on acetylcholine-stimulated coronary dynamics,[23] while another group showed post-CEE improvement in coronary endothelium-dependent vasodilator responsiveness.[24] Two groups from Australia reported vascular effects of chronic estrogen use in male-to-female transsexuals on estrogen preparations, with greater flow-mediated brachial artery dilator responses during postischemic hyperemia and greater dilator responses to nitroglycerin (a test of smooth muscle responsiveness to nitric oxide) than in control men.[25,26] This vascular effect of estrogen may relate in part to increased nitric oxide activity: in the pig, estrogen treatment increases nitric oxide synthase activity in male animals, although longer treatment is required for this effect than in female animals.[27] Further, estrogen has been shown to have lipoprotein effects in men similar to those seen in women on hormone replacement therapy, with reduction in LDL cholesterol levels and increases in HDL cholestrol levels.[28] However, despite the apparent vascular benefit of estrogen demonstrated in male transsexuals, the feminizing effects of estrogen would not be desirable for most men.

Because raloxifene shares some of the biologic properties of estrogen, including reduction in LDL cholesterol and lipoprotein(a) levels, which in turn may benefit vascular endothelial function through enhanced nitric oxide bioactivity, we reasoned that raloxifene therapy could provide a reasonable approach to the management of men who are at risk for atherosclerosis. Twenty-four healthy, nonsmoking, mild to moderately hypercholesterolemic (LDL cholesterol > 130 mg/dL) men (average age 48 years) who had not taken lipid-lowering therapies or antioxidant vitamins during the preceding two months were enrolled in this study.[29] Aspirin and nonsteroidal antiinflammatory drugs were stopped 10 days before starting the study and discontinued throughout the study. Subjects randomly took raloxifene 60 mg/day or an identical placebo, each for one month, with one month off therapy before crossover to the alternate treatment in this double-blind study. All subjects were placed on a nitrate-restricted diet for 72 hours before each study to reduce the contribution of dietary nitrates to oxidized products of nitric oxide in serum. Study participants underwent blood sampling and vascular studies at the end of each treatment period, one hour after the morning treatment. Vascular studies were performed by measuring brachial artery dilator responsiveness to hyperemia (flow-mediated dilation) as an index of endothelial nitric oxide release, and to nitroglycerin as an index of smooth muscle responsiveness to nitric oxide. Compared with placebo, raloxifene increased testosterone levels by approximately 20% and tended to lower levels of 17β-estradiol. This was not associated with significant changes in pituitary gonadotropin levels. Raloxifene caused a 5% decrease in total cholesterol, but only slight, nonsignificant reductions in LDL cholesterol and apolipoprotein B levels. Lipoprotein(a) levels were unchanged by raloxifene therapy. There was no effect of raloxifene on HDL cholesterol or apolipoprotein A-I levels. Raloxifene did not increase serum nitrogen oxide levels and did not improve brachial artery flow-mediated dilation or the dilator response to nitroglycerin. Soluble cell adhesion molecules regulated by nitric oxide in endothelial cell culture experiments were unchanged with raloxifene relative to placebo treatment. Thus, there was no evidence that raloxifene increased nitric oxide release from the endothelium in the study participants. We concluded from this study that despite appealing biologic properties of SERM therapy that could be of atheroprotective potential, raloxifene does not appear to confer such properties in men.

CONCLUSION

SERMs have biological effects on lipoproteins and nitric oxide bioactivity that would seem to be atheroprotective, although effects on atherosclerosis progression in animal models are conflicting. The potential benefit of raloxifene to prevention of cardiovascular events in postmenopausal women with risk factors for atherosclerosis or clinically established coronary artery disease is currently being tested in the Raloxifene Use in the Heart (RUTH) clinical trial.

REFERENCES

1. COLDITZ, G.A., W.C. WILLETT, M.J. STAMPFER, et al. 1987. Menopause and the risk of coronary heart disease in women. N. Engl. J. Med. **316:** 1105–1110.
2. STAMPFER, M.J. & G.A. COLDITZ. 1991. Estrogen replacement and coronary heart disease: a quantitative assessment of the epidemiologic evidence. Prev. Med. **20:** 47–63.
3. COLDITZ, G.A., S.E. HANKINSON, D.J. HUNTER, et al. 1995. The use of estrogens and progestins and the risk of breast cancer in postmenopausal women. N. Engl. J. Med. **332:** 1589–1593.
4. SATO, M., M.K. RIPPY & H.U. BRYANT. 1996. Raloxifene, tamoxifene, nafoxidine, and estrogen effects on reproductive and nonreproductive tissues in ovariectomized rats. FASEB J. **10:** 905–912.
5. YANG, N.N., M. VENUGOPALAN, S. HARDIKAR, et al. Identification of an estrogen response element activated by metabolites of 17β-estradiol and raloxifene. Science **275:** 1222–1225.
6. MITLAK, B.H. & F.J. COHEN. 1997. In search of optimal long-term female hormone replacement: the potential of selective estrogen receptor modulators. Horm. Res. **48:** 155–163.
7. GUETTA, V., R.M. LUSH, W.D. FIGG, et al. 1995. Effects of the antiestrogen tamoxifen on low-density lipoprotein concentrations and oxidation in postmenopausal women. Am. J. Cardiol. **76:** 1072–1073.
8. BLACK, L.J., M. SATO, E.R. ROWLEY, et al. 1994. Raloxifene (LY139481 HCl) prevents bone loss and reduce serum cholesterol without causing uterine hypertrophy in ovariectomized rats. J. Clin. Invest. **93:** 63–69.
9. DELMAS, P.D., N.H. BJARNASON, B.H. MITLAK, et al. 1997. Effects of raloxifene on bone mineral density, serum cholesterol concentrations, and uterine endometrium in postmenopausal women. N. Engl. J. Med. **337:** 1641–1647.

10. WALSH, B.W., L.H. KULLER, R.A. WILD, et al. 1998. Effects of raloxifene on serum lipids and coagulation factors in healthy postmenopausal women. JAMA **279:** 1445–1451.
11. BJARNASON, N.H., J. HAARBO, I. BYRJALSEN, et al. 1997. Raloxifene inhibits aortic accumulation of cholesterol in ovariectomized, cholesterol fed rabbits. Circulation **96:** 1964–1969.
12. CLARKSON, T.B., M.S. ANTHONY & C.P. JEROME. 1998. Lack of effect of raloxifene on coronary artery atherosclerosis of postmenopausal monkeys. J. Clin. Endocrinol. Metab. **83:** 721–726.
13. FIGTREE, G.A., L. YING-QING, C.M. WEBB, et al.1999. Raloxifene acutely relaxes rabbit coronary arteries in vitro by an estrogen receptor-dependent and nitric oxide-dependent mechanism. Circulation **100:** 1095–1101.
14. HERRINGTON, D.M., B.E. PUSSER, W.A. WILEY, et al. 2000. Cardiovascular effects of droloxifene, a new selective estrogen receptor modulator, in healthy postmenopausal women. Arterioscler. Thromb. Vasc. Biol. **20:** 1606–1612.
15. PENG, H.B., T.B. RAJARASHISTH, P. LIBBY, et al. 1995. Induction and stabilization of I kappa B alpha by nitric oxide mediates inhibition of NF-kappa B. J. Biol. Chem. **270:** 14214–14219.
16. DAVIES, M.J., J.L. GORDON, A.J.H. GEARING, et al. 1993. The expression of the adhesion molecules ICAM-1, VCAM-1, PECAM, and E-selectin in human atherosclerosis. J. Pathol. **171:** 223–229.
17. HWANG, S.J., C.M. BALLANTYNE, R. SHARRETT, et al. 1997. Circulating adhesion molecules VCAM-1, ICAM-1, and E-selectin in carotid atherosclerosis and incident coronary heart disease cases: the Atherosclerosis Risk in Communities (ARIC) study. Circulation **96:** 4219–4225.
18. RIDKER, P.M., C.H. HENNEKENS, B. ROITMAN-JOHNSON, et al. 1998. Plasma concentration of soluble intercellular adhesion molecule 1 and risks of future myocardial infarction in apparently healthy men. Lancet **351:** 88–92.
19. CAULIN-GLASER, T., W.J. FARRELL, S.E. PFAU, et al. 1998. Modulation of circulating cellular adhesion molecules in postmenopausal women with coronary artery disease. J. Am. Coll. Cardiol. **31:** 1555–1560.
20. KOH, K.K., C. CARDILLO, M.N. BUI, et al. 1999. Vascular effects of estrogen and cholesterol-lowering therapies in hypercholesterolemic postmenopausal women. Circulation **99:** 354–360.
21. BLUM, A., W.H. SCHENKE, L. HATHAWAY, et al. 2000. Effects of estrogen and the selective estrogen receptor modulator raloxifene on markers of inflammation in postmenopausal women. Am. J. Cardiol. **86:** 892–895.
22. RIDKER, P.M., C.H. HENNEKENS, J.E. BURING, et al. 2000. C-reactive protein and other markers of inflammation in the prediction of cardiovascular disease in women. N. Engl. J. Med. **324:** 836–843.
23. COLLINS, P., G.M. ROSANO, P.M. SARREL, et al. 1995. 17 beta-estradiol attenuates acetylcholine-induced coronary arterial constriction in women but not men with coronary heart disease. Circulation **92:** 24–30.
24. BLUMENTHAL, R.S., A.W. HELDMAN, J.A. BRINKER, et al. 1997. Acute effects of conjugated estrogens on coronary blood flow response to acetylcholine in men. Am. J. Cardiol. **80:** 1021–1024.
25. MCCROHON, J.A., W.A. WALTERS, J.T.C. ROBINSON, et al. 1997. Arterial reactivity is enhanced in genetic males taking high dose estrogens. J. Am. Coll. Cardiol. **29:** 1432–1436.
26. NEW, G., K.L. TIMMINS, S.J. DUFFY, et al. 1997. Long-term estrogen therapy improves vascular function in male to female transsexuals. J. Am. Coll. Cardiol. **29:** 1437–1444.
27. WEINER, C.P., I. LIZASOAIN, S.A. BAYLIS, et al. 1994. Induction of calcium-dependent nitric oxide synthases by sex hormones. Proc. Natl. Acad. Sci. USA **91:** 5212–5216.
28. DAMEWOOD, M.D., J.J. BELLANTONI, P.S. BACHORIK, et al. 1989. Exogenous estrogen effect on lipid/lipoprotein cholesterol in transsexual males. J. Endocrinol. Invest. **12:** 449–454.
29. BLUM, A., L. HATHAWAY, R. MINCEMOYER, et al. 2000. Hormonal, lipoprotein, and vascular effects of the selective estrogen receptor modulator raloxifene in hypercholesterolemic men. Am. J. Cardiol. **85:** 1491–1494.

Effects of Estrogen and Selective Estrogen Receptor Modulators on Hemostasis and Inflammation

Potential Differences among Drugs

MARY CUSHMAN

Department of Medicine, University of Vermont, Colchester, Vermont 05446, USA

ABSTRACT: Postmenopausal hormone replacement therapy (HRT), tamoxifen, and raloxifene all share an increase of about three-fold in the risk of venous thromboembolism (VTE). Currently, it is thought that HRT transiently increases the risk of myocardial infarction (MI), followed by subsequent reduction in risk, at least among women with established coronary heart disease. Raloxifene and tamoxifen are not known to share this apparent clinical effect. Study of hemostasis and inflammation factors, as surrogate end points, can be useful to form hypotheses concerning the pathophysiology related to clinical effects of these agents. Data presented here suggest differences among these agents that might relate to differences in clinical outcomes. From the vascular perspective, future studies need to focus on interactions of treatment with these biochemical parameters and their genetic correlates in order to define low- or high-risk subgroups for intervention with these therapies.

KEYWORDS: hormone replacement therapy (HRT); selective estrogen receptor modulators (SERMs); cardiovascular disease; women; thrombosis; myocardial infarction; inflammation; risk factors; menopause

Postmenopausal hormone replacement therapy (HRT), tamoxifen, and raloxifene all share an increase of about three-fold in the risk of venous thromboembolism (VTE). Currently, it is thought that HRT transiently increases the risk of myocardial infarction (MI), followed by subsequent reduction in risk, at least among women with established coronary heart disease[1] and possibly among healthy women. The effect of tamoxifen on risk of MI was neutral in the National Surgical Adjuvant Breast and Bowel Program Breast Cancer Prevention Trial (P-1 trial),[2] but other studies suggested risk reduction.[3,4] Detailed analysis from the P-1 trial did not identify an early increase in risk of MI.[5] Because of the clinical uncertainties regarding these therapies, study of the effects of these agents on hemostasis are useful, using blood biomarkers as surrogate end points. This paper will focus on potential differences in

Address for correspondence: Mary Cushman, M.D., M.Sc., Department of Medicine, University of Vermont, 208 South Park Drive, Suite 2, Colchester, VT 05446. Voice: 802-656-8968; fax: 802-656-8965.

mcushman@zoo.uvm.edu

effects on hemostasis and inflammation among these hormone therapies, first in relation to risk of MI and second in relation to venous thrombosis risk.

MYOCARDIAL INFARCTION (MI)

Several recent studies address the effects of HRT and selective estrogen receptor modulating drugs (SERMs) on inflammation, as assessed by high-sensitivity assays for C-reactive protein (CRP).[6–10] CRP is a recognized marker of increased risk of MI in general and in middle-aged women,[11] the group most likely to be considering hormone use. The effects of hormone therapies and SERMs on CRP may partly reflect underlying pathophysiology for alterations in coronary heart disease (CHD) risk with HRT; major differences among these drugs may exist.

A cross-sectional study of long-term (~15 years) HRT users ≥ age 65 in the Cardiovascular Health Study reported 59% higher CRP concentrations compared to nonusers, even after accounting for other differences between users and nonusers.[6] This association has been confirmed in experimental studies. The effects of four hormone preparations [conjugated equine estrogens, with or without continuous or cyclical medroxyprogesterone acetate (MPA) or micronized progesterone] on CRP were compared to placebo in a substudy of the Postmenopausal Estrogen/Progestin Interventions trial. In this analysis of 375 women, there was an 85% average increase in CRP over 3 years with all forms of HRT, with no differences among the drugs.[8] Similar findings were observed by others.[7,9] One small trial among diabetic women reported a small decline in CRP with transdermal estrogen; the authors suggested that the effects of orally administered estrogen might represent nonspecific first-pass liver effects rather than pro-inflammatory effects.[12] Synthesis of CRP in the liver is primarily regulated by interleukin-6 (IL-6), and adipocytes provide a major source of IL-6. One preliminary report confirmed a rise in CRP with estrogen and this was associated with a nonsignificant increase in plasma IL-6.[13] This suggests against a first-pass liver effect of HRT on CRP. Regardless, even if the mechanism of CRP raising with HRT is due to first-pass liver effects, several basic experiments support pathophysiologic roles for CRP in atherothrombosis.[14–17] Studies linking this biochemical effect of HRT with clinical outcomes are required.

Regarding the SERMs, two studies provide relevant data on CRP. In one large trial, compared to placebo, there was no effect of raloxifene on CRP.[9] By contrast, in a substudy of the P-1 trial, a CRP-lowering effect of tamoxifen was recently reported.[10] In this placebo-controlled study of 111 women, tamoxifen was associated with a 26% decline in CRP and a 9% decline in total cholesterol.

The effects of HRT and SERMs on other novel CHD risk factors have also been studied. HRT prevents the age-related rise in fibrinogen.[18] Tamoxifen was associated with a 21% reduction in fibrinogen in the P-1 trial substudy,[10] an effect previously observed[19] and similar to that of raloxifene.[20] HRT and tamoxifen also appear to differ in their effect on prothrombin fragment 1–2, a marker of procoagulant activity that has not been widely studied in relation to risk of MI. HRT has been associated with increases of fragment 1–2, and tamoxifen and raloxifene have neutral effects.[10,19–22] Any clinical relevance of fragment 1–2 changes with hormones is unknown. Higher levels of fibrin fragment D-dimer, as a marker of fibrin formation and reactive fibrinolysis, are associated with risk of MI.[23,24] Higher levels of plasminogen activation

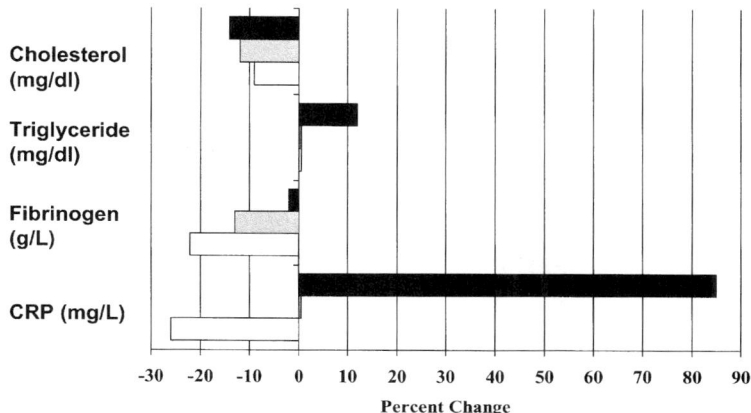

FIGURE 1. Differential effects of HRT, raloxifene, and tamoxifen on cardiac risk factors. Effects of different oral estrogen regimens (with or without progestin) were similar. HRT is indicated by the *dark bars*, raloxifene by the *stippled bars*, and tamoxifen by the *open bars*. Data are derived from Refs. 8–10 and 18.

inhibitor-1 (PAI-1), a marker of reduced fibrinolytic function, are inconsistently associated with risk of MI; HRT has been shown to substantially reduce PAI-1. While some have reported no influence of HRT, others have reported increased D-dimer with different forms of oral HRT.[25,26] This effect was variably associated with reduced PAI-1 and with increased coagulation activation,[25,26] although reduction of PAI-1 is consistently observed in different studies. Given the lack of clear association of PAI-1 with risk of MI, as well as the positive association of D-dimer with MI, a hypothesis may be made that the increase in D-dimer with HRT reflects increased fibrin formation and is associated with adverse cardiovascular effects.

Some biochemical effects of these drugs are summarized in FIGURE 1. Taken together, under the hypothesis that CRP or other novel markers of hemostasis either are markers of underlying vascular risk or are involved in the pathogenesis of atherosclerosis or its transition to clinical disease, the findings for HRT, raloxifene, and tamoxifen suggest differences among these drugs that may have implications in their evaluation for cardiovascular disease prevention. Clinical trials are required for confirmation.

VENOUS THROMBOSIS

The SERMs and HRT are associated with a similar 2- to 3-fold increase in the risk of VTE. Whether or not this is related to similar biochemical effects cannot be concluded from available data. Thrombosis of the veins appears to be precipitated by different components of the hemostatic system compared to thrombosis of the arteries. However, prospective data in this regard are sparse. Factors that might relate to both systems are fibrinogen and elevated coagulation factor VIII. Higher factor VIII is associated with both venous and arterial disease risk,[27–29] and heritability for

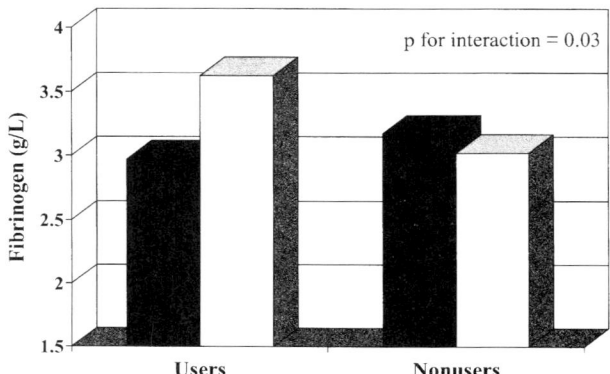

FIGURE 2. Association of HRT use with fibrinogen according to race. Data were from a cross-sectional analysis of 290 women ≥ age 65 using HRT compared to 196 nonusers in the same population.[6] White women are indicated by the *dark bars* and black women by the *open bars*; $P < 0.01$ within each race comparing users to nonusers.

higher factor VIII has been proposed. The SERMs, tamoxifen and raloxifene, appear to have a more favorable effect than HRT on fibrinogen lowering. One cross-sectional study reported differences by race for fibrinogen (FIG. 2). In this analysis, black women using HRT had higher fibrinogen levels than black nonusers, while the opposite association was observed among white women.[6] In one large trial, four estrogen preparations had no effect on factor VIIIc.[8] Findings were similar for tamoxifen[10] and there are no data available for raloxifene.

A common risk factor for venous thrombosis in the general population is resistance to activated protein C (APC). The majority of affected women have the associated factor V Leiden mutation (Arg506 → Gln). While there is an interaction of factor V Leiden and contraceptive use to increase the risk of VTE, there is limited data available on effects of postmenopausal hormone therapies on APC resistance or the interaction of HRT with factor V Leiden in this regard. One case-control study of the risk of VTE among women aged 45–64 reported an increased risk related to the joint presence of factor V Leiden and HRT use.[30] However, a single-arm study showed improved APC resistance in 17 women treated with cyclic transdermal 17β-estradiol combined with oral MPA (10 mg/day). We are not aware of other published data for HRT, tamoxifen, or raloxifene.

In families with thrombophilia, deficiencies of the natural anticoagulants, protein C, protein S, and antithrombin, are related to VTE, although only protein C deficiency was associated with risk in the general population.[31] Borderline low protein C has also been linked with VTE risk.[32] Few studies of hormone effects have measured all three of these proteins. Postmenopausal estrogen either has no effect or increases protein C (at higher dose), and appears to lower antithrombin and protein S. Tamoxifen has been associated with variable lowering of antithrombin and slight lowering of proteins C and S. Effects of raloxifene on anticoagulant function are unknown. Since both HRT and tamoxifen share more consistent effects on antithrombin, reduction of antithrombin might be key. *In vitro* studies suggest that, with other factors held constant, there is a large impact of antithrombin, through the normal range of its physiologic concentration, on thrombin generation.[33] However, there are no epidemiological data to confirm the clinical relevance of small changes in antithrombin concentration.

Another genetic trait associated with VTE is prothrombin 20210A, a polymorphism associated with higher levels of circulating prothrombin. In the heterozygous form, this disorder is associated with a 2- to 3-fold increase in risk. Again, while there is a reported interaction of oral contraceptives with the prothrombin polymorphism to increase this risk, there are no available data concerning HRT or SERMs and prothrombin 20210A or prothrombin levels.

In conclusion, further study is needed on the effects of SERMs and HRT on hemostasis and inflammation. Importantly, for VTE, the clinical interactions of these treatments, and their biochemical effects, with common inherited risk factors such as factor V Leiden and the prothrombin gene polymorphism need to be clarified. Randomized trials must collect the appropriate baseline and follow-up plasma and DNA to facilitate these studies and to link biochemical effects of hormones with clinical outcomes. Sufficient numbers of women from nonwhite races need to be included in these studies as limited data are available concerning these groups.

REFERENCES

1. HULLEY, S., D. GRADY, T. BUSH et al. 1998. Randomized trial of estrogen plus progestin for secondary prevention of coronary heart disease in postmenopausal women. JAMA **280:** 605–613.
2. FISHER, B., J.P. COSTANTINO, D.L. WICKERHAM et al. 1998. Tamoxifen for prevention of breast cancer: report of the National Surgical Adjuvant Breast and Bowel Project P-1 Study. J. Natl. Cancer Inst. **90:** 1371–1388.
3. RUTQVIST, L.E. & A. MATTSSON FOR THE STOCKHOLM BREAST CANCER STUDY GROUP. 1993. Cardiac and thromboembolic morbidity among postmenopausal women with early-stage breast cancer in a randomized trial of adjuvant tamoxifen. J. Natl. Cancer Inst. **85:** 1398–1406.
4. MCDONALD, C.C., F.E. ALEXANDER, B. WHYTE et al. 1995. Cardiac and vascular morbidity in women receiving adjuvant tamoxifen for breast cancer in a randomised trial. BMJ **311:** 977–980.
5. REIS, S.E., J.P. COSTANTINO, D.L. WICKERHAM et al. 2001. Cardiovascular effects of tamoxifen in women with and without heart disease: breast cancer prevention trial. J. Natl. Cancer Inst. **93:** 16–21.
6. CUSHMAN, M., E.N. MEILAHN, B.M. PSATY et al. 1999. Hormone replacement therapy, inflammation, and hemostasis in elderly women. Arterioscler. Thromb. Vasc. Biol. **19:** 893–899.
7. VAN BAAL, W.M., P. KENEMANS, M.J. VAN DER MOOREN et al. 1999. Increased C-reactive protein levels during short-term hormone replacement therapy in healthy postmenopausal women. Thromb. Haemostasis **81:** 925–928.
8. CUSHMAN, M., C. LEGAULT, E. BARRETT-CONNOR et al. 1999. Effect of postmenopausal hormones on inflammation-sensitive proteins: the Postmenopausal Estrogen/Progestin Interventions (PEPI) study. Circulation **100:** 717–722.
9. WALSH, B.W., S. PAUL, R.A. WILD et al. 2000. The effects of raloxifene compared with hormone replacement therapy on homocysteine and C-reactive protein in healthy postmenopausal women: a randomized controlled trial. J. Clin. Endocrinol. Metab. **85:** 214–218.
10. CUSHMAN, M., J.P. COSTANTINO, R.P. TRACY et al. 2001. Tamoxifen and cardiac risk factor in healthy women: suggestion of an anti-inflammatory effect. Arterioscler. Thromb. Vasc. Biol. **21:** 255–261.
11. RIDKER, P.M., J.E. BURING, J. SHIH et al. 1998. A prospective study of C-reactive protein and risk of future cardiovascular events among apparently healthy women. Circulation **98:** 731–733.

12. SATTAR, N., M. PERERA, M. SMALL et al. 1999. Hormone replacement therapy and sensitive C-reactive protein concentration in women with type-2 diabetes. Lancet **354:** 487–488.
13. COX, D.A., A. SASHEGYI, S. PAUL et al. 1999. Effects of raloxifene and hormone replacement therapy on markers of inflammation in healthy postmenopausal women [abstract]. Circulation **100**(suppl. 1): I-826.
14. CERMAK, J., N. KEY, R. BACH et al. 1993. C-reactive protein induces human peripheral blood monocytes to synthesize tissue factor. Blood **82:** 513–520.
15. BHAKDI, S., M. TORZEWSKI, M. KLOUCHE et al. 1999. Complement and atherogenesis: binding of CRP to degraded, nonoxidized LDL enhances complement activation. Arterioscler. Thromb. Vasc. Biol. **19:** 2348–2354.
16. PASCERI, V., J.T. WILLERSON & E.T.H. YEH. 2000. Direct proinflammatory effect of C-reactive protein on human endothelial cells. Circulation **102:** 2165–2168.
17. TORZEWSKI, M., C. RIST, R.F. MORTENSEN et al. 2000. C-reactive protein in the arterial intima: role of C-reactive protein receptor–dependent monocyte recruitment in atherogenesis. Arterioscler. Thromb. Vasc. Biol. **20:** 2094–2099.
18. THE WRITING GROUP FOR THE PEPI TRIAL. 1995. Effects of estrogen or estrogen/progestin regimens on heart disease risk factors in postmenopausal women: the Postmenopausal Estrogen/Progestin Interventions (PEPI) Trial. JAMA **273:** 199–208.
19. MANNUCCI, P.M., D. BETTEGA, V. CHANTARANGKUL et al. 1996. Effect of tamoxifen on measurements of hemostasis in healthy women. Arch. Intern. Med. **156:** 1806–1810.
20. WALSH, B.W., L.H. KULLER, R.A. WILD et al. 1998. Effects of raloxifene on serum lipids and coagulation factors in healthy postmenopausal women. JAMA **279:** 1445–1451.
21. CAINE, Y.G., K. BAUER, S. BARZEGAR et al. 1992. Coagulation activation following estrogen administration to postmenopausal women. Thromb. Haemostasis **68:** 392–395.
22. DE VALK–DE ROO, G.W., C.D.A. STEHOUWER, P. MEIJER et al. 1999. Both raloxifene and estrogen reduce major cardiovascular risk factors in healthy postmenopausal women: a 2-year, placebo-controlled study. Arterioscler. Thromb. Vasc. Biol. **19:** 2993–3000.
23. FOWKES, F.G.R., G.D.O. LOWE, E. HOUSELY et al. 1993. Cross-linked fibrin degradation products, progression of peripheral arterial disease, and risk of coronary heart disease. Lancet **342:** 84–86.
24. CUSHMAN, M., R.N. LEMAITRE, L.H. KULLER et al. 1999. Fibrinolytic activation markers predict myocardial infarction in the elderly: the Cardiovascular Health Study. Arterioscler. Thromb. Vasc. Biol. **19:** 493–498.
25. KOH, K.K., R. MINCEMOYER, M.N. BUI et al. 1997. Effects of hormone-replacement therapy on fibrinolysis in postmenopausal women. N. Engl. J. Med. **336:** 683–690.
26. TEEDE, H.J., B.P. MCGRATH, J.J. SMOLICH et al. 2000. Postmenopausal hormone replacement therapy increases coagulation activity and fibrinolysis. Arterioscler. Thromb. Vasc. Biol. **20:** 1404–1409.
27. KOSTER, T., A.D. BLANN, E. BRIET et al. 1995. Role of clotting factor VIII in effect of von Willebrand factor on occurrence of deep-vein thrombosis. Lancet **345:** 152–155.
28. FOLSOM, A.R., K.K. WU, W.D. ROSAMOND et al. 1997. Prospective study of hemostatic factors and incidence of coronary heart disease: the Atherosclerosis Risk in Communities (ARIC) study. Circulation **96:** 1102–1108.
29. TRACY, R.P., A.M. ARNOLD, W. ETTINGER et al. 1999. The relationship of fibrinogen and factors VII and VIII to incident cardiovascular disease and death in the elderly: results from the Cardiovascular Health Study. Arterioscler. Thromb. Vasc. Biol. **19:** 1776–1783.
30. LOWE, G., M. WOODWARD, M. VESSEY et al. 2000. Thrombotic variables and risk of idiopathic venous thromboembolism in women aged 45–64 years: relationships to hormone replacement therapy. Thromb. Haemostasis **83:** 530–535.
31. KOSTER, T., F.R. ROSENDAAL, E. BRIET et al. 1995. Protein C deficiency in a controlled series of unselected outpatients: an infrequent but clear risk factor for venous thrombosis (the Leiden Thrombophilia Study). Blood **85:** 2756–2761.
32. SPEK, C.A., T. KOSTER, F.R. ROSENDAAL et al. 1995. Genotypic variation in the promoter region of the protein C gene is associated with plasma protein C levels and thrombotic risk. Arterioscler. Thromb. Vasc. Biol. **15:** 214–218.
33. BUTENAS, S., C. VAN'T VEER & K.G. MANN. 1999. "Normal" thrombin generation. Blood **94:** 2169–2178.

Rationale and Overview of the Raloxifene Use for the Heart (RUTH) Trial

LORI MOSCA

Department of Medicine, Columbia University College of Physicians and Surgeons, and Department of Medicine, Weill Cornell Medical College, New York, New York, USA

ABSTRACT: Raloxifene is a selective estrogen receptor modulator (SERM) that has beneficial effects on several cardiovascular risk factors and has also been associated with a reduced risk of breast cancer in osteoporosis prevention trials. The Raloxifene Use for the Heart (RUTH) study was designed to test the hypothesis that, compared to placebo, raloxifene at 60 mg/day (1) lowers the risk of the combined end point of coronary death, nonfatal myocardial infarction (MI), and hospitalized acute coronary syndromes other than MI and (2) reduces the risk of invasive breast cancer (coprimary end point) in women at high risk for major coronary events based on established cardiovascular disease (CVD) or multiple risk factors. RUTH is a double-blind, placebo-controlled, randomized, clinical trial of 10,101 women aged 55 years or older from 26 countries and is expected to be completed in approximately 5 years.

KEYWORDS: selective estrogen receptor modulator; hormone replacement therapy; raloxifene; clinical trials; women; risk factors; menopause; breast cancer; osteoporosis

Raloxifene, a selective estrogen receptor modulator (SERM), has estrogen-agonist effects on lipoproteins,[1] homocysteine,[2] and bone[3] and estrogen-antagonist activity in the breast[4] and uterus,[5] positioning it as a potential agent for disease prevention in postmenopausal women. In preclinical studies, raloxifene inhibits atherogenesis,[6] vascular injury,[7] and low-density lipoprotein (LDL) oxidation.[8] Raloxifene also acutely relaxes rabbit coronary arteries *in vitro*[9] and enhances uterine and coronary artery blood flow *in vivo* in sheep,[10] at least partially via an endothelium- and nitric oxide–dependent mechanism. In postmenopausal women, raloxifene lowers LDL-cholesterol,[1,11,12] lipoprotein (a),[1] fibrinogen,[1] and homocysteine.[2] These various observations suggest that raloxifene may lower coronary heart disease (CHD) risk in women.

Estrogen replacement therapy (ERT) has been shown to have numerous beneficial effects on surrogate markers of cardiovascular disease (CVD) and has consistently been associated with a lower risk of CHD in observational epidemiological studies.[13] Despite this, the first large-scale randomized clinical trial of hormone replacement therapy (HRT), the Heart and Estrogen/Progestin Replacement Study

---

Address for correspondence: Lori Mosca, M.D., M.P.H., Ph.D., Preventive Cardiology Program, New York Presbyterian Hospital, PH 10-203B, 622 West 168th Street, New York, NY 10032. Voice: 212-305-4866; fax: 212-342-5238.

ljm10@columbia.edu

(HERS), showed no overall benefit after 4.1 years of treatment with conjugated equine estrogen (CEE) at 0.625 mg/day plus medroxyprogesterone acetate (MPA) at 2.5 mg/day versus placebo.[14] Several explanations for the unexpected result of HERS have been suggested, including the following: inadequate duration of follow-up; adverse effects of MPA; bidirectional effects of estrogen (early risk and late benefit); the population of women studied were too old to benefit from therapy (mean age = 66.7 years) or their disease was too advanced; the preparation of HRT was not ideal; the findings were due to chance; and possibly HRT is ineffective in preventing recurrent cardiovascular events in women with established disease.[15]

Results of HERS may not necessarily extrapolate to the RUTH trial for several reasons. Because raloxifene does not have stimulatory effects on the endometrium, there is no need for concomitant progestin therapy.[5] MPA has been shown to mitigate potentially beneficial effects of ERT on lipids, vascular reactivity, and atherosclerosis development in nonhuman primates.[13] The avoidance of the need for a progestational agent may therefore be advantageous for cardiovascular health. ERT has been associated with increases in C-reactive protein (CRP) levels,[16] which have been shown to be predictive of future cardiovascular events among healthy postmenopausal women.[17] In a multicenter randomized clinical trial of 390 postmenopausal women, raloxifene was not shown to increase CRP levels after 6 months of therapy, whereas HRT increased levels by 84%.[2] Although data are promising that SERMs may share some of the beneficial effects of ERT on intermediate end points, but may not have a pro-inflammatory effect, the clinical relevance of any differential effects on surrogate end points must be confirmed in randomized clinical trials. Risk for venous thromboembolic disease (VTE) is increased approximately 3-fold with ERT and the risk appears to be similar for raloxifene.[18] The absolute risk of VTE associated with HRT and raloxifene is low and it is not known if mechanisms that increase VTE risk also increase early CHD risk.

Unlike estrogen therapy, raloxifene has not been associated with an increased risk of breast cancer.[4] The Multiple Outcomes of Raloxifene Evaluation (MORE) trial included 7705 postmenopausal women with osteoporosis and demonstrated that the risk of invasive breast cancer was lowered by 76% during 3 years of treatment with raloxifene (60 mg/day) compared to placebo and cut the risk of vertebral fracture in half.[4] Although 1 in 2 women in the United States will die of CVD compared to 1 in 25 for breast cancer, women perceive the latter as a greater health threat.[19] The lack of awareness of actual CVD risk relative to concern about breast cancer and side effects of estrogen (bleeding and breast tenderness) may limit its use in clinical practice. Because of this, preventive therapies that have potential beneficial effects on osteoporosis and breast cancer, as well as CVD, may be associated with greater acceptance among postmenopausal women.

RUTH OBJECTIVES AND DESIGN OVERVIEW

Detailed methods and the design of the RUTH trial are published elsewhere.[20] Briefly, RUTH is an international, randomized, controlled, clinical trial that includes 10,101 postmenopausal women recruited from 26 countries. Enrollment was completed in 2.2 years (August 2000). The study was designed to test whether chronic oral treatment with raloxifene (60 mg/day) compared to placebo reduces the incidence of (1) the combined end point of coronary death, nonfatal myocardial infarction (MI), and hospitalized acute coronary syndromes other than MI (coronary primary end point) and (2) invasive breast cancer (breast cancer primary end point) in postmenopausal women at risk of major coronary events. Several secondary objectives will also be examined, including the effect of raloxifene compared with placebo on cardiovascular death, nonfatal MI, hospitalized acute coronary syndrome other than MI, myocardial revascularization, and stroke (each alone and combined). Other secondary end points include coronary death, all-cause mortality, hospitalized acute coronary syndromes, all-cause hospitalization, noncoronary arterial revascularization, nontraumatic lower-extremity amputation, and all breast cancers, fractures, and venous thromboembolic events.

The study is planned to end after 1670 participants experience a primary coronary end point. The sample size was calculated based on coronary end point assumptions of a 20% reduction in risk of coronary events with raloxifene, 89% power, and a two-sided alpha of 0.0417. For the breast cancer coprimary end point, assumptions included a two-sided alpha of 0.008 for the final analysis, yielding 80% power to detect a 58.5% reduction in risk of invasive breast cancer with raloxifene treatment. The projected average duration of follow-up is approximately 5 years.

Inclusion criteria were established to achieve an annual coronary event rate of 3.2% in the placebo group with the objective of including women with established CVD or at high risk for major coronary events owing to the presence of multiple risk factors. To be eligible, women had to be aged 55 years or older, at least 1 year postmenopausal, give informed consent, and accumulate a minimum of 4 points based on recent and/or history of CVD and/or documentation of CVD risk factors. Established CVD required a physician's prior written diagnosis of MI, a clinical history of angina or angina-like symptoms associated with a greater than 50% narrowing of one or more coronary arteries at angiography, lower-extremity arterial disease, or a documented coronary revascularization procedure. CVD risk factors included diabetes mellitus, age $\geq$ 65 years, MI or revascularization > 36 months prior to randomization, hyperlipidemia, current smoking, and hypertension. The RUTH trial was designed to be as generalizable as possible; therefore, exclusion criteria were chosen primarily to minimize adverse effects. Women with limited life expectancy, high risk of VTE, recent or suspicious cancer, menopausal symptoms, or use of hormone therapy or estrogen agonists/antagonists were not permitted in the study. Use of statins or other preventive therapies did not preclude a woman from being eligible for the trial.

Coronary end points are adjudicated by a central committee based on hospital records, ECG reports, cardiac enzymes, and troponin levels. Documentation of the coprimary end point, invasive breast cancer, is based on local pathology reports or equivalents, supplemented by mammogram films and other relevant reports. Estrogen receptor status is also determined.

COMPARISON WITH OTHER PREVENTION TRIALS

Given the null results of HERS, it is uncertain whether estrogen or SERMs will be useful for CVD prevention in postmenopausal women. However, the results of HERS may not apply to women without documented CHD. In RUTH, nearly equal numbers of women with and without existing CHD are enrolled, which will allow a subgroup analysis of the effect of raloxifene in the setting of primary and secondary prevention. HERS and the Women's Health Initiative (WHI)[21] are limited to the United States, where rates of concomitant cardiovascular therapy and revascularization procedures are much higher than in many countries participating in the RUTH trial. MPA, which may antagonize potential benefits of estrogen, was used in combination with estrogen in the HERS and also in the WHI and the Women's International Study of Long Duration of Oestrogen after Menopause (WISDOM)[22] trials. Raloxifene does not require the use of addition of a progestin.

The RUTH trial includes hospitalized acute coronary syndromes as a primary CHD end point, whereas many previous coronary prevention trials have limited the combined outcome to nonfatal MI and coronary death. The addition of this end point reflects the current trend to treat acute coronary syndromes of CHD aggressively before MI occurs. Moreover, acute coronary syndromes share a common pathophysiology and it is biologically plausible to include the spectrum of acute coronary syndromes in the primary CHD end point. The AFCAPS/TEXCAPS trial, conducted in men and women without CHD, with mild to moderate hyperlipidemia and low HDL-cholesterol, demonstrated that lipid-lowering therapy significantly reduces the incidence of the composite end point of unstable angina—nonfatal and fatal CHD.[23] Since the coronary protection associated with raloxifene is likely to be partly mediated through a reduction in LDL-cholesterol, use of CHD end points that are similar to contemporary lipid-lowering trials will more easily permit comparisons in the efficacy of these agents.

Adenocarcinoma of the breast is an important cause of morbidity and is the second leading cause of cancer death among women in the United States. The RUTH study is an appropriate cohort to assess the impact of raloxifene on breast cancer risk in a large population because RUTH includes a substantial number of older women who do not have established osteoporosis.

SUMMARY

RUTH is the first large-scale global clinical outcome trial of a SERM. The study will provide important information about the long-term efficacy and safety of raloxifene for the prevention of CHD and breast cancer among women at high risk for major coronary events. The geographical, ethnic, and cultural diversity of participants of the RUTH trial will enhance our understanding of the role of SERMs for the health of postmenopausal women.

REFERENCES

1. WALSH, B.W., L.H. KULLER, R.A. WILD et al. 1998. Effects of raloxifene on serum lipids and coagulation factors in healthy postmenopausal women. JAMA **279:** 1445–1451.
2. WALSH, B., S. PAUL, R.A. WILD et al. 2000. Effects of hormone replacement therapy and raloxifene on C-reactive protein and homocysteine in postmenopausal women: a randomized, controlled trial. J. Endocrinol. Metab. **85:** 214–218.
3. ETTINGER, B., D.M. BLACK, B.H. MITLAK et al. 1999. Reduction of vertebral fracture risk in postmenopausal women with osteoporosis treated with raloxifene: results from a 3-year randomized clinical trial. JAMA **282:** 637–645.

4. CUMMINGS, S., S. ECKERT, K. KRUEGER et al. 1999. The effect of raloxifene on risk of breast cancer in postmenopausal women. JAMA **281:** 2189–2197.
 5. GOLDSTEIN, S.R., W.H. SCHEELE, S.K. RAJAGOPALAN et al. 2000. A 12-month comparative study of raloxifene, estrogen, and placebo on the postmenopausal endometrium. Obstet. Gynecol. **95:** 95–103.
 6. BJARNASON, N.H., J. HAARBO, I. BYRJALSEN et al. 1997. Raloxifene inhibits aortic accumulation of cholesterol in ovariectomized, cholesterol-fed rabbits. Circulation **96:** 1964–1969.
 7. KAUFFMAN, R.F., J.S. BEAN, K.J. FAHEY et al. 2001. Raloxifene and estrogen inhibit neointimal thickening following balloon injury in the carotid artery of male and ovariectomized female rats. J. Cardiovasc. Pharmacol. In press.
 8. ZUCKERMAN, S.H. & N. BRYAN. 1996. Inhibition of LDL oxidation and myeloperoxidase dependent tyrosyl radical formation by the selective estrogen receptor modulator raloxifene (LY139481 HCl). Atherosclerosis **126:** 65–75.
 9. FIGTREE, G.A., Y. LU, C.M. WEBB & P. COLLINS. 1999. Raloxifene acutely relaxes rabbit coronary arteries *in vitro* by an estrogen receptor–dependent and nitric oxide–dependent mechanism. Circulation **100:** 1095–1101.
10. ZOMA, W.D., R.S. BAKER & K.E. CLARK. 2000. Coronary and uterine vascular responses to raloxifene in the sheep. Am. J. Obstet. Gynecol. **182:** 521–528.
11. DRAPER, M.W., D.E. FLOWERS, W.J. HUSTER et al. 1996. A controlled trial of raloxifene (LY139481) HCl: impact on bone turnover and serum lipid profile in healthy postmenopausal women. J. Bone Miner. Res. **11:** 835–842.
12. DELMAS, P.D., N.H. BJARNASON, B.H. MITLAK et al. 1997. Effects of raloxifene on bone mineral density, serum cholesterol concentrations, and uterine endometrium in postmenopausal women. N. Engl. J. Med. **337:** 1641–1647.
13. MOSCA, L. 2000. The role of hormone replacement therapy in the prevention of postmenopausal heart disease. Arch. Intern. Med. **160:** 2263–2272.
14. HULLEY, S., D. GRADY, T. BUSH et al. 1998. Randomized trial of estrogen plus progestin for secondary prevention of coronary heart disease in postmenopausal women: Heart and Estrogen/Progestin Replacement Study (HERS) Research Group. JAMA **280:** 605–613.
15. PETITTI, D.B. 1998. Hormone replacement therapy and heart disease prevention: experimentation trumps observation [editorial]. JAMA **280:** 650–652.
16. CUSHMAN, M., C. LEGAULT, E. BARRETT-CONNOR et al. 1999. Effect of postmenopausal hormones on inflammation-sensitive proteins: the Postmenopausal Estrogen/Progestin Interventions (PEPI) study. Circulation **100(7):** 717–722.
17. RIDKER, P., J.E. BURING, J. SHIH et al. 1998. Prospective study of C-reactive protein and the risk of future cardiovascular events among apparently healthy women. Circulation **98:** 731–733.
18. GRADY, D., N. WENGER, D. HERRINGTON et al. 2000. Postmenopausal hormone replacement therapy increases risk for thromboembolic disease: the Heart and Estrogen/Progestin Replacement Study. Ann. Intern. Med. **132:** 689–696.
19. MOSCA, L., W.K. JONES, K.B. KING et al. 2000. Awareness, perception, and knowledge of heart disease risk and prevention among women in the United States: American Heart Association Women's Heart Disease and Stroke Campaign Task Force. Arch. Fam. Med. **9:** 506–515.
20. MOSCA, L., E. BARRETT-CONNOR, N. WENGER et al. 2001. Design and methods of the Raloxifene Use for the Heart (RUTH) study. Am. J. Cardiol. **88:** 392–395.
21. WOMEN'S HEALTH INITIATIVE STUDY GROUP. 1998. Design of the Women's Health Initiative clinical trial and observational study. Control Clin. Trials **19:** 61–109.
22. VICKERS, M.R., T.W. MEADE & H.C. WILKES. 1995. Hormone replacement therapy and cardiovascular disease: the case for a randomized controlled trial. Ciba Found. Symp. **191:** 150–154.
23. DOWNS, J.R., P.A. BEERE, E. WHITNEY et al. 1997. Design and rationale of the Air Force/Texas Coronary Atherosclerosis Prevention Study (AFCAPS/TEXCAPS). Am. J. Cardiol. **80:** 287–293.

Prevention and Treatment of Osteoporosis

Introduction

SARALYN MARK AND JHUMKA GUPTA

United States Department of Health and Human Services' Office on Women's Health, Washington, District of Columbia 20201, USA

Osteoporosis has been defined by the World Health Organization as a "progressive systemic disease characterized by low bone mineral density (BMD) and microarchitectural deterioration of bone tissue, with a consequent increase in bone fragility and susceptibility to fracture." Osteoporotic fractures, commonly of the hip and spine, often result in secondary complications such as functional impairment, increased hospital stays that may be associated with additional morbidity, and increased dependence on others for living assistance. In the United States, approximately 10 million people are affected by osteoporosis, most of whom are postmenopausal women. Hence, the extent and severity of this public health issue are revealed by the millions of people affected by osteoporosis and the increasing health care costs to treat the disease and its associated complications. However, an array of prevention and treatment strategies that range from lifestyle modifications to therapeutic agents such as estrogen/hormone replacement therapy, selective estrogen receptor modulators (SERMs), and bisphosphonates are now available to reduce the devastating toll of this disease and its consequences.

The risk of fracture is determined by the interaction of several factors throughout an individual's life span. The changes in BMD with aging are among the most important of these factors. BMD in the elderly is determined by the amount of bone mass attained between the end of adolescence and young adulthood (peak bone mass) and then subsequent rates of bone loss during the aging process. The progressive loss of bone mass occurs in both men and women, but appears to accelerate at the time of menopause in women.

The therapeutic profiles of SERMs and bisphosphonates, two groups of pharmacological agents currently used to treat and prevent osteoporosis, are explored in this section. Both SERMs and bisphosphonates are antiresorptive agents that decrease the resorption of bone tissue by osteoclasts, thus inhibiting the process of bone loss. The first paper presents the current data available on the efficacy of these agents in the prevention and treatment of vertebral fractures and hip fractures, and outlines important research and clinical considerations for the future of SERMs and bisphosphonates. The conclusion supports the need for a greater understanding of the mech-

---

Address for correspondence: Saralyn Mark, M.D., Senior Medical Advisor, United States Department of Health and Human Services' Office on Women's Health, 200 Independence Avenue S.W., Room 719E, Washington, DC 20201. Voice: 202-690-7650; fax: 202-401-4005.
smark@osophs.dhhs.gov

anisms of these and other classes of agents, especially with respect to the differential between their effects on BMD and expected changes in fracture rates. For instance, while large-scale studies have demonstrated the efficacy of SERMs, such as raloxifene, and the bisphosphonates, including alendronate and risedronate, in preventing new vertebral fractures in osteoporotic women, only the bisphosphonates have been shown to be effective in reducing nonvertebral fractures in women with osteoporosis. Therefore, an increased understanding of the mechanisms of SERMs and bisphosphonates will enable clinicians to target therapeutic regimens more effectively to both premenopausal and postmenopausal women and to women with different fracture susceptibilities at different skeletal sites. Because raloxifene, in addition to its skeletal effects, promotes a lipid profile that is consistent with a cardioprotective effect and may also offer some protection against breast cancer, it offers an example of how an enhanced understanding of the effects of SERMs in different physiological systems will facilitate the refinement and development of future generations of SERMs.

The second paper discusses the paradoxical relationship between increments in BMD and the magnitude of expected versus observed decreases in vertebral fracture risk with different antiresorptive strategies such as a SERM like raloxifene and a bisphosphonate such as alendronate. While raloxifene functions to modestly improve bone mass in postmenopausal women, it reduces the risk of vertebral fractures in osteoporotic women by a magnitude that is much greater than expected from the change in BMD. This may be due to improved bone quality and microarchitecture, as well as changes in biomechanical forces. However, this hypothesis remains largely theoretical due to a lack of direct proof and an absence of appropriate testing methodologies. Further, while other antiresorptive therapies such as risedronate dramatically reduce the risk of vertebral fractures during the first year of treatment, there are indications that there may be a diminution of the effect with time. It has been suggested that the slowing of bone resorption may give rapid rise to biomechanical benefits that may wane in later years due to the detrimental effects of accumulating fatigue damage. Through a greater comprehension of the interactions between the biomechanical forces on bone and the physiological changes induced by antiresorptive agents, the rationale for more effective strategies to prevent vertebral and nonvertebral fractures will become evident. Successful prevention programs and treatment modalities will enhance the quality of life for millions of people at risk or who already have this debilitating disease.

Preventing and Treating Osteoporosis

Strategies at the Millennium

SHERRY SHERMAN

National Institute on Aging, National Institutes of Health, Gateway Building, Suite 3E327, Bethesda, Maryland 20892, USA

ABSTRACT: Osteoporosis has been defined as "a progressive systemic disease characterized by low bone density and microarchitectural deterioration of bone tissue, with a consequent increase in bone fragility and susceptibility to fracture." Osteoporosis and the consequences of compromised bone strength—particularly vertebral and hip fractures—are a significant cause of frailty, and increased morbidity and even mortality and hence are a serious and costly public health problem in the elderly population However, due to remarkable advances in basic and clinical research and in drug design, development, and testing, a number of efficacious, evidence-based options are available for the prevention and treatment of osteoporosis. These options extend far beyond estrogen/progestin therapy and include lifestyle and dietary changes such as increasing weight-bearing activity, enhancing calcium and vitamin D intake, as well as incorporating pharmacologic agents such as the bisphosphonates and selective estrogen receptor modulators (SERMs) such as raloxifene. In addition to its efficacy in increasing bone mineral density and reducing vertebral fractures by almost 40% in women with osteoporosis, the SERM raloxifene appears to promote a cardioprotective profile and to offer some protection against breast cancer. The potential of raloxifene to prevent or delay the development of a number of chronic diseases of aging such as osteoporosis, cardiovascular disease, and perhaps even Alzheimer's disease has stimulated the development and refinement of subsequent generations of SERMs aimed at maximizing beneficial effects in a wide variety of tissues while eliminating deleterious outcomes and side effects.

KEYWORDS: selective estrogen receptor modulators; SERMs; bone; osteoporosis; prevention of osteoporosis; treatment of osteoporosis; risk factors; fractures; menopause; bisphosphonates; alendronate; risedronate; estrogen replacement therapy

BACKGROUND

Osteoporosis has been defined as "a progressive systemic disease characterized by low bone density and microarchitectural deterioration of bone tissue, with a consequent increase in bone fragility and susceptibility to fracture."[1] Although the crucial clinical manifestation of osteoporosis is the occurrence of the fragility fracture,

---

Address for correspondence: Sherry Sherman, Ph.D., National Institute on Aging, NIH, Gateway Building, Suite 3E327, Bethesda, MD 20892-9205. Courier/express mail ZIP 20814. Voice: 301-435-3048; fax: 301-402-1784.

shermans@nia.nih.gov

the disease has been operationally defined by the World Health Organization (WHO) as bone mineral density (BMD) that is 2.5 standard deviations or more below the average value for peak adult bone mass. Commonly expressed relative to this young adult reference value as a T-score, the WHO criterion would be a T-score of ≤ -2.5. Because of the exponential age-related increase in fractures, advanced age and low BMD are the two most important risk factors for osteoporosis-related fractures. Osteoporosis and the consequences of compromised bone strength—particularly vertebral and hip fractures—are a significant cause of frailty and increased morbidity and even mortality, and hence are a serious public health problem in the elderly population. This disorder is also extremely costly, with direct expenditures in the United States for osteoporosis and fracture care estimated at $13.8 billion in 1995.[2] Hip fractures are among the most devastating of fractures, because they are commonly associated with substantial pain, hospitalization, serious morbidity and mortality, functional limitations, loss of independence, and the need for extended nursing home stays. Hip fractures alone numbered more than 350,000 cases per year in the mid-1990s and were responsible for 63% of the total expended costs of osteoporosis. Osteoporotic fractures exclusive of hip fractures are also of great concern, because they accounted for over 600,000 emergency room visits and two million physician outpatient visits.[2]

The progressive loss of bone mass, which can begin as early as the fourth decade in men and women, appears to accelerate at the time of menopause in women and to be responsible in large part for the enhanced prevalence of osteoporosis observed in women compared to men.[3] The striking contribution of gender to the risk of osteoporotic fractures is reflected by the observation that almost three-quarters of all hip fractures occur in postmenopausal women. In Caucasians, who have the highest rates of osteoporotic fractures, postmenopausal women have an estimated lifetime risk of hip fracture of 17.5% compared to 6.0% in men. In addition, at age 50 the lifetime risks of a clinically evident vertebral fracture are 15.6% vs. 5.0%; and the lifetime risks of a distal forearm fracture are 16% vs. 2.5% in women compared to men. Importantly, the estimated lifetime risk of all other fractures in Caucasian women is 31%.[2]

The risk of fracture is influenced by the interaction of a multiplicity of factors over time as individuals mature from youth to old age. Bone strength, which represents the amalgamation of bone density and bone quality, is one of key determinants of the propensity to fracture. Bone quality encompasses characteristics related to bone geometry and the distribution of bone mineral, architecture and connectivity, remodeling status, and the accumulation of microdamage. Since it is not currently possible to assess bone quality directly and BMD has been estimated to account for approximately 70% of bone strength, BMD, which is accurately and reliably assessed by bone densitometry technologies such as dual-energy X-ray absorptiometry (DEXA), is commonly used to assess the risk of fracture.[4]

Other important risk factors for low bone mass and increased risk of fracture include race/ethnicity, early menopause/estrogen deficiency, family history of osteoporotic fractures, low body mass index, history of previous fragility fractures, dietary factors (such as calcium nutrition and vitamin D status), lifestyle factors—including smoking and sedentary behavior, chronic use of medications (e.g., glucocorticoids, anticonvulsants, overreplacement of thyroxine), and malabsorption syndromes. For fractures of the hip, additional risk factors such as hip geometry, the increased propensity to fall (due to impairments in physical function, balance, muscle strength, reflexes, cognition, and vision) as well as the specifics of fall biomechanics become highly important.[4]

Bone mineral density in middle and old age is determined both by the level of bone mass attained between the end of adolescence and young adulthood (peak bone mass) and by subsequent rates of bone loss. Throughout life bone is continuously remodeled, a process whereby old bone is removed (or resorbed) and replaced with newly synthesized matrix, which is subsequently mineralized. The remodeling process(es) involved in bone turnover serve to prevent the accumulation of fatigue damage and microfractures, which are associated with activities of daily living, and thus promote bone health and quality. However, enhanced rates of remodeling can result from pathological conditions, drugs, aging, and—particularly in women—from the onset of the menopause transition. An increased remodeling rate can produce an imbalance such that the rate of bone resorption exceeds that of bone formation, leading to the loss of bone mass and architectural stability.[5] In untreated postmenopausal women, elevated levels of a number of biochemical indices of bone turnover are associated with increased risk of fractures.[6] Furthermore, after antiresorptive therapy, reductions in the levels of these "bone markers" have been associated with significant treatment-induced reductions in vertebral[7,8] and nonvertebral[8] fracture risk. However, the relationship(s) between the levels of a given biochemical marker at baseline or the magnitude of marker change (after treatment) with the reduction in fracture risk may be dependent on the specific pharmacologic agent tested.[6] Effects of treatment on specific bone markers will be discussed subsequently in the context of treatment interventions.

STRATEGIES FOR THE PREVENTION AND TREATMENT OF OSTEOPOROSIS

Calcium and Vitamin D

As a result of remarkable advances in basic and clinical research and in drug design, development, and testing, a number of efficacious, evidence-based options are available for the prevention and treatment of osteoporosis. These options include lifestyle and dietary alterations, such as increasing calcium and vitamin D intake; weight-bearing exercise; and pharmacologic therapies, such as the bisphosphonates, estrogen, and selective estrogen receptor modulators (SERMs), such as raloxifene. Because clinical intervention studies with calcium and vitamin D in healthy free-living elderly men and women[9] and in elderly women with suboptimal calcium and vitamin D status and hyperparathyroidism[10] have shown significant reductions in bone turnover with either preservation or increases in BMD, supplementation of both placebo and active treatment groups with vitamin D (in the presence of suboptimal vitamin D status) and calcium is now the norm in clinical trials. Supplementation with calcium and vitamin D has been shown to significantly reduce the risk of hip[10] and total nonvertebral[9] fractures and is inexpensive and well tolerated, with few unacceptable side effects.

Estrogen

Because the cessation of ovarian function and estrogen deficiency of menopause are associated with increased bone turnover and an acceleration in the rates of bone loss, menopause plays a major role in the development of postmenopausal osteoporosis.[3] Estrogen alone (or in combination with a progestin in women with a uterus) has long been the mainstay for the prevention and treatment of postmenopausal osteoporosis because of its widespread efficacy in the preservation (or enhancement) of bone density at all skeletal sites studied in both early and late menopausal women.[11–13] The primary mechanism of action of estrogen in reducing bone loss is believed to be the inhibition of excessive osteoclastic activation and activity which, in turn, results in a reduction of bone resorption and overall remodeling rates.[3] Although observational studies strongly support a role for estrogen in the prevention of hip (and other) fractures,[14] convincing findings from randomized controlled trials confirming the antifracture efficacy of estrogen are scarce.[4] Although estrogen has been used in the clinical setting for over 50 years, initially to relieve menopause-related symptomatology, side effects such as bleeding, breast tenderness, bloating, weight gain, and risk of breast cancer and venous thromboembolic events continue to limit acceptability and long-term adherence.

SERMs

Tamoxifen

Tamoxifen, initially developed as an antiestrogen for use in contraception, is a customary component of therapy for women with estrogen receptor–positive breast cancer in both the adjuvant and metastatic settings. Having been approved recently by the FDA for reduction of the risk of breast cancer in high-risk women, tamoxifen has now entered the arena of chemoprevention. Because long-term therapy (five years) was thought to be necessary to improve disease-free and overall survival, it has been important to identify potential adverse effects of tamoxifen on various systems throughout the body, given the possibility that, as in the breast, tamoxifen might have antiestrogenic effects in other estrogen-responsive tissues. To determine whether tamoxifen has estrogen agonist or antagonist effects in bone, Love *et al.*[15] conducted a two-year randomized, double-masked, placebo-controlled trial of tamoxifen (20 mg/day) in 140 postmenopausal women (mean age 48 years) with axillary node–negative breast cancer. In women randomized to tamoxifen, spine BMD increased by 0.61% per year ($P = 0.04$ compared to baseline); while in women receiving placebo, BMD declined by 1.00% per year ($P < 0.001$). However, the bone-sparing effect seen in the spine was not paralleled in the radius, where the BMD change of -0.88% per year in women on tamoxifen was not different from that of -1.29% per year in women on placebo. With respect to markers of bone turnover, which were assessed in subgroups of these women, serum osteocalcin declined by more than 50%, and serum alkaline phosphatase declined by 21% in the tamoxifen-treated group compared to those treated with placebo, indicating the potential of tamoxifen to have estrogen-like effects on the reduction of bone remodeling.

Preliminary data from Love *et al.*[15] also suggested that the positive effects of tamoxifen on spine BMD observed in postmenopausal women may not predominate in premenopausal women. To determine whether the skeletal effects in premenopausal women were comparable to those in postmenopausal women, Powles et al.[16] evaluated BMD changes (by dual-energy X-ray absorptiometry) in a subset of participants in the Royal Marsden Breast Cancer Prevention Trial, which was studying the effects of randomization to either placebo or tamoxifen (20 mg/day). The subset of 125 pre- and 54 postmenopausal women included in this analysis fulfilled the eligibility criteria of having a defined menopausal status and no hormone replacement therapy (HRT) use. Over the three-year study period, in postmenopausal women on tamoxifen BMD increased significantly (compared to baseline) by 1.17% and 1.71% per year in the spine and hip, respectively, in contrast to nonsignificant losses at these sites in women on placebo. However, tamoxifen had the opposite effect in premenopausal women. Lumbar spine BMD decreased progressively from baseline by 1.88% per year in tamoxifen-treated premenopausal women compared to premenopausal women on placebo, who had a modest gain in spine BMD of 0.24% per year. Also in premenopausal women, hip BMD declined in those who received tamoxifen such that BMD was significantly lower at 24 and 36 months compared to those treated with placebo ($P < 0.02$). Thus, the estrogen agonist effects on spine and hip BMD may be modulated by the endogenous estrogen milieu such that in the presence of premenopausal levels of estrogen the net effects of tamoxifen treatment are antiestrogenic in bone.[16]

The effect of tamoxifen on the prevention of hip, Colles', and spine fractures was evaluated as a secondary outcome in the P-1: BCPT (Breast Cancer Prevention Trial) randomized controlled trial of tamoxifen, which had as its primary end point the prevention of invasive breast cancer in women at increased risk. This study by the National Surgical Adjuvant Breast and Bowel Project (NSABP)[17] enrolled 13,388 women. Eligibility criteria required that a woman be age 60 years or older or, if between 35–59 years, have a five-year predicted breast cancer risk of at least 1.66% according to the Gail model criteria[18] or a history of lobular carcinoma in situ. In the tamoxifen-treated women, compared to those on placebo, there was a 19% reduction in the combined occurrence of fractures at the hip, spine, and lower radius that was nearly significant (RR = 0.81; 95% CI = 0.63–1.05). Although hip fractures were reduced by 45% in the women on tamoxifen, these fractures were rare (22 and 12 in the placebo and tamoxifen groups, respectively); therefore, this finding did not result in a statistically significant difference between the groups. The small total number of hip fractures is not surprising given the age distribution of the women. Because only 24% of the participants were 60–69 years of age and only 6% were older than 70, the overall population was relatively "young" in the trajectory of the exponential age-related rise in hip fractures. Furthermore, observational studies suggest that women at greater risk for breast cancer have greater bone density and thus are at reduced risk of osteoporotic fractures.[14] When stratified by age, the overall reduction in total fractures in women on tamoxifen compared to placebo was greater in women who were 50 years of age or older compared to those who were less than 50. Once again, in the older age group the 19% reduction in total fractures in the tamoxifen-treated women nearly reached significance (RR = 0.79; CI = 0.60–1.05).

Raloxifene

Raloxifene is a benzothiophene-derived SERM that possesses estrogen agonist effects on bone and serum lipids but, unlike tamoxifen, does not stimulate the uterus and breast.[19] Metabolic studies comparing raloxifene and estrogen have shown that raloxifene (60 mg/day) reduces bone resorption and reverses a negative calcium balance to a degree that is comparable to estrogen (0.625 mg/day) plus medroxyprogesterone (5 mg/day).[20] The longer-term implications of these positive effects have been evaluated in a two-year randomized controlled trial using three doses of raloxifene (30, 60, or 120 mg/day) in 601 healthy early postmenopausal women (45–60 years, mean age 55 years, and between 2–8 years postmenopause) who had a lumbar spine BMD between -2.5 SD below and 2.0 SD above the reference value for premenopausal women.[19] All women received 400–600 mg/day calcium. BMD of the lumbar spine, hip, and total body significantly increased with all three doses of raloxifene. In the group receiving 60 mg/day raloxifene, the increase in BMD relative to placebo was 2.4% in both the lumbar spine and the total hip. Biochemical markers of bone remodeling decreased, as indicated by 23% and 15% reductions in the concentration of bone-specific alkaline phosphatase and osteocalcin (both markers of bone formation) and by the 34% reduction in the urinary type I collagen C-telopeptide (CTx):creatinine ratio (an index of bone resorption). After 24 months on raloxifene, the biochemical markers of bone remodeling had fallen from elevated levels to values similar to those of premenopausal women. Subsequent follow-up of the participants of this European trial, combined with 544 women (for a total $N = 1145$) from an identical ongoing US trial (which was designed in parallel with the European trial), confirmed after 36 months that (1) the biochemical markers of bone turnover were still reduced and comparable to premenopausal values, and that (2) the gain in bone mass (although somewhat lower in magnitude in the combined populations than in the European population alone) persisted in women on raloxifene.[21] After 36 months, mean lumbar spine changes from baseline were -1.32% on placebo and $+0.71\%$, $+1.28\%$, and $+1.20\%$ on 30 mg/day, 60 mg/day, or 150 mg/day raloxifene, respectively, with comparable changes observed in the hip. However, there were significant (although attenuated compared to placebo) declines in BMD in the ultradistal radius and forearm with all doses of raloxifene. Although the incidence of hot flashes was greater in the raloxifene-treated women compared to placebo (25% vs. 18%), they were mild and did not increase study withdrawals; and tolerability of raloxifene was not different from that of the placebo. Thus, in a population of normal early postmenopausal women, treatment with raloxifene 30–150 mg/day suppresses bone resorption and bone turnover to levels characteristic of normal premenopausal women, while preserving bone mass in the hip, spine, and total body.[21]

The MORE (Multiple Outcomes of Raloxifene Evaluation) trial, a three-year randomized, double-masked placebo-controlled trial, was the first to demonstrate the antifracture efficacy of an estrogen-like drug or SERM in women with osteoporosis.[22] In this study, 7705 women (aged 31–80 years, mean age 67 years) with osteoporosis defined either by WHO criteria (i.e., BMD lower than -2.5 SD below the reference value, or a T-score < -2.5) or by the presence of low BMD and existing vertebral fractures were randomized to either 60 mg/day or 120 mg/day raloxifene or to placebo. All women received supplemental calcium and vitamin D. Relative to placebo, in the groups receiving 60 mg/day and 120 mg/day raloxifene, femoral neck BMD was increased by 2.1% and 2.4% and spine BMD was increased by 2.6% and 2.7%, respectively. Overall, fewer new spine fractures were observed in the raloxifene-treated women, regardless of the presence or absence of vertebral fractures at baseline. The risk of vertebral fracture was reduced by 30% in the group receiving

60 mg/day and by 50% in the group receiving 120 mg/day raloxifene. However, there was no effect of either dose of raloxifene on the rate of nonvertebral fractures.

Bisphosphonates

Bisphosphonate therapy includes drugs such as alendronate and risedronate—both of which have been approved, after rigorous randomized, placebo-controlled trials, for the prevention and treatment of postmenopausal osteoporosis. The mechanism of action leading to potent antiresorptive effects entails the binding of the bisphosphonate to the hydroxyapatite crystal of bone and subsequent inhibition of the production and/or activity of osteoclasts. As demonstrated in the Fracture Intervention Trial (FIT), alendronate provides substantial skeletal benefits to postmenopausal women in two categories: those with low bone mass and those with both low bone mass and existing vertebral fractures. In 2027 women, aged 55–81, with low BMD and at least one vertebral fracture at baseline, 36 months of alendronate significantly increased BMD (relative to placebo) by +6.2% in the lumbar spine, +4.7% in the total hip, and +4.1% in the femoral neck. Importantly, treatment with alendronate resulted in a significant 47% reduction in the risk of one or more new radiographic vertebral fractures. Hip and wrist fractures were also significantly reduced by approximately 50%. These effects were observed with an alendronate dose, which was initiated at 5 mg/day and then increased to 10 mg/day (for better efficacy) in the third year of the trial.[23]

The Fracture Intervention Trial also tested the efficacy of alendronate on BMD and fracture prevention in the category of women with low BMD but no existing vertebral fractures. In these 4432 women, whose femoral BMD was equal to or lower than 1.6 SD below the young adult reference value (T-score ≤ -1.6), four years of alendronate treatment increased BMD (relative to placebo) by 4.6% in the femoral neck, 5.0% in the total hip, and 6.6% in the spine.[24] The risk of a new radiographic vertebral fracture was reduced by 44% in alendronate-treated women. Alendronate also significantly reduced the risk of clinical fractures (i.e., fractures diagnosed by a doctor) by 36%, but only in women who had osteoporosis of the hip at baseline (i.e., femoral neck BMD T-score ≤ -2.5). Among women with higher bone mass, alendronate had no significant effect on the risk of clinical fractures.

Risedronate, the second bisphosphonate demonstrated to have antifracture efficacy, was evaluated in a three-year study of 2458 women under 85 years of age who were more than five years postmenopause and who had osteoporosis, as defined by the presence of one or more prevalent vertebral fractures at baseline.[8] Although the women were initially randomized to placebo and either 2.5 mg/day or 5 mg/day risedronate, the 2.5-mg/day arm was discontinued after the first year due to lack of efficacy in other trials. Treatment with 5 mg/day risedronate significantly reduced vertebral fractures by 65% in the first year. Compared to placebo, risedronate decreased the three-year cumulative incidence of new vertebral fractures by 41% and of nonvertebral fractures by 39%. Risedronate significantly improved BMD by 4.3% in the spine, 2.8% in the femoral neck, and 1.6% at the radius midshaft relative to placebo. The overall safety profile was reported to be similar to placebo. Importantly, in another study of 5445 elderly women (70–79 years old) with osteoporosis defined as the presence of baseline vertebral fractures and/or very low BMD (T-score

≤ −4 [or T-score ≤ −3 in the presence of additional nonskeletal risk factors]), risedronate significantly reduced hip fractures by 40%.[8]

Thus raloxifene and the bisphosphonates alendronate and risedronate are highly efficacious in reducing the risk of vertebral fractures in postmenopausal women with osteoporosis defined by prevalent vertebral fractures or by very low BMD (T-score ≤ −2.5). It is curious that, although the magnitude of the increases in BMD in the spine and hip in response to raloxifene is modest—usually under 2.5%, the magnitude of the reduction in risk of vertebral fractures is between 35 to 45%, which is not far from the 40–50% reduction observed in studies with either alendronate or risedronate, where the increases in BMD (especially in the spine) were much more substantial. In this volume, Dr. Cummings explores the significance of the lack of parallelism between the magnitude of the BMD response and that of the reduction in fracture risk observed with different antiresorptive therapies.[25]

CONCLUSION

As the new millennium unfolds, advances in bone biology, pharmacology, and clinical research have resulted in several highly efficacious options to prevent or treat osteoporosis in older women. Promising nonpharmacologic approaches for the maintenance of bone density and bone health include dietary modification (to achieve optimal calcium and vitamin D nutrition), lifestyle changes such as increased weight-bearing exercise, smoking cessation, monitoring effects of drugs that increase the risk of falls, and improving physical function and household safety.

Because preexisting vertebral fractures markedly increase the risk of subsequent vertebral, hip, and other fractures, identification of those at risk of their first osteoporotic vertebral fracture is key in preventing the downward spiral of alternating episodes and accumulating consequences of fracture and disability. Many questions need to be addressed in both the prevention and treatment arenas. Although large-scale studies have demonstrated the efficacy of alendronate, risedronate, and raloxifene in preventing new vertebral fractures in osteoporotic women, only the bisphosphonates are effective in reducing nonvertebral fractures and only in women with osteoporosis. The mechanisms mediating the broader nonvertebral antifracture efficacy of the bisphosphonates in osteoporotic women need to be elucidated in order to understand the lack of efficacy of raloxifene in preventing nonvertebral fractures and to develop new SERMs with greater antifracture efficacy.

In promoting primary prevention, the optimal agent and the timing and duration of therapy are unclear for women who are not osteoporotic but have low bone mass between one and two SD below the young adult reference value. This is particularly true in pre- and perimenopausal women, because few prospective studies have been designed to assess the efficacy of various strategies aimed at long-term maintenance of BMD and fracture risk reduction in women before the menopause transition. Given the paradoxical negative effects of tamoxifen on bone mass in premenopausal women compared to the positive effects in postmenopausal women, an enhanced research focus is needed to elucidate the mechanisms of action of raloxifene and other SERMs on bone and other estrogen-sensitive tissues in premenopausal women. This knowledge is particularly salient to those contemplating long-term SERM use in the setting of breast cancer prevention. In postmenopausal women taking tamoxifen in the breast cancer treatment or prevention setting (or, potentially, raloxifene, if proved efficacious for breast cancer prevention), those women who also have osteoporosis will need to explore additional strategies, including combination SERM-bisphosphonate therapy, to prevent nonvertebral fractures. Because men have been understudied in the SERM arena and little information exists on SERM effects in men, focus on the potential value of current and future SERMs on the prevention and treatment of osteoporosis, prostate cancer, and other chronic diseases of aging is highly desirable.

Studies of the skeletal effects of combination therapy using an antiresorptive drug (such as raloxifene or a bisphosphonate) with new emerging anabolic agents such as parathyroid hormone (PTH) may enhance our understanding of the mechanisms mediating the balance between, or coupling of, bone resorption and bone formation, as well as how to optimize skeletal dynamics and architecture.

The development and success of SERMs like tamoxifen and raloxifene constitute an important new stimulus in the advancement of strategies to combat not only breast cancer and osteoporosis but other chronic diseases of aging that may involve estrogen-responsive tissues. In assessing the place of new generations of SERMs in the arsenal of drugs to combat osteoporosis, future studies of new SERMs with greater skeletal potency should also evaluate the effects of these agents on a range of extra-skeletal tissues throughout the body in order to facilitate customized strategies that incorporate patient health profiles and value systems.

REFERENCES

1. GENANT, H.K., C. COOPER, G. POOR, et al. 1999. Interim report and recommendations of the World Health Organization Task Force for Osteoporosis. Osteoporosis Int. **10:** 259–264.
2. MELTON, L.J., III. 2000. Who has osteoporosis? A conflict between clinical and public health perspectives. J. Bone Miner. Res. **15:** 2309–2314.
3. RIGGS, B.L., S. KHOSLA & L.J. MELTON III. 1998. A unitary model for involutional osteoporosis: estrogen deficiency causes both type I and type II osteoporosis in postmenopausal women and contributes to bone loss in aging men. J. Bone Miner. Res. **13:** 763–773.
4. NIH CONSENSUS DEVELOPMENT PANEL ON OSTEOPOROSIS PREVENTION. 2001. Osteoporosis prevention, diagnosis, and therapy. JAMA **285:** 785–795.
5. EASTELL, R. 1998. Treatment of postmenopausal osteoporosis. N. Engl. J. Med. **11:** 736–746.
6. DELMAS, P.D. 2000. How does antiresorptive therapy decrease the risk of fracture in women with osteoporosis? Bone **27:** 1–3.
7. ETTINGER B., D.M. BLACK, B.H. MITLAK, et al. 1999. Reduction of vertebral fracture risk in postmenopausal women with osteoporosis treated with raloxifene. Results from a 3-year randomized clinical trial. JAMA **282:** 637–645.
8. HARRIS, S.T., N.B. WATTS, H.K. GENANT, et al. 1999. Effects of risedronate treatment on vertebral and nonvertebral fractures in women with postmenopausal osteoporosis. JAMA **282:** 1344–1352.
9. DAWSON-HUGHES, B., S.S. HARRIS, E.A. KRALL, et al. 1997. Effect of calcium and vitamin D supplementation on bone density in men and women 65 years of age or older. N. Engl. J. Med. **337:** 670–676.
10. CHAPUY, M.C., M.E. ARLOT, F. DUBOEUF, et al. 1992. Vitamin D3 and calcium to prevent hip fractures in elderly women. N. Engl. J. Med. **327:** 1637–1642.

11. THE WRITING GROUP FOR THE PEPI TRIAL. 1996. Effects of hormone therapy on bone mineral density: results from the Postmenopausal Estrogen/Progestin Interventions (PEPI) Trial. JAMA **276:** 1389–1396.
12. GREENDALE, G.A., B. WELLS, R. MARCUS & E. BARRETT-CONNOR. 2000. How many women lose bone mineral density while taking hormone replacement therapy? Results from the Postmenopausal Estrogen/Progestin Interventions Trial. Arch. Intern. Med. **160:** 3065–3071.
13. GALLAGHER, J.C., S.E. FOWLER, J.R. DETTER, et al. 2001. Combination treatment with estrogen and calcitriol in the prevention of age-related bone loss. J. Clin. Endocrinol. Metab. **86:** 3618–3628.
14. CAULEY, J.A., D.G. SEELEY, K. ENSRUD, K. et al. 1995. Estrogen replacement therapy and fractures in older women. Ann Intern. Med. **122:** 9–16.
15. LOVE, R., R.B. MAZESS, H.S. BARDEN, et al. 1992. Effects of tamoxifen on bone mineral density in postmenopausal women with breast cancer. N. Engl. J. Med. **326:** 852–856.
16. POWLES, T.J., T. HICKISH, J.A. KANIS, et al. 1996. Effect of tamoxifen on bone mineral density measured by dual-energy X-ray absorptiometry in healthy premenopausal and postmenopausal women. J. Clin. Oncol. **14:** 78–84.
17. FISHER, B., J.P. CONSTANTINO, D.L. WICKERHAM, et al. 1998. Tamoxifen for prevention of breast cancer: report of the National Surgical Adjuvant Breast and Bowel Project P-1 Study. J. Natl. Cancer Inst. **90:** 1371–1388.
18. GAIL, M.H., L.A. BRINTON, D.P. BYAR, et al. 1989. Projecting individualized probabilities of developing breast cancer for white females who are being examined annually. J. Natl. Cancer Inst. **81:** 1879–1886.
19. DELMAS, P.D., N.H. BJARNASON, B.H. MITLAK, et al. 1997. Effects of raloxifene on bone mineral density, serum cholesterol concentrations, and uterine endometrium in postmenopausal women. N. Eng. J. Med. **337:** 1641–1647.
20. HEANEY, R.P. & M.W. DRAPER. 1997. Raloxifene and estrogen: comparative bone remodeling kinetics. J. Clin. Endocrinol. Metab. **82:** 3425–3429.
21. JOHNSTON, C.C., JR., N.H. BJARNASON, F.J. COHEN, et al. 2000. Long-term effects of raloxifene on bone mineral density, bone turnover, and serum lipid levels in early postmenopausal women. Arch. Intern. Med. **160:** 3444–3450.
22. ETTINGER, B., D.M. BLACK, B.H. MITLAK, et al. 1999. Reduction of vertebral fracture risk in postmenopausal women with osteoporosis treated with raloxifene. Results from a 3-year randomized clinical trial. J. Amer. Med. Assn. **282:** 637–645.
23. BLACK, D.M., S.R. CUMMINGS, D.B. KARPF, et al. 1996. Randomised trial of alendronate on risk fo fracture in women with existing vertebral fractures. Lancet **348:** 1535–1541.
24. CUMMINGS, S.R., D.M. BLACK, D.E. THOMPSON, et al. 1998. Effect of alendronate on risk of fracture in women with low bone density but without vertebral fractures. Results from the Fracture Intervention Trial. JAMA **280:** 2077–2082.
25. CUMMINGS, S.R. 2001. The paradox of small changes in bone density and reductions in risk of fracture with raloxifene. Ann. N.Y. Acad. Sci. **949.** This volume.

The Paradox of Small Changes in Bone Density and Reductions in Risk of Fracture with Raloxifene

STEVEN R. CUMMINGS

Department of Epidemiology and Biostatistics, School of Medicine, University of California, San Francisco, San Francisco, California 94143, USA

KEYWORDS: antiresorptive drugs; raloxifene; vertebral fractures; bone density

As its name implies, antiresorptive therapy decreases the resorption of bone tissue by osteoclasts. Slowing the resorption of bone in postmenopausal women slows the loss of bone. Raloxifene and tamoxifen act in this fashion to improve bone mass in postmenopausal women, but this effect is of modest magnitude—about a 2% higher bone density in women randomly assigned to SERMs compared to those assigned to placebo. It is surprising, therefore, to see that raloxifene reduces the risk of vertebral fractures by 35–45% in women with osteoporosis. This implies that there must be some other mechanisms for reducing the risk of vertebral fracture that are not captured by standard measurements of hip and spine bone density.

Theoretically, slowing bone resorption may directly increase the biomechanical strength of bone. At sites of bone resorption, trabeculae are temporarily thinner. Increasing the number of resorption sites in trabecular bone would be expected to weaken the bone, probably to a degree that is out of proportion to what would be expected from the relatively small amount of bone that is lost. In addition, bone is constantly undergoing stress—forces placed on bone by ordinary daily activity. These forces are not evenly distributed in bone: they tend to focus at defects or depressions in a bone. So, theoretically, bone resorption both decreases mechanical strength at resorption sites and causes mechanical forces to increase disproportionately at the same sites. Therefore, slowing down the rate of resorption and the number of places that this occurs may improve the strength of bone to a degree that is not reflected in commensurate improvement in bone density. However, this remains theoretical and there is no direct proof or easy way to test this hypothesis. Studies of the relationship between change in markers of bone turnover and reduction in risk of fractures have not yet provided solid support for this hypothesis, but these markers are imperfect and highly variable indicators of bone resorption.

Address for correspondence: Steven R. Cummings, M.D., Suite 600, 74 New Montgomery St., San Francisco, CA 94105. Voice: 415-597-9114; fax: 415-597-9213.
scummings@psg.ucsf.edu

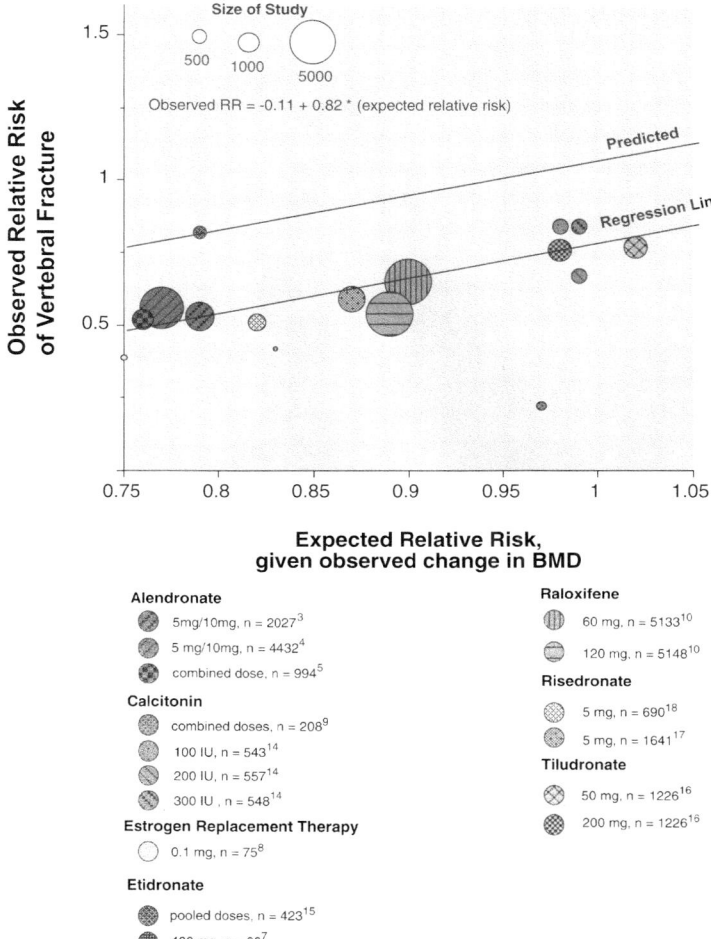

FIGURE 1. Relationship between improvement in spine bone mineral density versus change in risk of vertebral fracture.

This model of the action of antiresorptive drugs provides the best available explanation for the apparent paradox that raloxifene improved bone density by about 2.5%, but substantially reduced the risk of vertebral fractures. This hypothesis also helps explain a similar discrepancy seen with all antiresorptive drugs to date.

We conducted a metanalysis of all trials that measured spine bone density at baseline and assessed vertebral fracture. We plotted the relationship between improvement in spine BMD in those trials versus the change in risk of vertebral fracture observed in the same trials (FIG. 1).

To determine whether the reductions in risk of vertebral fracture were as large or larger than would be expected from the improvement in spine BMD, it is necessary to estimate just how much reduction in risk would be expected from a certain change in BMD. We used the placebo group of the Fracture Intervention Trial to calculate the relationship between spine BMD and risk of spine fracture. We confirmed that this relationship was very similar to that found in another large observational study, the Study of Osteoporotic Fractures. From this relationship, we estimated that each 1% improvement in spine BMD, as measured by dual-energy X-ray absorptiometry, would be expected to decrease the risk of vertebral fractures by about 4%. In other words, a 5% improvement in BMD would be expected to decrease the risk of vertebral fracture by about 20%.

As expected, in the trials of all antiresorptive drugs, we found that a 1% improvement in spine BMD was associated with a 4% decrease in the risk of vertebral fractures. However, all of the reductions in risk of vertebral fractures were greater than expected from the change in BMD. This is illustrated on the graph (FIG. 1) by the fact that all of the trials are below the line that represents the predicted reduction in risk of fractures. The two regression lines for the predicted effects and the observed effects on risk of fractures are 20–25% apart. In other words, antiresorptive treatment appears to be adding about a 20–25% reduction in the occurrence of vertebral fractures on top of that bone density effect. Thus, in the case of raloxifene, this model predicts that the 2.5% improvement in spine BMD observed with raloxifene would result in about a 10% decrease in risk of fractures as a result of improvement in spine BMD, but an additional 20–25% as a result of the "antiresorptive effect" of this class of drugs. This 30–35% is close to the observed 35% reduction seen with the FDA-approved dose of 60 mg a day.

There is one more twist to this story. It has recently been observed that risedronate reduces the risk of vertebral fracture by 65% during the first year of treatment! Similar early effects are seen with alendronate. This is much greater than predicted from the 2–3% improvments in BMD in the first year and suggests that most of this early effect is due to the rapid biomechanical benefits of slowing bone resorption.

The flip side of the coin of dramatic early reductions in risk is that reductions in the later years are much less. In other words, the effect of the bisphosphonates on risk of vertebral fractures seems to wane in later years of use. There is concern that this may be the result of accumulation of microscopic damage of bone—also known as fatigue damage. Bone turnover has the beneficial function of removing microdamage. Inhibiting turnvover might allow this damage to accumulate. There are other biolological explanations for this apparent waning of effect, including the possiblitity that the long-term effects of antiresorptives will eventually reflect their influence on bone mass. In this case, one would expect that antiresorptive drugs given long term would eventually have only modest effects on the risk of fractures, on the order of 15–40% of the reductions that would be predicted to result from 4–10% very long-term improvement in BMD.

This analysis has limitations. It is limited to spine bone density and vertebral fractures. The relationship between changes in bone density at any site in the occurrence of, or reduction of risk of, nonspine fractures is more complex because of the number of types of fractures involved. Furthermore, raloxifene did not reduce the risk of nonspine fractures during three years of treatment, so there is no "effect" to explain. In addition, current methods of densitometry do not fully reflect change in bone density in the important trabecular region of the vertebral body. It may be that more accurate and sensitive measurement methods, such as quantitative computed tomography (QCT), would find that most of the effects of antiresorptive drugs are due to changes in bone mass and structure in the spine that are missed by current methods.

In summary, antiresorptive drugs, including raloxifene, reduce vertebral fractures, at least in part, by improving bone density in a predictable fashion. There seems to be an additional and early reduction in risk of vertebral fractures that might be explained by the beneficial biomechanical effects of decreasing bone resorption. It will be very important to determine the effects of these agents when they are used beyond 5 or 10 years.

SERMs, Estrogen, and Cognitive Function
Introduction

ANDREW A. MONJAN

Neuroscience and Neuropsychology of Aging Program, National Institute on Aging, National Institutes of Health, Bethesda, Maryland 20892, USA

Over the last two to three decades, a number of observational and longitudinal studies have supported the concept that loss of estrogen associated with menopause results in a degree of cognitive decline. These human data were supported by animal studies showing that estrogens can mediate neurobiological mechanisms and pathways underlying cognitive functions. These exciting findings have led to the proposal that loss of estrogen, and its replacement, may be keys to the causes and treatments of Alzheimer's disease (AD). However, several recent large-scale clinical trials of the use of estrogen replacement therapy in postmenopausal women suggested that this treatment might not be effective in AD. The three papers in this section each critically review the human and animal studies on the effect of estrogen loss and replacement on cognitive and neural functioning in normal aging and AD. They also review the small number of studies using SERMS (raloxifene) that have produced varied and minimal to no effects on cognition in postmenopausal women. Problems in the clinical trials have been identified, including different measures to asses various cognitive domains; level of cognitive functioning at start of replacement therapy; length of postmenopausal status; and dose, type of preparation, duration, and temporal patterning of delivery. These papers also review new data, including the use of neuroimaging data, and ongoing and planned trials to further delineate and test the efficacy of hormone replacement therapy for cognitive functioning.

Address for correspondence: Andrew A. Monjan, Ph.D., M.P.H., Neuroscience and Neuropsychology of Aging Program, National Institute on Aging, 7201 Wisconsin Avenue, MSC 9205, Gateway Building, Suite 3C307, Bethesda, Maryland 20892-9205. Voice: 301-496-9350; fax: 301-496-1494.

am39m@nih.gov

Effects of Hormone Replacement Therapy on Cognitive and Brain Aging

SUSAN M. RESNICK AND PAULINE M. MAKI

Laboratory of Personality and Cognition, National Institute on Aging, National Institutes of Health, Baltimore, Maryland 21224, USA

ABSTRACT: Recent reports suggest that hormone therapy may be associated with a reduced risk for Alzheimer's disease and may offer some protection against age-associated declines in specific cognitive functions. The majority of these reports are based on observational studies, which are confounded by the "healthy user" bias—the tendency for women receiving hormone therapy to be younger, better educated, and have fewer medical problems. In one attempt to address these limitations, we conducted a series of studies examining effects of hormone therapy on cognitive and brain functioning in nondemented postmenopausal women in the Baltimore Longitudinal Study of Aging (BLSA). In this sample, women receiving hormone therapy and women who never received hormone therapy were comparable with respect to educational attainment, general medical health, and performance on a test of verbal knowledge. Despite these similarities, women receiving hormone therapy performed better on tests of verbal and visual memory compared to never-treated women. The two groups also differed in the patterns of regional brain activation evoked during performance of delayed verbal and figural memory tasks. Furthermore, longitudinal comparisons revealed greater relative blood flow increases over two years in women receiving hormone therapy for the hippocampus and other mesial temporal lobe structures that subserve memory. These observational findings from our studies in the BLSA have led to the development of a large-scale randomized clinical trial of hormone therapy and cognitive aging, the ancillary Women's Health Initiative Study of Cognitive Aging (WHISCA), and have important implications for studies of the effects of SERM's on cognitive and brain functioning.

KEYWORDS: hormone replacement therapy; estrogen replacement therapy; hormone therapy; cognitive aging; cognitive functioning; brain functioning

INTRODUCTION AND BACKGROUND

Recent reports suggest that estrogen replacement therapy (ERT) may have protective effects on cognitive aging in addition to its beneficial effects on certain aspects of physical health. A number of observational studies of postmenopausal women indicate that ERT, with or without adjuvant progestin treatment, is associated with a reduced risk for Alzheimer's disease[1,2] and may protect against age-associat-

Address for correspondence: Susan M. Resnick, Laboratory of Personality and Cognition, Box 03, National Institute on Aging, 5600 Nathan Shock Drive, Baltimore, MD 21224-6825. Voice: 410-558-8618; fax: 410-558-8108.

Susan.Resnick@nih.gov

ed memory decline in nondemented women.[3-5] Despite the increasing use of selective estrogen receptor modulators (SERMs), little is known about their effects on the central nervous system (CNS). The paucity of information is particularly troublesome as animal models have suggested that particular SERMs—for instance, tamoxifen—may antagonize some of the beneficial effects of estrogen on the CNS.[6] The purpose of this work is to review data on the effects of ERT on cognitive and brain aging in nondemented women, with a focus on a series of investigations we have been conducting on women in the Baltimore Longitudinal Study of Aging (BLSA). The findings of these studies can guide strategies for research on the effects of SERMs on cognitive and brain functioning.

There is a growing body of evidence, based on animal models, indicating a number of neurobiological mechanisms through which estrogens may exert neuroprotective and neurotrophic effects on the brain and influence memory functioning.[7] Estrogens have multiple effects on the CNS. On a cellular and molecular level, they have direct effects on neurons, regulating dendritic spine formation;[8,9] and they modulate neurotransmission in a variety of systems, including cholinergic,[10] dopaminergic,[11] serotonergic,[12] and noradrenergic effects.[13] Estrogens also help maintain normal lipoprotein synthesis and processing of the amyloid precursor protein, decreasing amyloid deposition in the brain.[14,15] On a global level, estrogens influence global and regional glucose metabolism.[16-18]

The results of animal studies provide support for the biological plausibility of a role of ERT in protecting against Alzheimer's disease and age-associated memory decline. A metanalysis of data published through 1997 on ERT and hormone replacement therapy (HRT) with adjuvant progestins and the risk of a diagnosis of dementia indicated a 29% reduction overall in the risk for dementia in women who had ever received hormone therapy compared with women who had never received such therapy.[1] The only two studies involving prospective assessment of hormone usage and diagnoses of Alzheimer's disease (one from the Baltimore Longitudinal Study of Aging[19]) indicated a risk reduction of more than 50%.[19,20] Moreover, a dose-response relationship was observed in one[20] of the two studies, with longer duration of ERT/HRT usage associated with greater risk reduction. Dose-response effects have also been reported in several, but not all, of the case-control studies.[2] These observational studies provide support for a beneficial role of hormone therapy in the *prevention* of dementia, whereas three recent randomized clinical trials[21-23] indicate that ERT is not effective in treating the symptoms of dementia in women with a diagnosis of Alzheimer's disease.

Studies of memory and other cognitive functions in postmenopausal women who are free of dementia present more mixed results. In general, two paradigms have been used to examine effects of HRT on cognitive functioning in nondemented women. A number of small randomized trials have been conducted on women who have undergone surgical menopause (hysterectomy and bilateral oophorectomy). These studies collectively indicate that estrogen treatment protects against cognitive decline following surgical induction of menopause, with the most consistent effects for verbal memory.[3,24] Estrogen-related enhancements in verbal memory have also been demonstrated in elderly women following two weeks of treatment with estradiol.[25] A recent randomized trial of a three-week treatment with transdermal estradiol provides additional support for a beneficial effect of estrogens on memory in postmenopausal women who have undergone natural menopause.[26] Compared with placebo, women receiving estradiol showed greater improvement relative to baseline on two tests of visual memory and in response times on a mental rotations task, but no significant differences on measures of executive functioning (i.e., self-monitoring and planning abilities). In summary, results from most, but not all,[27] of these small randomized trials provide considerably consistent evidence that ERT enhances verbal memory and preliminary evidence of beneficial effects on nonverbal memory and visuospatial functions.

The second paradigm involves observational studies—comparisons between women who choose to receive ERT/HRT and women who choose not to receive hormone treatment. Observational studies, many including larger numbers of women, have yielded somewhat inconsistent findings.[1] It is well known that women who choose to take ERT/HRT tend to be healthier, more highly educated, and have better access to medical care compared to women who choose not to receive HRT. This tendency, referred to as the "healthy user bias," is the most serious limitation of observational studies. Many observational studies employ statistical corrections to adjust for this bias, but the accuracy of these adjustments is uncertain. Another approach to address the healthy user bias is to study a group of women who are uniformly healthier and more highly educated. This is the approach we have followed in a series of investigations on women in the Baltimore Longitudinal Study of Aging (BLSA).

INVESTIGATIONS IN THE BALTIMORE LONGITUDINAL STUDY OF AGING

The BLSA study was initiated in 1958,[28] and women have been included since 1978. The BLSA involves a community-dwelling, highly educated sample. Participants return to the National Institute on Aging (NIA) on a routine basis (on average every two years) for a battery of physical and psychological assessments. One measure that has been administered as part of the psychological assessment since the early 1960s is the Benton Visual Retention Test (BVRT),[29] a measure of short-term figural memory and visuoperceptual and constructional skills. Studies in our laboratory[30,31] and elsewhere[32,33] have shown highly significant cross-sectional and longitudinal declines in BVRT performance with age.

ERT/HRT, MEMORY, AND OTHER COGNITIVE ABILITIES

To investigate the effects of ERT/HRT on cognitive function in nondemented postmenopausal women, we have been examining memory and other cognitive abilities in female participants in the BLSA. In our initial study,[4] we identified 116 women who were currently receiving ERT/HRT at the time of an assessment with the BVRT and compared their performance with a group of 172 women who had never received hormone therapy. Hormone use was primarily oral conjugated equine estrogens, and duration of use ranged from less than 6 months to more than 20 years. The groups were well matched on education (average of 15.2 years), but ERT/HRT users were younger (61.8 ± 9.1 years for current compared with 67.7 ± 11.1 years for never

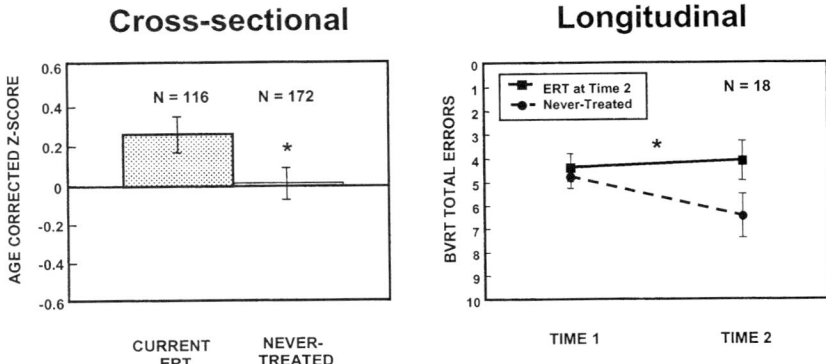

FIGURE 1. Cross-sectional *(left)* and longitudinal *(right)* studies of estrogen replacement therapy (ERT) on the Benton Visual Retention Test (BVRT) performance. Women receiving ERT at the time of testing perform significantly better (higher z-scores) than never-treated women (*$P < 0.05$, one-tailed). Initiation of ERT treatment between two assessments appears to protect against longitudinal age changes in memory over a six-year interval (group by time interaction, *$P < 0.05$). Note that higher numbers of errors are at the bottom of the y-axis.

users), consistent with prescribing practices during this time period. Therefore, BVRT scores were adjusted for age by calculating z-scores, using the mean and standard deviations for all female BLSA participants in each age decade for standardization.

Cross-sectional comparisons indicated that women currently receiving hormone treatment performed better than never-treated women (FIG. 1, left). Furthermore, from the original sample we were able to identify a subgroup of 18 women who began hormone treatment between two BVRT assessments on average six years apart. These women were matched on age, education, interval between testing, and baseline BVRT score to a group of 18 women who had never used hormone therapy and remained untreated at the second assessment. Analysis of BVRT performance revealed a significant treatment group by time interaction, $P < 0.05$. As shown in FIGURE 1 (right), women who began hormone treatment between the two assessments showed stable performance over the six-year longitudinal interval. In contrast, women who never received hormone treatment showed the expected age-associated decline in figural memory. (Note that higher numbers of errors are at the bottom of the y-axis.) These data provided the first demonstration of a possible protective effect of ERT/HRT on *longitudinal* decline in memory.

Our initial study of figural memory was based on cognitive evaluations performed through 1994. Since 1993, the California Verbal Learning Test (CVLT)[34] has been included in the cognitive battery administered to BLSA participants. The CVLT is a measure of verbal memory, comprised of a 16-item shopping list, and allows separate measures of encoding, free and cued recall following short and long (20-minute) delays, and recognition memory. Age differences on some CVLT measures are substantial, and women, on average, outperform men.[35] In a recently published paper,[36] we compared verbal learning and memory performance in 103 postmeno-

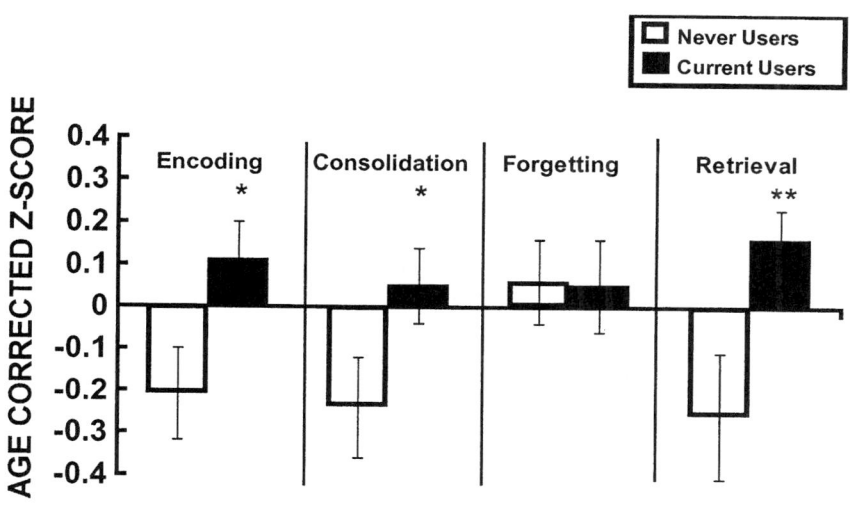

FIGURE 2. Women receiving hormone therapy show significantly better performance than those not receiving such therapy on specific aspects of verbal learning and memory, including encoding, consolidation, and retrieval of a word list on the California Verbal Learning Test (CVLT). ($*P < 0.05$, $**P < 0.01$, 1-tailed.)

pausal women receiving ERT/HRT at the time of the assessment with 81 never-treated women. Using diagnostic information from prospective follow-ups, only women who had remained free of a diagnosis of dementia for five years after the CVLT assessment were included in this sample. The uniformly high educational and health status of BLSA participants resulted in groups of hormone therapy users and never-users who were conveniently matched on education, vocabulary scores, self-rated depressive symptoms and health, and number of medical diagnoses. ERT/HRT users were, however, younger than never-treated women. Thus, age-adjusted z-scores were calculated for each CVLT measure using data from all female BLSA participants for standardization.

Compared with never-users, women who were currently receiving ERT/HRT showed better encoding, retrieval, and recognition of the word list. The ERT/HRT group showed enhanced initial learning and organization of the verbal material, better recall after short and long delays, and better recognition of previously learned words when mixed with unstudied distracters. On the other hand, there were no significant differences between groups under cued recall conditions or in the number of words forgotten between the short and long delay. These findings are summarized in FIGURE 2. Moreover, differences on other cognitive measures, including the BVRT, Digit Span tests of attention and memory, and the Card Rotations Test of spatial rotational ability, did not reach significance. Although these findings appear discrepant with our prior observations of enhanced BVRT performance in current users of hormone therapy,[4] differences in inclusion criteria and sample size are the likely source of the variance in findings. Reanalysis of the data from the CVLT sample, including individuals who are not demented at assessment but develop either dementia or mild cognitive impairment during the follow-up period, yields an effect size similar to that reported in our initial BVRT paper.

ERT/HRT AND REGIONAL CEREBRAL BLOOD FLOW

Since 1994, we have been conducting annual neuroimaging studies for a subgroup of BLSA participants, aged 55 and older and free of dementia at baseline assessment.[37] Magnetic resonance imaging (MRI) and positron emission tomography (PET) are performed to measure regional brain structure and function, respectively. PET studies use 15-oxygen–labeled water; and regional cerebral blood flow (rCBF) is measured under three conditions in a counter-balanced order, resting baseline and during performance of delayed verbal and figural recognition memory tasks.

Cross-sectional Effects of ERT/HRT

Imaging and concurrent neuropsychological test scores were compared for 15 women receiving ERT/HRT at baseline imaging assessment and 17 nonusers, matched on age, education, and vocabulary test scores.[38] On the neuropsychological tests, ERT/HRT users achieved significantly higher scores on the CVLT verbal mem-

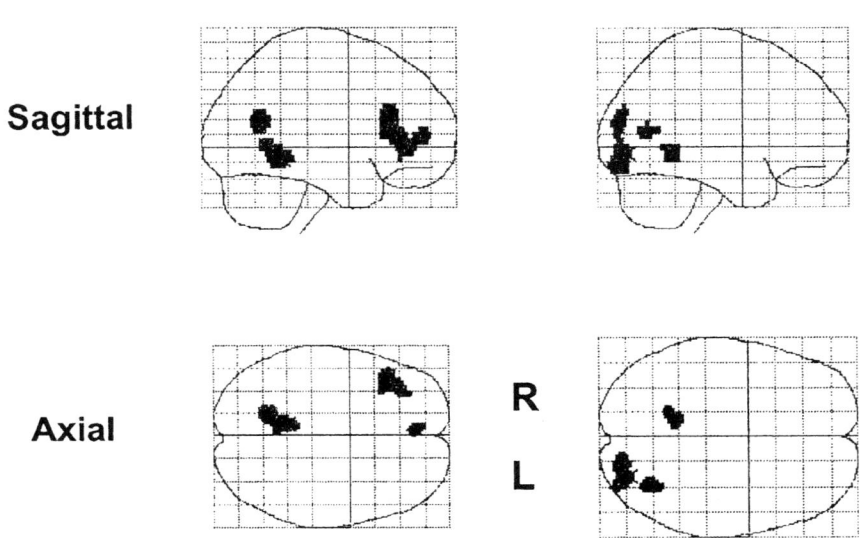

FIGURE 3. Brain regions showing differences in regional cerebral blood flow activation patterns for women receiving hormone therapy compared with nonusers. Sagittal *(top row)* and horizontal *(bottom row)* views are shown for the verbal and figural delayed memory tasks. Images depict group differences in task-related activation of the right frontal and parahippocampal regions during verbal memory *(left column)* and right parahippocampal and left visual association regions during figural memory *(right column)*.

ory and the BVRT figural memory tests, but did not differ significantly on other measures. There were no differences between groups in MRI measures of total brain, gray, white, or ventricular volumes. In contrast, PET scans revealed significant differences between women receiving hormone therapy and untreated women in the pattern of brain activation in response to both the verbal and figural memory tasks. As shown in FIGURE 3, brain regions showing different patterns of activation included the right inferior frontal region and the right parahippocampal gyrus for the verbal task and the right parahippocampal region and the right inferior parietal region for the figural task. Interestingly, right frontal and parahippocampal regions are known to be important in memory processing, and activation of these regions occurs during memory challenge.[39,40] Group differences as a function of hormone status in PET rCBF activation patterns occurred despite the absence of consistent behavioral differences on the PET memory tasks, suggesting that the physiological measures may be more sensitive indicators of hormonal influences.

Longitudinal Effects of ERT/HRT

From the group of participants in the cross-sectional analysis described in the previous section, we identified 12 women in the ERT/HRT group who continued treatment and 15 nonusers who remained untreated at the two-year follow-up evaluation.[41] The groups remained comparable with respect to age, education, and vocabulary performance. Across verbal and figural memory tests and both evaluations (baseline, two-year follow-up) combined, women receiving ERT/HRT had significantly better memory performance than untreated women. While there was no difference between groups in longitudinal change in memory performance, power to detect such an effect is extremely limited because little change is evident over this relatively brief interval. On the other hand, ERT/HRT and untreated women differed significantly in the pattern of longitudinal change in rCBF over time. Based on the results for all three scans (rest, verbal memory, figural memory) combined, ERT/HRT users showed relative increases in rCBF over time for the right hippocampus, right mesial temporal regions (entorhinal and posterior parahippocampal regions), bilateral middle temporal gyrus, right inferior frontal and insular regions, and the left medial frontal gyrus. These results provide the first demonstration that hormone therapy modulates changes in brain activity over a two-year interval. Importantly, the regions sensitive to the effects of hormone treatment were not random. ERT/HRT users showed relative increases in rCBF in brain regions that are important in the neural circuitry underlying memory processing and that show preclinical hypoperfusion in individuals at increased risk for Alzheimer's disease.[42–44]

SUMMARY AND CONCLUSIONS

In a series of investigations in the BLSA, we have shown that ERT/HRT reduces the risk for Alzheimer's disease[19] and offers some protection against cognitive aging in nondemented postmenopausal women. Our behavioral findings in nondemented women indicate that ERT/HRT offers a selective benefit to specific memory processes. ERT/HRT protects against age-associated decline in figural memory[4] and is associated with better encoding, retrieval, and recognition of verbal material.[36] Our results are consistent with other cross-sectional observational studies indicating an association between hormone therapy and enhanced memory on tests of verbal recall[5,45,46] and recall of proper names from visual face cues.[47] In the only other prospective study of longitudinal memory change, past use of hormone therapy was associated with less longitudinal decline in verbal memory over 2.5 years.[5]

In contrast to these findings, two large-scale observational studies reported no cross-sectional differences between ERT/HRT users and nonusers.[48,49] It is notable, however, that both investigations employed verbal memory tasks that require subjects to maximize how well they learn a list of words before their memory for those words is tested. We demonstrated that women who receive hormone therapy show better initial learning of word lists.[36] Procedures that eliminate this advantage may mask a beneficial effect of estrogen on verbal memory, because better initial learning contributes to better recall. In a third large-scale observational study,[50] women in the Nurses Health Study who reported use of hormone therapy obtained higher scores than never-treated women on a test of semantic memory (category fluency), but the groups obtained similar scores on tests of paragraph and word list recall. Note, however, that cognitive assessments in this study were performed by telephone, and hormone status was ascertained through biennial reports rather than concurrently with cognitive testing. The use of standardized memory tests and procedures that allow for assessments of different aspects of memory performance are important methodological considerations in studies of HRT and cognitive abilities.

The beneficial role of hormone therapy on memory is also supported by the results of neuroimaging studies. Our cross-sectional[38] and longitudinal[41] PET studies indicate that hormone therapy modulates the pattern of rCBF activation in brain regions that play critical roles in memory processing and that show hypoperfusion in individuals at increased risk for Alzheimer's disease[42–44] and in individuals in the early stages of the disease.[51] Consistent with these results, Shaywitz and colleagues reported ERT effects on fMRI activation patterns during performance of verbal and visual working memory tasks.[52] In a randomized, double-blind, placebo-controlled crossover trial of 46 postmenopausal women, estrogen treatment influenced frontal and inferior parietal lobe activation during storage of information and right frontal activation during retrieval. In a recent study,[53] relative values of frontal and temporal-parietal glucose metabolism in two groups of nondemented women (ERT/HRT and untreated) were compared with metabolic patterns in women with Alzheimer's disease. Women receiving hormone therapy had significantly higher relative metabolism in dorsolateral frontal and temporal-parietal regions compared to the patients with Alzheimer's disease, but untreated women did not differ significantly from patients. Although untreated women had metabolic values intermediate to the women receiving ERT and patients with Alzheimer's disease, the two groups of nondemented women did not appear to differ significantly in this small sample.

FUTURE DIRECTIONS

In summary, the cumulative results of small randomized trials and larger observational studies provide encouraging support for a beneficial effect of hormone therapy on memory and possibly other cognitive functions. However, additional research involving randomized clinical trials including larger numbers of subjects, a sensitive cognitive test battery, and prospective longitudinal follow-up assessments is required to provide more definitive information on the role of hormone therapy in the prevention of Alzheimer's disease and age-related cognitive decline. Several such studies are underway. The Women's Health Initiative Memory Study (WHIMS),[54] an ancillary study to the Women's Health Initiative randomized clinical trial, is following 8000 women to assess the effect of active hormone treatment versus placebo on the risk and progression of Alzheimer's disease. Active treatment consists of conjugated equine estrogen in women without a uterus or conjugated equine estrogen plus medroxyprogesterone acetate, administered continuously, for women with a uterus. Through an ancillary study to WHIMS, the Women's Health Initiative Study of Cognitive Aging (WHISCA) is following more than 2000 women annually. WHISCA was initiated by our group in 1999 and has been developed and performed in collaboration with the WHIMS investigators (Sally Shumaker, principal investigator). It is designed to assess the effects of hormone therapy on cognitive aging, particularly memory, in nondemented postmenopausal women. Other ongoing trials investigating hormone therapy, memory loss, and Alzheimer's disease include PREPARE (Preventing Memory Loss and Alzheimer's Disease) in the United States and WISDOM (Women's International Study of long-Duration Oestrogen after Menopause) in the United Kingdom.

These ongoing trials will not address additional important questions concerning hormone therapy and cognition. There is little information on the optimal timing, type, dose, and duration of hormone treatment necessary for beneficial effects on the CNS in humans. Observational studies indicating that "ever use" of estrogen protects against Alzheimer's disease suggest the possibility of a critical period for neuroprotection, since most use of hormone therapy in the past involved relatively short–duration treatment during menopause. Effects of estradiol versus conjugated equine estrogens, cyclic versus continuous administration regimens, and various adjuvant progestins on cognition are also unknown and may profoundly impact decisions about which hormone therapies are most effective clinically.[55] Finally, despite their widespread use, there is extremely limited information on the effects of SERMs on cognition and brain aging. There have been no studies of the effects of tamoxifen alone on cognition. Results of one relatively small trial of raloxifene found no effect on cognition,[56] and the recently published results of the Multiple Outcomes of Raloxifene Evaluation (MORE) trial indicated no significant effects of raloxifene on cognition in women with osteoporosis. However, in the latter study, raloxifene showed some beneficial effect on verbal memory in women age 70 and older, and the test battery may have lacked sensitivity in younger women.[57] Future studies of the effects of SERMs should include outcomes from functional neuroimaging assessments where possible, as preliminary information indicates that these measures may provide greater sensitivity to the effects of hormones.

Ongoing investigations in our laboratory are extending the imaging and neuropsychological studies to investigate the effects of ERT, various progestins, and SERMs on cognitive and brain function. As described above, WHISCA will provide information on the role of ERT and HRT in protecting against age-associated cognitive change. A parallel ancillary study to the STAR (Study of Tamoxifen and Raloxifene) trial has recently been initiated and will provide information on the effects of these SERMs on age-related changes in memory and other cognitive functions.

REFERENCES

1. YAFFE, K., G. SAWAYA, I. LIEBERBURG, et al. 1998. Estrogen therapy in postmenopausal women: effects on cognitive function and dementia. JAMA **279:** 688–695.
2. HENDERSON, V.W. 2000. Oestrogens and dementia. *In* Neuronal and Cognitive Effects of Oestrogens, Vol. 230. D.J. Chadwick & J.A. Goode, Eds: 254–265. John Wiley & Sons, Ltd., Novartis Foundation. London.
3. SHERWIN, B.B. 1997. Estrogen effects on cognition in menopausal women. Neurology **48:** S21–S26.
4. RESNICK, S.M., E.J. METTER & A.B. ZONDERMAN. 1997. Estrogen replacement therapy and longitudinal decline in visual memory: a possible protective effect? Neurology **49:** 1491–1497.
5. JACOBS, D.M., M.X. TANG, Y. STERN, et al. 1998. Cognitive function in nondemented older women who took estrogen after menopause. Neurology **50:** 368–373.
6. SIMPKINS, J.W., P.S. GREEN, B.S. GRIDLEY, et al. 1997. Role of estrogen replacement therapy in memory enhancement and the prevention of neuronal loss associated with Alzheimer's disease. Am. J. Med. **103:** 19S–25S.
7. MCEWEN, B.S., S.E. ALVES, K. BULLOCH, et al. 1997. Ovarian steroids and the brain: implications for cognition and aging. Neurology **48:** S8–S15.
8. GOULD, E., C.S. WOOLLEY, M. FRANKFURT, et al. 1990. Gonadal steroids regulate dendritic spine density in hippocampal pyramidal cells in adulthood. J. Neurosci. **10:** 1286–1291.
9. WOOLLEY, C.S., E. GOULD, M. FRANKFURT, et al. 1990. Naturally occurring fluctuation in dendritic spine density on adult hippocampal pyramidal neurons. J. Neurosci. **10:** 4035–4039.
10. LUINE, V.N. 1985. Estradiol increases choline acetyltransferase activity in specific basal forebrain nuclei and projection areas of female rats. Exp. Neurol. **89:** 484–490.
11. BECKER, J.B. 2000. Oestrogen effects on dopaminergic function in striatum. *In* Neuronal and Cognitive Effects of Oestrogens, Vol. 230. D.J. Chadwick & J.A. Goode, Eds: 134–145. John Wiley & Sons, Ltd., Novartis Foundation. London.
12. BETHEA, C.L., C. GUNDLAH & S.J. MIRKES. 2000. Ovarian steroid action in the serotonin neural system of macaques. *In* Neuronal and Cognitive Effects of Oestrogens, Vol. 230. D.J. Chadwick & J.A. Goode, Eds: 112–130. John Wiley & Sons, Ltd., Novartis Foundation. London.
13. HERBISON, A.E., S.X. SIMONIAN, N.R. THANKY, et al. 2000. Oestrogen modulation of noradrenaline neurotransmission. *In* Neuronal and Cognitive Effects of Oestrogens, Vol. 230. D. J. Chadwick & J.A. Goode, Eds: 74–85. John Wiley & Sons, Ltd., Novartis Foundation. London.
14. GANDY, S. 1999. Neurohormonal signaling pathways and the regulation of Alzheimer beta-amyloid precursor metabolism. Trends Endocrinol. Metab. **10:** 273–279.
15. PETANCESKA, S.S., V. NAGY, D. FRAIL, et al. 2000. Ovariectomy and 17beta-estradiol modulate the levels of Alzheimer's amyloid beta peptides in brain. Exp. Gerontol. **35:** 1317–1325.
16. NEHLIG, A., L.J. PORRINO, A.M. CRANE, et al. 1985. Local cerebral glucose utilization in normal female rats: variations during the estrous cycle and comparison with males. J. Cereb. Blood Flow Metab. **5:** 393–400.
17. NAMBA, H. & L. SOKOLOFF. 1984. Acute administration of high doses of estrogen increases glucose utilization throughout brain. Brain Res. **291:** 391–394.
18. BISHOP, J. & J.W. SIMPKINS. 1995. Estradiol enhances brain glucose uptake in ovariectomized rats. Brain Res. Bull. **36:** 315–320.
19. KAWAS, C., S. RESNICK, A. MORRISON, et al. 1997. A prospective study of estrogen replacement therapy and the risk of developing Alzheimer's disease: the Baltimore Longitudinal Study of Aging. Neurology **48:** 1517–1521.
20. TANG, M.X., D. JACOBS, Y. STERN, et al. 1996. Effect of oestrogen during menopause on risk and age at onset of Alzheimer's disease. Lancet **348:** 429–432.
21. HENDERSON, V.W., A. PAGANINI-HILL, B.L. MILLER, et al. 2000. Estrogen for Alzheimer's disease in women: randomized, double-blind, placebo-controlled trial. Neurology **54:** 295–301.

22. MULNARD, R.A., C.W. COTMAN, C. KAWAS, et al. 2000. Estrogen replacement therapy for treatment of mild to moderate Alzheimer disease: a randomized controlled trial. JAMA **283:** 1007–1015.
23. WANG, P.N., S.Q. LIAO, R.S. LIU, et al. 2000. Effects of estrogen on cognition, mood, and cerebral blood flow in AD: a controlled study. Neurology **54:** 2061–2066.
24. SHERWIN, B.B. 1988. Estrogen and/or androgen replacement therapy and cognitive functioning in surgically menopausal women. Psychoneuroendocrinology **13:** 345–357.
25. WOLF, O., B. KUDIELKA, D. HELLHAMMER, et al. 1999. Two weeks of transdermal treatment in postmenopausal elderly women and its effect on memory and mood: verbal memory changes are associated with the treatment induced estradiol levels. Psychoneuroendocrinology **24:** 727–741.
26. DUKA, T., R. TASKER & J.F. MCGOWAN. 2000. The effects of 3-week estrogen hormone replacement on cognition in elderly healthy females. Psychopharmacology (Berl.) **149:** 129–139.
27. POLO-KANTOLA, P., R. PORTIN, O. POLO, et al. 1998. The effect of short-term estrogen replacement therapy on cognition: a randomized double-blind, cross-over trial in postmenopausal women. Obstet. Gynecol. **91:** 459–466.
28. SHOCK, N.W., R.C. GREULICH, R. ANDRES, et al. 1984. Normal human aging: the Baltimore Longitudinal Study of Aging. *In* U.S. Public Health Service Publication No. 84-2450. U.S. Government Printing Office. Washington, D.C.
29. BENTON, A.L. 1963. The Revised Visual Retention Test: clinical and experimental applications (3rd edit.). Psychological Corporation. New York.
30. GIAMBRA, L.M., D. ARENBERG, A. B. ZONDERMAN, et al. 1995. Adult life span changes in immediate visual memory and verbal intelligence. Psychol. Aging **10:** 123–139.
31. RESNICK, S.M., K.M. TROTMAN, C. KAWAS, et al. 1995. Age-associated changes in specific errors on the Benton Visual Retention Test. J. Gerontol. Psychol. Sci. **50B:** P171–P178.
32. BENTON, A.L., P.J. ESLINGER & A.R. DAMASIO. 1981. Normative observations on neuropsychological test performances in old age. J. Clin. Neuropsychol. **3:** 33–42.
33. SCHICHITA, K., S. HATANO, Y. OHASHI, et al. 1986. Memory changes in the Benton Visual Retention Test between ages 70 and 75. J. Gerontol. **41:** 385–386.
34. DELIS, D.C., J.H. KRAMER, E. KAPLAN, et al. 1987. California Verbal Learning Test—Research Edition. The Psychological Corporation. New York.
35. NORMAN, M.A., J.D. EVANS, W.S. MILLER, et al. 2000. Demographically corrected norms for the California Verbal Learning Test. J. Clin. Exp. Neuropsychol. **22:** 80–94.
36. MAKI, P.M., A.B. ZONDERMAN & S.M. RESNICK. 2001. Enhanced verbal memory in nondemented elderly women receiving hormone-replacement therapy. Am. J. Psychiatry **158:** 227–233.
37. RESNICK, S.M., A.F. GOLDSZAL, C. DAVATZIKOS, et al. 2000. One-year age changes in MRI brain volumes in older adults. Cereb. Cortex **10:** 464–472.
38. RESNICK, S.M., P.M. MAKI, S. GOLSKI, et al. 1998. Estrogen effects on PET cerebral blood flow and neuropsychological performance. Horm. Behav. **34:** 171–184.
39. TULVING, E., S. KAPUR, F.I. CRAIK, et al. 1994. Hemispheric encoding/retrieval asymmetry in episodic memory: positron emission tomography findings. Proc. Natl. Acad. Sci. USA **91:** 2016–2020.
40. GRASBY, P.M., C.D. FRITH, K.J. FRISTON, et al. 1993. Functional mapping of brain areas implicated in auditory-verbal memory function. Brain **116:** 1–20.
41. MAKI, P.M. & S.M. RESNICK. 2000. Longitudinal effects of estrogen replacement therapy on PET cerebral blood flow and cognition. Neurobiol. Aging **21:** 373–383.
42. SMALL, G.W., J.C. MAZZIOTTA, M.T. COLLINS, et al. 1995. Apolipoprotein E type 4 allele and cerebral glucose metabolism in relatives at risk for familial Alzheimer disease. JAMA **273:** 942–947.
43. REIMAN, E.M., R.J. CASELLI, L.S. YUN, et al. 1996. Preclinical evidence of Alzheimer's disease in persons homozygous for the epsilon 4 allele for apolipoprotein E [see comments]. N. Engl. J. Med. **334:** 752–758.
44. FOX, N.C., E.K. WARRINGTON, A.L. SEIFFER, et al. 1998. Presymptomatic cognitive deficits in individuals at risk of familial Alzheimer's disease. A longitudinal prospective study. Brain **121:** 1631–1639.

45. KAMPEN, D.L. & B.B. SHERWIN. 1994. Estrogen use and verbal memory in healthy postmenopausal women. Obstet. Gynecol. **83:** 979–983.
46. VERGHESE, J., G. KUSLANSKY, M.J. KATZ, *et al.* 2000. Cognitive performance in surgically menopausal women on estrogen. Neurology **55:** 872–874.
47. ROBINSON, D., L. FRIEDMAN, R. MARCUS, *et al.* 1994. Estrogen replacement therapy and memory in older women. J. Am. Geriatr. Soc. **42:** 919–922.
48. BARRETT-CONNOR, E. & D. KRITZ-SILVERSTEIN. 1993. Estrogen replacement therapy and cognitive function in older women. JAMA **269:** 2637–2641.
49. SZKLO, M., J. CERHAN, A.V. DIEZ-ROUX, *et al.* 1996. Estrogen replacement therapy and cognitive functioning in the Atherosclerosis Risk in Communities (ARIC) study. Am. J. Epidemiol. **144:** 1048–1057.
50. GRODSTEIN, F., J. CHEN, D. POLLEN, *et al.* 2000. Postmenopausal hormone therapy and cognitive function in healthy older women. J. Am. Geriatr. Soc. **48:** 746–752.
51. JAGUST, W.J., J.L. EBERLING, B.C. RICHARDSON, *et al.* 1993. The cortical topography of temporal lobe hypometabolism in early Alzheimer's disease. Brain Res. **629:** 189–198.
52. SHAYWITZ, S.E., B.A. SHAYWITZ, K.R. PUGH, *et al.* 1999. Effect of estrogen on brain activation patterns in postmenopausal women during working memory tasks. JAMA **281:** 1197–1202.
53. EBERLING, J.L., B.R. REED, J.E. COLEMAN, *et al.* 2000. Effect of estrogen on cerebral glucose metabolism in postmenopausal women. Neurology **55:** 875–877.
54. SHUMAKER, S.A., B.A. REBOUSSIN, M.A. ESPELAND, *et al.* 1998. The Women's Health Initiative Memory Study (WHIMS): a trial of the effect of estrogen therapy in preventing and slowing the progression of dementia. Controlled Clin. Trials **19:** 604–621.
55. TORAN-ALLERAND, C.D. 2000. Estrogen as a treatment for Alzheimer disease. JAMA **284:** 307–308.
56. NICKELSEN, T., E.G. LUFKIN, B.L. RIGGS, *et al.* 1999. Raloxifene hydrochloride, a selective estrogen receptor modulator: safety assessment of effects on cognitive function and mood in postmenopausal women. Psychoneuroendocrinology **24:** 115–128.
57. YAFFE, K., K. KRUEGER, S. SARKAR, *et al.* 2001. Cognitive function in postmenopausal women treated with raloxifene. N. Eng. J. Med. **344:** 1207–1213.

Estrogens, Selective Estrogen Receptor Modulators, and Dementia: What Is the Evidence?

KRISTINE YAFFE

Departments of Psychiatry, Neurology and Epidemiology, University of California, San Francisco and the San Francisco VA Medical Center, San Francisco, California 94121, USA

ABSTRACT: At least 10% of people aged 65 or older have some form of cognitive impairment, increasing to around 50% by age 85. Several studies have suggested that estrogen may improve cognitive function or prevent the development of dementia, but other studies have not shown a benefit, and results from large randomized trials are lacking. Fortunately, further trials are currently being conducted. With the recognition that selective estrogen receptor modulators (SERMs) have differential tissue-dependent effects on estrogen receptor function, there is recent interest in the effects of raloxifene, tamoxifen, and other SERMs on cognition. In this paper, the current state of knowledge of the role of estrogen for preventing dementia in postmenopausal women will be reviewed. In addition, the status of ongoing and recently completed trials of estrogen and SERMs on cognitive function or on Alzheimer's disease severity will be summarized.

KEYWORDS: estrogens; selective estrogen receptor modulators; raloxifene; dementia

INTRODUCTION

At least 10% of persons over 65 years old and 50% of those over 85 have some form of cognitive impairment ranging from mild deficits to dementia.[1] Alzheimer's disease (AD), the most common cause of dementia, is estimated to currently affect 4 million people in the United States and to cost 70 billion dollars annually,[2] but is projected to affect 14 million by the year 2040. The importance of AD is highlighted by the "graying" of the U.S. population due both to increased life expectancy and demographic shifts in the population, with a consequent increasing incidence and prevalence of AD. AD affects women disproportionately to men with women having a slightly higher increased risk of AD, even after adjusting for age.[3] Despite the severity and prevalence of dementia and mild cognitive impairment, there are few effective treatments or prevention strategies. Recent studies have suggested that postmenopausal estrogen therapy might improve cognition in nondemented post-

Address for correspondence: Kristine Yaffe, M.D., University of California, San Francisco, Box 111G, 4150 Clement Street, San Francisco, California 94121. Voice: 415-750-6625; fax: 415-750-6641.

kyaffe@itsa.ucsf.edu

menopausal women, prevent the development of dementia, or improve the severity of dementia.

POSSIBLE BIOLOGICAL MECHANISMS OF ESTROGEN'S EFFECT ON COGNITION AND DEMENTIA

Estrogen receptors are found in the hypothalamus, the preoptic area, the anterior pituitary, the CA1 region of the hippocampus, and several other brain regions.[4] How estrogens may affect neuropsychologic function remains unknown, but several mechanisms have been suggested. One mechanism is the modulation of neurotransmitters, particularly acetylcholine. Estradiol administration to oophorectimized rats is associated with an increase in choline acetyltransferase and potassium-stimulated acetylcholine release in certain brain regions and an increase in the survival of cholinergic neurons.[5-7] Estrogen-treated rats have superior performance on behavioral memory tasks compared to estrogen-deprived animals, and performance is associated with increased choline uptake and higher levels of choline acetyltransferase in the hippocampus and frontal cortex.[8] Estradiol has also been found to affect other neurotransmitters such as serotonergic and dopaminergic activity.[9,10] These neurotransmitter alterations induced by estradiol have significant implications for AD prevention and treatment because reductions in acetylcholine, serotonin, dopamine, and norepinephrine are a hallmark feature of patients with AD.[11,12]

Another possible mechanism of estrogen's role in cognition is by promoting neuronal growth and synaptic reorganization. Estrogen regulates synaptic plasticity by stimulating axonal sprouting and dendritic spine formation in the adult rat hypothalamus and CA1 hippocampal pyramidal neurons.[4,13] Early neuron loss in the CA1 region of the hippocampus, a region associated with memory and learning, is found in patients with AD and age-related cognitive dysfunction. In addition to promoting neuronal circuitry, estrogen may prevent cerebral ischemia. Estrogens may protect against cerebral ischemia by inducing vasodilatation, reducing platelet aggregation, or limiting oxidative stress-related injury induced by excitotoxins and beta amyloid.[14,15] Postmenopausal estrogen therapy reduces serum LDL-cholesterol and increases HDL-cholesterol.[16] These lipoprotein changes may slow progression of cerebral atherosclerosis and prevent dementia and other cognitive decline. Estrogen also modulates the expression of the apolipoprotein E gene in rodent tissues and theoretically could reduce the risk of AD in humans via apolipoprotein E alterations.[17] Thus, estrogens may reduce the risk of AD and other forms of cognitive decline through a variety of mechanisms.

ESTROGEN THERAPY AND RISK OF DEMENTIA

The possible beneficial effects of estrogen on cognition in nondemented postmenopausal women, along with the observation that women may be at increased risk for AD, led to the hypothesis that estrogen deficiency associated with menopause may contribute to the development of dementia. There have been nine case-control studies, one cross-sectional population-based study, and two prospective cohort studies conducted to evaluate the association between AD and other dementias and postmenopausal estrogen therapy. The results of these studies are variable; some suggest a protective effect of estrogen on development of AD while others suggest an increased risk. Two of the case-control studies,[18,19] the cross-sectional study,[20] and the two prospective studies[21,22] found a statistically lower risk of developing dementia in postmenopausal women who had taken estrogen compared to those who had not. Of the seven other case-control studies, two showed a nonsignificant increased risk of dementia among estrogen users compared to nonusers,[23,24] two showed no difference in the risk of dementia,[25,26] and three found a nonsignificant decreased risk of dementia among estrogen users compared to nonusers.[27,28] Both prospective cohort studies found a decreased risk of AD in estrogen users. In one of the prospective studies, estrogen use was recorded among 1,124 elderly community-dwelling women who were evaluated for dementia 1–5 years later. Women who had ever used estrogen had a 50% reduction in risk of developing AD.[21] The other prospective study found a similar reduction in risk of developing AD among 472 postmenopausal women enrolled in the Baltimore Longitudinal Study of Aging who were followed for up to 16 years.[22] A metanalysis of most of these observational studies of estrogen and dementia was recently published.[29] The summary odds ratio for all types of dementia was 0.71 (95% CI 0.53–0.96, P for heterogeneity = 0.10), and for AD only the summary odds ratio was 0.71 (95% CI 0.52–0.98, P for heterogeneity = 0.11). This 29% decreased risk of developing dementia among estrogen users may be of major public health importance; however, the observational studies that were summarized are susceptible to confounding and compliance bias. For example, women who choose to take estrogen have been reported to have higher educations and to be healthier than nonusers,[30] differences that may contribute to a lower risk of developing AD.[31] Nonetheless, the results from the metanalysis support the hypothesis that postmenopausal estrogen use protects against the development of AD.

ESTROGEN AS A TREATMENT OF ALZHEIMER'S DISEASE SYMPTOMS

Epidemiologic evidence suggesting that estrogen use may prevent development of AD and improve cognitive function has sparked interest in estrogen as a treatment for AD. There have been eight trials of estrogen therapy in women with AD. In two uncontrolled trials that included 7 and 15 participants, severity of dementia was measured at baseline and after six weeks of estrogen therapy.[32,33] Each of these studies found improvement on some, but not all, measures of dementia severity after treatment. Because there was no control group for comparison, this improvement may represent a practice or learning effect. In addition, these two trials were not blinded, which may have biased the outcome. In another trial, 15 women with AD were treated with estrogen, and change in dementia severity was compared with 15 untreated controls matched for age and dementia severity at baseline.[34] While the control group did not improve, the treatment group improved on one cognitive scale and on one dementia rating scale compared to scores prior to treatment, but changes in the severity of dementia in the estrogen-treated group were not compared to changes in the untreated group. In the five placebo-controlled trials, results have been conflicting but predominantly negative. Honjo *et al.* randomly assigned 14 women with AD to conjugated estrogen or placebo and found greater improvement on one dementia scale but not on two other scales in the estrogen-treated group compared to the placebo-treated group.[35] In an eight-week randomized controlled trial of estradiol patch compared to placebo administered to 12 women with AD, improvements were observed for the estradiol group on tests of attention and verbal memory but not on the other seven cognitive tasks.[36] However, three larger (including 42 to 120 participants) controlled trials ranging from 3 to 12 months have recently been conducted. None of these trials found a statistically significant benefit of conjugated estrogen for any of the cognitive or functional assessments.[37–39] As this point, most clinicians and researchers are not optimistic that estrogen has an important role for treatment of Alzheimer's disease. Ongoing studies that are investigating whether different preparations of estrogens may be effective and whether estrogens may preferentially improve certain cognitive domains, such as verbal memory, will help clarify whether estrogens may be used in selected patients for treatment of Alzheimer's disease or for other types of dementia.

ESTROGEN AND APOLIPOPROTEIN E

The apolipoprotein E (ApoE) isoform e4 has recently been identified as a major biological risk factor for AD and preclinical cogntive decline.[40,41] Several lines of basic science evidence support the hypothesis that estrogen and ApoE may act synergistically. Estrogen modulates the expression of the ApoE gene in rodent tissues,[17] and the estradiol enhancement of synaptic sprouting in response to injury in rats may operate through an ApoE-dependent mechanism.[42] Another series of experiments using ApoE knockout mice has shown that transgenic e4 mice have marked behavioral and cognitive deficits and that these abnormalities are more pronounced in female rats.[43] In humans, women who are heterozygous for ApoE e4 have a greater risk of developing AD than do heterozygous men, especially those with the 2-4 genotype.[44,45] The effect of cholinesterase treatment for AD has been reported to vary for women according to their ApoE e4 status but not in men.[46] Compared to subjects without an e4 allele, women with an e4 allele had less of a treatment effect. The mechanism for this gender-specific ApoE genotype interaction is not clear but could be related to estrogen.

A recent study investigated whether estrogen use modifies the association between ApoE e4 and cognitive decline.[47] In that study, 3,393 older women, who were enrolled in the Cardiovascular Health Study, had cognitive testing annually with the Modified Mini-Mental State Exam (3MS). Over the six-year follow-up, women who were current estrogen users declined 1.5 points on 3MS, whereas women who never used estrogen declined 2.7 points ($P = 0.023$). Among e4-negative women, current estrogen use reduced the risk of developing cognitive impairment compared to never users by almost half, while it did not among e4-positive women (P for interaction = 0.037). Compared to never use, current estrogen use in e4-negative women was also associated with less internal and common carotid wall thickening, but not in e4-positive women (P for interaction < 0.05 for both). Thus, estrogen use was associated with less cognitive decline among e4-negative women, but not among e4-positive women. Potential mechanisms, including carotid atherosclerosis, by which e4 may interact with estrogen and cognition warrant further investigation.

SELECTIVE ESTROGEN RECEPTOR MODULATORS

Recently, several selective estrogen receptor modulators (SERMs) have been developed that have estrogen agonist and antagonist action in estrogen-responsive tissues. The two most widely recognized SERMS are tamoxifen and raloxifene. Both have estrogen-agonist properties on bone and lipids and estrogen-antagonist effects on breast, whereas raloxifene, unlike tamoxifen, has estrogen-antagonist effects on the uterus.[48] The identification of estrogen receptors in multiple brain regions, along with recognition that SERMs have differential tissue-dependent effects on estrogen receptor function, has prompted interest in the effects of raloxifene and other SERMs on cognition. Raloxifene has neurotrophic effects *in vitro*, stimulating neurite outgrown from cultured cells,[49] and increases the activity of choline acetyltransferase in some brain regions.[50] On the other hand, raloxifene and tamoxifen increase the incidence of hot flushes in some women, and hot flushes have been postulated to adversely affect cognitive performance.[51] The effects of raloxifene and other SERMs on central nervous system functions such as cognition and mood have not been well studied. No trials of tamoxifen for improvement of cognitive function or dementia prevention have been conducted. One small trial concluded that raloxifene had no consistent effect on cognitive function compared to placebo over 12 months in 143 postmenopausal women.[52] Recently, a large trial of raloxifene in osteoporotic postmenopausal women was completed. In this trial (the Multiple Outcomes of Raloxifene Evaluation trial), 7,478 women received either raloxifene (60 mg or 120 mg) or placebo for three years, and scores on six cognitive tests were evaluated. Mean cognitive scores improved slightly over the three years and were similar in the treatment groups at each visit. Compared to the placebo group, women assigned to raloxifene had a slightly lower risk of developing cognitive decline on an attention test and on a verbal memory test, but not on the other four tests.[53] Among women at greater risk for cognitive decline (aged >70 years), those assigned to raloxifene performed better compared to placebo on attention and verbal memory but not on the other tests. Reported hot flushes did not influence cognitive test scores or the effect of treatment on test performance ($P \geq 0.3$). Thus, raloxifene treatment for three years did not affect overall cognitive scores in postmenopausal women; however, it may lower the risk of decline in attention and memory domains. Further studies of raloxifene and other SERMs and cognitive outcomes are needed.

CONCLUSIONS AND FUTURE DIRECTIONS

There are plausible biological mechanisms that might account for a beneficial effect of estrogen therapy on cognition and dementia. Large, controlled, blinded trials are necessary to determine if estrogen therapy can reduce the risk of developing AD. The Women's Health Initiative Randomized Trial, which is currently under way, includes the Women's Health Initiative Memory Study (WHIMS). This ancillary trial will determine the effect of hormone replacement therapy on cognitive function and risk for developing AD and other dementias among approximately 8,000 postmenopausal women treated for 10 years. Another NIH-funded trial, Preventing Postmenopausal Memory Loss and AD with Replacement Estrogen (PREPARE) is enrolling approximately 1,000 older women with a family history of AD. This primary prevention trial will determine whether women who are randomized to receive estrogen for three years have less risk of developing AD than those receiving placebo. The trial will be completed in 2004. Based on the conflicting evidence and the potential side effects of estrogen therapy (endometrial abnormalities,[54] gallbladder disease,[55] venous thromboembolic events,[56] and breast cancer[57,58]), it is premature to recommend that estrogen be used as a prevention strategy for AD. Furthermore, most of the evidence does not support estrogen as a treatment for symptoms of AD; additional studies, however, are under way. Finally, the role of SERMs on cognitive function in older women and for dementia prevention also requires additional study.

REFERENCES

1. EVANS, D.A. 1990. Estimated prevalence of Alzheimer's disease in the United States. Milbank Q. **68:** 267–289.
2. ERNST, R.L. & J.W. HAY. 1994. The US economic and social costs of Alzheimer's disease revisited. Am. J. Public Health **84:** 1261–1264.
3. PAYAMI, H., K. MONTEE, *et al.* 1996. Increased risk of familial late–onset Alzheimer's disease in women. Neurology **46:** 126–129.
4. MCEWEN, B.S. & C.S. WOOLLEY. 1994. Estradiol and progesterone regulate neuronal structure and synaptic connectivity in adult as well as developing brain. Exp. Gerontol. **29:** 431–436.
5. HONJO, H., T. TAMURA, *et al.* 1992. Estrogen as a growth factor to central nervous cells. Estrogen treatment promotes development of acetylcholinesterase-positive basal forebrain neurons transplanted in the anterior eye chamber. J. Steroid Biochem. Mol. Biol. **41:** 633–635.
6. LUINE, V.N. 1985. Estradiol increases choline acetyltransferase activity in specific basal forebrain nuclei and projection areas of female rats. Exp. Neurol. **89:** 484–490.
7. GIBBS, R.B., A. HASHASH, *et al.* 1997. Effects of estrogen on potassium-stimulated acetylcholine release in the hippocampus and overlying cortex of adult rats. Brain Res. **749:** 143–146.
8. SIMPKINS, J.W., M. SINGH, *et al.* 1994. The potential role for estrogen replacement therapy in the treatment of the cognitive decline and neurodegeneration associated with Alzheimer's disease. Neurobiol. Aging **15** (Suppl. 2): S195–S197.
9. LUINE, V.N., R.I. KHYLCHEVSKAYA, *et al.* 1975. Effect of gonadal steroids on activities of monoamine oxidase and choline acetylase in rat brain. Brain Res. **86:** 293–306.
10. SUMMER, B.E. & G. FINK. 1995. Estrogen increases the density of 5-hydroxytryptamine(2A) receptors in cerebral cortex and nucleus accumbens in the female rat. J. Steroid Biochem. Mol. Biol. **54:** 15–20.
11. COYLE, J.T., D.L. PRICE, *et al.* 1983. Alzheimer's disease: a disorder of cortical cholinergic innervation. Science **219:** 1184–1190.
12. PALMER, A.M. & S.T. DEKOSKY. 1993. Monoamine neurons in aging and Alzheimer's disease. J. Neural Transm. Gen. Sect. **91:** 135–159.
13. GOULD, E., C.S. WOOLLEY, *et al.* 1990. Gonadal steroids regulate dendritic spine density in hippocampal pyramidal cells in adulthood. J. Neurosci. **10:** 1286–1291.
14. GOODMAN, Y., A.J. BRUCE, *et al.* 1996. Estrogens attenuate and corticosterone exacerbates excitotoxicity, oxidative injury, and amyloid beta-peptide toxicity in hippocampal neurons. J. Neurochem. **66:** 1836–1844.
15. GANGAR, K.F., S. VYAS, *et al.* 1991. Pulsatility index in internal carotid artery in relation to transdermal oestradiol and time since menopause. Lancet **338:** 839–842.
16. APPLEBAUM-BOWDEN, D., P. MCLEAN, *et al.* 1989. Lipoprotein, apolipoprotein, and lipolytic enzyme changes following estrogen administration in postmenopausal women. J. Lipid Res. **30:** 1895–1906.
17. SRIVASTAVA, R.A., N. SRIVASTAVA, *et al.* 1997. Estrogen up-regulates apolipoprotein E (ApoE) gene expression by increasing ApoE mRNA in the translating pool via the estrogen receptor alpha-mediated pathway. J. Biol. Chem. **272:** 33360–33366.

18. HENDERSON, V.W., H.A. PAGANINI, et al. 1994. Estrogen replacement therapy in older women. Comparisons between Alzheimer's disease cases and nondemented control subjects. Arch. Neurol. **51:** 896–900.
19. WARING, S.C., W.A. ROCCA, et al. 1999. Postmenopausal estrogen replacement therapy and risk of AD: a population-based study. Neurology **52:** 965–970.
20. BALDERESCHI, M., A. DI CARLO, et al. 1998. Estrogen-replacement therapy and Alzheimer's disease in the Italian Longitudinal Study on Aging. Neurology **50:** 996-1002.
21. TANG, M.X., D. JACOBS, et al. 1996. Effect of oestrogen during menopause on risk and age at onset of Alzheimer's disease. Lancet **348:** 429–432.
22. KAWAS, C., S. RESNICK, et al. 1997. A prospective study of estrogen replacement therapy and the risk of developing Alzheimer's disease: the Baltimore Longitudinal Study of Aging. Neurology **48:** 1517–1521.
23. HEYMAN, A., W.E. WILKINSON, et al. 1984. Alzheimer's disease: a study of epidemiological aspects. Ann. Neurol. **15:** 335–341.
24. AMADUCCI, L.A., L. FRATIGLIONI, et al. 1986. Risk factors for clinically diagnosed Alzheimer's disease: a case-control study of an Italian population. Neurology **36:** 922–931.
25. GRAVES, A.B., E. WHITE, et al. 1990. A case-control study of Alzheimer's disease. Ann. Neurol. **28:** 766–774.
26. BRENNER, D.E., W.A. KUKULL, et al. 1994. Postmenopausal estrogen replacement therapy and the risk of Alzheimer's disease: a population-based case-control study. Am. J. Epidemiol. **140:** 262–267.
27. PAGANINI-HILL, A. & V.W. HENDERSON. 1994. Estrogen deficiency and risk of Alzheimer's disease in women. Am. J. Epidemiol. **140:** 256–261.
28. MORTEL, K.F. & J.S. MEYER. 1995. Lack of postmenopausal estrogen replacement therapy and the risk of dementia. J. Neuropsychiatry Clin. Neurosci. **7:** 334–337.
29. YAFFE, K., G. SAWAYA, et al. 1998. Estrogen therapy in postmenopausal women: effects on cognitive function and dementia. JAMA **279:** 688–695.
30. CAULEY, J.A., S.R. CUMMINGS, et al. 1990. Prevalence and determinants of estrogen replacement therapy in elderly women. Am. J. Obstet. Gynecol. **163:** 1438–1444.
31. MORTIMER, J.A. & A.B. GRAVES. 1993. Education and other socioeconomic determinants of dementia and Alzheimer's disease. Neurology **43**(Suppl. 4): S39–44.
32. FILLIT, H., H. WEINREB, et al. 1986. Observations in a preliminary open trial of estradiol therapy for senile dementia-Alzheimer's type. Psychoneuroendocrinology **11:** 337–345.
33. HONJO, H., Y. OGINO, et al. 1989. In vivo effects by estrone sulfate on the central nervous system-senile dementia (Alzheimer's type). J. Steroid Biochem. **34:** 521–525.
34. OHKURA, T., K. ISSE, et al. 1994. Evaluation of estrogen treatment in female patients with dementia of the Alzheimer type. Endocr. J. **41:** 361–371.
35. HONJO, H., Y. OGINO, et al. 1993. An effect of conjugated estrogen to cognitive impairment in women with senile dementia-Alzheimer's type: a placebo-controlled double blind study. J. Jpn. Menopause Soc. **1:** 167–171.
36. ASTHANA, S., S. CRAFT, et al. 1999. Cognitive and neuroendocrine response to transdermal estrogen in postmenopausal women with Alzheimer's disease: results of a placebo-controlled, double-blind, pilot study. Psychoneuroendocrinology **24:** 657–677.
37. HENDERSON, V.W., A. PAGANINI-HILL, et al. 2000. Estrogen for Alzheimer's disease in women: randomized, double-blind, placebo-controlled trial. Neurology **54:** 295–301.
38. MULNARD, R.A., C.W. COTMAN, et al. 2000. Estrogen replacement therapy for treatment of mild to moderate Alzheimer disease: a randomized controlled trial. Alzheimer's Disease Cooperative Study. JAMA **283:** 1007–1015.
39. WANG, P.N., S.Q. LIAO, et al. 2000. Effects of estrogen on cognition, mood, and cerebral blood flow in AD: a controlled study. Neurology **54:** 2061–2066.
40. ROSES, A.D. 1995. Apolipoprotein E genotyping in the differential diagnosis, not prediction, of Alzheimer's disease. Ann. Neurol. **38:** 6–14.
41. YAFFE, K., J. CAULEY, et al. 1997. Apolipoprotein E phenotype and cognitive decline in a prospective study of elderly community women. Arch. Neurol. **54:** 1110–1114.
42. STONE, D.J., I. ROZOVSKY, et al. 1998. Increased synaptic sprouting in response to estrogen via an apolipoprotein E-dependent mechanism: implications for Alzheimer's disease. J. Neurosci. **18:** 3180–3185.

43. RABER, J., D. WONG, et al. 1998. Isoform-specific effects of human apolipoprotein E on brain function revealed in ApoE knockout mice: increased susceptibility of females. Proc. Natl. Acad. Sci. USA **95:** 10914–10919.
44. PAYAMI, H., S. ZAREPARSI, et al. 1996. Gender difference in apolipoprotein E-associated risk for familial Alzheimer disease: a possible clue to the higher incidence of Alzheimer disease in women. Am. J. Hum. Genet. **58:** 803–811.
45. FARRER, L.A., L.A. CUPPLES, et al. 1997. Effects of age, sex, and ethnicity on the association between apolipoprotein E genotype and Alzheimer disease. A meta-analysis. APOE and Alzheimer Disease Meta Analysis Consortium. JAMA **278:** 1349–1356.
46. FARLOW, M.R., D.K. LAHIRI, et al. 1998. Treatment outcome of tacrine therapy depends on apolipoprotein genotype and gender of the subjects with Alzheimer's disease. Neurology **50:** 669–677.
47. YAFFE, K., M. HAAN, et al. 2000. Estrogen use, APOE, and cognitive decline: evidence of gene-environment interaction. Neurology **54:** 1949–1954.
48. BRYANT, H.U. & W.H. DERE. 1998. Selective estrogen receptor modulators: an alternative to hormone replacement therapy. Proc. Soc. Exp. Biol. Med. **217:** 45–52.
49. NILSEN, J., G. MOR & F. NAFTOLIN. 1998. Raloxifene induces neurite outgrowth in estrogen receptor positive PC12 cells. Menopause **5:** 211–216.
50. WU, X., M.A. GLINN, et al. 1999. Raloxifene and estradiol benzoate both fully restore hippocampal choline acetyltransferase activity in ovariectomized rats. Brain Res. **847:** 98–104.
51. BIRGE, S.J. 1998. Hormones and the aging brain. Geriatrics **53** (Suppl. **1**): S28–30.
52. NICKELSEN, T., E.G. LUFKIN, et al. 1999. Raloxifene hydrochloride, a selective estrogen receptor modulator: safety assessment of effects on cognitive function and mood in postmenopausal women. Psychoneuroendocrinology **24:** 115–128.
53. YAFFE, K., K. KRUEGER, et al. 2001. Cognitive function in postmenopausal women receiving raloxifene therapy for three years: results from the Multiple Outcomes of Raloxifene Trial. N. Engl. J. Med. **344:** 1207–1213.
54. GRADY, D., S.M. RUBIN, et al. 1992. Hormone therapy to prevent disease and prolong life in postmenopausal women. Ann. Intern. Med. **117:** 1016–1037.
55. PETITTI, D.B., S. SIDNEY, et al. 1988. Increased risk of cholecystectomy in users of supplemental estrogen. Gastroenterology **94:** 91–95.
56. DALY, E., M.P. VESSEY, et al. 1996. Risk of venous thromboembolism in users of hormone replacement therapy. Lancet **348:** 977–980.
57. GRADY, D. & V. ERNSTER. 1991. Does postmenopausal hormone therapy cause breast cancer? Am. J. Epidemiol. **134:** 1396–1400.
58. COLDITZ, G.A, S.E. HANKINSON, et al. 1995. The use of estrogens and progestins and the risk of breast cancer in postmenopausal women. N. Engl. J. Med. **332:** 1589–1593.

Estrogen Replacement Therapy for the Potential Treatment or Prevention of Alzheimer's Disease

MARILYN M. MILLER, ANDREW A. MONJAN, AND NEIL S. BUCKHOLTZ

Neuroscience and Neuropsychology of Aging Program, National Institute on Aging, National Institutes of Health, Bethesda, Maryland 20892, USA

> ABSTRACT: Alzheimer's disease (AD) is an irreversible, progressive brain disorder that occurs gradually and results in memory loss, behavior and personality changes, and a decline in cognitive abilities. Although basic biological data suggest that estrogen may have neuroprotective and neuroenhancing functions, a number of studies have produced conflicting findings on the use of estrogen for maintaining cognitive function in older people. This review summarizes clinical studies that have examined the effects of estrogen in women with AD.
>
> KEYWORDS: Alzheimer's disease; estrogen; cognitive function; clinical trials; epidemiology; memory

INTRODUCTION

It has been estimated that about four million people aged 65 and older have probable Alzheimer's disease (AD), and the numbers are projected to grow.[1] Since estrogen decreases precipitously at menopause and the risk of AD increases with postmenopausal age, it has been proposed that estrogen's loss, based upon plausible biological mechanisms, might be associated with a decrease in cognitive function and an increased incidence of dementias including AD in women; however, the epidemiological data are inconsistent.[2,3] Several studies have suggested both increased incidence[4] and prevalence of AD with increasing age[2,5–7] in women compared to men. Furthermore, the Bronx Aging Study, a large-scale prospective analysis,[8] showed that very old women had a 2.7 times higher risk for developing AD than men, as compared to other types of dementia, where incidences were similar between sexes. In contrast, other studies report no increased age-adjusted incidence or prevalence of AD in women compared to men.[9–12] Since these data are not in agreement, whether women are at increased risk of AD compared to men is not yet clear. Nevertheless, whether long-term estrogen treatment is of benefit to cognitive func-

---

Address for correspondence:, Neil S. Buckholtz, Ph.D., Neuroscience and Neuropsychology of Aging Program, National Institute on Aging, 7201 Wisconsin Avenue, Gateway Building Suite 3C307 MSC 9205, Bethesda, Maryland 20892-9205. Voice: 301-496-9350; fax: 301-496-1494.

BuckholN@nia.nih.gov

tion has emerged as an important clinical question: whether estrogen may be a preventive or treatment approach for AD has become a controversial issue.[13] This paper reviews clinical studies on the effects of estrogen in women with AD.

ESTROGEN AND THE ETIOLOGY OF AD

There are plausible mechanisms whereby estrogen might retard neurodegenerative changes in AD that may be linked to the pathophysiology of the disease. Amyloid precursor protein (APP) is the source of amyloid beta (β); the insoluble (plaque forming) form of amyloid β accumulates in brains of AD patients and may damage or kill neurons.[14] First, estrogen may play an important role in reducing the synthesis[15] or reducing the tissue levels of amyloid[16,17] (the extracellular deposits in the parenchyma of amygdala, hippocampus, and neocortex that are major histopathological markers for AD[18]). Increased amyloid deposition (amyloid load) may be linked to the decline in memory function in mice.[19,20] Second, estrogen may mediate APP processing;[21] an alternative APP processing route yields soluble APP,[22] which does not form amyloid plaques. Secretion of the soluble form of APP is stimulated by protein kinase C (PKC) activation,[23,24] which can be upregulated by estrogen *in vitro*.[25] Another means by which estrogen may help alleviate AD symptoms is via action through the cholinergic system. When tacrine (a cholinesterase inhibitor) and estrogen were given together to women with AD, cognitive function was significantly improved, suggesting an interaction of estrogen and the cholinergic system in AD.[26] Estrogen increases the amount of the enzyme for synthesis of acetylcholine[27] and the number of cholinergic neurons[28] in animal models. The mechanism of this effect is not known, but it may involve both direct and indirect effects of estrogen on acetylcholine-,[28–30] nerve growth factor-,[31] and/or brain-derived nerve growth factor–containing neurons.[29] Finally, estrogen may act by upregulating a presynaptic protein, synaptophysin, which is involved in neurotransmitter release;[32] by modulating levels of antiapoptotic proteins such as Bcl-xL;[33] by improving cerebral blood flow;[34–36] or by acting in an antiinflammatory capacity.[37]

Another potential contributor to AD pathology is oxidative stress and associated free radical–mediated oxidative damage. Amyloid β induces lipid peroxidation, and hydrogen peroxide may mediate amyloid β toxicity. Estrogens, in contrast to all other natural steroids, are antioxidants of membrane phospholipid peroxidation because of their phenolic structure.[38] Under some circumstances 17-β estradiol and 17-α estradiol can prevent intracellular peroxide accumulation, and this could lessen neuronal degeneration caused by free radicals. The neuroprotectant antioxidant activity of estrogens is dependent upon the presence of the hydroxyl group in the C3 position on the A ring of the steroid molecule.[38]

Genetic variance may also be a factor in the influence of estrogen on cognitive function. For example, one form of the apolipoprotein (APO) E gene on chromosome 19 (APOE-ε 4) is associated with increased risk of late-onset AD.[39] A study has examined the effects of estrogen on normally aging women without clinically diagnosed AD who did or did not have the APOE-ε 4 marker. In this analysis, which was part of the Cardiovascular Health Study, 2,716 women over the age of 65 at four trial centers across the United States were evaluated for measures of thickening of the carotid artery. Women were given estrogen for six years and were compared to women who had never used estrogen replacement therapy (ERT). After this long course of treatment, there was a significantly decreased risk of cognitive decline in women who did not carry the APOE-ε 4 allele, even when adjustments were made for age, education, and having had a stroke. Furthermore, ERT had no effect on the cognitive function of women who had an APOE-ε 4 allele; these women had as much thickening of the carotid wall as those who did not take estrogen, indicating that increased arteriosclerosis was not a differential risk factor.[40] Thus, genetic factors may play a role in how a woman will respond cognitively to ERT.

EPIDEMIOLOGY STUDIES

At menopause, which occurs between the ages of 45 and 55 in American women, the ovary stops secreting estrogen. Based upon these putative biological processes, withdrawal of estrogen at menopause may have an important impact upon the etiology of AD. Several epidemiological studies have been done to determine whether there is an association between the loss of estrogen at menopause and the risk of AD. These studies have produced conflicting results.

Three early studies were done with small numbers of patients. A population-based case-control analysis using computerized pharmacy records from the period of 1977–1992 examined the effects of ERT in 107 female AD patients with age- and sex-matched controls. Women with AD were as likely as controls to have used ERT,[41] suggesting that estrogen use might not be of benefit as protection against the risk of AD. In a retrospective study of 143 women, estrogen use (Premarin, Ogen, or other) was more prevalent among nondemented patients than among those with dementia,[42] although interpretation of the data is limited by the fact that estrogen use was reported by caregivers, so that one must allow for possible reporting errors. In a study using a case-control method, cognitively impaired women ($n = 93$ with probable AD and $n = 65$ with other types of dementia) were compared to matched normally aging women ($n = 148$). Although "use" was not defined as "current use" or "ever use" and type and duration of treatment were not stated, there were significantly fewer estrogen users in the dementia group than in the normally aging group.[43]

Subsequent larger studies have linked estrogen use to a decreased risk of AD. The Baltimore Longitudinal Study of Aging is a multidisciplinary study of normal aging with a cognitive component. After adjusting for education, the relative risk for AD in women ($n = 472$ post- or perimenopausal healthy women followed for up to 16 years) taking ERT was significantly reduced, but there was no effect of duration of ERT usage.[44] These data are supported by another longitudinal study of 1,124 elderly women who were initially free of AD. The age at onset for AD was significantly later in women who had taken oral estrogen than in those who did not. The relative risk of the disease was also significantly reduced in estrogen users, even after adjustment for education, ethnic origin, and APOE genotype. Women using oral estrogen longer than one year had a greater reduction in risk of developing AD.[45] In general, then, these latter larger studies tend to support a role for estrogen for prevention of AD.

CLINICAL TRIALS OF ERT ON PROGRESSION OF AD

The first clinical trials of estrogen treatment for AD provided a broad spectrum of results but tended to suggest that estrogen use is not of benefit for maintenance or improvement of cognitive function in women with AD. Some of these studies involved small numbers of subjects and short treatment intervals. For example, a treatment trial was done on seven women with AD[46] who were tested for cognitive function and then placed on estradiol for six weeks. Subsequent psychometric tests, including Mini-Mental Status Examination (MMSE), Blessed Dementia Scale, Mattis Dementia Rating Scale, selected subtests of the Wechsler Adult Intelligence Scale, as well as a measure of depression (Hamilton Depression Rating Scale) were done at 3, 6, and 9 weeks after treatment was completed. At the end of the trial, MMSE scores improved over baseline only on items involving attention and orientation in just three of the seven women.

Another small treatment study was done in Japan using 0.625 mg Premarin treatment twice daily for 5–45 months in women with AD (56–77 years of age).[47] Five of seven of the women were individuals who had previously responded well to short-term ERT (1.25 mg/day conjugated equine estrogens for six weeks). In this study, psychometric assessment was done once every 2–4 weeks. In four of seven patients, the MMSE and Hasegawa Dementia Scale (HDS) scores improved above pretreatment levels while patients were on estrogen. The HSD, which is commonly used in Japan and is similar to the MMSE, assesses orientation, registration, attention, calculation, recall, and verbal fluency. Termination of ERT resulted in a decrease in both scores. There were no placebo controls in either of the above studies.

In a second Japanese study,[48] seven women with AD were given conjugated estrogen (mainly estrone sulfate) at a dose of 1.25 mg /day over a six-week period. Cognitive status was examined every three weeks using the "New Screening Test for Dementia" (NS, developed by the Japanese National Institute of Mental Health to evaluate sampling memory, orientation, general knowledge, judgment, and calculations) and the HSD. By the end of the six-week trial, six women showed improvements ($P \leq 0.05$) in the NS and five women showed improvements ($P \leq 0.05$) on the HSD. Seven untreated women with AD showed no improvement. Three weeks after the end of the trial (at week 9), the authors noted improvement in test scores from baseline for six of the seven estrogen-treated women, despite the fact that estradiol levels had returned to pretreatment levels. The seven women who were not treated did not show any changes in test scores over the trial period.

Findings from three large placebo-controlled, double-blinded clinical trials were reported in 2000. A large clinical trial testing the effects of estrogen on cognitive and other functions was reported by Mulnard and co-workers as a component of the Alzheimer's Disease Cooperative Study.[49] The goal of this trial was to determine whether or not ERT could improve cognitive, affective, or functional decline in postmenopausal women with AD. This study involved 120 women (mean age 74) with mild to moderate AD who were previously hysterectomized (allowing for treatment with unopposed estrogen) and not already receiving hormone replacement therapy (HRT). The interventions chosen were placebo or conjugated estrogens (Premarin) 0.625 or 1.25 mg per day to examine dose effect. This form of estrogen was chosen because over eight million postmenopausal women taking hormone replacement therapy in the United States use this preparation (www.fda.gov/cder/news/ceqa.htm). The primary outcome measure of this study was the Alzheimer Disease Cooperative Study—Clinical Global Impression of Change (ADCS-CGIC), developed as a semistructured interview from the traditional CGIC Scale. Secondary outcome measures included measurements of mood, memory, attention, language function, motor speed, and activities of daily living. Broad instrumentation was used because the brain region(s) that might be affected by estrogen replacement in the postmenopausal woman are not yet known. In both the Intent to Treat (ITT) and the completers' analyses, comparing either all women on estrogen to placebo or the dose response analysis, there were no differences in the rate of decline on the primary outcome measure. Similarly, there were no significant differences in rate of decline on any of the secondary outcome measures. Premarin, when given unopposed by progesterone for one year, neither slowed disease progression nor improved global, cognitive, or functional outcomes in these women with mild to moderate AD. Interestingly, the authors did find a benefit of low-dose estrogen on change in the MMSE score after two months of exposure (low dosage = -0.36; placebo = -1.64, $P < 0.05$). Thus, Premarin given for two months in this study helped to prevent worsening of AD symptoms. This effect was lost at time points beyond two months. This study did not support the role of long-term use of estrogen in the slowing of cognitive decline in AD.

A second clinical trial was done by Henderson and co-workers, who studied 42 women with mild to moderate AD.[50] The subjects were in their late 70s and most had experienced menopause around the age of 50; therefore, they had been without estrogen for about 25 years. Women with or without a uterus were given 1.25 mg of Premarin for four months, providing unopposed physiological levels of steroid that would be present in young women during a normal menstrual cycle. At one month and four months, women were assessed using the cognitive subscale of the Alzheimer's Disease Assessment Scale, clinical-rated global impression of change, or caregiver-rated functional status, as well as measures of mood and specific aspects of cognitive performance. In this short-term study, there were no significant differences or statistical trends between treatment groups on primary outcome measures. This study suggests that short-term use of oral estrogen at a high dose in women who already have mild to moderate AD is not of benefit to memory function.

A third clinical trial examined the effects of estrogen on cognition, mood, and blood flow to the brain of women 60 years and older who had a diagnosis of mild to moderate AD.[51] Unfortunately the numbers of women who did or did not have uteri were not stated. This study tested the effect of physiological levels of three months of unopposed estrogen (1.25 mg given as Premarin) in women in Taipei, Taiwan. The primary outcome measures were the Cognitive Ability Screening Instrument, Clinical Dementia Rating, and Clinical Interview–based Impression of Change. Secondary outcomes were Behavioral Pathology in AD, the Hamilton Anxiety Rating Scale, and the Hamilton Depression Rating Scale. Brain blood flow was measured using ^{99m}Tc hexamethylpropylene amine oxime SPECT. There was no beneficial effect of oral estrogen in women who already had mild to moderate AD. The findings are of interest because they examine a population of women in another part of the world. When taken with data from United States clinical trials, this study suggests that the negative estrogen findings are not unique to the American population.

These three recent clinical trials indicate that conjugated equine estrogen (0.625 or 1.25 mg daily), if given alone (i.e., without progesterone) continuously and for durations ranging from 1–12 months, is not of benefit for cognitive function in women who already have mild to moderate AD. We need to be somewhat cautious in our conclusions about these studies, because they apply only to a total small population of less than 200 patients with AD and include women of advanced age only who have already had the disease for some time. It is important to note that even when a patient has AD, there are other potential benefits to taking estrogen, which include prevention of osteoporosis and benefits for the cardiovascular system (reviewed in Ref. 52), although this has recently been questioned.[53]

While the three larger clinical trials using oral estrogen have provided discouraging outcomes, a small clinical trial reported in 1999 that used the estrogen patch was somewhat more positive.[54] This randomized, placebo controlled, double-blind parallel-group pilot study was done in 12 women with probable AD of mild-moderate severity and employed an eight-week treatment period. Estradiol 17-β was delivered by a skin patch that provided 0.05 mg/day to six women. The remaining six women wore a placebo skin patch. Cognition was assessed using a battery of neuropsychological tests. Statistically significant improvements in estrogen-treated women were reported on attention (Stroop: number of self-corrections in the interference condition) and verbal memory (Busche: delayed cued recall). Positive effects of estrogen were on measures of attention and executive function but not on other measures. Effects were observed as soon as the first week of treatment and diminished when treatment was withdrawn. In the control group there were no significant effects of placebo on measures of cognition. This study was of short duration (two months of estrogen) and suggests that estrogen replacement may enhance cognition for postmenopausal women with AD when given in the patch form, bypassing the metabolism in the liver that occurs with oral estrogen administration. A longer clinical trial of the effects of estradiol 17-β delivered by the patch on cognition in patients with AD is in progress.

FACTORS THAT MAY BE IMPORTANT IN THE COGNITIVE RESPONSE TO ERT

When examined together, the results of the clinical trial studies of estrogen treatment in women who have AD are mixed. Many factors affect cognitive function, and several issues remain unresolved. Important elements that could affect study outcome may include: (1) whether estrogen is given in a constant or cyclic fashion; (2) the dose of estrogen that is administered; (3) the temporal parameters of estrogen administration; (4) the form of estrogen given; (5) the route of estrogen administration; (6) the role of progestins; (7) the role of phytoestrogens; and (8) the role of newly developed selective estrogen receptor modulators in cognitive function.

Tonic or Cyclic Administration of Estrogen

Whether estrogen is administered in a tonic or cyclic fashion may be important. It may be that the female brain is "programmed" to understand varying rather than constant levels of estrogen. It is unknown whether administration of estrogen in a cyclic fashion, with incremental increases, peaks, and decreases of the steroid, such as is found in the menstrual cycle of the younger woman, might be of benefit to cognitive function in the peri- or postmenopausal woman. In the estrogen replacement studies done so far, only constant levels of either high- (1.25 mg) or low- (0.625) dose estrogen have been studied. Short-term (30 days) treatment of estrogen followed by removal (3 days) to allow "recovery" of the estrogen receptors and subsequent readministration of the steroid might be a another possible treatment approach for women with AD.[55] The effects on cognition of varying the dose of estrogen either on a long-term or short-term basis beginning at menopause are completely unknown.

Dose of Estrogen

The dose of estrogen may be an important factor in maintaining cognitive function. While only constant levels of either high- (1.25 mg) or low- (0.625) dose estrogen have been studied, it is possible that an even lower dose may be efficacious.

Temporal Parameters of Estrogen Administration

The temporal parameters of administering estrogen may also be key factors in maintaining or improving cognitive function during aging. It is important to understand the optimal time for starting estrogen to help women at high risk of getting AD. The length of time of estrogen administration may be an important issue. Will continuous exposure to estrogen for as many as 30 years after menopause be of benefit to cognition? Estrogen receptors in rodents downregulate after prolonged exposure to estrogen; this may also occur in the human.[55] Alternatively, would a woman who has not been exposed to exogenous estrogens at the time of menopause or thereafter benefit from ERT 20 years after menopause?

Form of Estrogen Given

The form of estrogen given may have effects on cognitive function. Systematic and standardized comparisons of the effects of various forms of estrogen (e.g., estradiol 17-β, conjugated equine estrogens, estrone) on cognitive function need to be done. As noted in a recent report by the U.S. Food and Drug Administration Center for Drug Evaluation and Research, conjugated equine estrogen (CEE), or Premarin, contains a number of biologically active steroids other than estradiol 17-β that can act at the estrogen receptor. These include δ (8,0) dehydroestrone sulfate (DHES); the full spectrum of estrogenic compounds present in Premarin has not yet been identified, despite the fact that most women on ERT take this form of estrogen and have done so since the mid-1970s (http://www.fda.gov/cder/news/cebackground.htm). The long-term effects of the different types of estrogens that are not endogenous to the human reproductive system are unknown, as are their effects on the aging CNS.

Route of Estrogen Administration

The extent of estrogen metabolism may affect cognitive function. Since the way the body metabolizes estrogen depends upon how it is administered, another important issue is the route of administration. The route of delivery, oral versus transdermal via a patch, may be an important factor in the response of target tissues to the steroid. While the patch delivers estradiol 17-β to its target via the blood stream, orally administered estrogens are metabolized by the liver before arrival at their target tissue, with the dose at the target being determined in part by metabolism by the liver. Liver function can vary significantly in the aged individual.

Role of Progestins

How do the different forms of progesterone that are given to postmenopausal women affect cognitive function? While it is necessary for women who have a uterus and who are taking estrogen to also take progesterone in order to reduce the risk of developing uterine cancer, an additional confounding factor is, in fact, the presence of progestins in many preparations of hormone replacement therapy. Progesterone has been shown in some studies to have a negative effect on cognitive function.[56]

Role of Phytoestrogens

Many women are now consuming dietary supplements containing phytoestrogens. Little is known about the efficacy of binding of these unique steroids to the estrogen receptor, how their binding may change with age, or how phytoestrogens may affect cognitive function in either normally aging women or those at risk for developing AD, and how dietary supplements may interact with estrogens and progestins.

Role of Newly Developed SERMs in Cognitive Function

As important as these issues are, the situation is becoming more complex. A number of very specific synthetic estrogen-like drugs and estrogen antagonists are becoming available. Do they cross the blood-brain barrier? What will be the effect of these drugs on cognition? Raloxifene is a selective estrogen receptor modulator (SERM) with estrogen agonist effects on bone and lipid metabolism and antagonist effects on reproductive tissues. This agent is used clinically to prevent and treat bone loss. A recent phase 2, two-site, parallel-group, placebo-controlled, randomized, double-blind 12-month study assessed cognitive function in cognitively normal postmenopausal women 45–75 years of age employing 60 and 120 mg/day raloxifene. The Memory Assessments Clinical Battery, Walter Reed Performance Battery, and Geriatric Depression Scale were used. After 12 months of treatment, there were no significant differences between study groups. Thus it appears that raloxifene has no effect on cognitive decline in normally aging women.[57] A study is in progress as part of the Multiple Outcomes of Raloxifene Health (MORE) Study to determine whether elderly women treated with raloxifene have differences in cognitive scores and differences in the incidence of dementia as compared to women treated with placebo.

STUDIES IN PROGRESS

While considerable progress has been made over the past decade in our understanding of the etiology of AD and how estrogen might impact upon the progress of the disease, more studies are urgently needed to address the unanswered questions relating to the use of estrogen replacement therapy in the postmenopausal woman.

One prevention study is presently in progress in cognitively normal women with a family history of AD. This study will examine whether estrogen replacement therapy in women who have been hysterectomized or whether estrogen with progesterone therapy in women who have not been hysterectomized can prevent AD. Another clinical trial of women with AD is in progress to test whether estradiol 17-β administered via a patch can be effective as a treatment for AD. A large ongoing study funded by Wyeth Ayerst is a component of the NIH-funded Women's Health Initiative. It is following cognitively normal women receiving conjugated estrogens with or without progesterones for six years. Each woman suspected to have dementia will undergo clinical and laboratory testing. The overall goal of the study is to determine whether women receiving hormone replacement therapy will have a lower risk of developing AD.

CONCLUSIONS

It is clear that there are several factors that could account for the differences in results of the studies on the effectiveness of estrogen in preventing or treating cognitive decline and dementia, including the level of cognitive deficit the individual was experiencing at the start of the study. Are we using the right instruments for measuring cognitive function to allow comparisons among clinical trials? The application of standardized measures of cognitive function across a number of cognitive domains in order to compare the outcomes of multiple studies will be an important aspect of the next generation of analyses of the effects of estrogen on cognitive function.

A large segment of the female population is entering the postmenopausal years, when life-changing decisions about the use of estrogen need to be made. Epidemiological and observational clinical data on the use of estrogen to maintain cognitive function with normal aging have been somewhat encouraging. Studies involving small numbers of women and short-term (two months) first-pass replacement via the patch provide some positive evidence that estrogen may be efficacious in women with mild to moderate AD. On the other hand, placebo-controlled double-blind studies of larger numbers of women with established AD showed no benefit of long-term ERT. Neurons and pathways that mediate cognitive function may have already been damaged or lost due to the cascade of events associated with the neuropathology of the disease. It may be that the window of opportunity has been missed in these women. For women at high risk for AD, our next challenge is to assess the best types of estrogens and progestins, the routes and doses of administration, the most efficacious pattern of dosing, and the optimal time for initiation of ERT or HRT; and to learn how the brain responds and how long the brain will continue to respond.

REFERENCES

1. EVANS, D.A., H.H. FUNKENSTEIN, M.S. ALBERT, et al. 1989. Prevalence of Alzheimer's disease in a community population of older persons. Higher than previously reported. JAMA **262:** 2551–2556.
2. HASKELL, S.G., E.D. RICHARDSON & R.I. HORWITZ. 1997. The effect of estrogen replacement therapy on cognitive function in women: a critical review of the literature. J. Clin. Epidemiol. **50:** 1249–1264.

3. YAFFE, K., G. SAWAYA, I. LIEBERBURG, et al. 1998. Estrogen therapy in postmenopausal women—effects on cognitive function and dementia. JAMA **279:** 688–695.
4. KOKMEN, E., V. CHANDRA & B.S. SCHOENBERG. 1988. Trends in incidence of dementing illness in Rochester, Minnesota, in three quinquennial periods, 1960–1974. Neurology **38:** 975–980.
5. ROCCA, W.A. & L. AMADUCCI. 1989. The etiology of Alzheimer's disease: an epidemiologic point of view. Neurobiol. Aging **10:** 440–441.
6. JORM, A.F., A.E. KORTEN & A.S. HENDERSON. 1987. The prevalence of dementia: a quantitative integration of the literature. Acta Psychiatr. Scand. **76:** 465–479.
7. HOFMAN, A., W.A. ROCCA, C. BRAYNE, et al. 1991. The prevalence of dementia in Europe: a collaborative study of 1980–1990 findings. Eurodem. Prevalence Research Group. Int. J. Epidemiol. **20:** 736–748.
8. ARONSON, M.K., W. LOOI, H. MORGENSTERN, et al. 1990. Women, myocardial infarction, and dementia in the very old. Neurology **40:** 1102–1106.
9. SCHOENBERG, B.S., E. KOKMEN & H. OKAZAKI. 1987. Alzheimer's disease and other dementing illnesses in a defined United States population: incidence rates and clinical features. Ann. Neurol. **22:** 724–729.
10. HAGNELL, O., L. ÖJESJÖ & B. RORSMAN. 1992. Incidence of dementia in the Lundby Study. Neuroepidemiology **11** (Suppl. 1): 61–66.
11. TREVES, T., A.D. KORCZYN, N. ZILBER, et al. 1986. Presenile dementia in Israel. Arch. Neurol. **43:** 26–29.
12. NILSSON, L.V. 1984. Incidence of severe dementia in an urban sample followed from 70 to 79 years of age. Acta Psychiatr. Scand. **70:** 478–486.
13. LEBLANC, E.S., J. JANOWSKY, B.K. CHAN & H.D. NELSON. 2001. Hormone replacement therapy and cognition: systematic review and meta-analysis. JAMA **285:** 1489–1499.
14. MATTSON, M.P. 1997. Cellular actions of beta-amyloid precursor protein and its soluble and fibrillogenic derivatives. Physiol. Rev. **77:** 1081–1132.
15. PETANCESKA, S.S., V. NAGY, D. FRAIL, et al. 2000. Ovariectomy and 17beta-estradiol modulate the levels of Alzheimer's amyloid beta peptides in brain. Neurology **54:** 2212–2217.
16. NASLUND, J., V. HAROUTUNIAN, R. MOHS, et al. 2000. Correlation between elevated levels of amyloid beta-peptide in the brain and cognitive decline. JAMA **283:** 1571–1577.
17. LI, R., Y. SHEN, L.B. YANG, et al. 2000. Estrogen enhances uptake of amyloid beta-protein by microglia derived from the human cortex. J. Neurochem. **75:** 1447–1454.
18. PRICE, D.L., S.S. SISODIA & S.E. GANDY. 1995. Amyloid beta amyloidosis in Alzheimer's disease. Curr. Opin. Neurol. **8:** 268–274.
19. MORGAN, D., D.M. DIAMOND, P.E. GOTTSCHALL, et al. 2000. A beta peptide vaccination prevents memory loss in an animal model of Alzheimer's disease. Nature **408:** 982–985.
20. JANUS, C., J. PEARSON, J. MCLAURIN, et al. 2000. A beta peptide immunization reduces behavioural impairment and plaques in a model of Alzheimer's disease. Nature **408:** 979–982.
21. XU, H.X., G.K. GOURAS, J.P. GREENFIELD, et al. 1998. Estrogen reduces neuronal generation of Alzheimer β-amyloid peptides. Nature Med. **4:** 447–451.
22. JAFFE, A.B., C.D. TORAN-ALLERAND & P.GREENGARD. 1994. Estrogen regulates metabolism of Alzheimer amyloid beta precursor protein. J. Biol. Chem. **269:** 13065–13068.
23. KOO, E.H. 1997. Phorbol esters affect multiple steps in beta-amyloid precursor protein trafficking and amyloid beta-protein production. Mol. Med. **3:** 204–211.
24. SLACK, B.E., J. BREU, L. MUCHNICKI, et al. 1997. Rapid stimulation of amyloid precursor protein release by epidermal growth factor: role of protein kinase C. Biochem J. **327** (Pt. 1): 245–249.
25. JAFFE, A.B., C.D. TORAN-ALLERAND, P. GREENGARD, et al. 1994. Estrogen regulates metabolism of Alzheimer amyloid β precursor protein. J. Biol. Chem. **269:** 13065–13068.
26. SCHNEIDER, L.S., M.R. FARLOW, V.W. HENDERSON, et al. 1996. Effects of estrogen replacement therapy on response to tacrine in patients with Alzheimer's disease. Neurology **46:** 1580–1584.

27. GIBBS, R.B. 1996. Fluctuations in relative levels of choline acetyltransferase mRNA in different regions of the rat basal forebrain across the estrous cycle: effects of estrogen and progesterone. J. Neurosci. **16:** 1049–1055.
28. MILLER, M.M., S.M. HYDER, R. ASSAYAG, et al. 1999. Estrogen modulates spontaneous alternation and the cholinergic phenotype in the basal forebrain. Neuroscience **91:** 1143–1153.
29. SIMPKINS, J.W., P.S. GREEN, K.E. GRIDLEY, et al. 1997. Role of estrogen replacement therapy in memory enhancement and the prevention of neuronal loss associated with Alzheimer's disease. Am. J. Med. **103:** 19S–25S.
30. MILLER, M.M., H.P. BENNETT, R.B. BILLIAR, et al. 1998. Estrogen, the ovary, and neutotransmitters: factors associated with aging. Exp. Gerontol. **33:** 729–757.
31. TORAN-ALLERAND, C.D., R.C. MIRANDA, W.D. BENTHAM, et al. 1992. Estrogen receptors colocalize with low-affinity nerve growth factor receptors in cholinergic neurons of the basal forebrain. Proc. Natl. Acad. Sci. USA **89:** 4668–4672.
32. STONE, D.J., I. ROZOVSKY, T.E. MORGAN, et al. 1998. Increased synaptic sprouting in response to estrogen via an apolipoprotein E–dependent mechanism: implications for Alzheimer's disease. J. Neurosci. **18:** 3180–3185.
33. PIKE, C.J. 1999. Estrogen modulates neuronal Bcl-xL expression and beta-amyloid–induced apoptosis: relevance to Alzheimer's disease. J. Neurochem. **72:** 1552–1563.
34. MAKI, P.M. & S.M. RESNICK. 2000. Longitudinal effects of estrogen replacement therapy on PET cerebral blood flow and cognition. Neurobiol. Aging **21:** 373–383.
35. DUBAL, D.B. & P.M. WISE. 2001. Neuroprotective effects of estradiol in middle-aged female rats. Endocrinology **142:** 43–48.
36. THOMAS, T., J.A. RHODIN, E.T. SUTTON, et al. 1999. Estrogen protects peripheral and cerebral blood vessels from toxicity of Alzheimer peptide amyloid-beta and inflammatory reaction. J. Submicrosc. Cytol. Pathol. **31:** 571–579.
37. BRUCE-KELLER, A.J., J.L. KEELING, J.N. KELLER, et al. 2000. Antiinflammatory effects of estrogen on microglial activation. Endocrinology **141:** 3646–3656.
38. BEHL, C., T. SKUTELLA, F. LEZOUALC'H, et al. 1997. Neuroprotection against oxidative stress by estrogens: structure-activity relationship. Mol. Pharmacol. **51:** 535–541.
39. STRITTMATTER, W.J., A.M. SAUNDERS, D. SCHMECHEL, et al. 1993. Apolipoprotein E: high-avidity binding to β-amyloid and increased frequency of type 4 allele in late-onset familial Alzheimer disease. Proc. Natl. Acad. Sci. USA **90:** 1977–1981.
40. YAFFE, K., M. HAAN, A. BYERS, et al. 2000. Estrogen use, APOE, and cognitive decline: evidence of gene-environment interaction. Neurology **54:** 1949–1954.
41. BRENNER, D.E., W.A. KUKULL, A. STERGACHIS, et al. 1994. Postmenopausal estrogen replacement therapy and the risk of Alzheimer's disease: a population-based case-control study. Am. J. Epidemiol. **140:** 262–267.
42. HENDERSON, V.W., A. PAGANINI-HILL, C.K. EMANUEL, et al. 1994. Estrogen replacement therapy in older women. Comparisons between Alzheimer's disease cases and nondemented control subjects. Arch. Neurol. **51:** 896–900.
43. MORTEL, K.F. & J.S. MEYER. 1995. Lack of postmenopausal estrogen replacement therapy and the risk of dementia. J. Neuropsychiatry Clin. Neurosci. **7:** 334–337.
44. KAWAS, C., S. RESNICK, A. MORRISON, et al. 1997. A prospective study of estrogen replacement therapy and the risk of developing Alzheimer's disease: the Baltimore Longitudinal Study of Aging. Neurology **48:** 1517–1521.
45. TANG, M.X., D. JACOBS, Y. STERN, et al. 1996. Effect of oestrogen during menopause on risk and age at onset of Alzheimer's disease. Lancet **348:** 429–432.
46. FILLIT, H., H.WEINREB, I. CHOLST, et al. 1986. Observations in a preliminary open trial of estradiol therapy for senile dementia–Alzheimer's type. Psychoneuroendocrinology **11:** 337–345.
47. OHKURA, T., K. ISSE, K. AKAZAWA, et al. 1995. Long-term estrogen replacement therapy in female patients with dementia of the Alzheimer type: 7 case reports. Dementia **6:** 99–107.
48. HONJO, H., Y. OGINO, K. NAITOH, et al. 1989. *In vivo* effects by estrone sulfate on the central nervous system–senile dementia (Alzheimer's type). J. Steroid Biochem. **34:** 521–525.

49. MULNARD, R.A., C.W. COTMAN, C. KAWAS, *et al.* 2000. Estrogen replacement therapy for treatment of mild to moderate Alzheimer disease: a randomized controlled trial. Alzheimer's Disease Cooperative Study. JAMA **283:** 1007–1015.
50. HENDERSON, V.W., A. PAGANINI-HILL, B.L. MILLER, *et al.* 2000. Estrogen for Alzheimer's disease in women: randomized, double-blind, placebo-controlled trial. Neurology **54:** 295–301.
51. WANG, P.N., S.Q. LIAO, R.S. LIU, *et al.* 2000. Effects of estrogen on cognition, mood, and cerebral blood flow in AD: a controlled study. Neurology **54:** 2061–2066.
52. MILLER, M.M. & K.B. FRANKLIN. 1999. Theoretical basis for the benefit of postmenopausal estrogen substitution. Exp. Gerontol. **34:** 587–604.
53. HERRINGTON, D.M., D.M. REBOUSSIN, K.B. BROSNIHAN, *et al.* 2000. Effects of estrogen replacement on the progression of coronary-artery atherosclerosis. N. Engl. J. Med. **343:** 522–529.
54. ASTHANA, S., S. CRAFT, L.D. BAKER, *et al.* 1999. Cognitive and neuroendocrine response to transdermal estrogen in postmenopausal women with Alzheimer's disease: results of a placebo-controlled, double-blind, pilot study. Psychoneuroendocrinology **24:** 657–677.
55. TORAN-ALLERAND, C.D. 2000. Estrogen as a treatment for Alzheimer disease. JAMA **284:** 307–308.
56. RICE, M.M., A.B. GRAVES, S.M. MCCURRY, *et al.* 1997. Estrogen replacement therapy and cognitive function in postmenopausal women without dementia. Am. J. Med. **103:** 26S–35S.
57. NICKELSEN, T., E.G. LUFKIN, B.L. RIGGS, *et al.* 1999. Raloxifene hydrochloride, a selective estrogen receptor modulator: safety assessment of effects on cognitive function and mood in postmenopausal women. Psychoneuroendocrinology **24:** 115–128.

Reproductive and Related Endocrine Considerations

Introduction

ESTELLA C. PARROTT

National Institute of Child Health and Human Development, National Institutes of Health, Bethesda, Maryland 20892, USA

Selective estrogen receptor modulators (SERMs) are a growing class of therapeutic agents that bind with high affinity to estrogen receptors and mimic the effect of estrogens in some tissues, but act as estrogen antagonists in others. SERMs, such as raloxifene and tamoxifen, produce beneficial estrogen-like effects on bone and lipid metabolism. While tamoxifen exhibits estrogen agonist effects on the endometrium, raloxifene antagonizes estrogen effects on reproductive tissue. Estrogenic hormones play critical roles in many aspects of women's reproductive health. Thus, the impact of any hormonal manipulation must be carefully considered. Steroid hormones are known to stimulate a variety of short- and long-term effects leading to growth, differentiation, maturation, and specialization in target tissues. Elucidating the mechanisms by which estrogens, other steroid hormones, and SERMs regulate steroid-sensitive cells is critical for increasing the knowledge of basic reproductive function and potential disease states. Further understanding of the hormonal mechanisms governing reproductive processes in men and women will provide the foundation for clinical therapies directed toward reproductive disorders.

Much of the research targeting SERMs has concentrated on the breast, endometrium, skeletal system, and cardiovascular system. Recent progress in the relationship of SERMs to reproductive tissues and other nontraditional target tissues is explored in this section. The first paper presents the ongoing discussions concerning the type of endometrial surveillance, if any, that women on tamoxifen therapy require to ensure timely recognition of pathological conditions. Studies demonstrate the appearance of high- and low-risk groups for the development of atypical hyperplasia based on the presence or absence of underlying endometrial abnormalities prior to tamoxifen therapy. The data presented support the conclusion that potential screening strategies or guidelines to evaluate the effects of SERMs on the endometrium will have to be determined in the context of future clinical trials. The second paper focuses on SERMs and their potential impact on pelvic organ prolapse, ovarian

---

Address for correspondence: Estella C. Parrott, M.D., M.P.H., Program Director, Reproductive Medicine Gynecology Program, Reproductive Sciences Branch, Center for Population Research, National Institute of Child Health and Human Development, National Institutes of Health, 6100 Executive Boulevard, Room 8B01, Bethesda, MD 20892-7510. Voice: 301-496-6515; fax: 301-496-0962.

ep61h@nih.gov

cyst formation, and increased growth of uterine fibroids. While tamoxifen has been primarily associated with these findings, the impact that current and future SERMs have on the pelvic floor and other genital tissues will be important to understanding their long-term clinical application. The final paper highlights the effects of selected SERMs on the hypothalamic-pituitary-gonadal (HPG) axis in women (both pre- and postmenopausal) and men. Since the clinical profile of SERMs may be influenced by the prevalent hormonal environment, it concludes that future research should focus on further characterizing potential differences between SERMs on a wide range of hormonal parameters.

The future of SERMs in the management of estrogen-dependent gynecological conditions, such as endometriosis, dysfunctional bleeding, and uterine fibroids, will be important in developing therapeutic designs and future clinical applicability. An important effect of research on SERMs will be an expanded basic understanding of the mechanisms that govern the effects of these drugs on the endometrium and on reproductive structures outside of the endometrium. Once these possibilities are explored, we may be able to fully appreciate the influence of SERMs on the reproductive milieu in women and men.

The Effect of SERMs on the Endometrium

STEVEN R. GOLDSTEIN

Department of Obstetrics and Gynecology, New York University School of Medicine, New York, New York 10016, USA

ABSTRACT: Tamoxifen, the first clinically available SERM, was developed in 1966 and approved by the FDA (United States Food and Drug Administration) in 1978. It is the most prescribed antineoplastic drug in the world, with approximately 10 million women-use-years of experience. Tamoxifen has proved efficacious in all settings of breast cancer. However, in the mid-to-late 1980s, a series of letters to the editor and case reports announced an association between tamoxifen therapy in women with breast cancer and the development of endometrial carcinoma. Subsequently, in 1998, the observation of a significant 49% reduction in invasive breast cancer relative to placebo in a cohort of women at increased risk for the disease resulted in the early stopping of the National Surgical Adjuvant Breast and Bowel Project's (NSABP) P-1: Breast Cancer Prevention Trial (BCPT). Importantly, this was the first time that information became available about the effects of tamoxifen in healthy women, that is, women who did not already have breast cancer. In this healthy population, the relative risk of developing endometrial carcinoma in the tamoxifen arm was 2.54, although when stratified by age, in women over 50, the risk grew to 4.01. Thus, the risk appears to be confined to women over 50 because, in contrast, in women under 50 there was no statistically significant increase in the risk of endometrial carcinoma.

KEYWORDS: selective estrogen receptor modulators (SERMs); endometrium; uterus

Controversy exists about the extent of uterine surveillance, if any, that women on tamoxifen therapy require. The American College of Obstetricians and Gynecologists (ACOG) in its committee opinion concluded that no more than annual pelvic exams with Pap smears are needed in asymptomatic women. Others have advocated periodic blind endometrial sampling. We have employed a regimen of transvaginal ultrasound and saline infusion sonohysterography when the image generated by an initial transvaginal ultrasound is of poor, indistinct quality or suggestive of thickening of the endometrial wall. Recent data seem to point to a high- and low-risk group that can be identified before treatment with tamoxifen by screening with transvaginal ultrasound. Patients with no uterine abnormalities on transvaginal ultrasound appear to be at very low risk of developing atypical hyperplasia. However, patients with any

Address for correspondence: Steven R. Goldstein, M.D., Professor of Obstetrics/Gynecology, New York University Medical Center, 530 First Avenue, Suite 10N, New York, NY 10016. Voice: 212-263-7416; fax: 212-263-6259.
Steven.Goldstein@Med.Nyu.Edu

lesions on the initial screen (although most are usually benign polyps) appear to have an 18-fold increased risk and, even if asymptomatic, may be appropriate candidates for ongoing surveillance.

Raloxifene, a second-generation SERM, was initially approved for prevention of osteoporosis in 1997. In October 1999, this indication was extended to include treatment of existing osteoporosis based on the results of the Multiple Outcomes of Raloxifene Evaluation (MORE) trial. In another study in which the primary end point was the effect of drug on the uterus, transvaginal ultrasound, sonohysterography, and endometrial histology showed no differences between the raloxifene and placebo groups when these drugs were administered to healthy postmenopausal women with normal uteri over a 12-month period. In this study, no malignancies and no hyperplasia were observed. A 3% incidence of proliferation was seen only in women whose BMI (body mass index) exceeded 29 kg/m^2. However, this study was done on what would have to be considered a low-risk group since women with any endometrial lesions on the initial screen were excluded. The MORE trial, which addressed a broader cohort and which had no eligibility exclusions based on endometrial criteria, showed that there were no differences in the risk of endometrial carcinoma with raloxifene compared to placebo over a 3-year time period. Interestingly, there was a 20% reduction in the number of endometrial carcinomas in the raloxifene group, although this was not statistically significant.

TAMOXIFEN

Tamoxifen, a triphenylethylene derivative, was developed in 1966 and approved by the FDA (United States Food and Drug Administration) in 1978. It is the most prescribed antineoplastic drug in the world, with approximately 10 million women-use-years of experience. Tamoxifen has proved efficacious in all settings of breast cancer. In 1985, the first report of its association with endometrial neoplasia appeared.[1] Numerous letters and case reports followed.[2–5] The first data obtained from a prospective study, carried out without a baseline endometrial assessment, reflected a 7.5-fold increase in risk of endometrial carcinoma (average annual hazard rate of 0.2/1000 for placebo vs. 1.6/1000 for tamoxifen).[6] The first prospective study that included a baseline uterine evaluation showed that, among women treated with tamoxifen, there was a 6% incidence of carcinoma, a 25% incidence of polyp formation, and a 44% incidence of proliferation. After 3 years, only 50% of these postmenopausal patients maintained an inactive, atrophic endometrium.[7] Other investigators found an 18% incidence in the development of hyperplasia with a tamoxifen treatment duration of 12 months.[8]

The early studies documenting an association of endometrial carcinoma with tamoxifen use employed either hysteroscopy[7] or blind endometrial office sampling.[8] Simultaneously, transvaginal ultrasound was introduced to evaluate uterine bleeding in postmenopausal women.[9,10] Numerous tamoxifen patients were evaluated with transvaginal ultrasound.[11] With the introduction of saline infusion sonohysterography[12] came the first reports of microcystic changes on ultrasound. Such changes represent glandular cystic atrophy and can be present in the basalis of the endometrium, in the proximal myometrium, or even within polyps. Similar findings have been reported with just 3 months of treatment with idoxifene.[13]

The published data demonstrating an association between tamoxifen and the development of benign as well as malignant endometrial lesions would appear to suggest a need for routine screening for endometrial neoplasms in women taking this drug. Yet, the standard test for detecting endometrial disease, that is, endometrial biopsy, is fraught with difficulties and is of limited utility in screening women treated with tamoxifen.[14,15] The endometrial biopsy procedure leaves uncertainty about the origin of the tissue, which is obtained in a blind fashion. Because the endometrial abnormalities seem to be more heterogeneous in women taking tamoxifen than in other settings, blind endometrial biopsy leads to a false-negative rate that is higher than usual.[16,17] Furthermore, the presence of cervical stenosis in a high percentage of patients can preclude outpatient sampling and can require dilatation curettage under anesthesia.[8,17–19] Hysteroscopy has been used for screening,[17,20,21] but it is expensive and operator-dependent and has limited sensitivity in terms of revealing positive endometrial pathologic findings.[22]

Alternative approaches to endometrial screening among women taking tamoxifen have therefore been explored. As an example, an algorithm of uterine surveillance using transvaginal ultrasound and saline infusion sonohysterography has been described to overcome the shortcomings of blind endometrial sampling and hysteroscopy.[23] In that observational study of asymptomatic postmenopausal breast cancer patients on tamoxifen that employed this algorithm, there was a 4% incidence of carcinoma, a 9% incidence of proliferation or hyperplasia, and a 27% incidence of endometrial polyps. Furthermore, unenhanced transvaginal ultrasound revealed that only 25% of these tamoxifen-treated patients had a thin linear endometrial echo predictive of inactive atrophic endometrium. However, both procedures together (transvaginal ultrasound and saline infusion sonohysterography, where indicated according to the algorithm) showed that 59% of the patients exhibited inactive surface epithelium. Thus, controversy exists regarding which, if any, method of endometrial surveillance is appropriate for patients receiving tamoxifen therapy. The ACOG Committee Opinion No. 169 (February 1996) recommends that evaluations be limited to an annual pelvic exam and Pap smear unless there is any abnormal bleeding. However, the opinion also acknowledges the following: "Practitioners should be alert to the increased incidence of endometrial malignancy. Screening procedures or diagnostic tests should be performed at the discretion of the individual gynecologist."[24]

More recently, data have suggested that, prior to the initiation of tamoxifen therapy for breast cancer, patients at higher risk of endometrial abnormalities may be distinguished from those at lower risk on the basis of initial endometrial lesions.[25] In an update, Berliere et al.[26] reported on pretreatment screening of 575 postmenopausal patients with breast cancer. Endometrial polyps were present in 16.6% of patients at baseline, prior to tamoxifen therapy. After their polyps were removed, these patients were followed, as were those patients who had no initial endometrial lesions. Of the group with no initial lesions, 12.9% developed polyps and 0.7% developed atypical hyperplasia. In the group with initial lesions, 17.6% developed polyps and 11.7% developed atypical hyperplasia. This represents an 18-fold increase in incidence rate of atypical lesions in the high-risk group (those with initial benign inactive polyps) relative to the low-risk group (apparent absence of uterine abnormalities).

The only data on the endometrial effects of tamoxifen in healthy women (i.e., not with a diagnosis of breast cancer) were generated from the BCPT.[27] In women under

50 (who were presumed to be premenopausal), there was no statistically significant difference in the incidence of endometrial carcinoma between the tamoxifen and placebo arms. However, in women over 50 (who were presumed to be postmenopausal), the rate of endometrial carcinoma per 1000 women was 0.76 for placebo and 3.05 for tamoxifen (RR = 4.01; CI = 1.70–10.90). Because the study design lacked entry or exit data regarding endometrial end points, there was no way to objectively assess the incidence of benign endometrial changes (either proliferative endometrium or polyps) or atypical hyperplasia. However, other gynecologic symptoms that could be evaluated noninvasively were followed up. Thus, the incidence of vaginal discharge classified as moderately bothersome or worse was 29% in the tamoxifen group and 13% in the placebo group (no statistical analysis provided).

RALOXIFENE

Raloxifene, a benzothiophene derivative, does not stimulate the endometrium in ovariectomized rats.[28,29] Furthermore, raloxifene completely inhibits estrogen-induced endometrial proliferation in ovariectomized rats.[30,31] In the MORE trial, an osteoporosis treatment study,[32] raloxifene therapy was not associated with an increased risk of vaginal bleeding, endometrial proliferation, or endometrial carcinoma. However, among 2262 women who underwent transvaginal ultrasound, 8% of raloxifene-treated patients had endometrial fluid versus 6% in the placebo group ($P = 0.02$). In a clinical trial of raloxifene with uterine effects as the primary end point,[33] treatment for 1 year with raloxifene at 60 mg/day resulted in no increase in endometrial thickness (assessed by transvaginal ultrasound and saline infusion sonohysterography), no hyperplasia, and no malignancy. Although the incidence of proliferative tissue was 3.6% in the raloxifene (60 mg/day) group and 2.1% in the placebo group at the end of the study, the finding of proliferative tissue was limited to women who had a BMI > 29 kg/m^2. Two polyps were observed in the placebo group and four polyps in the raloxifene (60 mg/day) group, but the difference was not statistically significant.

CONCLUSIONS

In summary, whether used for breast cancer therapy or prevention in postmenopausal women, tamoxifen results in an increase in endometrial proliferation, polyp formation, hyperplasia, and carcinoma. Interestingly, tamoxifen appears not to have that effect in premenopausal women. Furthermore, at least in some patients, it is associated with an unusual ultrasound appearance on saline infusion sonohysterography, suggesting that simple transvaginal ultrasound without fluid enhancement may be less reliable as a screening modality. The high incidence of focal abnormalities makes blind endometrial sampling unreliable as well. Finally, it appears that women may be identified as being at higher or lower risk for the development of atypical hyperplasia based on the presence or absence of endometrial lesions prior to initiating tamoxifen therapy. The effects of raloxifene on the uterus appear to differ from those of tamoxifen. However, one limitation of the study with endometrial safety as the primary end point is that women with preexisting endometrial lesions—who have been shown to constitute a high-risk group for subsequent abnormalities after treatment with tamoxifen therapy—were excluded from the study. Future clinical studies with tamoxifen, raloxifene, and newer SERMs should be designed to determine the incidence of various endometrial pathologies, both malignant and benign, as well as other gynecologic disorders (e.g., vaginal dryness, discharge, prolapse, and incontinence). Studies should also be designed so as not to exclude women with previous benign lesions. Such studies may require larger cohorts than those involving prescreened populations. Nevertheless, the results of the nonexclusionary type of study with regard to the effects of SERMs on reproductive tissues can be generalized to a larger group of patient—namely, those who in practice do not undergo such rigorous prescreening prior to commencement of tamoxifen therapy.

REFERENCES

1. KILLACKEY, M.A., T.B. HAKES & V.K. PIERCE. 1985. Endometrial adenocarcinoma in breast cancer patients receiving antiestrogens. Cancer Treat. Rep. **69:** 237–238.
2. HARDELL, L. 1988. Tamoxifen as risk factor for carcinoma of corpus uteri [letter]. Lancet **2:** 563.
3. JORDAN, V.C. 1989. Tamoxifen and endometrial cancer [letter]. Lancet **2:** 117–120.
4. MATHEW, A., A.B. CHABON, B. KABAKOW et al. 1990. Endometrial carcinoma in five patients with breast cancer on tamoxifen therapy. N.Y. J. Med. **90:** 207–208.
5. ATLANTA, G., M. POZZI, C. VINCENZONI & G. VOCATURO. 1990. Four case reports presenting new acquisitions on the association between breast and endometrial carcinoma. Gynecol. Oncol. **37:** 378–380.
6. FORNANDER, T., L.E. RUTQVIST, B. CEDERMARK et al. 1989. Adjuvant tamoxifen in early breast cancer: occurrence of new primary cancers. Lancet **1:** 117–120.
7. NEVEN, P., X. DE MUYLDER, Y. VAN BELLE et al. 1990. Hysteroscopic follow-up during tamoxifen treatment. Eur. J. Obstet. Gynecol. Reprod. Biol. **35:** 235–238.
8. GAL, D., S. KOPEL, M. BASHEVKIN et al. 1991. Oncogenic potential of tamoxifen on endometria of postmenopausal women with breast cancer—preliminary report. Gynecol. Oncol. **42:** 120–123.
9. GOLDSTEIN, S.R., M. NACHTIGALL, J.R. SNYDER & L. NACHTIGALL. 1990. Endometrial assessment by vaginal ultrasonography before endometrial sampling in patients with postmenopausal bleeding. Am. J. Obstet. Gynecol. **163:** 119–123.
10. NASRI, M.N., J.H. SHEPARD, M.E. SETCHELL et al. 1991. The role of vaginal scan in measurement of endometrial thickness in postmenopausal women. Br. J. Obstet. Gynaecol. **98:** 470–475.
11. ANTEBY, E., S. YAGEL et al. 1992. False sonographic appearance of endometrial neoplasia in postmenopausal women treated with tamoxifen. Lancet **340:** 433.
12. THE WRITING GROUP FOR THE PEPI TRIAL. 1996. Effects of hormone replacement therapy on endometrial histology in postmenopausal women: the Postmenopausal Estrogen/Progestin Interventions (PEPI) Trial. JAMA **275:** 370–375.
13. FLEISCHER, A.C., J.E. WHEELER et al. 1999. Sonographic assessment of the endometrium in osteopenic postmenopausal women treated with idoxifene. J. Ultrasound Med. **18:** 503–512.
14. LANGER, R.D., J.J. PIERCE, K.A. O'HANLAN et al. FOR THE POSTMENOPAUSAL ESTROGEN/ PROGESTIN INTERVENTIONS TRIAL. 1997. Transvaginal ultrasonography compared with endometrial biopsy for the detection of endometrial disease. N. Engl. J. Med. **337:** 1792–1798.
15. BARAKAT, R.R., T.A. GILEWSKI, L. ALMADRONES et al. 2000. Effect of adjuvant tamoxifen on the endometrium in women with breast cancer: a prospective study using office endometrial biopsy. J. Clin. Oncol. **18:** 3459–3463.

16. COHEN, I., M.M. ALTARAS, J. SHAPIRA et al. 1997. Different coexisting endometrial histological features in asymptomatic postmenopausal breast cancer patients treated with tamoxifen. Gynecol. Obstet. Invest. **43:** 60–63.
17. SUH-BERGMAN, E.J. & A. GOODMAN. 1999. Surveillance for endometrial cancer in women receiving tamoxifen. Ann. Intern. Med. **131:** 127–135.
18. BERTELLI, G., M. VENTURINI, L. DEL MASTRO et al. 1998. Tamoxifen and the endometrium: findings of pelvic ultrasound examination and endometrial biopsy in asymptomatic breast cancer patients. Breast Cancer Res. Treat. **47:** 41–46.
19. BARAKAT, R.R. 1999. Endometrial cancer and tamoxifen. Primary Care Cancer **19**(suppl. 1): 27–30.
20. MARCONI, D., C. EXACOUSTOS, B. CANGI et al. 1997. Transvaginal sonographic and hysteroscopic findings in postmenopausal women receiving tamoxifen. J. Am. Assoc. Gynecol. Laparosc. **4:** 331–339.
21. NEVEN, P. & H. VERNAEVE. 2000. Guidelines for monitoring patients taking tamoxifen treatment. Drug Saf. **22:** 1–11.
22. COHEN, I., R. AZARIA, R. AVIRAM et al. 1999. Postmenopausal endometrial pathologies with tamoxifen treatment: comparison between hysteroscopic and hysterectomy findings. Gynecol. Obstet. Invest. **48:** 187–192.
23. SCHWARTZ, L.B., J. SNYDER et al. 1998. The use of transvaginal ultrasound and saline infusion sonohysterography for the evaluation of asymptomatic postmenopausal breast cancer patients on tamoxifen. Ultrasound Obstet. Gynecol. **11:** 48–53.
24. ACOG COMMITTEE OPINION (NO. 169). 1996. Tamoxifen and endometrial cancer: Committee on Gynecologic Practice, American College of Obstetricians and Gynecologists. Int. J. Gynaecol. Obstet. **53:** 197–199.
25. BERLIERE, M., A. CHARLES, C. GALANT & J. DONNEZ. 1998. Uterine side effects of tamoxifen: a need for systematic pretreatment screening. Obstet. Gynecol. **91:** 40–44.
26. BERLIERE, M., G. RADIKOV, C. GALANT et al. 2000. Identification of women at high risk of developing endometrial cancer on tamoxifen. Eur. J. Cancer **36:** S35–S36.
27. FISHER, B., J.P. COSTANTINO, D.L. WICKERHAM et al. 1998. Tamoxifen for prevention of breast cancer: report of the National Surgical Adjuvant Breast and Bowel Project P-1 Study. J. Natl. Cancer Inst. **90:** 1371–1388.
28. BLACK, L.J., M. SATO, E.R. ROWLEY et al. 1994. Raloxifene (LY139481 HCl) prevents bone loss and reduces serum cholesterol without causing uterine hypertrophy in ovariectomized rats. J. Clin. Invest. **93:** 63–69.
29. SATO, M., J. KIM, L.L. SHORT et al. 1995. Longitudinal and cross-sectional analysis of raloxifene effects on tibiae from ovariectomized aged rats. J. Pharmacol. Exp. Ther. **272:** 1252–1259.
30. BLACK, L.J., C.D. JONES & J.F. FALCONE. 1983. Antagonism of estrogen action with a new benzothiophene-derived antiestrogen. Life Sci. **32:** 1031–1036.
31. FUCHS-YOUNG, R., A.L. GLASEBROOK, L.L. SHORT et al. 1995. Raloxifene is a tissue-selective agonist/antagonist that functions through the estrogen receptor. Ann. N.Y. Acad. Sci. **761:** 355–360.
32. CUMMINGS, S.R., S. ECKERT, K.A. KRUEGER et al. 1999. The effect of raloxifene on risk of breast cancer in postmenopausal women: results from the MORE randomized trial. JAMA **316:** 2189–2197.
33. GOLDSTEIN, S.R., W.H. SHEELE, S.K. RAJAGOPALAN et al. 2000. A 12-month comparative study of raloxifene, estrogen, and placebo on the postmenopausal endometrium. Obstet. Gynecol. **95:** 95–103.

Effect of Selective Estrogen Receptor Modulators on Reproductive Tissues Other Than Endometrium

SUSAN L. HENDRIX AND S. GENE McNEELEY

Department of Obstetrics and Gynecology, Wayne State University/Hutzel Hospital, Detroit, Michigan 48201, USA

ABSTRACT: The objective of this paper is to review the published and unpublished knowledge of the effect of selective estrogen receptor modulators on reproductive tissues other than endometrium. Pharmaceutical companies developing or marketing selective estrogen receptor modulators (SERMs) were identified. The investigators at each company responsible for the conduct of investigational trials were contacted and queried about reports of adverse events in any ongoing or completed trials involving SERMs produced by their company. Levormeloxifene and idoxifene trials noted a higher proportion of surgery for pelvic organ prolapse in treated versus untreated women. The development of these pharmaceutical agents was discontinued, primarily for endometrial concerns. However, pelvic organ prolapse was reported to the FDA as an adverse event associated with both drugs. Study weaknesses preclude a definitive association between the agents and pelvic organ prolapse. The treated groups were not necessarily similar for confounding factors such as age, parity, obesity, cigarette smoking, and other risk factors for pelvic organ prolapse. Tamoxifen and raloxifene increase hot flash intensity and frequency. Ovarian cyst formation and uterine fibroid growth have also been reported with some SERMs. The identification and assessment of the impact of current and future SERMs on the pelvic floor and other genital tissues will be important to understanding their potential long-term application in disease treatment and prevention.

KEYWORDS: selective estrogen receptor modulators; pelvic organ prolapse; hot flashes; vagina; ovary; fallopian tube; myometrium; tamoxifen; raloxifene; idoxifene

INTRODUCTION

Selective estrogen receptor modulators (SERMs) make up a class of pharmacologic agents that have both estrogenic and antiestrogenic properties. Only three SERMs: raloxifene (Evista), tamoxifen (Nolvadex), and toremifene (Fareston), are

Address for correspondence: Susan L. Hendrix, D.O. Department of Obstetrics and Gynecology, Wayne State University/Hutzel Hospital, 4707 St. Antoine, Detroit, MI 48201. Voice: 313-966-910; fax: 313-993-8504.

shendrix@med.wayne.edu

approved by the Food and Drug Administration (FDA) for clinical use in women in various settings, but ongoing clinical trials are investigating new agents with a similar mechanism of action. Raloxifene is indicated for the prevention and treatment of osteoporosis; tamoxifen is indicated for the treatment of metastatic breast cancer, for use as an adjuvant therapy for the treatment of localized breast cancer, and for the reduction of risk of breast cancer in high-risk women; and toremifene is indicated for the treatment of advanced breast cancer.[1,2] Clomiphene citrate (Clomid, Serophene) is a SERM indicated for the treatment of anovulation.[3] It is prescribed for premenopausal women wishing to become pregnant. It is used intermittently for short segments of each month. Consequently, potential stimulatory effects on reproductive tissues that might result from long-term or continuous administration are unlikely to be observed in the context of its current clinical use. Therefore, it will not be reviewed in this paper.

SERMs are classified by their chemical structures. Among the SERMs, benzothiophenes form a class of compounds that have estrogen-antagonistic effects in both the breast and uterus and estrogen-like agonistic effects in bone and on serum lipid levels. Currently, raloxifene is the only FDA-approved drug in this class. Another class of SERMs, the triphenylethylenes, includes tamoxifen and its derivatives—i.e., toremifene, idoxifene, droloxifene, and miproxifene. Development of idoxifene, droloxifene, and miproxifene has been discontinued because of adverse effects on the uterus and endometrium. Triphenylethylenes are estrogen antagonistic in breast tissue, but, unlike benzothiophenes, they appear to be stimulatory in the endometrium.[4] Other SERMs in development include centchroman and various other chemical compounds that are still identified by their compound names. Centchroman (ormeloxifene), a nonsteroidal estrogen antagonist, is widely used in India as an oral antifertility drug that is taken once a week.[5] It has also been reported to have a beneficial effect on bone[6] and has been in development for the treatment of advanced breast cancer.[7]

Despite similar mechanisms of action, raloxifene, tamoxifen, and toremifene each has a unique pharmacologic profile. Numerous clinical trials have demonstrated not only the efficacy of each agent within its specific indications, but also the different effects that each SERM has on cardiovascular risk factors and the endometrium. These results have led to increased interest in finding a single agent that would have beneficial effects on the cardiovascular system, on breast tissue, and on bone density without excessively increasing the thickness of the endometrial lining, which is sometimes associated with endometrial cancer.[8]

Those drugs that are now known as SERMs were initially categorized as antiestrogens. However, after SERMs were discovered to have tissue-specific effects that were both estrogenic and antiestrogenic, drugs belonging to this class were reclassified as "selective estrogen receptor modulators." The mechanisms of action that control the selectivity of SERMs are multifaceted and not fully understood. However, preclinical and clinical evidence have led to the consensus that each SERM has a unique profile with regard to tissue specificity, allowing it to exert multiple benefits simultaneously. Because of this multiplicity of effects, it is important to consider monitoring the effect of these drugs on all reproductive tissues, not just the endometrium. This paper will review the effect of selective estrogen receptor modulators on reproductive tissues other than endometrium.

SERM EFFECTS IN REPRODUCTIVE TISSUES

Pelvic Organ Prolapse

The possibility of a risk of pelvic organ prolapse with SERMs first came to light in the clinical trials of levormeloxifene (Novo). This agent is the L-enantiomer of centrochroman (ormeloxifene). In a clinical trial of healthy postmenopausal women, levormeloxifene exhibited positive effects on bone mineral density and markers of bone turnover as well as strong, beneficial estrogenic effects on the serum concentrations of various cholesterol subfractions.[9] It has also been shown to have anti-atherogenic properties in preclinical experiments using rabbits.[10] The most important adverse clinical effect of this pharmaceutical agent has been the induction of increased endometrial thickness.[9] Ultimately, the development of levormeloxifene was discontinued, primarily because of the concerns regarding the endometrium. However, pelvic organ prolapse was reported to the FDA as an adverse event associated with the drug.

Idoxifene (Smith-Kline-Beecham, SKB) was the second SERM for which a preponderance of prolapse cases in treated versus untreated women was observed. Of 1436 nonhysterectomized women enrolled in two clinical trial groups, there were 9 uterine prolapses, 3 cystoceles (bladder prolapse), and 3 cystocele/rectocele (bladder/rectal prolapse) combinations, all identified in the treated group (14 cases total; 1 subject had uterine prolapse and cystocele/rectocele) and 0 cases in the untreated group.[11] The cohorts were evenly matched for body mass index (BMI) (a stratification variable) and age. Heavy cigarette smoking was an exclusion criterion, and data on parity were not collected. The difference between the treated and untreated groups was statistically significant by Fisher's exact test, $P \leq 0.0001$. As mentioned earlier, idoxifene has been discontinued from development for concerns regarding not only pelvic organ prolapse but also its effect on the endometrium.

Droloxifene, a structural analogue of tamoxifen (3-hydroxytamoxifen), behaves as an estrogen agonist in terms of its relation to bone as well as its impact on certain components of the lipid and coagulation profiles.[12] Its potential for use in advanced breast cancer was suggested by its ability to modulate plasma sex hormone levels in a direction resembling that seen during tamoxifen treatment in postmenopausal women with breast cancer.[13] In the phase 2 studies of droloxifene, the prevalence of all prolapse disorders in over 1000 women was 10%, the same in both the treatment and control arms.[14] In phase 3 studies involving 300 osteoporotic women on four different doses of droloxifene, the incidence of prolapse was the same in all groups. Clinical trials with this drug have been closed because of endometrial stimulation. Finally, to this author's knowledge, no increase in the incidence of pelvic prolapse has been reported with raloxifene (Lilly)[15] or tamoxifen (Astra Zeneca).[16]

While only levormeloxifene and idoxifene showed a problem with prolapse, all SERMs must be evaluated for this adverse effect. Yet, there are many questionable findings in the observations of adverse events in the clinical trials of these agents that have precipitated a more careful examination of the results. Thus, (1) although in the idoxifene study described above the prevalence of pelvic organ prolapse was higher in the group treated with idoxifene, the overall (both arms together) incidence of prolapse was extraordinarily low (0% in the untreated group, 1.5% in the treated group)—that is, considerably lower than that commonly reported in the general population. While pelvic organ prolapse is one of the most common indications for gynecologic surgery, there is little epidemiologic information regarding the condition. In one report from Quebec, it accounted for 13% of all hysterectomies in all age groups.[17] (2) Non–drug-related factors could account for the difference in the incidence of prolapse. Because the arms in the idoxifene study were not necessarily similar with regard to confounding factors such as age, parity, obesity, cigarette smoking, and other risk factors for pelvic organ prolapse, the relative incidence of prolapse in the two arms might have been skewed by imbalance in one or more of these etiologic factors, rather than by idoxifene per se. Additional biases, rather than drug intervention, might have contributed to the difference in incidence of prolapse between the groups. (3) The majority of the case reports on idoxifene occurred after rumors surfaced of problems with pelvic organ prolapse in the levormeloxifene phase 3 trial. The possibility exists that these revelations about levormeloxifene sensitized investigators to the need to look for prolapse.

Additional questions can be asked regarding the conduct of these clinical studies, and the same questions should be addressed in future trials incorporating pelvic organ prolapse as an end point. For example, (4) was the assessment for pelvic organ prolapse different among examiners? This question arises because a high probability exists that the women in these trials were examined by nongynecologists inexperienced in pelvic examination, as these were osteoporosis trials. If so, this could lead to an underestimate of the incidence of pelvic prolapse. Along the same lines, (5) were the changes mild and possibly no different from previous exams, but not previously assessed? (6) How was prolapse defined? Was it defined according to symptoms, examination, or the requirement for surgery? (7) Was the increase in prolapse severe enough to trigger surgical intervention that otherwise would not have been required? (8) Were the anatomic changes accompanied by functional changes or symptoms, such as urinary incontinence or dyspareunia? All of these questions should be addressed in future studies if a more thorough understanding of the clinical manifestation of pelvic prolapse in the setting of SERM therapy is to be clarified.

The mechanistic basis for SERM induction of pelvic prolapse also remains to be elucidated. Thus, preclinical studies should be conducted to investigate whether some SERMs modify or otherwise affect collagen, thereby increasing the elasticity of the pelvic floor tissues and increasing the risk for pelvic organ prolapse. If they do increase the elasticity of collagen, there may be a role for these medications in the treatment of diseases involving excessive production of collagen, such as scleroderma. There has been speculation that some SERMs may cause tissue edema, increasing the risk for prolapse by increasing the weight of the uterus. Perhaps some other mechanism that we do not yet understand accounts for the increased risk of pelvic organ prolapse.

In summary, the lessons learned from idoxifene and levormeloxifene should be incorporated into future clinical trial research on SERMs. Important modifications include the use of a standardized pelvic exam administered by gynecologists or other clinicians trained in a uniform approach. In addition, consideration should be given to excluding those women with moderate to severe prolapse until the effect of SERMs on the risk of prolapse are better known. Not only should the worsening of the condition of pelvic prolapse be assessed by examination, but the degree of clinical significance—that is, whether there is a requirement for further testing or surgical intervention—should also be addressed. Finally, the notation of anatomic worsening should be accompanied by an assessment of functional changes, such as urinary incontinence or dyspareunia.

Hot Flashes, Cognition, and Other Central Nervous System Effects of SERMs

All studies of tamoxifen have shown an increase in hot flashes in the majority of women treated. In the Breast Cancer Prevention Trial, 47.5% of women reported the increase as quite a bit or extremely bothersome, compared to 28.7% in the placebo group.[16] In clinical trials an increased incidence of new or an exacerbation of existing hot flashes has been observed among women treated with raloxifene; however, this effect appears to resolve after six months.[18] These events occurred in a minority of women (7/100) and were mild to moderate. Although idoxifene did not cause worsening in the frequency or severity of hot flashes in phase 2 studies,[19] effects resembling those observed with raloxifene were seen in the phase 3 trials.[11]

The link between estrogen withdrawal, hot flashes, and a negative effect on cognitive function has been empirically noted in the clinical setting.[20] Although there is an association between restoring estrogen and improving cognitive function, this link has not been definitively attributed to direct effects of estrogen on mentation. Rather, clinicians have observed that hormone replacement therapy (HRT) alleviates many menopausal symptoms, such as hot flashes and sleep interruption, that are associated with a diminution in cognitive function.[21] While these clinical observations support an indirect effect of estrogen on the improvement of cognitive function, recent evidence for a more direct role for estrogen has emerged from the discovery that there is a connection between estrogen receptors found in immune cells and brain function. Microglia, or brain macrophages, affect brain function, development, and injury. Studies on macrophage activity in aging rats showed that estrogen is an activator of macrophage activity and that repeated activation produces free radicals. These free radicals contribute to the development of hypothalamic failure due to neuronal and astroglial damage. The same study showed that the pathologic changes that accompanied the aging process in rats were directly attributable to estrogen receptor activity. The investigators found that treatment with raloxifene produced an estrogen-antagonistic effect in the estrogen receptors found in the microglia of rats and prevented hypothalamic failure.[22] Conversely, in another experimental study that looked at the effect of raloxifene on the brain in order to evaluate the effect of selective estrogenic/antiestrogenic activity on neuronal activity, raloxifene acted in an estrogenic fashion with respect to neuronal outgrowth.[23] The data are therefore inconsistent, and further study is required if we are to understand the true effect(s) of estrogen and SERMs on brain activity.

Ovary and Fallopian Tube

Tamoxifen was associated with an 81% increased risk of ovarian cyst formation in women still having menstrual cycles.[24] Those receiving high-dose chemotherapy did not develop ovarian cysts. Conflicting information exists on postmenopausal women. Although Mourits et al.[24] did not find an association, Schwartz et al.[25] showed an increase in both ovarian cyst formation and uterine fibroid growth. Droloxifene was associated with hydrosalpinx in a woman with a previous tubal ligation.[26] A mild cystocele/rectocele was reported in the same patient. Hydrosalpinx was also seen in some women in the idoxifene trial.[11]

Because we do not routinely assess the ovary ultrasonographically outside of clinical trials, we do not fully understand the clinical significance of conditions like ovarian cyst formation and hydrosalpinx found incidentally in postmenopausal women. We do not know if the increase in ovarian cyst formation is associated with an increase in the risk of endometriomas or ovarian cancer. The concern is that ovarian stimulation may increase the risk of malignant transformation. Even if the ovarian enlargement is benign, the growth of cysts may trigger surgical intervention, with its incumbent morbidity, that otherwise would not have been required. Future studies should examine these changes in the ovary and fallopian tube to better understand their consequence.

Vagina

Twenty-nine percent of the women in the Breast Cancer Prevention Trial reported moderately bothersome or worse vaginal discharge, compared to 13% on placebo.[16] There were no significant differences in the reported adverse events associated with vaginal atrophy (vaginitis, leukorrhea, decreased libido, or dyspareunia) in eight clinical studies of 2789 postmenopausal women randomized to raloxifene or placebo or ERT/HRT.[18,27–30] Urinary incontinence was also not significantly different among the raloxifene, placebo, and HRT groups, but was greater in women treated with estrogen alone (estrogen 4.3%; raloxifene 0%; $P < 0.05$).

The clinical relevance of vaginal discharge seen in these clinical trials is unknown. The concern is that the discharge might represent infection. The pH, and along with it the microflora, changes with menopause. SERMs may have an impact on these factors. The possibility exists that some SERMs might improve sexual function in sexually active women, by increasing vaginal lubrication.

Myometrium

Tamoxifen has been implicated in the increased growth of uterine fibroids.[31] Fibroid growth was also seen in a few participants in the idoxifene trial.[11] This increase in fibroid growth might well trigger surgical intervention that otherwise would not have been required. Furthermore, as in the case of ovarian stimulation, the increase in myometrial cell proliferation might increase the risk for malignant transformation.

GOALS FOR THE FUTURE

There are other SERMs still in development. Two SERMs that are nearing, or have recently entered, the clinical trial phase of development are TSE424 (Wyeth) and SERM 3 (Lilly). The identification and assessment of the impact that current and future SERMs have on the pelvic floor and other genital tissues will be important to envisioning their long-term application in disease treatment and prevention.

REFERENCES

1. JORDAN, V.C. & M. MORROW. 1999. Raloxifene as a multifunctional medicine? [editorial]. Br. Med. J. **319:** 331–332.

2. MITLAK, B.H. & F.J. COHEN. 1999. Selective estrogen receptor modulators: a look ahead. Drugs **57:** 653–663.
3. Clomid® (clomiphene citrate tablets USP). 2000. *In* Physicians' Desk Reference: 1366–1368. Medical Economics Co. Montvale, NJ.
4. BRYANT, H.U. & W.H. DERE. 1998. Selective estrogen receptor modulators: an alternative to hormone replacement therapy. Proc. Soc. Exp. Biol. Med. **217:** 45–52.
5. SINGH, M.M. 2001. Centchroman, a selective estrogen receptor modulator, as a contraceptive and for the management of hormone-related clinical disorders. Med. Res. Rev. **21:** 302–347.
6. WILLIAMS, J.P., J.M. MCDONALD, M.A. MCKENNA, *et al.* 1997. Differential effects of tamoxifen-like compounds on osteoclast bone degradation, H(+)-ATPase activity, calmodulin-dependent cyclic nucleotide phosphodiesterase activity, and calmodulin binding. J. Cell. Biochem. **66:** 358–369.
7. MISRA, N.C., P.K. NIGAM, R. GUPTA, *et al.* 1989. Centchroman—a non-steroidal anticancer agent for advanced breast cancer: phase-II study. Int. J. Cancer **43:** 781–783.
8. FISHER, B., J.P. COSTANTINO, D.L. WICKERHAM, *et al.* 1998. Tamoxifen for prevention of breast cancer: report of the National Surgical Adjuvant Breast and Bowel Project P-1 Study. J. Natl. Cancer Inst. **90:** 1371–1388.
9. ALEXANDERSEN, P., B.J. RIIS, J.A. STAKKESTAD, *et al.* 2001. Efficacy of levormeloxifene in the prevention of postmenopausal bone loss and the lipid profile compared to low dose hormone replacement therapy. J. Clin. Endocrinol. Metab. **86:** 755–760.
10. HOLM, P., M. SHALMI, N. KORSGAARD, *et al.* 1997. A partial estrogen receptor agonist with strong antiatherogenic properties without noticeable effects on reproductive tissue in cholesterol-fed female and male rabbits. Arterioscler. Thromb. Vasc. Biol. **17:** 2264–2272.
11. B. MACDONALD. Personal communication. Smith-Klein-Beecham.
12. HERRINGTON, D.M., B.E. PUSSER, W.A. RILEY, *et al.* 2000. Cardiovascular effects of droloxifene, a new selective estrogen receptor modulator, in healthy postmenopausal women. Arterioscler. Thromb. Vasc. Bio. **20:** 1606–1612.
13. GEISLER, J., H. HAARSTAD, S. GUNDERSEN, *et al.* 1995. Influence of treatment with the anti-oestrogen 3-hydroxytamoxifen (droloxifene) on plasma sex hormone levels in postmenopausal patients with breast cancer. J. Endocrinol. **146:** 359–363.
14. A. LEE. Personal communication. Pfizer.
15. L. PLOUFFE. Personal communication. Lilly.
16. FISHER, B., J.P. COSTANTINO, D.L. WICKERHAM, *et al.* 1998. Tamoxifen for prevention of breast cancer: report of the National Surgical Adjuvant Breast and Bowel Project P-1 Study. J. Natl. Cancer Inst. **90:** 1371–1388.
17. ALLARD P. & L. ROCHETTE. 1991. The descriptive epidemiology of hysterectomy, Province of Quebec, 1981–1988. Ann. Epidemiol. **1:** 541–549.
18. DAVIES, G.C., W.J. HUSTER, Y. LU, *et al.* 1999. Adverse events reported by postmenopausal women in controlled trials with raloxifene. Obstet. Gynecol. **93:** 558–565.
19. HENDRIX, S., D. FITTS, M. WATTROUS, B. MACDONALD. 1997. Idoxifene improves menopausal symptoms in a short term dose ranging study. Proc. North Am. Menopause Soc. (Abstr. no. 97.099).
20. PHILLIPS, S.M. & B.B. SHERWIN. 1992. Effects of estrogen on memory function in surgically menopausal women. Psychoneuroendocrinology **17:** 485–495.
21. NAFTOLIN, F. 1997. Menopause and cognition: short-term memory impairment. Menopause Management. September/October: 17–19.
22. SEIFER, D., L. ROA-PEOA, D. KEEFE, *et al.* 1994. Increasing hypothalamic arcuate nucleus glial peroxidase activity in aging female rats is reduced by antiestrogen and gonadotropin releasing hormone agonist. Menopause **1:** 83–90.
23. NILSEN, J., G. MOR & F. NAFTOLIN. 1998. Raloxifene induces neurite outgrowth in receptor positive PC12 cells. Menopause **5:** 211–216.
24. MOURITS, M.J., E.G. DE VRIES, P.H. WILLEMSE, *et al.* 1999. Ovarian cysts in women receiving tamoxifen for breast cancer. Br. J. Cancer **79:** 1761–1764.
25. SCHWARTZ, L.B., N. RUTKOWSKI, C. HORAN, *et al.* 1998. Use of transvaginal ultrasonography to monitor the effects of tamoxifen on uterine leiomyoma size and ovarian cyst formation. 1998. J. Ultrasound Med. **17:** 699–703.

26. PFIZER PHARMACEUTICALS. 1999. MedWatch FDA Adverse Event Report on Droloxifene, no. 9045434.
27. JOHNSTON, C.C., N.H. BJARNASON, F.J. COHEN, et al. 2000. Long-term effects of raloxifene on bone mineral density, bone turnover, and serum lipid levels in early postmenopausal women. Three-year data from two double-blind, randomized, placebo-controlled trials. Arch. Intern. Med. **160:** 3444–3450.
28. MEUNIER, P.J., E. VIGNOT, P. GARNERO, et al. 1999. Treatment of postmenopausal women with osteoporosis or low bone density with raloxifene. Raloxifene Study Group. Osteoporos. Int. **10:** 330–336.
29. GLUSMAN, J.E., W.J. HUSTER & S. PAUL. 1998. Raloxifene effects on vasomotor and other climacteric symptoms in postmenopausal women. Primary Care Update. Obstet. Gynecol. **5:** 166.
30. ETTINGER, B., D.M. BLACK, B.H. MITLAK, et al. FOR THE MULTIPLE OUTCOMES OF RALOXIFENE EVALUATION (MORE) INVESTIGATORS. 1999. Reduction of vertebral fracture risk in postmenopausal women with osteoporosis treated with raloxifene: results from a 3-year randomized clinical trial. JAMA **282:** 637–645.
31. LEO, L., A. LANZA, A. RE, et al. 1994. Leiomyomas in patients receiving tamoxifen. Clin. Exp. Obstet. Gynecol. **21:** 94–98.

The Effect of Selective Estrogen Receptor Modulators on Parameters of the Hypothalamic-Pituitary-Gonadal Axis

LEO PLOUFFE, JR. AND SURESH SIDDHANTI

Lilly Research Laboratories, Eli Lilly and Company, Indianapolis, Indiana 46284, USA

ABSTRACT: The SERMs currently in clinical practice or in late stages of clinical development have been studied primarily for their effects on the breast, cardiovascular, bone, and reproductive systems. The effect of SERMs on the hypothalamic-pituitary-gonadal (HPG) axis has not been the primary focus of the studies conducted thus far. However the effect of SERMs on the HPG axis and the associated regulation of endocrine parameters may play an important role in their overall clinical profile. In this review the effects of selected SERMs on the HPG axis in premenopausal women, postmenopausal women, and men are summarized.

KEYWORDS: selective estrogen receptor modulators; hypothalamic-pituitary-gonadal axis; premenopause; postmenopause; males

INTRODUCTION

By definition, a selective estrogen receptor modulator (SERM) is a compound that can act as an estrogen agonist or antagonist, depending on the specific target tissue.[1] At present, four SERMs are approved by regulatory agencies for clinical use (TABLE 1). Three of these compounds belong to the triphenylethylene family: clomiphene (CLOM), tamoxifen (TAM) and toremifene (TOR).[2] Raloxifene (RAL), the other SERM in clinical use, belongs to the benzothiophene family.

Clomiphene is indicated for use in premenopausal women only, while TAM and TOR may be used in premenopausal or postmenopausal women.[2] The clinical use of RAL is restricted to postmenopausal women.[2] In addition, many other SERMs are in various stages of clinical development for a number of indications, including arzoxifene, EM-800 and 652, and lasofoxifene.[3–6]

To date, relatively little attention has been paid to the effects of SERMs on the hypothalamic-pituitary-gonadal (HPG) axis in the development of these compounds. However, these effects actually may represent an important dimension of the profile of SERMs. The ability to use SERMs for an expanding number of indications will relate, in large part, to the ability to modulate the effect of SERMs on the HPG axis.

Address for correspondence: Leo Plouffe, Jr., M.D., C.M., Medical Director, U.S. Women's Health and Reproductive Medicine, Lilly Research Laboratories, Eli Lilly and Company, Indianapolis, IN 46285. Phone: 317-277-6284; fax: 317-277-3743.
lplouffe@lilly.com

TABLE 1. SERMs approved for use in the United States

SERM	Indication for use
Clomiphene	treatment of ovulatory dysfunction in women desiring pregnancy
Raloxifene	treatment and prevention of osteoporosis in postmenopausal women
Tamoxifen	treatment of metastatic breast cancer in women and men reduction in risk of breast cancer in women at high risk of breast cancer
Toremifene	treatment of metastatic breast cancer in postmenopausal women with estrogen receptor positive or unknown tumors

TABLE 2. Effects of estrogenic compounds on selected components of hypothalamic-pituitary-gonadal axis

Factor	Premenopause/reproductive years	Postmenopause
GnRH	inhibitory/stimulatory	inhibitory
FSH	↓	↓
LH	↓	↓
Estradiol	NA	NA
Testosterone	↓	↓
SHBG	↑	↑

SYMBOLS AND ABBREVIATIONS: ↓ = decrease; ↑ = increase; GnRH = gonadotropin-releaseing hormone; FSH = follicle-stimulating hormone; LH = luteinizing hormone; SHBG = sex hormone–binding globulin; NA = not available.

We present here a review about some of the known effects of selected SERMs on the HPG axis in premenopausal women, postmenopausal women, and men.

BACKGROUND CONSIDERATIONS

The hypothalamic-pituitary-gonadal axis is an intricately regulated endocrine system that involves the interplay of a large number of steroid and peptide hormones.[7] For the purpose of this presentation, we will examine the effect of selected SERMs on gonadotropin-releasing hormone (GnRH), follicle-stimulating hormone (FSH), luteinizing hormone (LH), prolactin (PRL), the gonadal hormones including estradiol (E2), testosterone (T), and sex hormone–binding globulin (SHBG), the primary binding protein for circulating sex steroids.

In order to assess the effects of SERMs on the parameters outlined above, it is helpful to review the effect of estrogenic compounds on them. These effects are summarized in TABLE 2.[8] As the table outlines, the overall effects are qualitatively similar during the reproductive years and the postmenopausal period.

The gonadotropin axis displays an additional level of complexity relating to ovulation in women. At midcycle, high sustained serum levels of estradiol lead to in-

TABLE 3. Relative effects of equal doses of estrogenic compounds on sex hormone–binding globulin (SHBG) and follicle-stimulating hormone (FSH)[a]

Equal dosage of estrogen	Relative effect on SHBG	Relative effect on FSH
Conjugated equine estrogen	32	1.4
Micronized E2 (oral)	1.0	1.3
Piperazine estrone sulfate	1.0	1.1
Ethinyl estradiol	614	200

[a]Modified from Mashchak et al.[9]

creased levels of GnRH, FSH and LH.[8] This stimulatory effect of estrogens on the gonadotropins is seen only at the time of midcycle corresponding to ovulation and is not truly relevant to the current discussion, which focuses on chronic exposure to SERMs.

While all estrogens act qualitatively the same, the efficacy of different estrogen preparations has been compared through studies in postmenopausal women. The data, although limited, clearly indicate differences between various estrogens for their action profile on specific targets (TABLE 3).[9] For example, on a per mg basis, conjugated equine estrogens increase SHBG 32-fold compared with oral micronized estradiol, whereas both compounds have nearly comparable effects in reducing serum FSH levels. The differential effects of various SERMs on serum levels of individual target gonadotropins highlight the need to generate compound-specific data for each parameter.

Finally, it must be remembered that since the effect of SERMs may be influenced by the prevalent hormonal environment, the effects of SERMs must be examined separately for premenopausal and postmenopausal women.

EFFECTS IN PREMENOPAUSAL WOMEN

Clomiphene citrate (CC) was introduced in the early 1960s for the purpose of ovulation induction.[10] Over the past 30 years, CC has remained the most widely used medication in the management of anovulatory infertility.[11] Its use, therefore, is limited to premenopausal women.

Tamoxifen (TAM) and toremifene (TOR) are both approved for clinical use in premenopausal women. Tamoxifen is used extensively throughout the world in the management of breast cancer as well as in risk reduction of breast cancer in women over age 35 who are at high risk for breast cancer.[2] Toremifene is another SERM in use for the management of breast cancer patients.[2]

In contrast, there is no indication to use raloxifene (RAL) in premenopausal women.[12] Its clinical development was focused entirely on indications related to postmenopausal women.[2] The data in premenopausal women with RAL comes from phase 2 studies focusing on the pharmacologic and physiologic properties of the compound. Similar to raloxifene, the majority of new SERMs in clinical development are targeting postmenopausal indications.

TABLE 4. Reported effects of selected SERMs in premenopausal women[a]

Parameter assessed	Clomiphene citrate	Tamoxifen citrate	Raloxifene HCl
GnRH	stimulatory	probably stimulatory	probably stimulatory
FSH	↑	↑	↑
LH	↑	↑	↑
Estradiol	↑↑↑	↑↑↑	↑↑
Other estrogens	↑	↑	↑
Testosterone	NA	NA	NA
SHBG	↑	↑	↑

[a]Adapted from Adashi,[11] Bernades et al.,[13] and Baker et al.[12]

SYMBOLS AND ABBREVIATIONS: ↑ = increase; GnRH = gonadotropin-releasing hormone; FSH = follicle-stimulating hormone; LH = luteinizing hormone; SHBG = sex hormone–binding hormone; NA = not available.

To our knowledge, there are no head-to-head trials comparing different SERMs specifically for their effects on the hypothalamic-pituitary-ovarian (HPO) axis or SHBG in premenopausal women. The available data for individual SERMs do support a dose-related effect for most compounds in terms of their action on FSH and other parameters.[11–12] Furthermore, the directional impact of various SERMs on parameters of the HPO axis and SHBG in premenopausal women shows a degree of similarity (TABLE 4).[11–13]

As outlined in TABLE 4, at least three SERMs have been shown to increase circulating levels of FSH and LH in premenopausal women. The exact mechanism for this rise is postulated to result from estrogen antagonist activity of the SERMs at the level of the hypothalamus and pituitary,[11] and the rise in estradiol is attributed to the increases in FSH. Total testosterone levels remain relatively unchanged, but all compounds increase SHBG in premenopausal women, which is an important consideration with respect to the levels of circulating free hormone. We are unaware of any data generated on the effects of SERMs on the circulating levels of free hormones, such as estradiol or testosterone.

Taken together, the current data indicate that, in varying degrees, many SERMs stimulate or enhance the hormonal changes that accompany ovulation in premenopausal women. Depending on the context, this can be a desired effect (e.g., ovulation induction in women with chronic anovulation), or it may be perceived as an undesirable side effect. Clomiphene citrate is used specifically for its ability to induce ovulation or to increase the number of follicles produced in a given cycle, in the hope of achieving a pregnancy.[11]

In contrast, in women being treated for breast cancer the occurrence of ovarian cysts and high circulating levels of estradiol that may occur with the use of tamoxifen in reproductive age women is a well-documented adverse event.[14] The ovarian cysts may cause discomfort and, rarely, result in conditions requiring surgical intervention. Recent reports have proposed that the ovarian stimulation from tamoxifen in premenopausal women can be blocked or reversed by the concurrent use of a long-acting GnRH agonist.[15]

A number of challenges remain in our understanding the effect of SERMs in premenopausal women. The effect on FSH and LH, shown in the table as an increase,

TABLE 5. Reported effects of selected SERMs in postmenopausal women

Parameter	Tamoxifen	Toremifene	Raloxifene	Droloxifene	Overall
GnRH	inhibitory	inhibitory	inhibitory	inhibitory	inhibitory[a]
FSH	↓↓	↓	↓	↓	↓
LH	↓↓	↓	↔	↔	↓
Estradiol	↓ / ↔ / ↑	↓	↔	↔	↔
Other estrogens	↔ / ↑	↔	↔	↔	↔
Testosterone	↔ / ↓	?	?	?	?
SHBG	↑	↑	↑	↑	↑

[a]Primarily suspected on the basis of FSH/LH effects.
SYMBOLS AND ABBREVIATIONS: ↓ = decrease; ↑ = increase; ↔ = no change; GnRH = gonadotropin-releasing hormone; FSH = follicle-stimulating hormone; LH = luteinizing hormone; SHBG = sex hormone–binding globulin.

is actually much more complex and represents changes in pulsatile release of these two hormones. This in turn could indicate a significant impact of SERMs on the GnRH pulse generator, which deserves more in-depth study.

The increased understanding of the mechanism of action of SERMs gives rise to a number of possibilities for the further development of compounds targeted to reproductive-age women. The ideal SERM would have different effects on the HPO axis based on the target indication. For example, in the context of ovulation induction, an ideal SERM would be a potent stimulator of FSH release while having a neutral effect on LH and prolactin. In contrast, a SERM designed for the treatment of endometriosis would have a neutral or even inhibitory effect on FSH and LH while being neutral on the other parameters. Finally, the ideal SERM for breast cancer risk reduction or treatment should be neutral on the HPO axis in premenopausal women. Much additional research is required to reach this high level of selectivity.

EFFECTS IN POSTMENOPAUSAL WOMEN

The clinical use of SERMs in postmenopausal women has been limited to RAL, TAM, and TOR.[2] Raloxifene HCl is indicated for the prevention and treatment of postmenopausal osteoporosis.[16,17] The indications for TAM and TOR relate to breast cancer, either in the context of treatment (TAM and TOR) or risk reduction (TAM).[2]

The known effects of SERMs on the HPO axis in postmenopausal women are shown in TABLE 5.[18–21] These data indicate that SERMs demonstrate an overall partial estrogen agonist effect in postmenopausal women. This contrasts with the primarily antagonistic activity on FSH and LH seen in reproductive-age women, as discussed above. As with premenopausal women, there are no head-to-head studies comparing these agents for their effects on the HPO axis. Results from studies examining tamoxifen, toremifene, raloxifene, or other SERMs alone suggest that differences may exist between the various compounds in terms of their effects on the HPO axis (Refs. 18–21 and data on file).

The clinical consequences of the effects of SERMs on the HPO axis in postmenopausal women have rarely been the focus of attention. For example, one report discusses the occasional association of TAM use and the development of benign ovarian cysts in postmenopausal women.[22] Overall, these effects are currently felt to have less clinical importance in postmenopausal women than in reproductive-age women. Further insights into the dynamics of the HPO axis, such as that of controlling circulating testosterone levels in postmenopausal women, may change the level of attention given to SERM effects in postmenopausal women.

EFFECTS IN MALES

There have been relatively few studies of SERMs in males. Clomiphene citrate and TAM have been proposed in the literature for the management of male-related infertility.[23–25] One study of TAM in males documented increased levels of FSH and LH with an accompanying increase in testosterone levels.[25] More recently, the principles of evidence-based medicine have fueled an extensive review of the literature around SERMs and male infertility.[26] This comprehensive review of the data supports the consistent stimulation of FSH and LH release by CC and TAM but fails to find definite evidence of improved fertility with these treatments.[26] Further studies are indicated to define the role of existing SERMs in the management of male infertility and explore the potential of new SERMs in this therapeutic area.

FUTURE RESEARCH EFFORTS

Most of the clinical research around SERMs has focused on their effect on primary target tissues, such as the breast, skeletal, and cardiovascular systems.[2] Except for investigations on fertility, studies investigating the effects of SERMs on the HPG axis have been limited and, in general, have been a secondary focus of the investigation and clinical development of the compound. Yet, these effects are of clear relevance to women of reproductive age, and may well be for postmenopausal women and men.

Future research in women should focus on further characterizing potential differences between SERMs on a wide range of hormonal parameters. Changes in the HPO axis in response to SERMs relative to the recent onset of menopause should be explored. Effects in males relative to aging should also be evaluated.

While there are a number of differences in the effects of these compounds on various target tissues, at present the data are too limited to suggest significant differences in terms of activity on the hypothalamic-gonadal axis. Further studies are needed to sort out potential differences and to introduce new compounds with more selective activity for these parameters.

As was stated before, a new focus of SERM research will need to be the development of compounds that have selective activity on components of the HPG axis, including variable modulation of the GnRH pulse generator and differential effects on FSH and LH. The overall impact on circulating levels of estradiol, testosterone, other sex steroids, and SHBG should also be the focus of targeted efforts in developing new SERMs.

REFERENCES

1. SATO, M., A.L. GLASEBROOK & H.U. BRYANT. 1994. Raloxifene: a selective estrogen receptor modulator. J. Bone Miner. Metab. **12**(2): S9–S20.
2. PLOUFFE, L., JR. 2000. Selective estrogen receptor modulators (SERMs) in clinical practice. [Review] J. Soc. Gynecol. Invest. **7**: S38–S46.
3. SATO, M., C.H. TURNER, T. WANG, et al. 1998. LY353381 HCl: a novel raloxifene analog with improved SERM potency and efficacy in vivo. J. Pharmacol. Exp. Ther. **287**(1): 1–7.
4. LUO, S., C. LABRIE, A. BELANGER, et al. 1998. Prevention of development of dimethylbenz(a)anthracene (DMBA)–induced mammary tumors in the rat by the new nonsteroidal antiestrogen EM-800 (SCH57050). Breast Cancer Res. Treat. **49**(1): 1–11.
5. KE, H.Z., H. QI, D.T. CRAWFORD, et al. 2000. Lasofoxifene (CP-336,156), a selective estrogen receptor modulator, prevents bone loss induced by aging and orchidectomy in the adult rat. Endocrinology **141**(4): 1338–1344.
6. LABRIE, F., C. LABRIE, A. BELANGER, et al. 1999. EM-652 (SCH 57068), a third generation SERM acting as pure antiestrogen in the mammary gland and endometrium. [Review] J. Steroid Biochem. **69**(1–6): 51–84.
7. DANIELS, G. & J. MARTIN. 1991. Neuroendocrine regulation and diseases of the anterior pituitary and hypothalamus. In Harrison's Principles of Internal Medicine, Part 12. J. Wilson, E. Braunwald, J. Isselbacher, et al., Eds.: 1655–1679.
8. FERIN, M.J. 1996. The menstrual cycle: an integrative view. In Reproductive Endocrinology, Surgery, and Technology. E.Y. Adashi, J.A. Rock & Z. Rosenwaks, Eds: 103–121. Lippincott-Raven. Philadelphia.
9. MASHCHAK, C.A., R.A. LOBO, R. DOZONO-TAKANO, et al. 1982. Comparison of pharmacodynamic properties of various estrogen formulations. Am. J. Obstet. Gynecol. **144**(5): 511–518.
10. GREENBLATT, R.B., W.E. BARFIELD, E.C. JUNGCK & A.W. RAY. 1961. Induction of ovulation with MRL/41. JAMA **178**: 101–104.
11. ADASHI, E.Y. 1996. Ovulation induction: clomiphene citrate. In Reproductive Endocrinology, Surgery, and Technology. E.Y. Adashi, J.A. Rock & Z. Rosenwaks, Eds: 1181–1206. Lippincott-Raven. Philadelphia.
12. BAKER, V.L., M. DRAPER, S. PAUL, et al. 1998. Reproductive endocrine and endometrial effects of raloxifene hydrochloride, a selective estrogen receptor modulator, in women with regular menstrual cycles. J. Clin. Endocrinol. Metab. **83**(1): 6–13.
13. BERNARDES, J.R., JR., S. NONOGAKI, M.T. SEIXAS, et al. 1999. Effect of a half dose of tamoxifen on proliferative activity in normal breast tissue. Int. J. Gynecol. Obstet. **67**: 33–38.
14. COHEN, I., A. FIGER, R. TEPPER, et al. 1999. Ovarian overstimulation and cystic formation in premenopausal tamoxifen exposure: comparison between tamoxifen-treated and nontreated breast cancer patients. Gynecol. Oncol. **72**(2): 202–207.
15. COHEN, I., R. TEPPER, A. FIGER, et al. 1999. Successful co-treatment with LHRH-agonist for ovarian over-stimulation and cystic formation in premenopausal tamoxifen exposure. Breast Cancer Res. Treat. **55**(2): 119–125.
16. DELMAS, P., N. BJARNASON, B. MITLAK, et al. 1997. Effects of raloxifene on bone mineral density, serum cholesterol concentration, and uterine endometrium in postmenopausal women. N. Engl. J. Med. **337**(23): 1641–1647.
17. ETTINGER, B. 1999. Reduction of vertebral fracture risk in postmenopausal women with osteoporosis treated with raloxifene. JAMA **282**(7): 638–645.
18. LONNING, P.E., D.C. JOHANNESSEN, E.A. LIEN, et al. 1995. Influence of tamoxifen on sex hormones, gonadotrophins and sex hormone binding globulin in postmenopausal breast cancer patients. J. Steroid Biochem. **52**: 491–496.
19. KOSTOGLOU-ATHANASSIOU, I., K. NTALLES, J. GOGAS, et al. 1997. Sex hormones in postmenopausal women with breast cancer on tamoxifen. Horm. Res. **47**(3): 116–120.
20. SZAMEL, I., I. HINDY, B. BUDAI, et al. 1998. Endocrine mechanism of action of toremifene at the level of the central nervous system in advanced breast cancer patients. Cancer Chemother. Pharmacol. **42**(3): 241–246.

21. GEISLER, J., D. EKSE, S. HOSCH & P.E. LONNING. 1995. Influence of droloxifene (3hydroxytamoxifen), 40 mg daily, on plasma gonadotrophins, sex hormone binding globulin and estrogen legels in postmenopausal breast cancer patients. J. Steroid Biochem. **55:** 193–195.
22. SHUSHAN, A., T. PERETZ, B. UZIELY, *et al.* 1996. Ovarian cysts in premenopausal and postmenopausal tamoxifen-treated women with breast cancer. Am. J. Obstet. Gynecol. **175**(3 Pt. 1): 752–753.
23. GONZALES, G.F., A. SALIRROSAS, D. TORRES, *et al.* 1998. Use of clomiphene citrate in the treatment of men with high sperm chromatin stability. Fertil. Steril. **69**(6): 1109–1115.
24. HAMMAMI, M.M. 1996. Hormonal evaluation in idiopathic oligozoospermia: correlation with response to clomiphene citrate therapy and sperm motility. Arch. Androl. **36**(3): 225–232.
25. KADIOGLU, T.C., I.T. KOKSAL & M. TUNC. 1999. Treatment of idiopathic and postvaricocelectomy oligozoospermia with oral tamoxifen citrate. Br. J.Urol. Int. **83**(6): 646–648.
26. VANDEKERCKHOVE, P., R. LILFORD, A. VAIL & E. HUGHES. 2000. Clomiphene or tamoxifen for idiopathic oligo/asthenospermia. Cochrane Database Syst. Rev. **45**(2): CD000151.

Translation of Basic Research: Finding the Perfect SERM

Introduction

FRANCIS L. BELLINO[a] AND LORETTA FINNEGAN[b]

[a]*National Institute on Aging, National Institutes of Health, Bethesda, Maryland 20892, USA*

[b]*Office of Research on Women's Health, National Institutes of Health, Bethesda, Maryland 20892, USA*

Is a single compound that mimics all of the beneficial effects of estradiol in peri- and postmenopausal women, with none of the potentially harmful effects, that is, the "perfect SERM", an achievable goal or so utopian as to be unrealistic to pursue? Can this goal be achieved with a single compound or a judicious choice of compounds tailored to the needs of the individual woman? What resources and support can the NIH provide to facilitate achievement of effective treatment options for peri- and postmenopausal women that accommodate their specific health protective needs without exacerbating health problems for which they may be at risk?

To develop improved SERMs, future research should focus on understanding the biology of SERM action. For example, results from the Heart and Estrogen/Progestin Replacement Study[1] and the Estrogen Replacement and Atherosclerosis Trial,[2] as well as early findings from the Women's Health Initiative,[3] suggested that the estrogen-responsive health-related issues need to be addressed in the cardiovascular system. Thus, we require a better understanding of the biology of estrogen action in specific tissues under normal, predisease, and disease conditions. Are SERMs and estrogens acting in a similar manner? By focusing on research conducted in young adult animals, can we gain insight into age-related changes in the biology of estrogen and/or SERM action that would enhance our understanding of the use of these compounds in middle-aged and older women?

One approach to addressing the question of whether SERMs and estrogen act in a similar fashion is to utilize gene expression microarrays and proteomics targeting estrogen action in specific tissues. Another approach is to develop model systems, both human primary cells from various tissues as well as animal models (including increasing numbers of nonhuman primates) specific for primary and secondary prevention research.

The logic and performance of preclinical testing protocols are paramount to the development of the perfect SERM or optimal combination of therapies. Preclinical

Address for correspondence: Francis L. Bellino, Ph.D., Biology of Aging Program, National Institute on Aging, 7201 Wisconsin Avenue, Suite 2C231, Bethesda, MD 20892-9205. Voice: 301-496-6402; fax: 301-402-0010.

bellinof@nia.nih.gov

testing should be sensitive to the validity and limitations of whatever animal models and other model systems (such as cell culture systems) are employed and should take into consideration the process and consequences of aging. Pharmacokinetics and short- and long-term toxicity of the parent drug and major metabolites are key issues that need to be considered. Valid surrogate end points should be established for long-term consequences such as breast or uterine cancer. Eliminating an unsuccessful candidate drug at an earlier stage of development will leave more funds available for additional drug discovery and testing of more promising agents, leading to successful drugs. A lesson learned from the unsuccessful SERM drug, levormeloxifene, for which uterine prolapse occurred when tested in monkeys, but not in earlier rodent-based studies, was that candidate drugs showing promise in rodent studies should be tested in large animals, particularly nonhuman primates, before being moved to the clinic.

Should SERM therapy utilize a single broadly acting compound or utilize several compounds to target specific health problems? On the one hand, women prefer a single agent with multiple benefits, potentially enhancing compliance, and use of a single drug may minimize problems related to drug interactions. On the other hand, a combination of drugs targeted to specific health problems is more likely to be effective than a single compound designed to have a broad spectrum of health-protective effects. For example, the combination of estrogen replacement therapy (ERT) plus a SERM may allow the brain-protective effects of estrogen, which is believed to cross the blood-brain barrier more readily than SERMs, while utilizing the estrogen antagonist properties of the SERM to protect peripheral target organs (endometrium and breast). However, in another example, although the combination of ERT plus a pure estrogen antagonist may protect against uterine and breast actions of estrogen, the protective effect of ERT on bone may also be prevented.

In summary, provision of appropriate resources for SERM research could target the following objectives:

- Continue toward a better understanding of the underlying biology of estrogen and SERM action.

- Develop appropriate models, on the molecular, cellular, and whole animal level, to evaluate estrogen and SERM action.

- Assess a single multitarget compound as well as combination therapy utilizing the strengths of several therapeutic compounds.

REFERENCES

1. HULLEY, S., D. GRADY, T. BUSH et al. 1998. Randomized trial of estrogen plus progestin for secondary prevention of coronary heart disease in postmenopausal women: Heart and Estrogen/Progestin Study (HERS) Research Group. JAMA **280:** 605–613.
2. HERRINGTON, D.M., D.M. REBOUSSIN, K.B. BROSNIHAN et al. 2000. Effects of estrogen replacement on the progression of coronary artery atherosclerosis. N. Engl. J. Med. **343:** 522–529.
3. NIH. 2001. Women's Health Initiative (www.nhlbi.nih.gov/whi/hrt-en.htn). National Institutes of Health/National Heart, Lung, and Blood Institute. Bethesda, MD.

What Would Be the Properties of an Ideal SERM?

MARIETTA ANTHONY,[a] J. KOUDY WILLIAMS,[b] AND BARBARA K. DUNN[c]

[a]*Georgetown University Medical Center, Washington, DC 20007, USA*
[b]*Wake Forest University School of Medicine, Winston-Salem, North Carolina 27157, USA*
[c]*National Cancer Institute, National Institutes of Health, Bethesda, Maryland 20892, USA*

ABSTRACT: Selective estrogen receptor modulators (SERMs) are drugs that bind to the estrogen receptor (ER); in some tissues they act like estrogen (agonists), while in other tissues they oppose the action of estrogen (antagonists). The SERM tamoxifen acts as an estrogen antagonist in the breast in that it prevents and treats breast cancer, but it acts as an estrogen agonist in the endometrium, where it can induce cancer. Estrogen, and to a lesser extent SERMs, are effective in preventing and treating osteoporosis. Contrary to the prevalent hypothesis that estrogen provides benefit to women with regard to secondary prevention of coronary heart disease (CHD), randomized clinical trials have demonstrated that estrogen is associated with an increased risk of CHD in this population of women. Conflicting results have been reported on the effect of estrogens on cognitive function. The latest and largest randomized clinical trials have demonstrated a beneficial role in short-term memory in nondemented women, in contrast to the absence of such benefit in improving symptoms in women with Alzheimer's disease. Although estrogens have been used successfully to treat some menopausal symptoms such as hot flashes, the SERMs tamoxifen and raloxifene actually induce or increase hot flashes. Data on the beneficial and adverse effects of estrogen and SERMs are reported along with an elaboration of the constellation of properties that would characterize an ideal SERM working through the ER.

KEYWORDS: SERM; estrogen; HRT; cancer; cardiovascular; osteoporosis

INTRODUCTION

Selective estrogen receptor modulators (SERMs) act via a mechanism that is based on binding to the estrogen receptor (ER). The clinical observation that tamoxifen has estrogenic and antiestrogenic effects in different tissues was the impetus for the development of other chemicals that would have desirable agonistic or antagonistic properties in selective tissues. In addition, this dichotomy of actions has motivated an extensive investigation of the role of the estrogen receptor and molecular signaling in this process. Two types of ERs have been discovered and found to be

Address for correspondence: Barbara K. Dunn, M.D., Ph.D., Basic Prevention Science Research Group, Division of Cancer Prevention, National Cancer Institute, National Institutes of Health, EPN 2056, 6130 Executive Boulevard, Rockville, MD 20852. Voice: 301-496-8541; fax: 301-480-4110.
 bd62y@nih.gov

widely, but differentially, distributed in cells of major systems. Knowledge of the chemical structure of the ligands that bind to the ER has led to targeted drug development—that is, designing a drug (SERM) to bind to a designated receptor (ER) to cause a specific reaction in a selected tissue (breast, bone, heart and blood vessels, brain).

Drug development targeted to the ER has also led to a new paradigm in menopause-related diseases/conditions. The traditional use of drugs has been to treat these diseases. The new paradigm is that drugs, specifically estrogens and subsequently SERMs, could be used to prevent future disease. In fact, SERMs have been shown to prevent breast cancer and osteoporosis. Could they also be used in other systems—for example, to prevent cardiovascular disease and dementia?

However, the clinical scenario has been much more complex than the theoretical construct. While estrogen has historically been taken by women for relief of menopausal symptoms, unwanted side effects such as irregular bleeding have led to declining usage. For women with a uterus, estrogen use has necessitated the inclusion of a progestin, which, in turn, has potential for other unwanted side effects and attenuation of some of the benefits of estrogen. In terms of risk, both estrogen and SERMs have the potential for serious and life-threatening risks such as endometrial cancer and thromboembolic complications.

An additional challenge in SERM research is the development and validation of biomarkers that are surrogates for meaningful clinical outcomes. Biomarkers are not always predictive of their clinical counterparts—that is, they are not truly surrogates. In cardiovascular disease, for example, presumed surrogate biomarkers such as cholesterol do not always predict clinical outcomes such as myocardial infarction. In the skeletal system, bone density alone does not completely predict the risk of fracture.

In this paper, we have explored some of the research on estrogens and SERMs and their impact on the major diseases/conditions/systems in terms of benefits and risks. Our goal is to put in perspective the properties that one would expect of the ideal SERM acting through an ER.

CANCER

Background

SERMs have been shown to antagonize cancer in certain target tissues and to promote cancers in others. Individual SERMs differ from one another with respect to their cancer-inhibiting/promoting profile. In this sense, cancer serves as a model disease for demonstrating the concept of "selectivity" in selective estrogen receptor modulators.

Estrogen

Breast cancer is the most prominent disease/site for which a beneficial effect of SERMs has been shown. This is not at all surprising since estrogen has been implicated as a risk factor for breast cancer in postmenopausal women in multiple studies.[1] A statistically significant positive association between the circulating levels of endogenous estrogens and the subsequent risk of breast cancer has been observed.[2,3]

Similarly, exogenous estrogen use, specifically estrogen (ERT) and estrogen-progestin (HRT) replacement therapy, increases the risk of breast cancer with the combined regimen increasing the risk to a greater extent than estrogen alone.[4–6] The increase in risk appears to be related to the duration of use. The development of an agent that selectively antagonizes this undesirable effect of estrogen in the breast has served as a motivating force behind SERM development.

SERMs

Beneficial Effects: Breast Cancer

Tamoxifen, a first-generation SERM and the first SERM to be used in clinical practice, has had as its major application the treatment of all stages and the prevention of breast cancer.[7,8] During the past 25 years, over 10 million woman-years of clinical experience have accumulated with this important agent in this disease. This extensive clinical application, together with the abundant preclinical evidence for tamoxifen's beneficial effect on the breast,[9,10] has drawn attention to the breast and specifically to breast cancer, as a disease/site to be targeted in the development of later SERMs. Thus, breast cancer has to a large extent been the motivating force behind SERM development in general, serving as a fulcrum around which research on SERM activity at other diseases/sites has revolved.

A second-generation SERM, raloxifene, showed promise in preclinical studies for its activity in breast cancer.[11,12] However, in early clinical studies involving metastatic breast cancer raloxifene failed to prove efficacious.[13] Interestingly, more recent data have suggested that high-dose raloxifene has modest activity in highly selected postmenopausal women with advanced breast carcinoma.[14] Raloxifene's activity in breast cancer continues to be of interest and has been followed as a secondary end point in postmenopausal women without breast cancer in the osteoporosis study the Multiple Outcomes of Raloxifene Evaluation (MORE) trial.[15–17] The results of the MORE trial showed that raloxifene reduced the incidence of all invasive breast cancers by 76% and of ER-positive breast cancers by 90%.[16] These promising observations of breast cancer prevention provided a beneficial outcome to a secondary end point that led to the hypothesis that raloxifene is an effective chemopreventive agent for breast cancer. That hypothesis is now being tested in the NSABP's (National Surgical Adjuvant Breast and Bowel Project) P-2: Study of Tamoxifen and Raloxifene (STAR) trial.[18,19] In STAR, raloxifene is being compared to tamoxifen, the recently established standard for chemoprevention of breast cancer in high-risk women,[20] for efficacy as well as toxicity.

The only other SERM, in addition to tamoxifen, that is approved for breast cancer is toremifene, with its use being limited to the metastatic setting.[21,22]

Adverse Effects: Cancer Induction

Unfortunately, at certain nonbreast sites, specific SERMs have exhibited an agonistic effect with regard to cancer, the most noteworthy example being the uterus. In animal models the induction of endometrial cancer occurs in response to tamoxifen and toremifene.[23] In humans, an increased rate of endometrial cancer, relative risk two- to sevenfold in various studies, is a well-documented outcome of tamoxifen treatment. The data supporting this association have emerged from observational studies as well as prospective randomized trials.[20, 24–29]

Tamoxifen has been shown to induce other cancers such as hepatocellular carcinomas and granulosa cell tumors of the ovary in laboratory animals, both occurring at high doses.[7] Similar outcomes in humans have not been substantiated in either cohort studies or clinical trials.

OSTEOPOROSIS

Background

Osteoporosis has been defined by the NIH Consensus Conference on Osteoporosis Prevention, Diagnosis, and Therapy[30] as a skeletal disorder characterized by compromised bone strength that predisposes to increased risk of fracture. Osteoporosis is a major health problem, with 10 million people with the disease and another 18 million with low bone mass in the United States alone. Eighty percent of those affected are postmenopausal women. Three categories of bone end points have been addressed: bone mineral density (BMD), metabolic—that is, biochemical—and histologic markers of bone turnover, and bone fracture—mostly of the hip, spine, and wrist. Whereas BMD and bone turnover are surrogates, the end point of most significance is the clinical outcome of fracture.[30]

Estrogen

Estrogen deficiency has been determined to be associated with osteoporosis[31] and an increased risk of hip and vertebral fractures.[32] Furthermore, studies have shown that ERT has been associated with a reduction in the risk of osteoporotic fractures in postmenopausal women,[33,34] although some of this data have been called into question. Estrogen can be used both to prevent and to treat osteoporosis.[35] Importantly, however, in a study of HRT (estrogen and progestin) in postmenopausal women with coronary disease (Heart Estrogen/progestin Replacement Study, or HERS), there was no evidence of a reduction in the incidence of fractures or rate of height loss with HRT.[36]

SERMs

In addition to estrogen, several other drugs, including the SERM raloxifene, can be used to prevent and treat osteoporosis. BMD has been measured in women taking tamoxifen. In postmenopausal women with breast cancer on tamoxifen, BMD of the spine increased; but fracture risk was not assessed in these studies.[37,38] In the NSABP's P-1: Breast Cancer Prevention Trial, women who were at increased risk for breast cancer and given tamoxifen for prevention of this disease were evaluated for the rate of fracture. The results of the P-1 trial showed a 19% reduction (relative risk [RR] = 0.81; 95% CI = 0.63–1.05) in osteoporotic fracture events (combined hip, spine, and lower radius) in women on tamoxifen compared to women on placebo.[20] Daily treatment of postmenopausal women with raloxifene was shown by Delmas et al.[39] to increase BMD of the lumbar spine, hip, and total body and by Ettinger *et al.* in the MORE trial [15] to reduce the rate of vertebral fracture risk. To date, although SERM therapy with raloxifene has demonstrated benefits in increasing BMD and significantly decreasing fracture risk, the magnitude of BMD increases appears to be considerably smaller than that of estrogen.[40]

THE CARDIOVASCULAR SYSTEM

Background

Cardiovascular disease (CVD), including stroke, is the leading cause of mortality among women in industrialized countries.[41]

Estrogen

Based on observational studies that employed biomarker and clinical end points such as myocardial infarction, estrogen was thought to provide benefit to the cardiovascular system. Estrogens have been shown to improve the lipid profile by raising serum high-density lipoproteins and lowering total cholesterol and low-density lipoproteins. When estrogen is combined with medroxyprogesterone acetate, the beneficial HDL-raising effects are attenuated.[42] ERT and HRT have been associated with an increase in expression of another biomarker, the inflammation factor C-reactive protein, in postmenopausal women.[43] While the full clinical significance of increased C-reactive protein remains to be clarified, those at the greatest risk of future cardiovascular events have higher levels of C-reactive protein.[44,45] Higher levels of C-reactive protein may reflect upregulation of mediators or markers of inflammation involved with atherosclerosis and/or thrombosis.[43]

While observational studies examining the role of ERT/HRT in postmenopausal women without established coronary heart disease (CHD) have found a reduction in CHD events among users versus nonusers, bias may well have contributed to these outcomes.[46–49] Estrogens were thought to reduce the risk of CHD, possibly by inhibiting atherogenesis, promoting vasodilation, and reducing the risk of coronary artery thrombosis.[50]

In contrast to the epidemiologic data, the HERS[51] and the Estrogen Replacement and Atherosclerosis (ERA) trial,[52] both randomized, double-blinded, placebo-controlled trials (RCT), raise doubt about the cardioprotective effects of ERT and HRT in postmenopausal women with existing coronary disease—that is, for secondary prevention. In the HERS trial, the relation between hormone use and risk for coronary events appeared to be time dependent, with the hormone-treated group showing a 52% higher risk in the first year but a 33% lower risk in the fourth and fifth years.[53] A large-scale RCT is being conducted on ERT/HRT in postmenopausal women without preexisting coronary disease—that is, primary prevention—in the Women's Health Initiative (WHI).[54] WHI participants were recently informed that there was an early increased risk of cardiovascular events in women on ERT or HRT compared to placebo.[55] Therefore, the early adverse effect of estrogen on the cardiovascular system may apply to primary as well as secondary prevention, but at this time in the former setting the data are even less clear regarding overall benefits and risks. In view of these reports from RCTs, the American Heart Association recommends that decisions to use ERT and HRT should be based on known benefits in systems other than the cardiovascular system, potential risks and patient preference.[56] HRT should not be initiated for the secondary prevention of cardiovascular disease (CVD), while clinical recommendations for the use of HRT for primary prevention of CVD await the results of ongoing RCTs.

SERMs

In the NSABP's P-1: BCPT, C-reactive protein was reduced by 26% in healthy women taking tamoxifen, showing that this drug has an effect on inflammatory markers consistent with reduced cardiovascular risk.[57] Yet, the P-1: BCPT results revealed no association between tamoxifen and either beneficial or adverse cardiovascular events.[58] It should be remembered, however, that these effects on the cardiovascular system were evaluated as a secondary end point in women with and without CHD as part of an RCT for which the primary end point was the prevention of breast cancer.

When compared to conjugated equine estrogen + medroxyprogesterone acetate, another SERM, raloxifene, had a somewhat similar effect in lowering low-density lipoproteins; but it did not change high-density lipoproteins, triglycerides, or plasminogen activator inhibitor–1.[40] Raloxifene is currently being evaluated in a clinical trial in postmenopausal women at high risk for CVD (Raloxifene Use for The Heart, or RUTH).[59]

COGNITIVE FUNCTION

Background

As the population ages, decline in cognitive function has evolved into a major public health concern as there are no effective strategies for its prevention or treatment. Approximately 10% of people over 65 years and 50% of those over 85 years have dementia.[60] Because it is known that estrogen receptors are located throughout the brain, especially in regions involved with learning and memory,[61] SERMs, acting as estrogen agonists, might be expected to have an impact on cognitive function.

Estrogen

Animal models have provided support for plausible, biological mechanisms of estrogen's effect on the brain, such as promotion of neuronal survival and dendritic sprouting,[62] and modulation in several systems, including the cholinergic,[63] serotonergic,[64] dopaminergic,[65] and noradrenergic.[66] Estrogen has been reported to aid in the prevention of cerebral ischemia.[67]

Many studies have assessed cognitive function of nondemented women in relation to endogenous and exogenous estrogens; they have yielded mixed results. First, a prospective study of women over 65 years with an average follow-up of five years reported that endogenous estrogen levels did not correlate with cognitive function.[68] Observational studies on cognitive function and estrogen use reported conflicting results. In three cross-sectional studies, it was reported that estrogen use was associated with somewhat better cognitive function than nonuse, but there was no adjustment for the strong predictors of age, education, and depression.[69–71] Two other observational studies, a prospective cohort study with 15 years of follow-up of 800 women[72] and a nested case-control study of 214 women,[73] did not show an association between estrogen use and cognitive function. However, a small RCT in 19 women after hysterectomy found that estrogen had some positive affect on immediate recall.[74] In more recent reports from small randomized trials in nondemented women taking ERT over 2–3 weeks, an improvement in visuospatial abilities was reported in one study,[75] while two other studies[76,77] failed to demonstrate the superiority of ERT to placebo in any test of cognitive function. It must be emphasized that all of the above studies were done with small numbers (18–70) of women. Data from the Baltimore Longitudinal Study of Aging (BLSA) involving 288 postmenopausal women demonstrated a better performance of short-term memory and, in a subgroup of 18 women, protective effects of ERT on longitudinal change in memory.[78]

The role of estrogen in preventing, delaying, and treating dementia has also been evaluated. A subset of 472 women from the BLSA was followed for up to 16 years and exhibited a RR of 0.46 (95% CI, 0.209–0.997) of developing Alzheimer's disease (AD) among ERT users compared to nonusers.[79] A metanalysis of the observational studies on the effect of estrogen on the risk of developing AD reported a 29% decreased risk among estrogen users, but these studies are subject to confounding and compliance bias.[80] Regarding treatment of AD, three recent RCTs indicated that ERT is not an effective treatment in women diagnosed with AD.[81–83] In the largest of these studies, ERT for one year did not slow disease progression nor improve cognitive or functional outcomes in 120 women with mild to moderate AD.[82]

SERMs

Limited information is available on the effect of SERMs on cognition and aging. A retrospective analysis of women with primary breast cancer reported little difference between women who had used tamoxifen in the past and controls on three cognitive tests. However, while using tamoxifen these women reported memory problems.[84] A secondary analysis of residents in a long-term care facility reported that women who had received tamoxifen were less likely to have a diagnosis of AD but more likely to have a diagnosis of depression.[85] Cognitive assessment performed as part of a small short-term phase 2 osteoporosis trial[86] and the MORE trial[87] showed that raloxifene compared to placebo had no effect on cognitive function or mood in postmenopausal women with osteoporosis. Therefore, evidence regarding the role of SERMs in preventing, delaying, or treating AD is limited.

MENOPAUSAL SYMPTOMS

Background

Menopause is the permanent cessation of menstruation resulting from the loss of ovarian follicular activity. Natural menopause is recognized to have occurred after 12 consecutive months of amenorrhea for which there is no other obvious pathologic or physiologic cause. The average age of natural menopause in the Western world is

51 years. In 2000 in the United States, there were an estimated 41.75 million women over age 50.[88]

Estrogen

Many different menopausal symptoms have been documented (listed in order of decreasing frequency): stiffness and soreness in joints, neck, and shoulders; headache; forgetfulness; difficulty sleeping; hot flashes; night sweats; heart pounding; urine leakage; and vaginal dryness.[89] Depression has also been associated with menopause.[90] Since estrogen levels are reduced with menopause,[91] estrogen replacement is effective in treating some menopausal symptoms, particularly hot flashes.[92] Conjugated equine estrogen was approved by the FDA in 1942 for treatment of vasomotor symptoms (hot flashes) associated with menopause.[93] Since then, many different products (estrogen, combination estrogen and progestins, and progestins) that have different formulations and routes of administration have become available.[94]

While women choose to take ERT or HRT primarily for relief of postmenopausal symptoms, they stop taking it mainly because of its unwanted side effects, mainly bleeding.[95–98] In a study of 3395 women taking ERT, only 43% continued their estrogen treatment beyond the first year.[99]

SERMs

In contrast to estrogen, which is used to treat hot flashes, the SERMs tamoxifen and raloxifene induce or increase the menopausal symptom of hot flashes.[100,101]

Combination SERM and ERT or HRT

In an effort to overcome these difficulties, the combined use of HRT and SERMs has been examined in studies involving women at increased risk for breast cancer. In the Italian Tamoxifen Prevention Study, which permitted HRT use, subset analysis showed a borderline-significant reduction of breast cancer among women who took HRT and received tamoxifen. In contrast, analysis of all women in the study did not show such a decrease in breast cancer incidence.[102,103] Furthermore, the beneficial effect of tamoxifen on cardiovascular risk factors, including lipid levels, was unaffected in current HRT users, although this benefit was slightly attenuated in women who started transdermal HRT while on tamoxifen.[104] These data therefore suggest that there is no adverse effect and possibly a beneficial effect from simultaneous use of HRT and tamoxifen. Based on this and on the observation that some women left the study secondary to menopausal symptoms, the possibility was proposed that the combination of HRT and tamoxifen might reduce the side effects of tamoxifen and thereby enhance compliance to the intervention.[103,105] This proposal, in turn, provided the rationale for the ongoing HOT (HOrmone Replacement Therapy and Tamoxifen) study—namely, that compliance with SERMs implemented to target other diseases/sites (e.g., tamoxifen to decrease breast cancer risk or to positively alter lipid levels) may be improved by concurrent administration of HRT (updated trial results to be published in the near future; A. Decensi, personal communication).

The issue of whether estrogens (ERT and HRT) should be used concomitantly with tamoxifen intersects another controversial area—namely, whether estrogens should be used in women who have had breast cancer and, by extrapolation, in women who are at increased risk for breast cancer. Women who take tamoxifen will, by definition, belong to one of these two breast cancer categories. The standard of care in the United States has been to view a history of breast cancer as a relative contraindication to estrogen therapy.[106–108] This position has evolved from the observed association between exogenous estrogen use and breast cancer risk among healthy women, discussed above.[4–6] On the other hand, a systematic review of observational data suggests that estrogen therapy does not significantly affect breast cancer recurrence.[108] However, only minimal data exist that specifically address the effects of HRT in women already diagnosed with breast cancer.[109] It is premature to conclude that there is no increase risk related to ERT/HRT in this setting.[110] In an ongoing debate over the issue, some authors have encouraged the implementation of randomized trials to address the effect of estrogen replacement therapy in women with breast cancer.[111] Ongoing and proposed studies include: HABITS, a multicenter study in Scandinavia that will employ HRT for two years as the intervention in 1300 women with early-stage breast cancer, some of whom will be taking concurrent tamoxifen;[109,110] and an ECOG study in which randomization will also be to tamoxifen plus placebo versus tamoxifen plus ERT or HRT, depending on the hysterectomy status of the woman.[109]

With regard to high-risk women, the inclusion of HRT/ERT in conjunction with tamoxifen is believed by some to be counterproductive, since estrogens might be expected to negate the beneficial effect of tamoxifen in preventing breast cancer. Thus, the NSABP has maintained HRT/ERT as an exclusion criterion for its BCPT and STAR participants.[18,20] In contrast, the British Royal Marsden Trial[112] and, as elaborated above, the Italian Tamoxifen Prevention Study [103] and the newer HOT trial have permitted HRT/ERT use among their randomized high-risk participants.

ADDITIONAL ADVERSE REACTIONS

Background

SERMs have been and will continue to be used to treat existing cancers and to prevent cancers, mainly breast cancer. It is vital that one distinguish between (1) reduction of the burden of disease (existing or at increased risk for occurring) by an active intervention with a SERM or other drug and (2) the absence of an adverse outcome from this intervention. These two attributes should coexist as properties of an ideal SERM. In the case of cancer, a SERM should antagonize breast cancer while not inducing endometrial cancer. The same principle should apply to other diseases/sites in which SERM intervention is applied. From the clinical perspective, avoiding an adverse outcome due to an intervention is not the same as prospectively antagonizing or preventing that outcome. Specifically, in the absence of the intervention this adverse outcome would not have been induced in the first place.

Increased Adverse Outcomes

In addition to the induction of endometrial cancer and increase in menopausal symptoms discussed above, SERMs have other adverse effects. Estrogen,[113–119] tamoxifen,[20,120,121] and raloxifene[15,16] all increase the risk of venous thromboembolic events such as deep vein thrombosis and pulmonary embolism. In the P-1: BCPT, women taking tamoxifen had an increased incidence of stroke (RR = 1.59, 95% CI 0.93–2.77), an increase in deep vein thrombosis (RR = 1.60, 95% CI = 0.91–2.86), and a threefold higher rate of pulmonary emboli (RR = 3.01, 95% CI = 1.15–9.27). It should be noted that the risk of these adverse events was greater in women age 50 and older.[20] Raloxifene, too, was shown to increase the risk of deep venous thromboembolic (VTE) disease (RR = 3.1; 95% CI 0.26–3.0). There was also a higher rate of pulmonary embolus in the raloxifene groups (0.3%) than in the placebo group (0.1%).[15,16] The tendency of SERMs to induce thromboemboli is probably a reflection of their estrogen agonist properties, since both oral contraceptives[113,114] and HRT[115–117] have been associated with an increased risk of VTE. The increased risk of VTE was documented in a prospective RCT in postmenopausal women receiving estrogen with progestin.[118] In addition, the first controlled clinical trial to study estrogen therapy among postmenopausal women with a history of stroke reported that ERT was not effective for secondary prevention of this thromboembolic disease end point. In fact, women on ERT had a higher risk of fatal stroke and more severe impairment after stroke than women who took a placebo (The Women's Estrogen for Stroke Trial, or WEST).[119]

PROPERTIES OF AN IDEAL SERM

Risks

In addition to providing benefits in treating or preventing a disease, drugs have side effects. Treatment decisions involve consideration of benefits and risks that, in turn, depend on the profile of both the drug and the patient. For example, consideration of the disease state is critical to the patient/consumer in making treatment decisions. Intolerance of drug toxicity is especially acute in the prevention setting where at-risk, but healthy, individuals have a much lower acceptance of drug side effects than do individuals who have cancer and may willingly tolerate severe adverse effects of chemotherapy in the hope of cure, or at least control, of existing life-threatening disease.[19]

Endometrial cancer is clearly an undesirable and potentially dangerous side effect that should be avoided in the ideal SERM profile. The underlying mechanisms in SERM (e.g., tamoxifen) induction of endometrial cancer (see above) suggest that efforts to eliminate this carcinogenic outcome from the ideal SERM profile should target nongenotoxic mechanisms of carcinogenesis, specifically ER-mediated cellular proliferation. The unacceptability of any side effects, even those that are merely uncomfortable, is amplified by the long duration of therapy (sometimes indefinite) that characterizes intervention with drugs for the purpose of preventing disease. Thromboembolism is another undesirable and potentially fatal side effect of both estrogen and SERMS. Thus, the ideal SERM should have a decreased risk profile relative to estrogen and existing SERMS in this procoagulant activity.

Attempts have been made to analyze the risk:benefit ratio of an intervention, specifically tamoxifen in the preventive setting, by attaching quantifiable values to the specific benefits and risks of this SERM.[120] This effort has met with mixed reactions,[121] however. Such a quantitative approach should be regarded as merely a tool in the overall decision making process. A woman's final decision as to whether she should take a SERM, such as tamoxifen, especially for the purpose of disease prevention, requires discussions with her physician and other knowledgeable health professionals and interested parties.[19,122,123]

Benefits

Breast Cancer

For breast cancer, an ideal SERM would have to provide superior efficacy relative to tamoxifen or an improvement in the toxicity profile. With regard to cancer outcomes, for example, extensive prior experience with tamoxifen has shown us that an ideal SERM should reduce the burden of breast cancer while not increasing the burden of endometrial cancer. With regard to the beneficial effect of breast cancer reduction, even if the elimination of adverse effects, such as endometrial cancer and thromboembolic disease, is accomplished, the degree of efficacy still needs to be improved. Future efforts in SERM development should therefore be directed at (1) clarifying/defining specific subgroups of breast cancer (e.g., ER-positive) that are SERM responsive (and expanding the repertoire of SERM-responsive subgroups, if possible) and (2) enhancing the degree of activity in that responsive subgroup of breast cancers until 100% can be eliminated.

Osteoporosis

The ideal SERM should aid in the prevention and treatment of osteoporosis. Since room exists for improvement in effectiveness, the ideal SERM should approximate or surpass estrogen in treating and preventing osteoporosis without having estrogen's risk profile. However, on the molecular level, we do not know the mechanism to target for improved efficacy for prevention or treatment of osteoporosis. Should a SERM's desirable properties be to reduce bone turnover, increase bone formation, both, or should it perhaps act by some other mechanism? We do know that the most meaningful assessment of SERM efficacy for treating and preventing osteoporosis is the clinical outcome of reducing fracture risk, rather than solely the measurement of biochemical markers of bone turnover and bone density.

Cardiovascular Disease

In evaluating SERMs with regard to cardiovascular end points at both the molecular and clinical levels, the question emerges as to whether SERMs are cardioprotective and, if so, for which population of women. If SERMs can provide significant benefit in cancer prevention and treatment and in osteoporosis prevention and treatment, then a minimum requirement would be to cause no harm to the cardiovascular system. The question of a cardioprotective benefit of SERMs may hinge on the role of estrogen in the cardiovascular system. Certainly, a property of an ideal SERM would be to provide beneficial effects for the cardiovascular system in women with and without preexisting CHD. However, results from the HERS, ERA, and WHI trials have provided discouraging results in women taking ERT or HRT. And since their mechanism of action is through the ER, the extension of these results to SERMs seems likely.

Cognitive Function

Molecular and animal research have shown a beneficial effect of estrogen on nerve cells. Desirable effects of the ideal SERM would be to maintain or improve cognitive function and delay or, if possible, prevent the development of dementia in nondemented women. If some of these goals are attainable with estrogen, they should be achievable for SERMs. However, clinical research has not supported a role for either estrogens or SERMs in the treatment of Alzheimer's disease.

Menopausal Symptoms

The existing options for treatment of menopausal symptoms are ERT for hysterectomized women and HRT for women with a uterus; both of these have unwanted side effects. Current SERMs increase or induce hot flashes and therefore cannot be used to treat menopausal symptoms. A property of an ideal SERM would be to provide relief from menopausal symptoms and, certainly, not to exacerbate these symptoms. If normal healthy women will be using SERMs for relief of menopausal symptoms, it is extremely important that the ideal SERM have a reduced risk profile of serious and life-threatening complications, such as endometrial cancer and thromboembolic complications.

CONCLUSIONS

Current thinking is that the ideal SERM should provide enhanced benefit over existing ERT, HRT, and SERMs, and/or a decreased risk profile. In terms of risk, the ideal SERM should not increase the risk of serious and life-threatening events and of chronic diseases/conditions associated with aging. Nor should an ideal SERM induce less serious, but debilitating, side effects (e.g., hot flashes) that might compromise compliance. At a minimum, a SERM should be an estrogen antagonist in the breast with efficacy superior to, or less serious side effects than, tamoxifen. It would be desirable for an ideal SERM not to induce or increase menopausal symptoms. SERMs already have some role in reducing bone fracture risk, and it would be desirable to increase this activity to at least that of estrogen without the risk profile of the latter. While additional desirable properties would be to prevent and treat cardiovascular diseases and to maintain or improve cognitive function or delay dementia, at a minimum a SERM should not cause harm in these systems.

Until we have more data on the potential mechanisms by which SERMs can affect cells, organs, and systems in beneficial or harmful ways, the progress in SERM development may be limited. And perhaps the goal of developing one compound that has a beneficial effect on all these major systems is unrealistic. Nevertheless, the achievement of a drug profile encompassing the tissue-specific agonistic and antagonistic properties outlined above should continue to govern our search for the ideal SERM.

REFERENCES

1. CLEMONS, M. & P. GOSS. 2001. Estrogen and the risk of breast cancer. N. Engl. J. Med. **344:** 276–285.

2. HANKINSON, S.E., W.C. WILLETT, J.E. MANSON, et al. 1998. Plasma sex steroid hormone levels and risk of breast cancer in postmenopausal women. J. Natl. Cancer Inst. **90:** 1292–1299.
3. CAULEY, J.A., F.L. LUCAS & L.H. KULLER FOR THE STUDY OF OSTEOPOROTIC FRACTURES RESEARCH GROUP. 1999. Elevated serum estradiol and testosterone concentrations are associated with a high risk for breast cancer. Ann. Intern. Med.**130:** 270–277.
4. COLDITZ, G.A., S.E. HANKINSON, D.J. HUNTER, et al. 1995. The use of estrogens and progestins and the risk of breast cancer in postmenopausal women. N. Engl. J. Med. **332:** 1589–1593.
5. COLLABORATIVE GROUP ON HORMONAL FACTORS IN BREAST CANCER. 1997. Breast cancer and hormone replacement therapy: collaborative reanalysis of data from 51 epidemiological studies of 52,705 women with breast cancer and 108,411 women without breast cancer. Lancet **350:** 1047–1059.
6. SCHAIRER, C., J. LUBIN, R. TROISI, et al. 2000. Menopausal estrogen and estrogen-progestin replacement therapy and breast cancer risk. JAMA **283:** 485–491.
7. INTERNATIONAL AGENCY FOR RESEARCH ON CANCER (IARC). WORLD HEALTH ORGANIZATION. 1996. Tamoxifen. *In* IARC Monographs on the Evaluation of Carcinogenic Risks to Humans, Vol. 66. Some Pharmaceutical Drugs: 253–365. IARC. Lyon, France.
8. JORDAN, V.C. & M. MORROW. 1999. Tamoxifen for breast cancer prevention. *In* Tamoxifen for the Treatment and Prevention of Breast Cancer. V.C. Jordan, Ed.: 207–223. PRR. Melville, NY.
9. GOTTARDIS, M.M. & V.C. JORDAN. 1987. Antitumor actions of keoxifene and tamoxifen in the N-nitrosomethylurea–induced rat mammary carcinoma model. Cancer Res. **47:** 4020–4024.
10. JORDAN, V.C., M.K. LABABIDI & S. LANGAN-FAHEY. 1991. Suppression of mouse mammary tumorigenesis by long-term tamoxifen therapy. J. Natl. Cancer Inst. **83:** 492–496.
11. THOMPSON, E.W., R. REICH, T.B. SHIMA, et al. 1988. Differential regulation of growth and invasiveness of MCF-7 breast cancer cells by antiestrogens. Cancer Res. **48:** 6764–6868.
12. ANZANO, M.A., C.W. PEER, J.M. SMITH, et al. 1996. Chemoprevention of mammary carcinogenesis in the rat: combined use of raloxifene and 9-cis-retinoic acid. J. Natl. Cancer Inst. **88:** 1234–125.
13. BUZDAR, A.U., C. MARCUS, F. HOLMES, et al. 1988. Phase II evaluation of Ly156758 in metastatic breast cancer. Oncology **45:** 344–345.
14. GRADISHAR, W., J. GLUSMAN, Y. LU, et al. 2000. Effects of high dose raloxifene in selected patients with advanced breast carcinoma. Cancer **88:** 2049–2053.
15. ETTINGER, B., D.M. BLACK, B.H. MITLAK, et al. 1999. Reduction of vertebral fracture risk in postmenopausal women with osteoporosis treated with raloxifene. Results from a 3-year randomized clinical trial. JAMA **282:** 637–645.
16. CUMMINGS, S.R., S. ECKERT, K.A. KRUEGER, et al. 1999. The effect of raloxifene on risk of breast cancer in postmenopausal women: results from the MORE randomized trial. JAMA **16:** 2189–2197.
17. LIPPMAN, M.E., K.A. KRUEGER, S. ECKERT, et al. 2001. Indicators of lifetime estrogen exposure: effect on breast cancer incidence and interaction with raloxifene therapy in the Multiple Outcomes of Raloxifene Evaluation study participants. J. Clin. Oncol. **19:** 3111–3116.
18. WOLMARK, N. 1999. The Breast Cancer Prevention Trial, and the woman at high risk for breast cancer. Primary Care Cancer **19** (Suppl. 1): 11–16.
19. DUNN, B.K. & L.G. FORD. 2000. Prevention of breast cancer. Semin. Breast Dis. **3:** 90–99.
20. FISHER, B., J.P. COSTANTINO, D.L. WICKERHAM, et al. 1998. Tamoxifen for prevention of breast cancer: report of the National Surgical Adjuvant Breast and Bowel Project P-1 Study. J. Natl. Cancer Inst. **90:** 1371–1378.
21. BUZDAR, A.U. & G.N. HORTOBAGYI. 1998. Tamoxifen and toremifene in breast cancer: comparison of safety and efficacy. J. Clin. Oncol. **26:** 348–353.

22. WISEMAN, L.R. & K.L. GOA. 1997. Toremifene. A review of its pharmacological properties and clinical efficacy in the management of advanced breast cancer. Drugs **54:** 141–160.
23. O'REGAN, R.M., A. CISNEROS, G.M. ENGLAND, *et al.* 1998. Effects of the antiestrogens tamoxifen, toremifene, and ICI 182,780 on endometrial cancer growth. J. Natl. Cancer Inst. **90:** 1552–1558.
24. FISHER, B., J.P. COSTANTINO, C.K. REDMOND, *et al.* 1994. Endometrial cancer in tamoxifen-treated breast cancer patients: findings from the National Surgical Adjuvant Breast and Bowel Project (NSABP) B-14. J. Natl. Cancer Inst. **86:** 527–537.
25. VAN LEEUWEN, F.E., J. BENRAADT, J.W. COEBERGH & L.A.L.M. KIEMENEY. 1994. Risk of endometrial cancer after tamoxifen treatment of breast cancer. Lancet **343:** 448–452.
26. BARAKAT, R.R. 1995. The effect of tamoxifen on the endometrium. Oncology **9:** 129–139.
27. RUTQVIST, L.E., H. JOHANSSON & T. SIGNOMKLAO. 1995. Adjuvant tamoxifen therapy for early stage breast cancer and second primary malignancies. J. Natl. Cancer Inst. **87:** 645–651.
28. BERNSTEIN, L., D. DEAPEN, J.R. CERHAN & S.M. SCHWARTZ. 1999. Tamoxifen therapy for breast cancer and endometrial cancer risk. J. Natl. Cancer Inst. **91:** 1654–1662.
29. SHAPIRO, C.L. & A. RECHT. 2001. Side effects of adjuvant treatment of breast cancer. N. Engl. J. Med. **344:** 1997–2008.
30. NIH CONSENSUS DEVELOPMENT PANEL ON OSTEOPOROSIS PREVENTION, DIAGNOSIS AND THERAPY. 2001. Osteoporosis prevention, diagnosis, and therapy. JAMA **285:** 785–795
31. RIGGS, B.L., S. KHOSLA & L.J. MELTON III. 1998. A unitary model for involutional osteoporosis: estrogen deficiency causes both type I and type II osteoporosis in postmenopausal women and contributes to bone loss in aging men. J. Bone Miner. Res. **13:** 763–773
32. CUMMINGS, S.R., W.S. BROWNER, D. BAUER, *et al.* FOR THE STUDY OF OSTEOPOROTIC FRACTURES RESEARCH GROUP. 1998. Endogenous hormones and the risk of hip and vertebral fractures among older women. N. Engl. J. Med. **339:** 767–768.
33. LUFKIN, E.G., H.W. WAHNER, W.M. O'FALLON, *et al.* 1992. Treatment of postmenopausal osteoporosis with transdermal estrogen. Ann. Intern. Med. **117:** 1–9.
34. CAULEY, J.A., D.G. SEELEY, K. ENSRUD, *et al.* FOR THE STUDY OF OSTEOPOROTIC FRACTURES RESEARCH GROUP. 1995. Estrogen replacement therapy and fractures in older women. Ann. Intern. Med. **122:** 9–16.
35. Drugs for prevention and treatment of postmenopausla osteoporosis. Med. Lett. Drugs Therapeutics 2000. **42:** 97–100
36. CAULEY, J.A., D.M. BLACK, E. BARRETT-CONNOR, *et al.* 2001. Effects of hormone replacement therapy on clinical fractures and height loss: the Heart and Estrogen/Progestin Replacement Study (HERS). Am. J. Med. **110:** 442–450.
37. LOVE, R.R., R.B. MAZESS, H.S. BARDEN, *et al.* 1992. Effects of tamoxifen on bone mineral density in postmenopausal women with breast cancer. N. Engl. J. Med. **326:** 885–886.
38. KRISTENSEN, B., B. EJLERTSEN, P DALGAARD, *et al.* 1994. Tamoxifen and bone metabolism in postmenopausal low-risk breast cancer patients: a randomized study. J. Clin Oncol **12:** 992–997.
39. DELMAS, P.D., N.H. BJARNASON, B.H. MITLAK, *et al.* 1997. Effects of raloxifene on bone mineral density, serum cholesterol concentrations, and uterine endometrium in postmenopausal women. N. Engl. J. Med. **337:** 1641–1647.
40. WALSH, B.W., L.H. KULLER, R.A. WILD, *et al.* 1998. Effects of ralox̄fiene on serum lipids and coagulation factors in healthy postmenopausal women. JAMA **279:** 1445–1451.
41. HOYERT, D.L., K.D. KOCHANEK, S.L. MURPHY. 1999. Deaths: final data for 1997. Natl. Vital Stat. Rep. **47:** 1–104.
42. THE WRITING GROUP FOR THE PEPI TRIAL. 1995. Effects of estrogen or estrogen/progestin regimens on heart disease risk factors in postmenopausal women: the Postmenopausal Estrogen/Progestin Interventions (PEPI) Trial. JAMA **273:** 199–208.

43. CUSHMAN, M., C. LEGAULT, E. BARRETT-CONNOR, et al. 1999. Effect of postmenopausal hormones on inflammation-sensitive proteins: the Postmenopausal Estrogen/Progestin Interventions (PEPI) Study. Circulation **100**: 717–722
44. RIDKER, P.M., M. CUSHMAN, M.J. STAMPFER, et al. 1997. Inflammation, aspirin, and the risk of cardiovascular disease in apparently healthy men. N. Eng. J. Med. **336**: 973–979.
45. TRACY R.P., R.N. LEMAITRE, P.M. PSATY, et al. 1997. Relationship of C-reactive protein to risk of cardiovascular disease in the elderly: results from the Cardiovascular Health Study and the Rural Health Promotion Project. Arterioscler. Thromb. Vasc. Biol. **17**: 1121–1127.
46. STAMPFER, M.J. & G.A. COLDITZ. 1991. Estrogen replacement therapy and coronary heart disease: a quantitative assessment of the epidemiologic evidence. Prev. Med. **20**: 47–63.
47. GRADY, D., S.M. RUBIN, D.B. PETITTI, et al. 1992. Hormone therapy to prevent disease and prolong life in post-menopausal women. Ann. Intern. Med. **117**: 1016–1037.
48. PSATY, B.M., S.R. HECKBRT, D. ATKINS, et al. 1994. The risk of myocardial infarction associated with the combined use of estrogens and progestins in postmenopausal women. Arch. Intern. Med. **154**: 1333–1339.
49. SIDNEY, S., D.B. PETITTI & C.P. QUESENBERRY, JR. 1997. Myocardial infarction and the use of estrogen and estrogen-progestogen in postmenopausal women. Ann. Intern. Med. **127**: 501–508.
50. MENDELSOHN, M. & R.H. KARAS. 1999. The protective effects of estrogen on the cardiovascular system. N. Engl. J. Med. **340**: 1801–1811.
51. HULLEY, S., D. GRADY, T. BUSH, et al. 1998. Randomized trial of estrogen plus progestin for secondary prevention of coronary heart disease in postmenopausal women. JAMA **280**: 605–613.
52. HERRINGTON, D.M., D.M. REBOUSSIN, K.B. BROSNIHAN, et al. 2000. Effects of estrogen replacement on the progression of coronary-artery atherosclerosis. N. Engl. J. Med. **343**: 522–529.
53. GRODSTEIN, F., J.E. MANSON & M.J. STAMPFER. 2001. Postmenopausal hormone use and secondary prevention of coronary events in the Nurses' Health Study: a prospective, observational study. Ann. Intern. Med. **135**: 1–8.
54. THE WOMEN'S HEALTH INITIATIVE STUDY GROUP. 1998. Design of the Women's Health Initiative clinical trial and observational study. Control Clin. Trials. **19**: 61–109.
55. NATIONAL INSTITUTES OF HEALTH. NATIONAL HEART LUNG AND BLOOD INSTITUTE. 2000. http://www.NHLBI.NIH.GOV/WHI/HRT-EN.HTM.
56. MOSCA, L., P. COLLINS, D.M. HERRINGTON, et al. 2001. Hormone replacement therapy and cardiovascular disease. a statement for healthcare professionals from the American Heart Association. Circulation **104**: 499–503.
57. CUSHMAN, M., J. COSTANTINO & R.T. TRACEY. 2001. Tamoxifen and cardiac risk factors in healthy women. Suggestion of an anti-inflammatory effect. Artheriosclerosis Thromb. Vasc. Biol. **21**: 255–261. Feb. [http://www.atvbaha.org].
58. REIS, S.E., J.P. COSTANTINO, D.L. WICKERHAM, et al. FOR THE NATIONAL SURGICAL ADJUVANT BREAST AND BOWEL PROJECT BREAST CANCER PREVENTION TRIAL INVESTIGATORS. 2001. Cardiovascular effects of tamoxifen in women with and without heart disease: Breast Cancer Prevention Trial. J. Natl. Cancer Inst. **93**: 16–21.
59. MOSCA, L.E., E. BARRETT CONNOR, N. WENGER, et al. 2001. Design and methods of the Raloxifene Use for The Heart (RUTH) Study. Am. J. Cardiol. In press.
60. EVANS, D.A. 1990. Estimated prevalence of Alzheimer's in the United States. Milbank Q. **68**: 267–289.
61. SHUGHRUE, P.J., M.V. LANE & I. MERCHENTHALER. 1997. Comparative distribution of estrogen receptor–alpha and –beta mRNA in the rat central nervous system. J. Comp. Neurol. **388**: 507–525.
62. MCEWEN, B.S. & C.S. WOOLEY. 1994. Estradiol and progesterone regulate neuronal structure and synaptic connectivity in adult as well as developing brain. Exp. Gerontol. **29**: 431–436.
63. TORAN-ALLERAND, C.D., R.C. MIRANDA, W.D. BETHAM, et al. 1992. Estrogen receptors co-localize with low-affinity nerve growth factor receptors in cholinergic neurons of the basal forebrain. Proc. Natl. Acad. Sci. USA **89**: 4668–4672.

64. SUMMER, B.E. & G. FINK. 1995. Estrogen increases the density of 5-hydroxytryptamine (2A) receptors in cerebral cortex and nucleus accumbens in the female rat. J. Steroid Biochem. Mol. Biol. **54:** 15–20.
65. BECKER, J.B. 2000. Oestrogen effects on dopaminergic function n striatum. In Neuronal and Cognitive Effects of Oestrogens, Vol. 230. D.J. Chadwick & J.A. Goode, Eds.: 134–145. John Wiley & Sons, Ltd. Novartis Foundation. London.
66. HERBISON, E.E., S.X. SIMONIAN, N.R. THANKY, et al. 2000. Oestrogen modulation of noradrenaline neurotransmission. In Neuronal and Cognitive Effects of Oestrogens, Vol. 230. D.J. Chadwick & J.A. Goode, Eds.: 74–85. John Wiley & Sons, Ltd. Novartis Foundation. London.
67. SULLIVAN, T.J., R.H. KARAS, M ARONOVITZ, et al. 1995. Estrogen inhibits the response-to-injury in a mouse carotid artery model. J. Clin. Invest. **96:** 2482–2488.
68. YAFFE, K., D. GRADY, A. PRESSMAN & S. CUMMINGS. 1998. Serum estrogen levels, cognitive performance, and risk of cognitive decline in older community women. J. Am. Geriatr. Soc. **46:** 816–821.
69. KAMPEN, D.L. & B.B. SHERWIN. 1994. Estrogen use and verbal memory in healthy postmenopausal women. Obstet. Gynecol. **83:** 979–983.
70. ROBINSON, D., L. FRIEDMAN, R. MARCUS, et al. 1994. Estrogen replacement therapy and memory in older women. J. Am. Geriatr. Soc. **42:** 919–922.
71. KIMURA, D. 1994. Estrogen replacement therapy may protect against intellectual decline in postmenopausal women. Horm. Behav. **29:** 312–321
72. BARRETT-CONNOR, E. & D. KRITZ-SILVERSTEIN. 1993. Estrogen replacement therapy and cognitive function in older women. JAMA **26:** 2637–2641.
73. PAGANINI-HILL, A. & V.W. HENDERSON. 1996. The effects of hormone replacement therapy, lipoprotein cholesterol levels, and other factors on a clock drawing task in older women. J. Am. Geriatr. Soc. **44:** 818–822.
74. PHILLIPS, S.M. & B.B. SHERWIN. 1992. Effects of estrogen on memory function in surgically menopausal women. Psychoneuroendocrinology **17:** 485–495.
75. DUKA, T., R. TASKER & J.F. MCGOWAN. 2000. The effects of 3-week estrogen hormone replacement on cognition in elderly healthy females. Psychopharmacology (Berl.) **149:** 129–139.
76. POLO-KANTOLA, P., R. PORTIN, O. POLO, et al. 1998. The effect of short-term estrogen replacement therapy on cognition: a randomized double-blind, cross-over trial in postmenopausal women. Obstet. Gynecol. **91:** 459–466.
77. WOLF, O., B. KUDIELKA, D. HELLHAMMER, et al. 1999. Two weeks of transdermal treatment in postmenopausal elderly women and its effect on memory and mood: verbal memory changes are associated with the treatment induced estradiol levels. Psychoneuroendocrinology **24:** 727–741.
78. RESNICK, S.M., E.J. METTER & A.B. XONDREMAN. 1997. Estrogen replacement therapy and longitudinal decline in visual memory: a possible protective effect? Neurology **49:** 1491–1497.
79. KAWAS, C., S. RESNICK, A. MORRISON, et al. 1997. A prospective study of estrogen replacement therapy and the risk of developing Alzheimer's disease: the Baltimore Longitudinal Study of Aging. Neurology **48:** 1517–1521.
80. YAFFE, K., G. SAWAYA, I. LIEBERBURG & D. GRADY. 1998. Estrogen therapy in postmenopausal women. Effects on cognitive function and dementia. JAMA **279:** 688–695.
81. HENDERSON, V.W., A. PAGANINI-HILL, B.L. MILLER, et al. 2000. Estrogen for Alzheimer's disease in women: randomized, double-blind, placebo-controlled trial. Neurology **54:** 295–301.
82. MULNARD, R.A., C.W. COTMAN, C. KAWAS, et al. 2000. Estrogen replacement therapy for treatment of mild to moderate Alzheimer disease: a randomized controlled trial. JAMA **283:** 1007–1015.
83. WANG, P.N., S.Q. LIAO, R.S. LIU, et al. 2000. Effects of estrogen on cognition, mood, and cerebral blood flow in AD: a controlled study. Neurology **54:** 2061–2066.
84. PAGANINI-HILL, A. & L.J. CLARK. 2000. Preliminary assessment of cognitive function in breast cancer patients treated with tamoxifen. Breast Cancer Res. Treat. **64:** 165–176.

85. BREUER, B. & R. ANDERSON. 2000. The relationship of tamoxifen with dementia, depression, and dependence in actvities of daily living in elderly nursing home residents. Women Health **31:** 71–85.
86. NICKELSEN, T., E.G. LUFKIN, B.L.RIGGS, et al. 1998. Raloxifene hydrochloride, a selective estrogen receptor molulator: safety assessment of effects on cognitive function and mood in postmenopausal women. Psychoneuroendocrinology **24:** 115–128.
87. YAFFE, K., K. KRUEGER, S. SARKAR, et al. 2001. Cognitive function in postmenopausal women treated with raloxifene. N. Engl. J. Med. **344:** 1207–1213.
88. NORTH AMERICAN MENOPAUSE SOCIETY. 2001. www.menopause.org
89. GOLD, E.B., B. STERNFELD, J.L. KELSEY, et al. 2000. The relation of demographic and lifestyle factors to symptoms in a multi-ethnic population of 40–55 year old women. Am. J. Epidemiol. **152:** 463–473.
90. HAY, A.G., J. BANCROFT & E.C. JOHNSTONE. 1994. Affective symptoms in women attending a menopause clinic. Br. J. Psychiatry **164:** 513–516.
91. SHERMAN, B.M. & S.G. KORENMAN. 1975. Hormonal characteristics of the human menstrual cycle throughout reproductive life. J. Clin. Invest. **55:** 699–706.
92. TATARYN, I.V., P. LOMAX, D.R. MELDRUM, et al 1981. Objective techniques for the assessment of hot flashes. Obstet. Gynecol. **57:** 340–344.
93. U.S. FOOD AND DRUG ADMINISTRATION. 1997. Backgrounder on conjugated estrogens: http://www.fda.gov/cder/news/cebackground.htm
94. U.S. FOOD AND DRUG ADMINISTRATION. OFFICE OF WOMEN'S HEALTH. 2001. Health topics. http://www.fda.gov/womens/HealthTopics/hrt.htm
95. GOLDMAN, G.A., B. KAPLAN, D.M. LEISEROWITZ, et al. 1998. Compliance with hormone replacement therapy in postmenopausal women. A comparative study. Clin. Exp. Obstet. Gynecol. **25:** 18–19.
96. NACHTIGALL, L.E. 1990. Enhancing patient compliance with hormone replacement therapy at menopause. Obstet. Gynecol. **75:** 77S–83S.
97. HAHN, R.G., R.D. NACHTIGALL & T.C. DAVIES. 1984. Compliance difficulties with progestin supplemented estrogen replacement therapy. J. Fam. Pract. **18:** 411–414.
98. HAMMOND, C.B. 1994. Women's concerns with hormone replacement therapy–compliance issues. Fertil. Steril. **62** (Suppl 2): 157S–160S.
99. PILON, D., A. CASTILLOUX & J. LELORIER. 2001. Estrogen replacement therapy: determinants of persistence with treatment. Obstet. Gynecol. **97:** 97–100.
100. LOVE, R.R., L. CAMERON, B.L. CONNELL & H. LEVENTHAL. 1991. Symptoms associated with tamoxifen treatment in postmenopausal women. Arch. Intern. Med. **151:** 1842–1847.
101. DAVIES G.C., W.J. HUSTER, Y. LU, et al. 1999. Adverse events reported by postmenopausal women in controlled trials with raloxifene. Obstet. Gynecol. **93:** 558–565.
102. VERONESI, U., P. MAISONNEUVE, A. COSTA, et al. 1998. Prevention of breast cancer with tamoxifen: preliminary findings from the Italian randomised trial among hysterectomised women. Lancet **352:** 93–97.
103. DECENSI, A., B. BONANNI, N. ROTMENSZ, et al. ON BEHALF OF THE ITALIAN INVESTIGATORS. 2000. Update on tamoxifen to prevent breast cancer. The Italian Tamoxifen Prevention Study. Eur. J. Cancer **36:** S49–S56.
104. DECENSI, A., C. ROBERTSON, N. ROTMENSZ, et al. ON BEHALF OF THE ITALIAN CHEMOPREVENTION GROUP. 1998. Effect of tamoxifen and transdermal hormone replacement therapy on cardiovascular risk factors in a prevention trial. Br. J. Cancer **78:** 572–578.
105. BONANNI, B., A. GUERRIERI-GONZAGA, N. ROTMENSZ, et al. 2000. Hormonal therapy and chemoprevention. Breast J. **6:** 317–323.
106. COBLEIGH, M.A. 2000. Managing menopausal symptoms. *In* Diseases of the Breast, 2nd edit. J.R. Harris et al., Eds.: 1041–1050. Lippincott Williams & Wilkins. Philadelphia.
107. SWAIN, S., R. SANTEN, H. BURGER & K. PRITCHARD. 1999. Treatment of estrogen deficiency symptoms in women surviving breast cancer. Part 1: Defining the problem. Proceedings of a conference held at the Boar's Head Inn, Charlottesville, Virginia, September 21–23, 1997. Oncology **13** (1): 109–136.

108. COL, N.F., L.K. HIROTA, R.K. ORR, *et al.* 2001. Hormone replacement therapy after breast cancer: a systematic review and quantitative assessment of risk. J. Clin. Oncol. **19:** 2357–2363.
109. SWAIN, S., R. SANTEN, H. BURGER & K. PRITCHARD. 1999. Treatment of estrogen deficiency symptoms in women surviving breast cancer. Part 2: Hormone replacement therapy and breast cancer. Proceedings of a conference held at the Boar's Head Inn, Charlottesville, Virginia, September 21–23, 1997. Oncology **13** (2): 245–267.
110. PRITCHARD, K.I. 2001. Hormone replacement in women with a history of breast cancer. Oncologist **6:** 353–362.
111. COLDITZ, G.A. 1997. Estrogen replacement therapy for breast cancer patients. Oncology **11:** 1491–1497.
112. POWLES, T.J., R. EELES, S. ASHLEY, *et al.* 1998. Interim analysis of the incidence of breast cancer in the Royal Marsden Hospital tamoxifen randomised chemoprevention trial. Lancet **352:** 98–101.
113. VESSEY, M., D. MANT, A. SMITH & D. YEATES. 1986. Oral contraceptives and venous thromboembolism; findings in a large prospective study. Br. Med. J. (Clin. Res. Ed.) **292:** 526–530.
114. WORLD HEALTH ORGANIZATION COLLABORATIVE STUDY OF CARDIOVASCULAR DISEASE AND STEROID HORMONE CONTRACEPTION. 1995. Venous thromboembolic disease and combined oral contraceptives: results of an international multicentre case-control study. Lancet **346:** 1575–1582.
115. DALY, E., M.P. VESSEY, M.M. HAWKINS, *et al.* 1996. Risk of venous thromboembolism in users of hormone replacement therapy. Lancet **348:** 977–980.
116. JICK, H., L.E. DERBY, M.W. MYERS, *et al.* 1996. Risk of hospital admission for idiopathic venous thromboembolism among users of postmenopausal oestrogens. Lancet **348:** 981–983.
117. GRODSTEIN, F., M.J. STAMPFER, S.Z. GOLDHABER, *et al.* 1996. Prospective study of exogenous hormones and risk of pulmonary embolism in women. Lancet **348:** 983–987.
118. GRADY, D., N.K. WENGER, D. HERRINGTON, *et al.* FOR THE HEART AND ESTROGEN/PROGESTIN REPLACEMENT STUDY RESEARCH GROUP. 2000. Postmenopausal hormone therapy increases risk for venous thromboembolic disease. The Heart and Estrogen/progestin Replacement Study. Ann. Intern. Med. **132:** 689–696.
119. VISCOLI, C.M., L.M. BRASS & W.N. KERNAN. 2001. Estrogen after ischemic stroke: effect of estrogen replacement on risk of recurrent stroke and death. In the Women's Estrogen for Stroke Trial (WEST). (Abstr.) Stroke **32:** 329.
120. GAIL, M.H., J.P COSTANTINO, J. BRYANT, *et al.* 1999. Weighing the risks and benefits of tamoxifen treatment for preventing breast cancer. J. Natl. Cancer Inst. **91:** 1829–1846.
121. TAYLOR, A.L., L.L. ADAMS-CAMPBELL, J.T. WRIGHT, JR. 1999. Risk/benefit assessment of tamoxifen to prevent breast cancer— still a work in progress? J. Natl. Cancer Inst. **91:** 1792–1793.
122. CHLEBOWSKI, R.T., D. COLLYAR, M.R. SOMERFIELD, *et al.* 1999. American Society of Clinical Oncology technology assessment on breast cancer risk reduction strategies: tamoxifen and raloxifene. J. Clin. Oncol. **17:** 1939–1955.
123. NEVEN, P. & I. VERGOTE. 1998. Should tamoxifen users be screened for endometrial lesions? (Commentary) Lancet **351:** 155–556.

Weighing the Benefits and Risks in Clinical Trials and Practice
Introduction

WORTA McCASKILL-STEVENS

Division of Cancer Prevention, National Cancer Institute, Bethesda, Maryland 20892, USA

The ability of the SERMs to affect multiple organs presents challenges to clinical trialists and clinicians who weigh risks and benefits of their use in treatment and prevention. The delicate balance between risks and benefits is especially acute in the prevention setting. In prevention, SERMs are weighed not only for their intrinsic risks and benefits, but for potential interactions with other drugs and with comorbid conditions. Results from studies of SERMs have not been easily interpreted by clinicians, making them uncomfortable discussing risks and benefits in clinical practice. Paramount to public health concerns is the communication of benefit and risk to the general population.

The papers in this section explore an innovative, yet developing area of work that attempts to measure risks and benefits of SERM interventions by focusing upon the applications of current methodologies (e.g., risk assessment tools) in clinical research and clinical practice. Key elements of such risk/benefit methodologies are identified in order that they can be incorporated into the design of clinical trials. Suggestions are also made as to how available risk/benefit methodologies can be better translated from outcomes of clinical trials to outcomes that are meaningful to individual patients. Problems inherent with the decision-making process are discussed, including a comparison of the role of relative risk versus absolute risk versus net effect (with regard to risk) in communicating to patients and high-risk individuals about SERM use. Constraints of the existing tools and databases required to provide accurate and useful information about risks and benefits to all populations (e.g., different ages, racial/ethnic groups, gender) are also critically reviewed. The papers in this section span the gamut from the development of statistical models of risk/benefit assessment to application of such models in the clinical setting, with its inherent psychological and sociological components. Perspectives are provided from different clinical specialties/disciplines in which SERMs are frequently used, and areas of research needs (e.g., how to incorporate the perspective and values of the potential user of SERMs) are identified.

Address for correspondence: Worta McCaskill-Stevens, M.D., M.S., Program Director, Community Oncology and Prevention Trials Research Group, Division of Cancer Prevention, National Cancer Institute, 6130 Executive Boulevard, Room 2014, Bethesda, MD 20892. Voice: 301-496-8541; fax: 301-496-8667.

wm57h@nih.gov

Benefit/Risk Assessment of SERM Therapy

Clinical Trial versus Clinical Practice Settings

JOSEPH P. COSTANTINO

Department of Biostatistics, Graduate School of Public Health, University of Pittsburgh, Pittsburgh, Pennsylvania 15213, USA

ABSTRACT: Benefit/risk assessment (B/rA) can be used in a variety of circumstances encompassing clinical practice and research settings. Subsequent to the reporting of the results from the Breast Cancer Prevention Trial (BCPT), methodology was developed to perform B/rA for the use of the selected estrogen receptor modulator (SERM), tamoxifen. Although the methodology was specifically developed and applied to the use of tamoxifen, it is a generalized procedure that can be readily modified and applied to other forms of therapy including other SERMs. Recently, the methodology has been incorporated into the Study of Tamoxifen and Raloxifene (STAR) trial, a randomized clinical trial designed to compare the chemopreventive effects of two SERMs—tamoxifen and raloxifene. The B/rA of SERMs is complex because SERMs are known to exhibit properties that can reduce or increase the incidence of several health outcomes. This paper summarizes the uses of B/rA in the clinical practice and clinical trial settings and describes the constraints of the methodology as it is being applied to the assessment of therapy with SERMs.

KEYWORDS: benefit/risk assessment (B/rA); tamoxifen

APPLICATIONS OF BENEFIT/RISK ASSESSMENT OF SERM THERAPY

The methodology developed for the benefit/risk assessment (B/rA) of tamoxifen therapy was proposed as a tool for use in clinical practice.[1] In this setting, it is employed to provide information regarding the potential trade-offs of benefits and risks from therapy for an individual who may be contemplating the use of tamoxifen to reduce the risk of breast cancer. In the research setting, B/rA can be employed for several purposes. It can be used to (a) justify the importance of a trial by demonstrating the potential for a net benefit of therapy in terms of the general public health, (b) provide information to support the informed consent process of participant recruitment, and (c) supplement the methods for monitoring the safety of trial participants by determining the net effect of beneficial and detrimental outcomes experienced within the study cohort. A key aspect that differentiates between the application of B/rA in these two settings is the nature of the unit upon which the assessments are based. In the clinical practice setting, the assessment unit is an individual patient. In the research setting, the assessment unit is not always an individual, but rather the

---

Address for correspondence: Joseph P. Costantino, University of Pittsburgh, Graduate School of Public Health, 103 DeSoto Street, Room 516, Pittsburgh, PA 15213. Voice: 412-624-5379; fax: 412-624-2183.

costan@nsabp.pitt.edu

TABLE 1. End points affected by tamoxifen therapy

Nature of therapy effect	
Beneficial—reduces risk	*Detrimental—increases risk*
Invasive breast cancer	Endometrial cancer
In situ breast cancer	Pulmonary embolism
Hip fracture	Deep vein thrombosis
Spine fracture	Stroke
Colles' fracture	Cataracts

assessment unit is the general population or a subset of the population that has some particular characteristic or set of characteristics. This distinction regarding the unit of assessment is important in terms of understanding the limitations of the B/rA being used for tamoxifen and raloxifene. This issue will be discussed in addition to the general methods of B/rA used for these SERMs and the tools used to communicate the results of a B/rA to an individual.

There are ten different health end points that are potentially affected by therapy with tamoxifen (TABLE 1). Five end points are affected in a beneficial manner and five are affected in a detrimental manner. The end points for which the risk will be reduced by tamoxifen therapy include invasive breast cancer, *in situ* breast cancer, hip fracture, spine fracture, and Colles' fracture. Those for which the risk will be increased include endometrial cancer, pulmonary embolism (PE), deep vein thrombosis (DVT), stroke, and cataracts. The end points potentially affected by raloxifene are the same as those for tamoxifen, with one exception. The currently available evidence indicates that raloxifene does not affect the risk of endometrial cancer. Also, based on preliminary evidence from studies among women with osteoporosis, it is assumed that the effect of raloxifene on breast cancer is similar to that of tamoxifen. The verification of this potential effect is the primary objective of the Study of Tamoxifen and Raloxifene (STAR) trial. The B/rA method used to assess these SERMs includes procedures for estimating the treatment effects for each of the ten end points. To accomplish this, estimates of the expected incidence rate for each of the end points are multiplied by the end point–specific risk ratios seen in the Breast Cancer Prevention Trial (BCPT) population.[2] These risk ratios were obtained by dividing the incidence rates among those in the BCPT tamoxifen group by the incidence rates among those in the BCPT placebo group.

LIMITATIONS OF B/rA FOR SERM THERAPY

The existing B/rA methodology for SERM use is well conceived and is considered to be state of the art. While it is applicable in a variety of settings, it is not universally ideal for all types of application. A B/rA methodology that would be considered as universally ideal for use in all settings would be one that incorporates (as measures of expected baseline risk) broad-based, age- and race-specific incidence rates for each of the end points potentially affected (in a beneficial or detrimental way) by therapy. The ideal methodology would also be one that incorporates the con-

TABLE 2. Example of data presentation tool for communicating the benefits and risks of tamoxifen therapy

Severity of event	Type of event	Expected number of cases among 10,000 untreated women	Expected effect among 10,000 women if they all take tamoxifen for 5 years
			Potential benefits:
Life-threatening events	invasive breast cancer	$N_{0,1}$ cases expected	$N_{1,1}$ of these cases may be prevented
	hip fracture	$N_{0,2}$ cases expected	$N_{1,2}$ of these cases may be prevented
			Potential risks:
	endometrial cancer	$N_{0,3}$ cases expected	$N_{1,3}$ more cases may be caused
	stroke	$N_{0,4}$ cases expected	$N_{1,4}$ more cases may be caused
	pulmonary embolism	$N_{0,5}$ cases expected	$N_{1,5}$ more cases may be caused
			Potential benefit:
Other severe events	*in situ* breast cancer	$N_{0,6}$ cases expected	$N_{1,6}$ of these cases may be prevented
			Potential risk:
	deep-vein thrombosis	$N_{0,7}$ cases expected	$N_{2,7}$ more cases may be caused
Other events	*Potential benefits*: Tamoxifen use may reduce the risk of a certain type of wrist fracture called Colles' fracture by about 39% and also may reduce the risk from fractures of the spine by about 26%.		
	Potential risk: Tamoxifen use may increase the occurrence of cataracts by about 14%.		

NOTE: Shown are the number of certain events that would be expected during the next 5 years among 10,000 untreated women of your age (age_X), race ($race_Y$), and 5-year breast cancer risk ($risk_Z$). To help understand the potential benefits and risks of treatment, these numbers can be compared with the number of expected cases that would be prevented or caused by 5 years of tamoxifen use.

sideration of how the baseline risk for each of the potentially affected end points may be modified by the presence or absence of important risk factors. Unfortunately, due to deficiencies in the information that is available for incorporation, it is currently impossible to develop the universally ideal B/rA methodology.

Data from the Surveillance, Epidemiology, and End Results (SEER) Project provide an excellent source of broad-based, age- and race-specific incidence rates for the estimates of baseline breast and endometrial cancer risks.[3] However, for the other end points shown in TABLE 2, such rates are not available or are available for only limited segments of the population. While the SEER Project is an excellent source of cancer incidence data, population-based cohort studies are potential sources for expected rates of the end points of bone fracture, cataracts, DVT, PE, and stroke. To date, most of the representative cohort studies that include assessment of these end points have been restricted to the study of males. As a result, appropriate baseline incidence rates for females are sparse or nonexistent. This deficiency is most severe for non-Caucasian females. A similar problem exists regarding the availability of validated, multivariate models that could be used to incorporate key risk factors into the determination of expected baseline risks for most of the end points potentially affected by SERM therapy. This latter problem is not an issue for invasive and *in situ* breast cancer. The expected incidence rates used in the B/rA methodology for these end points are specific for an individual's profile of breast cancer risk factors, determined from the Gail *et al.* model.[4] This model includes the multivariate consideration of eight breast cancer risk factors. However, for the other end points of interest, there are no validated, multivariate models available that can be used to predict risk among females as a function of their risk factor profile. The inclusion of such models would be most important for the vascular-related end points (DVT, PE, and stroke), where risk factors such as diabetes, hypertension, obesity, exercise habits, and smoking history are important modifiers of risk. Since there are no models currently available to estimate baseline risk as a function of all key risk factors for these other end points, the expected incidence rates used in the B/rA for these end points are a function of only race and age group, with age classified into 10-year intervals.

Due to the aforementioned deficiencies of the available information, the B/rA methodology is more ideal for some settings than for others. As described earlier in this paper, the intended use of B/rA in the clinical trial setting is usually as a population-based assessment. In contrast, in the clinical practice setting, the intended use of B/rA is as an individual-based assessment. As the B/rA algorithms for determining the baseline risks of the vascular-related end points do not include the consideration of the full risk factor profile, the estimates of the treatment effect for these end points represent the average effects for all women within a race and age group-specific population and not the specific effects for a particular individual within that population. As such, the B/rA methodology is ideal for use to estimate the benefits and risks of therapy among a population as a whole, as is the case for most clinical trial applications. The methodology, though, is not ideal for use as an individual-based assessment, the typical clinical practice application. Despite this limitation, the B/rA methodology provides a very useful tool for use in the clinical practice setting, providing information to facilitate the understanding of the complicated interplay of potential gains and losses for the numerous end points potentially affected by the use of therapy. However, when a clinician uses B/rA as a tool to provide information to a woman who may be considering the use of therapy to reduce her risk of breast cancer, it should be recognized that the actual effects of therapy expected for the individual being assessed may be quite different than that expected as the average effect experience among all women who are within the same race and age category as the individual. The clinician should make it a point to qualify the estimates of the vascular-related effects in light of the individual's personal profile of risk factors for these end points. If the woman being assessed does not smoke, does not have diabetes, is normotensive, is not obese, and is physically active, the detrimental effects that she may experience are likely to be substantially less than that estimated by the B/rA. On the other hand, if the woman's profile includes several risk factors, the detrimental effects that she may experience are likely to be greater than that estimated by the B/rA.

COMMUNICATING THE RESULTS OF B/rA TO THE INDIVIDUAL

With such a complicated interplay of numerous potential beneficial and detrimental effects of SERMs like tamoxifen, the communication of the results of a B/rA to an individual woman can be a difficult task. A tool has been developed for use with the B/rA to aid in the communication process (TABLE 2). The tool is the product of a panel of experts who participated in a national workshop sponsored by the National Cancer Institute that was convened for the purpose of developing such a tool.[1] When designing the tool, the workshop panel had established a list of desired properties that an ideal benefit/risk communication tool should possess. These properties of an ideal tool were identified as a tool that (a) avoids to the extent possible the use of probabilities or relative risks as these are entities that can be confusing to those not familiar with such statistical measures, (b) includes information on all potentially affected end points with consideration of effects grouped by the relative severity of the different end points, and (c) provides a presentation that summarizes the results of the B/rA that is limited to one page. The approach to providing information in the tool is based on describing the effects of therapy in terms of the number of cases expected to occur over 5 years of follow-up among 10,000 women of the same race, age group, and predicted breast cancer risk as the individual being assessed. The tool provides a comparison of the number of cases expected if none of the 10,000 women was treated to the number of cases that may be prevented or caused if all 10,000 women were treated. Subsequent to the publication of the workshop panel's recommendations, a version of the B/rA communication tool has been incorporated into the informed consent process of the STAR trial as a tool to explain the potential benefits and risks associated with trial participation.

An additional distinction to be made on the unit of assessment when the B/rA is population-based is to develop an index of net effect, that is, a mechanism to describe the overall net effect of therapy. This index is obtained by summing, across all end points, the difference between the number of cases potentially prevented by therapy and the number of cases potentially caused by therapy. This is a valid approach in the population-based application of B/rA because, in the population as a whole, one would expect to actually observe the effect on the occurrence of all ten of the end points of interest. In contrast, the observation of the effect on the occurrence of all 10 end points in any one individual is not possible. If the individual experiences any of the end points, it is likely that she will experience only one. Thus, it is recommended that a net index not be used as part of the communication of B/rA results to an individual. Instead, the communication should focus on a description of the magnitude of effects for each separate end point. In addition to avoiding the use of a net index that is nonintuitive in this setting, the latter approach provides the woman being assessed with more specific information to use as input to decide which end points are most relevant to her concerns, and it allows her to apply her own weighing of the end points to decide which risks she finds acceptable.

REFERENCES

1. GAIL, M.H., J.P. COSTANTINO & J. BRYANT. 1999. Weighing the risks and benefits of tamoxifen for preventing breast cancer. J. Natl. Cancer Inst. **91:** 1829–1846.
2. FISHER, B., J.P. COSTANTINO, D.L. WICKERHAM *et al.* 1998. Tamoxifen for prevention of breast cancer: report of the National Surgical Adjuvant Breast and Bowel Project P-1 Study. J. Natl. Cancer Inst. **90:** 1371–1388.
3. NCI. 1999. Surveillance, Epidemiology, and End Results (SEER) Program Public-Use CD-ROM (1973–1997). DCCPS, Cancer Surveillance Research Program, Cancer Statistics Branch, National Cancer Institute. Bethesda, MD.
4. COSTANTINO, J.P., M.H. GAIL & D. PEE. 1999. Validation studies for models to project the risk of invasive and total breast cancer incidence. J. Natl. Cancer Inst. **91:** 1541–1548.

The Estimation and Use of Absolute Risk for Weighing the Risks and Benefits of Selective Estrogen Receptor Modulators for Preventing Breast Cancer

MITCHELL H. GAIL

National Cancer Institute, Bethesda, Maryland 20892, USA

ABSTRACT: In order to weigh the risks and benefits of intervention with selective estrogen response modifiers for preventing breast cancer, one needs to consider the effects of intervention on several health outcomes. For example, tamoxifen was shown to reduce the risks of breast cancer and hip fracture while increasing the risks of endometrial cancer and cardiovascular end points, including stroke. One approach to weighing risks and benefits is to estimate the net effect of the intervention on the absolute risk of each of the relevant health outcomes. To estimate this net effect, one needs to know not only the relative risk from the intervention, but also the absolute risk of the health outcome in the absence of intervention. Intervention trials yield unbiased estimates of intervention relative risks, but data are usually too limited to estimate these relative risks precisely for subgroups or for rare health outcomes. Moreover, intervention trials are usually too small to provide data for developing a model for estimating the individualized absolute risk of various health outcomes in the absence of intervention. The model of Gail *et al.* for projecting the individualized risk of breast cancer, as modified for use in the Breast Cancer Prevention Trial, has been validated. To weigh various risks and benefits of interventions, there is a need for research to develop such models for a range of health outcomes.

KEYWORDS: risks, benefits, breast cancer prevention, SERMs

The decision to use selective estrogen receptor modulators (SERMs) to prevent, treat, and reduce the risk of breast cancer is complicated by the fact that SERMs influence many health outcomes. For example, the Breast Cancer Prevention Trial (BCPT), also known as P-1,[1] demonstrated that tamoxifen reduced the risks of invasive and noninvasive breast cancer and of hip fractures, while increasing the risks of endometrial cancer, stroke, pulmonary embolism, and deep vein thrombosis. A woman deciding whether to take tamoxifen needs to weigh the various risks she faces in the presence and the absence of tamoxifen. An essential ingredient in this decision process is an estimate of the absolute risks of the various outcomes in the presence and the absence of tamoxifen. In this paper we discuss the role of absolute

---

Address for correspondence: M.H. Gail, M.D., Ph.D., National Cancer Institute, EPS/8032, 6120 Executive Blvd., Bethesda, MD 20892-7244. Voice: 301-496-4156; fax: 301-402-0081.
Gailm@exchange.nih.gov

TABLE 1. Numbers of events expected in five years in a population of 10,000 40-year-old white women with a projected risk of breast cancer of 2% in the absence of tamoxifen

	Expected without tamoxifen $I_j \times 10^4$	Expected with tamoxifen $R_j I_j \times 10^4$	Prevented (or caused) by tamoxifen $I_j(1 - R_j) \times 10^4$
Invasive breast cancer	200	102	98
Hip fracture	2	1	1
Endometrial cancer	10	26	(16)
Stroke	22	35	(13)
Pulmonary embolism	7	22	(15)

risk and its estimation. Although we illustrate these ideas with data from the BCPT and rely heavily on a publication aimed at measuring the risks and benefits of tamoxifen,[2] our comments apply more broadly to the evaluation of SERMs and to other interventions to prevent or reduce the risk of disease.

The absolute risk of developing breast cancer over a period of five years, for example, is just the probability that a woman who is free of breast cancer at age "a" will be observed to develop breast cancer at or before age "$a + 5$." Suppose that there are "J" adverse health outcomes of interest, "$j = 1, 2, ..., J$." Suppose that, in the absence of tamoxifen, outcome "j" has a 5-year absolute risk "I_j." We call "I_j" the baseline absolute risk of outcome "j." Suppose the effect of tamoxifen is to multiply this risk by a relative risk factor "R_j," which is less than one for a protective effect of tamoxifen and greater than one for an adverse effect of tamoxifen. Then, to a good approximation, the net effect of tamoxifen is to reduce (or increase) the absolute risk of outcome "j" by the net amount

$$I_j - R_j I_j = I_j(1 - Rj), \qquad (1)$$

which is positive when tamoxifen is beneficial and negative otherwise. More complicated expressions are needed for longer time periods in which competing risks from the various health outcomes and other causes of death must be taken into account,[2–3] but Eq.(1) is quite adequate for 5-year time intervals.

BCPT was a randomized intervention study and provided excellent estimates of relative risks R_j for various health outcomes, including those in TABLE 1. Estimates of "I_j" are more problematic, as we shall discuss in subsequent sections, and often must be based on data sources outside a particular intervention trial.

To make the idea of absolute risk easier to understand, we tabulate the number of women expected to have a given event in a population of 10,000 women followed for five years (TABLE 1). Thus, in the absence of tamoxifen, an absolute risk of breast cancer of 0.02 or 2% over five years would correspond to an expected 0.02 × 10,000 = 200 women who develop breast cancer in that population.

In such a population of white women, data from the BCPT indicate[1,2] that tamoxifen would prevent 98 invasive breast cancers and one hip fracture, while causing an additional 16 endometrial cancers, 13 strokes, and 15 pulmonary embolisms (TABLE 1). In counseling, each woman might react to these data differently, depending on her concerns about the various health outcomes. In putting these numbers in perspective, it might be useful to note that 92 white women would be expected to die from any cause in this population during this 5-year period. Gail et al.[2] presented a more elaborate version of TABLE 1 with more health outcomes, and they summarized the benefits and losses from tamoxifen by taking the weighted average of the various net outcomes (column 4, TABLE 1). But whether one summarizes the results in TABLE 1 or discusses each outcome separately, the basic ingredients in the decision include the absolute risks in columns 2 and 3 of TABLE 1, the net effect of intervention on each outcome (column 4) and the importance the woman attaches to each outcome. In implementing this approach to assessing risks and benefits, we found that there is substantial uncertainty, not only concerning R_j, but also especially concerning I_j. We discuss these uncertainties in the following sections.

UNCERTAINTIES IN THE ESTIMATION OF TREATMENT RELATIVE RISKS, R_j

A carefully designed and conducted randomized intervention trial is an ideal study to estimate treatment relative risks, R_j. Randomization protects against selection bias and yields unbiased estimates of the relative risk associated with treatment. Even a large and well-executed study such as the BCPT will often provide only limited information on R_j for some of the rarer outcomes, however. For example, the BCPT was designed to yield precise results for the effects of tamoxifen on invasive breast cancer. The relative risk for invasive breast cancer, based on 264 events in the trial, was $R = 0.51$ with 95% confidence interval (CI) 0.39–0.66, indicating a substantial protective effect. Data on endometrial cancer were comparatively sparse; the relative risk for endometrial cancer was 2.53 with a fairly wide 95% CI of 1.35–4.97 based on 51 events. For stroke, the relative risk was 1.59 with 95% CI 0.93–2.77 based on 62 events. Thus, although the BCPT yielded unbiased estimates of R_j for various outcomes, the precision of the estimates varied, depending on how rare or common the outcome was.

The data from BCPT are too limited to permit reliable estimates of tamoxifen effects for small subgroups of the population. One usually assumes that the treatment effects are homogeneous across subgroups, unless there is evidence to the contrary. Indeed, Fisher et al.[1] found very consistent effects of tamoxifen on the risk of invasive breast cancer in subgroups defined by baseline predicted breast cancer risk, age, history of carcinoma in situ, and number of first-degree relatives with breast cancer. Only 1.7% of the women in BCPT were African American. Thus, there is little power to demonstrate whether tamoxifen's effects differ between African-American women and other trial participants. In practice, one will often be forced to assume that treatment effects observed for the entire trial population apply to various subgroups of the population.

ESTIMATING ABSOLUTE RISKS I_j IN THE ABSENCE OF TAMOXIFEN

Absolute risk, in the absence of tamoxifen, depends strongly on a number of individual characteristics such as age, medical history, ethnicity, and selection factors used to define eligibility for participation in an intervention study. In counseling a woman on her risk of breast cancer in the absence of tamoxifen, it is important to individualize the risk projection to the extent possible. Data from an intervention trial, such as the BCPT, will usually be insufficient to define baseline absolute risk within subgroups defined by age and various medical factors. For example, only 89 women in the placebo arm of the BCPT developed invasive breast cancer; thus it would not be feasible to estimate baseline risk precisely, even in subgroups defined only by age. Instead, one must rely on larger studies to provide information on baseline absolute risk.

To project baseline risk for invasive breast cancer for BCPT, statisticians Stewart Anderson and Carol Redmond of the University of Pittsburgh modified the model for projecting breast cancer risk developed by Gail et al.,[3] which was based on data from the Breast Cancer Detection Demonstration Project (BCDDP). Gail et al. analyzed case-control data from BCDDP of 2,852 white women who developed breast cancer and 3,146 white women without breast cancer to develop a multivariate relative risk model that took into account age, age at menarche, age at first live birth, number of previous breast biopsies, the presence of atypical hyperplasia on any biopsy, and the number of first-degree relatives (mothers and sisters) with breast cancer. Gail et al. showed how to combine this relative risk information with age-specific breast cancer incidence rates from the entire BCDDP population of 243,221 white women to estimate the absolute risk of developing disease over particular time intervals, such as a 5-year age interval, for a woman with a given age and set of risk factors. Drs. Anderson and Redmond modified the calculations by substituting for BCDDP age-specific rates the age-specific incidence rates from the National Cancer Institute's Surveillance, Epidemiology and End Results (SEER) Program. They also adapted the model to project risks for African-American women, as described in Costantino et al.[4]

This modification of the model by Gail et al.[3] was used to characterize women who were eligible for the BCPT. Indeed, women under age 60 who had a projected 5-year risk less than 1.66% were ineligible. The predictions from this model for women in various age groups proved to be quite accurate, as was seen by comparing expected and observed cancer incidence in subgroups of the placebo arm of the BCPT.[4] A recent validation analysis on data from the Nurses Health Study confirmed the good calibration of this model.[5] This model is available at the National Cancer Institute's web site hppt://cancernet.nci.nih.gov/genetics_prevention.html.

Thus, one has a well-calibrated model for projecting the 5-year risk of breast cancer for white women with particular risk factors. The net benefits of tamoxifen for preventing invasive breast cancer depend directly on the level of baseline absolute risk, as indicated in Eq. 1. For example, if a woman with particular risk factors has a baseline risk $I = 0.02$, as in TABLE 1, her net benefit is $0.02 (1-0.51) \times 10,000 = 98$. In contrast, a woman with more risk factors and a higher baseline risk of $I = 0.04$ stands to benefit by $0.04 (1-0.51) \times 10,000 = 196$ events. This calculation illustrates the importance of having individualized estimates of baseline incidence rates, I_j, for each of the health outcomes of interest.

Unfortunately, models to project individualized absolute risk are not available for many important health outcomes. This is because registries are not available to gather data on the incidence of many of these diseases and because few investigators have published data on individualized absolute risk from cohort studies.

As an important example, Gail et al.[2] estimated the age-specific risk of stroke in white women from population-based studies in Rochester, Minnesota.[6] Rochester, Minnesota probably has lower incidence rates than rates in other parts of the United States, however. Indeed, age-adjusted stroke mortality rates for white women were 69.8 per 10^5 woman-years for women aged 35–84 years in Olmstead County, Minnesota, compared to a rate of 92.2 for the United States. In addition, these data could not be used directly to obtain individualized estimates depending on medical factors such as blood pressure, weight, and the presence of a cardiac arrhythmia. Incidence data were not even available on ethnicity, because Rochester, Minnesota has a predominantly white population. Yet it is known that African-American women have stroke mortality rates considerably higher than white women in the U.S., and, as reviewed by Gail et al.,[2] the literature indicates similar elevation in stroke incidence among African-American women. Thus, Gail et al.[2] individualized stroke baseline incidence rates for age and ethnicity, but were unable to find validated models for absolute risk that incorporated important features of the medical history. This can be problematic when advising a black woman, for example, who is in excellent physical condition and has no health problems. Her baseline risk of stroke may be considerably lower than the average black woman in her age group, and she may therefore have a lower risk of stroke than one would find in tables individualized only for age and ethnicity, such as Table 3 in Gail et al.[2]

To project individualized absolute risk in the absence of tamoxifen, one needs a multivariate relative risk model to take various prognostic factors into account, and one needs to obtain absolute rates from following a cohort or from registry data.[3] Cohort or case-control studies can be used to estimate the multivariate relative risk function, but only cohorts or registries provide the additional ingredients needed to compute individualized absolute risk. Many analyses of cohort studies have focused on the relative risk features of the model, which may be applicable in various populations, rather than on modeling individualized absolute risk. For whatever reason, there is a dearth of validated individualized models for absolute risk for most health outcomes, and there is a need to develop such models. Large cohorts, such as the Women's Health Initiative cohort, can provide valuable information on absolute risk. Volunteers for such studies, however, tend to be healthier than the general population and to have lower incidence and mortality rates from cardiovascular diseases.

DISCUSSION

The assessment of intervention with SERMs to prevent breast cancer is complicated by their effects on multiple health outcomes. The important role of individualized absolute risk in the absence of intervention, as well as the treatment relative risk from intervention, in assessing the net gains and losses from intervention for each health outcome affected by intervention has been highlighted. These gains and losses can be examined individually (TABLE 1) or can be summarized to assist in decision making. Although unbiased estimates of treatment relative risks can be obtained from randomized intervention studies, there will typically be insufficient information to estimate treatment effects precisely within subgroups or for uncommon health outcomes. To permit more reliable assessment of the risks and benefits of preventive interventions, there is a pressing need for research to develop models for projecting individualized absolute risks of various health outcomes in the absence of intervention.

REFERENCES

1. FISHER, B., J.P. COSTANTINO, D.L. WICKERHAM, *et al.* 1998. Tamoxifen for prevention of breast cancer: report of the National Surgical Adjuvant Breast and Bowel Project P-1 Study. J. Natl. Cancer Inst. **90:** 1371–1388.
2. GAIL, M.H., J.P. COSTANTINO, V. VOGEL, *et al.* 1999. Weighing the risks and benefits of tamoxifen treatment for preventing breast cancer. J. Natl. Cancer Inst. **91:** 1829–1846.
3. GAIL, M.H., L.A. BRINTON, C. SCHAIRER, *et al.* 1989. Projecting individualized probabilities of developing breast cancer for white females who are being examined annually. J. Natl. Cancer Inst. **81:** 1879–1886.
4. COSTANTINO, J.P., M.H. GAIL, D. PEE, *et al.* 1999. Validation studies for models projecting the risk of invasive and total breast cancer incidence. J. Natl. Cancer Inst. **91:** 1541–1548.
5. ROCKHILL, B., D. SPIEGELMAN, G.A. COLDITZ, *et al.* 2001. Validation of the Gail *et al.* model of breast cancer risk prediction and implications for chemoprevention. J. Natl. Cancer Inst. **93:** 358–366.
6. BRODERICK, J.P., S.J. PHILLIPS, E.J. BERGSTRALH, *et al.* 1998. Incidence rates of stroke in the eighties: the end of the decline in stroke? Stroke **20:** 577–582.

SERMs, Ethnicity, and Clinical Trials
Opportunities and Challenges

ANNE L. TAYLOR

Division of Cardiology, Mayo Medical School, Minneapolis, Minnesota 55455, USA

> ABSTRACT: Selective estrogen receptor modulators (SERMs) are an exciting new class of pharmacotherapeutics that may have application in a wide variety of disease states. The science, both basic and clinical, that would guide the usage of these agents is in some respects at a relatively early developmental stage. Thus, the research community has an opportunity, before their use becomes widespread, to structure clinical trials such that the most complete profiles of benefits and risks are described. Tamoxifen is the SERM that has been most extensively studied and for which there are indications for both treatment and prevention of breast cancer based on trials involving more than 50,000 women. Despite this seemingly adequate sample size, an extremely important question remains unanswered—namely, whether there are ethnic differences in benefit and adverse effects of SERMs. It has generally been the case that new pharmacologic agents are tested in relatively small numbers of subjects, often only male, in North America and western Europe. While the populations are multi-ethnic, clinical trial subjects are most often not representative of the ethnic variability of these areas. Guidelines for usage of new drugs based on data from small, ethnically limited population groups are then generalized to other population groups, without consideration that differences in drug metabolism and/or responsiveness might exist.
>
> KEYWORDS: ethnicity; SERMs; clinical trials

Ethnicity as well as sex/gender are well-recognized important variables in pharmacokinetics and/or pharmacodynamics (i.e., biologic responsiveness to drug, including drug-tissue interaction, biomarker modulation, etc.) and may have important effects on clinical outcomes.[1–5] In clinical trials, it has been shown that women are at higher risk for lethal cardiac arrhythmias (e.g., torsades de pointes) when treated with drugs blocking cardiac potassium channel sites.[2–4] Similarly, ethnic differences in drug pharmacokinetics and pharmacodynamics have been well documented[5] and shown to be clinically important. For example, the prevalence of slow or rapid drug acetylation of antituberculous drugs is well characterized. Rapid acetylation occurs in 80% to 90% of subjects of Asian origin, but in only 40% to 50% of Caucasians.[6] Differ-

---

Address for correspondence: Anne L. Taylor, M.D., Professor of Medicine, Division of Cardiology, Associate Dean for Faculty Affairs, Office of the Dean—Medical School, C694 Mayo Memorial Building, Mayo Mail Code 293, 420 Delaware Street S.E., Minneapolis, MN 55455. Voice: 612-624-5442; fax: 612-626-4911.
  taylo135@umn.edu

ences in acetylation of these drugs can be associated with either treatment failure or toxicity. In another example, patients with high renin hypertension have an enhanced hypotensive response when treated with angiotensin-converting enzyme (ACE) inhibitors and beta-blockers. In African-American populations, a low prevalence of high renin hypertension exists and, consequently, a lesser hypotensive response to monotherapy with these classes of agents has been demonstrated.[7] This difference, in effect, disappears when a diuretic is added to the therapeutic regimen, thus permitting African-American patients to have adequate blood pressure control as well as other therapeutic benefits from these drugs, so recognition of this difference has important treatment implications.

Reduction of risk of breast cancer with tamoxifen[8–11] is the signal event for an era in which prevention by means other than lifestyle modifications, in addition to screening with treatment, will be effective in reducing the morbidity and mortality from cancer.[10] It is thus critically important to accurately define risk/benefit ratios for use of chemopreventive agents such as tamoxifen as there are adverse effects, including increases in endometrial cancer and venous thromboembolic events associated with use of the drug. This is particularly true when prevention in small numbers of patients requires large numbers of patients to be exposed to the risks of treatment. Additionally, risk/benefit profiles have important health policy implications as they may be used to construct physician care paths and may influence physician education and insurance reimbursements for medications. In an era of evidence-based medicine, published guidelines derived from large clinical trials may powerfully influence who receives or is denied preventive treatments with tamoxifen. An analysis of the risk-to-benefit ratio of tamoxifen use for the prevention of breast cancer has been performed.[12] In this work, it was suggested that differences existed between African-American and Caucasian women in the risks of stroke, endometrial cancer, and venous thrombotic events that would have an impact on the use of the drugs in these groups of women. Data from the Breast Cancer Prevention Trial (BCPT)[9] and epidemiologic databases were used by these authors to construct ratios of the risks and benefits resulting from tamoxifen use, and then guidelines were developed for use in women at increased risk of breast cancer.[12,13] It was suggested that African-American women were at higher risk for the thromboembolic complications associated with tamoxifen usage and therefore had a different risk-to-benefit ratio from Caucasian women of comparable age. As a corollary of this analysis, it was suggested that African-American women be counseled against (and potentially denied) preventive therapy with tamoxifen at ages approximately 10 years younger than white women.[12] While it is critically important to define risk/benefit ratios for preventive therapies, particularly when there may be significant undesirable side effects, the BCPT and subsequent publications highlight an important and ongoing problem in clinical trials: the underrepresentation of minority groups in the large cancer prevention trials, leading to an inability to generate results that are statistically valid for such minority subgroups.[13,14] The BCPT, for example, had more than 13,000 participants; however, only 220 were African-American and 249 were of other unspecified ethnicities. With such a small sample size, it is clearly impossible to assess either positive or negative effects of tamoxifen therapy in minority women and it is also impossible to determine whether any adverse effects of tamoxifen might be better defined by components of risk profiles other than race.

Thus, guidelines for tamoxifen use derived from these data should be applied only to subjects similar to the population studied.[15] Where population data are inadequate, development of guidelines for the underrepresented populations should be deferred. Opportunities to repeat trials such as the BCPT in women of ethnicities that are initially poorly represented are nonexistent. Such trials are therefore missed opportunities to fully understand the biology and the applications of these new therapies and are certain to contribute to continuing ethnic disparities in health care. As new SERMs are developed and tested, it is critically important that minority women be included in sufficient numbers to be able to definitively describe any variability in risk to benefit attributable to ethnicity.

REFERENCES

1. LIU, X. *et al.* 1998. Gender difference in the cycle length–dependent QT and potassium currents in rabbits. J. Pharmacol. Exp. Ther. **285:** 672–679.
2. LEHMANN, M.H. *et al.* 1999. JTc prolongation with *d,l*-Sotalol in women versus men. Am. J. Cardiol. **83:** 354–359.
3. LEHMANN, M.H. *et al.* 1996. Sex difference in risk of torsades de pointes with *d,l*-Sotalol. Circulation **94:** 2534–2541.
4. MAKKAR, R.R. *et al.* 1992. Female gender as a risk factor for torsades de pointes associated with cardiovascular drugs. JAMA **270**(21): 2590–2597.
5. WOOD, A.J.J. & H.H. ZHOU. 1991. Ethnic differences in drug disposition and responsiveness. Clin. Pharmacokinet. **20**(5): 350–373.
6. WEBER, W. 1987. Genetics of drug response. *In* The Acetylator Genes and Drug Response. Oxford University Press. London/New York.
7. GILLUM, R.F. 1979. Pathophysiology of hypertension in blacks and whites. Hypertension **1:** 468–475.
8. EARLY BREAST CANCER TRIALISTS' COLLABORATIVE GROUP. 1998. Tamoxifen for early breast cancer: an overview of the randomised trials. Lancet **351:** 1451–1467.
9. FISHER, B., J.P. COSTANTINO, D.L. WICKERHAM *et al.* 1998. Tamoxifen for prevention of breast cancer: report of the National Surgical Adjuvant Breast and Bowel Project P-1 Study. J. Natl. Cancer Inst. **90:** 1371–1388.
10. LIPPMAN, S.M. & P.H. BROWN. 1999. Tamoxifen prevention of breast cancer: an instance of the fingerpost. J. Natl. Cancer Inst. **91:** 1809–1819.
11. OSBORNE, C.K. 1998. Tamoxifen in the treatment of breast cancer. N. Engl. J. Med. **339:** 1609–1618.
12. GAIL, M.H. *et al.* 1999. Weighing the risks and benefits of tamoxifen treatment for preventing breast cancer. J. Natl. Cancer Inst. **91:** 1829–1846.
13. TAYLOR, A.L., L.L. ADAMS-CAMPBELL & J.T. WRIGHT, JR. 1999. Risk/benefit assessment of tamoxifen to prevent breast cancer—still a work in progress? J. Natl. Cancer Inst. **91**(21): 1792–1793.
14. HAYNES, M.A. & B.D. SMEDLEY, Eds. 1999. The Unequal Burden of Cancer: An Assessment of NIH Research and Programs for Ethnic Minorities and the Medically Underserved. Committee on Cancer Research among Minorities and the Medically Underserved. Institute of Medicine. National Academy Press. Washington, D.C.
15. GLEITER, C.H. & R. GUNDERT-REMY. 1996. Gender differences in pharmacokinetics. Eur. J. Drug Metab. Pharmacokinet. **21**(2): 123–128.

Raloxifene: Risks and Benefits

ELIZABETH BARRETT-CONNOR

Division of Epidemiology, Department of Family and Preventive Medicine, University of California, San Diego, La Jolla, California 92093, USA

ABSTRACT: Raloxifene, a selective estrogen receptor modulator (SERM), was designed to have the expected benefits of long-term estrogen replacement therapy without the risks. This paper reviews the clinical trial evidence for raloxifene benefits and risks, and how they compare with those of hormone replacement therapy (HRT) and relate to the choices of postmenopausal women.

KEYWORDS: selective estrogen receptor modulators (SERMs); raloxifene; risks; benefits

INTRODUCTION

Estrogen receptors bind with multiple ligands, eliciting tissue-specific responses. Selective estrogen receptor modulators (SERMs) are designed to have both estrogen agonist and antagonist effects. Raloxifene is the first SERM approved for osteoporosis prevention and treatment. This paper summarizes the evidence for raloxifene's benefits and risks based on results from randomized placebo-controlled clinical trials. Unless otherwise indicated, only data related to the now-recommended dose, 60 mg/day, are reviewed.

BENEFITS

Osteoporosis Prevention and Treatment

Osteoporosis is a major cause of morbidity and mortality in elderly women. The largest completed clinical trial of raloxifene and fractures is the Multiple Outcomes of Raloxifene Evaluation (MORE), in which 5,153 postmenopausal women were randomized to either placebo or raloxifene at the 60 mg daily dose.[1] At baseline, all participants (mean age 67 years) had osteoporosis as defined by bone mineral density or prior vertebral fracture criteria. At 36 months of treatment, raloxifene had no significant effect on the risk of nonvertebral fractures, but the risk of radiographic vertebral fractures was reduced significantly in women with and without prevalent fractures at baseline. As shown in FIGURE 1, the 3-year risk of a vertebral fracture in women without prior spine fractures was reduced by 50% (4.5% on placebo and 2.3% on raloxifene); for women with prior vertebral fractures, the risk of new vertebral fractures was

---

Address for correspondence: Elizabeth Barrett-Connor, M.D., Professor of Family and Preventive Medicine, Chief, Division of Epidemiology, 9500 Gilman Drive #0607, University of California, San Diego, La Jolla, CA 92093.
ebarrettconnor@ucsd.edu

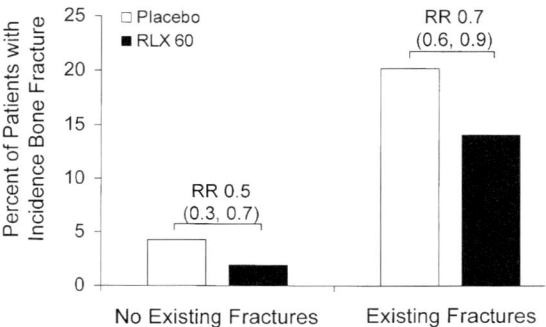

FIGURE 1. The risk of vertebral fracture in women without prior spine fractures was reduced by 50% and by 30% for women with prior spine fractures. (Adapted from Ettinger et al.[1])

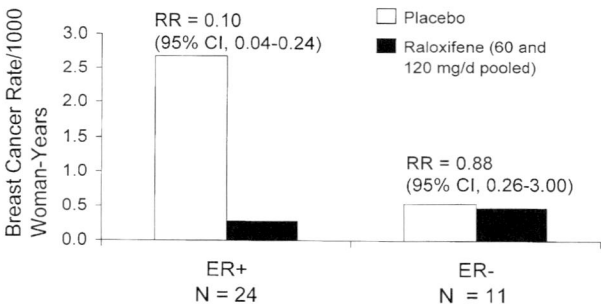

FIGURE 2. Estrogen receptor (ER) positive breast cancers were reduced by 90% in women assigned to raloxifene. (Adapted from Cummings et al.[3])

reduced by 30% (21.2% on placebo and 14.7% on raloxifene). Raloxifene reduced the risk of symptomatic vertebral fractures by 61% within the first year.[2]

Breast Cancer

Breast cancer is the most common cause of cancer death in women worldwide. In the MORE trial,[3] invasive breast cancers were reduced by 76% in women assigned to raloxifene (3.6 cancers per 1,000 woman-years in the placebo group vs. 0.9 cancers per 1,000 woman-years in the pooled raloxifene 60 mg/day and 120 mg/day group). Estrogen receptor (ER) positive cancers were reduced by 90%, as shown in FIGURE 2. The overall reduction in breast cancer risk was maintained for at least 48 months.[4] Although MORE women were selected for osteoporosis, and might therefore be expected to be at a reduced risk of breast cancer, breast cancer incidence in the MORE placebo group was similar to that expected in the general population of the same age.

Because the observed breast cancer risk reduction in MORE was based on few cases and was not a planned primary outcome, the trial has been extended with a new name, Continuing Outcomes Relevant to Evista (CORE), with invasive breast cancer as a designated outcome. CORE will enroll approximately 4,000 MORE participants for an additional four years, extending the total trial duration to eight years. Invasive breast cancer is also a co-primary outcome in the Raloxifene Use and The Heart (RUTH) trial (see below) and in the Study of Tamoxifen and Raloxifene (STAR).[5] The latter will compare raloxifene with tamoxifen in 22,000 postmenopausal women at high risk for breast cancer.

Endometrial Bleeding, Hyperplasia, and Cancer

In the MORE trial, bleeding rates were the same in women assigned to raloxifene (3.1%) or placebo (3.1%).[3] Fluid in the endometrial cavity (observed on transvaginal ultrasound) was present in more women assigned to raloxifene (2.4%) than placebo; the clinical significance of this finding is unknown.

In clinical trials of up to five years' duration, there were very low rates of endometrial hyperplasia and cancer in women treated with raloxifene or placebo, with no significant differences between treatment groups.[3,6-8] The STAR breast cancer prevention trial is also designed to determine whether raloxifene reduces the risk of endometrial cancer.

Cardiovascular Disease

Heart disease is the most common cause of death in women in most of the western world. For this reason, the largest potential benefit for a SERM is the prevention of coronary heart disease. No clinical trial data show an altered risk of heart disease in women taking raloxifene. The large clinical trial Raloxifene Use for The Heart (RUTH) was designed to determine whether raloxifene will reduce the risk of coronary heart disease in women at high risk of heart disease. Among the 10,101 women enrolled, about half have known coronary heart disease and about half have heart disease risk factors, most commonly diabetes. In RUTH, the primary cardiovascular end point is a combined outcome of myocardial infarction, coronary heart disease–related death, or hospitalization for acute coronary syndrome. The rationale for this study was the observation that raloxifene improves several heart disease risk factors, lowering LDL cholesterol and apolipoprotein B level without raising triglycerides, and lowering homocysteine and fibrinogen levels.[9,10]

RISKS

Venous Thromboembolic Events

To date, the only serious adverse event clearly associated with raloxifene is a tripling of the risk of venous thromboembolic events (VTE).[3] By 40 months of follow up, deep vein thrombosis had occurred in 7/1,000 MORE women assigned to raloxifene versus 2/1,000 assigned to placebo, and pulmonary embolus in 3/1,000 assigned to raloxifene versus 1/1,000 assigned to placebo.

Hot Flashes

Raloxifene increases hot flashes. In pooled analyses of trial data including 1,165 younger postmenopausal women (average age 55 years), those assigned to raloxifene reported more hot flashes (24.6%) than did women assigned to placebo (18.3%).[11] In similar comparisons in the older MORE women (average age 67 years), hot flashes were much less common but still reported by more women taking raloxifene (9.7%) than by women taking placebo (6.4%).[1] In both age groups, hot flashes tended to be mild and led to discontinuation of raloxifene by less than 2%,[12] but trials excluded women with severe vasomotor symptoms.

Miscellaneous Adverse Events

Leg cramps were more common in MORE women assigned to raloxifene than placebo (7.0 vs. 3.7%).[3] Compared to women assigned to placebo, MORE women assigned to raloxifene also reported a significantly higher incidence of an influenza-like syndrome (2.1%); peripheral edema (0.8%); and worsening of diabetes (0.7%).[3]

Central Nervous System

In a 12-month randomized clinical trial of 143 women (mean age 68 years), the incidence of depressive symptoms, emotional lability, insomnia, anxiety, dizziness, malaise, and memory loss did not differ between women assigned to raloxifene or placebo.[13] In the MORE trial, overall performance on cognitive function tests did not differ between postmenopausal women assigned to raloxifene or placebo for three years. In an age-stratified analysis, however, women aged 70 or older performed better on two of six tests after taking raloxifene than did women taking placebo.[14]

RALOXIFENE VERSUS ESTROGEN

Osteoporosis. No head-to-head comparisons of estrogen versus raloxifene have been published. In the Postmenopausal Estrogen/Progestin Intervention (PEPI) trial, there was an average 4–5% increase in vertebral bone density after two years of HRT,[15] more than the 2–3% two-year increase with raloxifene.[16] No large clinical trials of estrogen designed to evaluate fracture risk in osteoporotic women have been reported. The Heart and Estrogen/Progestin Replacement Study (HERS), the largest clinical trial with nearly complete follow-up, studied women selected for heart disease, not low bone density.[17] Nevertheless, there were more than 250 new clinical fractures during the trial and no difference in clinical fracture rates between HRT-treated and untreated women. Unfortunately, vertebral X-rays were not obtained, so a reduction in subclinical spine fractures could have been missed.

Breast Cancer. Unlike raloxifene, there are no clinical trial data showing an increased or decreased risk of breast cancer after hormone replacement therapy (HRT). The 33% increase observed in HERS women on hormones was not statistically different from the placebo rate.[17] Data from the PEPI trial have shown that HRT increases breast pain and breast density on mammography, with a higher incidence after combined therapy than with estrogen alone (about 45 vs. 15%).[18] Radiographic breast density is a risk factor for breast cancer.[19] Unlike estrogen, raloxifene does not increase breast pain[11] or breast density.[20]

Endometrial Pathology. Unlike raloxifene, HRT in standard doses commonly causes bleeding during the first year of treatment; lower doses appear to reduce the

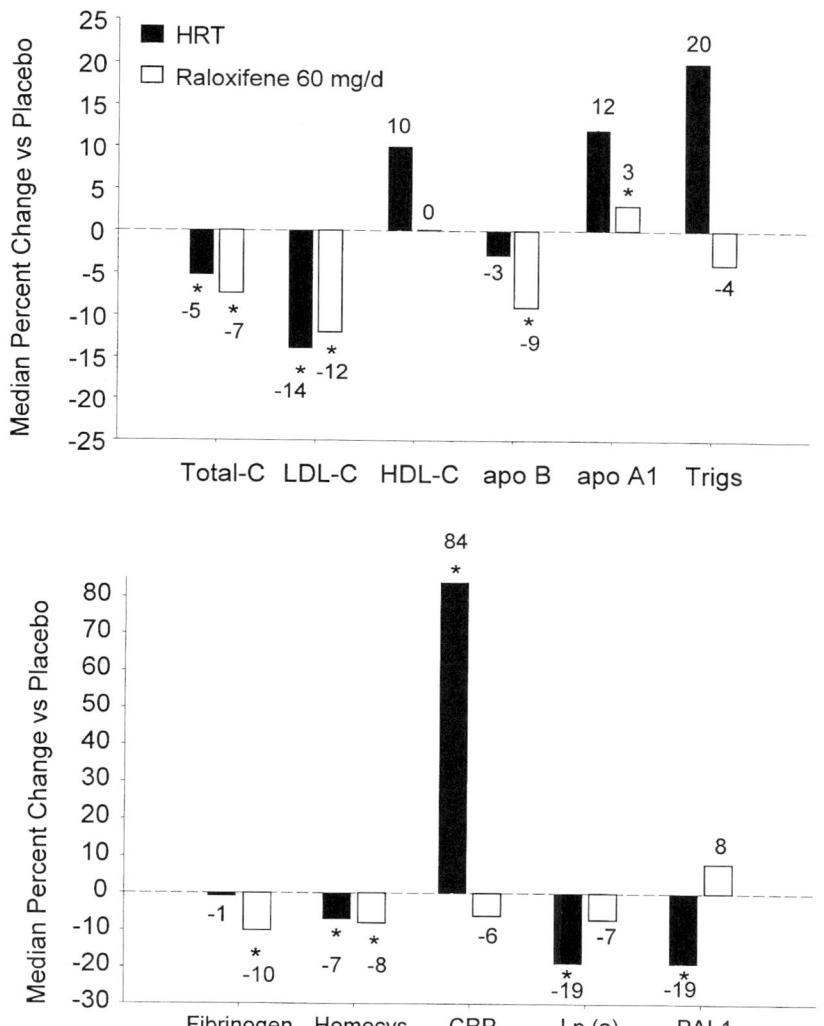

FIGURE 3. Effects of raloxifene and estrogen (HRT) on heart disease risk factors: raloxifene was better than estrogen in lowering fibrinogen and apolipoprotein B (apo B) levels, and in not raising triglycerides (Trigs) or C reactive protein (CRP); only estrogen reduced Lp (a) and PAI-1 and raised HDL cholesterol (HDL-C) and apolipoprotein A-1 (apo A1). (Adapted from Walsh et al.[9,10])

frequency and duration of bleeding. Unopposed estrogen caused endometrial hyperplasia at a rate of 10% per year in PEPI women.[21]

Heart Disease. The effects of raloxifene and estrogen on heart disease risk factors have been studied in clinical trials with head-to-head comparisons. As shown in FIGURE 3, raloxifene and estrogen (HRT) similarly improved total and LDL cholesterol

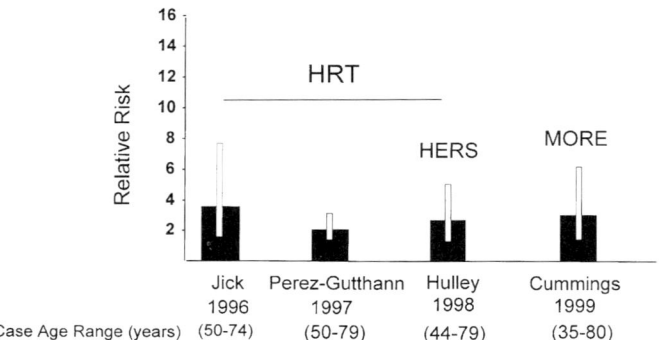

FIGURE 4. Comparing women in HERS and in MORE, the risk of VTE (venous thromboembolic disease) with raloxifene is similar to that with HRT (hormone replacement therapy).

and homocysteine levels. Raloxifene was better than estrogen in lowering fibrinogen and apolipoprotein B levels, and in not raising triglycerides or C reactive protein, but only estrogen was effective in reducing Lp(a) and PAI-1, and in raising HDL cholesterol and apolipoprotein A-1.[9–10,22] Changes in heart disease risk factors do not necessarily translate to favorable changes in the risk of heart disease, as illustrated by the failure of HRT to reduce CHD or stroke risk in primary and secondary prevention trials.[17,23–26]

Cognitive Function. Despite several small clinical trials showing that estrogen improved cognition in young women soon after bilateral oophorectomy, no large clinical trials have shown improved mood or cognition in older women without menopausal symptoms. In HERS, cognitive function test performance was slightly poorer in women on HRT compared to placebo. In another clinical trial, when women with early dementia were assigned to estrogen, they scored more poorly on the Clinical Dementia Rating Scale than did women assigned to placebo.[27]

Venous Thromboembolic Disease. Based on a comparison between women in HERS and women in MORE, the risk of VTE with raloxifene is similar to that with HRT. These risks are also similar to those found in observational studies of women not selected for osteoporosis or CHD risk (FIG. 4).[28,29]

Menopause Symptoms. Estrogen is the treatment of choice for vasomotor symptoms and urogenital dryness, in contrast to raloxifene which may worsen hot flashes and has no effect on vaginal dryness. In a randomized trial of 187 women with vaginal atrophy, raloxifene did not reduce the beneficial effects of vaginal estrogen cream or moisturizer.[30,31]

DISCUSSION

Weighing risks and benefits is necessary if we are to help patients make intelligent choices. Women can understand that their risk of breast cancer without hormone therapy varies based on age, body size, reproductive history, family history, and other factors. Yet relative and absolute risk can be confusing. Consider a disease that affects 2/1,000 people without treatment and 4/1,000 with treatment—the relative risk is 2 but the absolute excess risk is only 2/1,000 treated people. Absolute risk is preferable to relative risk, because only the former estimates the probability of the condition without the intervention. On average, using hormone therapy for 15 years is associated with a relative risk of breast cancer of 1.5 (a 50% increase in risk), but adds only an additional 5–20 cases per 1,000 women.[32]

The absolute risk can be translated into the number needed to treat (NNT). For example, based on the data shown in FIGURE 1, 46 women without prevalent fractures would need to be treated for 36 months to prevent one vertebral fracture, compared to 16 women with prevalent vertebral fractures. FIGURE 1 also illustrates one of the problems with NNT: despite the smaller number of women with prevalent fractures who need to be treated to prevent one new fracture, the number of fractures occurring despite treatment is larger in this group than in women with no fractures at baseline. Thus, more women will suffer new fractures despite treatment, if one waits for a vertebral fracture as an indication to treat.

Similar calculations can be made for breast cancer. Based on MORE data, 126 women unselected for breast cancer risk would need to be treated to prevent one breast cancer. No data are yet available for women at particularly high risk for breast cancer. Calculations cannot be made for cardiovascular disease: the MORE data suggest no benefit (or risk) for women with osteoporosis (presumably at low risk of heart disease), but estimates for high-risk women will have to wait for the RUTH results.

Finally, with regard to serious risk, the best estimate is that one excess VTE will occur for every 155 women treated with raloxifene for three years.

The idea of absolute risk with and without treatment is relatively easy to understand. But none of the numbers, relative risk, absolute risk, or NNT, deal with individual women and their personal concerns. All medications have side effects, which may be more or less unacceptable to different women. Women who are most concerned about breast cancer will rarely accept a medication thought to increase breast cancer risk—even if the drug is shown to reduce the risk of a more common condition such as heart disease. Women's decisions are also influenced by their age and their personal experience. Women less than 60 are more likely to have friends with breast cancer than heart disease or osteoporosis. Women with symptoms are more apt to initiate and continue HRT, trading demonstrated current well-being for future possible risk. Social class is another determinant of medication initiation and continuation—even when the medicine is provided at no cost. It may be that those with a weekly paycheck will be less likely to begin or continue medication, with possible benefits in the far future, than women with a more stable income and (presumably) more predictable future.

Finally, risk benefit estimates from clinical trials may be misleading. Although clinical trials are needed to document the efficacy of a new drug, they cannot guarantee these findings will apply in clinical practice. Poor adherence by patients and physicians can undermine the benefits demonstrated in clinical trials. And sometimes post-marketing surveillance is necessary to see a rare but serious side effect.

At present, the following conclusions about raloxifene risks and benefits can be made. Raloxifene has effects on several heart disease risk factors—in some instances more favorable than estrogen and in others less favorable. Whether raloxifene can reduce heart disease risk is being studied now. Because heart disease is such a common cause of morbidity and mortality in older women, heart disease prevention would greatly enhance the risk-benefit ratio for raloxifene. However, given the documented fracture prevention, and if the breast cancer risk reduction is confirmed, the overall risk-benefit ratio for raloxifene should be favorable even if raloxifene does not reduce the risk of heart disease. An unfavorable risk-benefit ratio would emerge only if raloxifene causes an early excess risk of cardiovascular disease, as has been observed with HRT.

REFERENCES

1. ETTINGER, B., D.M. BLACK, B.H. MITLAK, et al. 1999. Reduction of vertebral fracture risk in postmenopausal women with osteoporosis treated with raloxifene: results from a 3-year randomized clinical trial. Multiple Outcomes of Raloxifene Evaluation (MORE) Investigators. JAMA **282:** 637–645.
2. EASTELL, R., J. ADACHI, K. HARPER, et al. 2000. The effects of raloxifene on incident vertebral fractures in postmenopausal women with osteoporosis: 4-year results from the MORE trial. Abstr. 492. The American Society of Bone and Mineral Research 22nd Annual Meeting. Toronto, Canada.
3. CUMMINGS, S.R., S. ECKERT, K.A. KRUEGER, et al. 1999. The effect of raloxifene on risk of breast cancer in postmenopausal women: results from the MORE randomized trial. Multiple Outcomes of Raloxifene Evaluation. JAMA **281:** 2189–2197.
4. CAULEY, J., N. NORTON, M.E. LIPPMAN, et al. 2001. Continued breast cancer risk reduction in postmenopausal women treated with raloxifene: 4-year results from the MORE trial. Breast Cancer Res. Treat. **65:** 125–134.
5. JORDAN, V.C. & M. MORROW. 1999. Tamoxifen, raloxifene, and the prevention of breast cancer. Endocr. Rev. **20:** 253–278.
6. COHEN, F.J., S. WATTS, A. SHAH, et al. 2000. Uterine effects of 3-year raloxifene therapy in postmenopausal women younger than age 60. Obstet. Gynecol. **95:** 104–110.
7. GOLDSTEIN, S.R., W.H. SCHEELE, S.K. RAJAGOPALAN, et al. 2000. A 12-month comparative study of raloxifene, estrogen, and placebo on the postmenopausal endometrium. Obstet. Gynecol. **95:** 95–103.
8. JOLLY, E.E., J.T. O'GORMAN, R.J. AKERS, et al. 2000. Effect of raloxifene therapy for 5 years on endometrial hyperplasia and endometrial cancer in postmenopausal women under the age of 60. Abstr. 2318. The Endocrine Society's 82nd Annual Meeting, Toronto, Canada.
9. WALSH, B.W., L.H. KULLER, R.A. WILD, et al. 1998. Effects of raloxifene on serum lipids and coagulation factors in healthy postmenopausal women. JAMA **279:** 1445–1451.
10. WALSH, B.W., S. PAUL, R.A. WILD, et al. 2000. The effects of hormone replacement therapy and raloxifene on C-reactive protein and homocysteine in healthy postmenopausal women: a randomized, controlled trial. J. Clin. Endocrinol. Metab. **85:** 214–218.
11. DAVIES, G.C., W.J. HUSTER, Y. LU, et al. 1999. Adverse events reported by postmenopausal women in controlled trials with raloxifene. Obstet. Gynecol. **93:** 558–565.
12. KRUEGER, K.A., T.S. EVANS, S. ECKERT, et al. 2000. Characteristics of hot flushes with raloxifene in postmenopausal osteoporotic women in the MORE trial: Abstr. P-69. North American Menopause Society 11th Annual Meeting. Orlando, FL.
13. NICKELSEN, T., E.G. LUFKIN, B.L. RIGGS, et al. 1999. Raloxifene hydrochloride, a selective estrogen receptor modulator: safety assessment of effects on cognitive function and mood in postmenopausal women. Psychoneuroendocrinology **24:** 115–128.
14. KRUEGER, K.A., K. YAFFE, S. SARKAR, et al. 2000. Effects of raloxifene on cognitive function in postmenopausal women without dementia. J. Am. Geriatr. Soc. **48:** S106.
15. PEPI WRITING GROUP. 1996. Effects of hormone therapy on bone mineral density: results from the postmenopausal estrogen/progestin interventions (PEPI) trial. JAMA **276:** 1389–1396.

16. DELMAS, P.D., N.H. BJARNASON, B.H. MITLAK, et al. 1997. Effects of raloxifene on bone mineral density, serum cholesterol concentrations, and uterine endometrium in postmenopausal women. N. Engl. J. Med. **337:** 1641–1647.
17. HULLEY, S., D. GRADY, T. BUSH, et al. 1998. Randomized trial of estrogen plus progestin for secondary prevention of coronary heart disease in postmenopausal women. Heart and Estrogen/Progestin Replacement Study (HERS) Research Group. JAMA **280:** 605–613.
18. GREENDALE, G.A., B.A. REBOUSSIN, A. SIE, et al. 1999. Effects of estrogen-progestin on mammographic parenchymal density. Postmenopausal Estrogen/Progestin Interventions (PEPI) Investigators. Ann. Intern. Med. **130:** 262–269.
19. BOYD, N.F., J.W. BYING, R.A. JONG, et al. 1995. Quantitative classification of mammographic densities and breast cancer risk: results from the Canadian National Breast Screening Study. J. Natl. Cancer Inst. **87:** 670–675.
20. FREEDMAN, M., J.S. SAN MARTIN, J. O'GORMAN, et al. 2001. Digitized mammography: a clinical trial of postmenopausal women randomly assigned to receive raloxifene, estrogen, or placebo. J. Natl. Cancer Inst. **93:** 51–56.
21. PEPI WRITING GROUP. 1996. Effects of hormone replacement therapy on endometrial histology in postmenopausal women. The Postmenopausal Estrogen/Progestin Interventions (PEPI) Trial. JAMA **275:** 370–375.
22. DE VALK-DE ROO, G.W., C.D. STEHOUWER, P. MEIJER, et al. 1999. Both raloxifene and estrogen reduce major cardiovascular risk factors in healthy postmenopausal women. Arterioscler. Thromb. Vasc. Biol. **19:** 2993–3000.
23. HEMMINKI, R. & K. MCPHERSON. 2000. Value of drug-licensing documents in studying the effect of postmenopausal hormone therapy on cardiovascular disease. Lancet **355:** 566–569.
24. HERRINGTON, D., D.M. REBOUSSIN, K.B. BROSNIHAN, et al. 2000. Effects of estrogen replacement on the progression of coronary artery atherosclerosis. N. Engl. J. Med. **343:** 522–529.
25. LENFANT, C. 2000. Statement on preliminary trends in the Women's Health Initiative. NHLBI Communications Office; http://www.nhlbi.nih.gov/whi/index.html
26. VISCOLI, C.M., L.M. BRASS, W.N. KERNAN, et al. 2001. A clinical trial of estrogen-replacement therapy after ischemic stroke. N. Engl. J. Med. **345:** 1243–1249.
27. MULNARD, R.A., C.W. COTMAN, C. KAWAS, et al. 2000. Estrogen replacement therapy for treatment of mild to moderate Alzheimer's Disease: Alzheimer's Disease Cooperative Study. JAMA **283:** 1007–1015.
28. JICK, H., L.E. DERBY, M.W. MYERS, et al. 1996. Risk of hospital admission for idiopathic venous thromboembolism among users of postmenopausal oestrogens. Lancet **348:** 981–983.
29. PEREZ GUTTHANN, S., L.A. GARCIA RODRIGUEZ, J. CASTELLSAGUE, et al. 1997. Hormone replacement therapy and risk of venous thromboembolism: population based case-control study. BMJ **314:** 796–800.
30. PARSONS, A.K., L.E. NACHTIGALL, P. SULAK, et al. 1999. Vaginal Premarin vs. Replens in women with pre-existing vaginal atrophy receiving oral placebo or raloxifene: effects on subjective endpoints. Menopause **6:** 340, P33.
31. PARSONS, A. L. NACHTIGALL, D. MERRITT, et al. 1999. Vaginal Premarin vs. Replens in women with pre-existing vaginal atrophy receiving oral placebo or raloxifene: effects on objective endpoints. Menopause **6:** 341, P34.
32. COLLABORATIVE GROUP ON HORMONAL FACTORS IN BREAST CANCER. 1997. Breast cancer and hormone replacement therapy: collaborative reanalysis of data from 51 epidemiological studies of 52,705 women with breast cancer and 108,411 women without breast cancer. Lancet **350:** 1047–1059.

Defining Benefits and Risks for SERMs in Clinical Trials and Clinical Practice

SUSAN R. JOHNSON,[a] BARBARA K. DUNN,[b] AND MARIETTA ANTHONY[c]

[a]*University of Iowa Colleges of Medicine and Public Health, Iowa City, Iowa 52242, USA*

[b]*Division of Cancer Prevention, National Cancer Institute, National Institutes of Health, Bethesda, Maryland 20892, USA*

[c]*Department of Pharmacology, Georgetown University Medical Center, Washington, District of Columbia 20007, USA*

ABSTRACT: Differences between clinical trials and clinical practice with respect to defining benefits and benefit/risk ratios for SERMs are discussed. These differences stem from the perception that there is discordance between the statistical significance and the "clinical meaningfulness" of research data in the minds of the practitioner and patient. One way that we can obtain data that are more clinically meaningful is to solicit input in the planning stages of clinical trials from practicing community clinicians and their patients. However, there are drawbacks to community input, such as potentially unrealistic expectations. A further issue is the need to characterize clinically meaningful drug benefits and acceptable benefit/risk ratios for a drug. Individual patients have differences regarding their views of optimal benefits and acceptable risks, so a method or tool for determining what is clinically meaningful would be helpful in presenting comprehensive information to the patient. To present useful information to clinicians, head-to-head comparisons of a new drug with a standard agent should be undertaken. NIH's support in this area of comparator trials is critical to their implementation. Estrogen has been considered the standard for comparison of agents for conditions associated with menopause in clinical trials. Estrogen has been the "gold standard" in clinical practice as well. In fact, challenging the position of estrogen, even where scientifically supported, has proven to be an uphill battle. In the practice setting, we elaborate the challenges of keeping up with the scientific literature and of then communicating this information in a fashion that is relevant to the individual patient.

KEYWORDS: benefits; benefit/risk; estrogen; SERMs; statistically significant; clinically meaningful

INTRODUCTION

This presentation addresses the following question: "Are there differences between clinical trials and clinical practice with respect to defining benefits and risks of interventions for conditions associated with menopause?" The focus will be on

Address for correspondence: Susan R. Johnson, M.D., M.S., University of Iowa College of Medicine, 206 CMAB, Iowa City, IA 52242.
susan-johnson@uiowa.edu

real and perceived differences between the statistical and clinical significance of data from clinical research. The perspective that we have tried to take is that of a practicing gynecologist dedicated both to implementing evidence-based medicine and to presenting scientific data in a manner designed to help advise patients. The typical patient in a gynecologic practice is healthy with respect to the sites that are targeted by selective estrogen receptor modulators (SERMs)—that is, the woman does not have breast cancer or osteoporosis. Thus, her perception of any benefits to be reaped and of any benefit/risk balance from a SERM intervention will be colored by the fact that she does not have a life-threatening disease as a starting point.

Our premise is as follows: unless a drug, even though approved by the FDA (Food and Drug Administration), is actually prescribed and used by women, it can't have any personal or public health benefit. It will just sit on the shelf. SERMs are to some extent in this unused category at the present time. Based on conversations by one of us (S. Johnson) with gynecologists and her own patients, both groups are somewhat skeptical of the available SERMs, despite all the evidence from randomized trials showing statistically significant benefits. Thus, the issue of knowing what matters to real people in terms of meaningful drug benefits and acceptable benefits/risks is an important one.

HOW CAN CLINICAL TRIAL DATA BE MADE "CLINICALLY MEANINGFUL" TO PATIENTS?

What Quantitative Level in a Clinical Trial Is "Clinically Meaningful"?

What Is a "Clinically Meaningful" Benefit for a Drug?

The almost exclusive focus on statistical outcomes, as opposed to "clinically meaningful" outcomes, in the analysis of clinical trials applies to most trials and not just those of SERMs. If we think this emphasis on statistics is inadequate, leading to nonacceptance of drugs in practice settings, we need to ask what the alternatives are. Statisticians involved in the design of clinical trials attempt to incorporate clinically meaningful end points prospectively into their power calculations for estimating sample size. However, this intention is not always perceived as successful by patients who ultimately may be candidates for the drug. In essence, there is often a disjunction between statistical significance and clinical meaningfulness.

One solution is to incorporate the perspective of future users of a drug a priori, before starting a trial, as to what level of clinical benefit would be meaningful to them. The success of a trial would then be judged based on user-influenced statistical significance rather than on data that are statistically significant, but clinically not meaningful. Thus, in a hypothetical example, it might be decided that a new therapeutic agent would only be of real benefit if it reduced the rate of a disorder by 30%. In such a situation, if the trial showed that the benefit yielded instead only a 20% reduction, the drug would be assessed as "not effective enough." This scenario might happen even in the face of a highly statistically significant difference from placebo at the level of a 20% reduction. However, some potential users of this drug might be satisfied with the lesser 20% reduction in disease rate. In such a case, they will be deprived of access to an agent that they would willingly use. Conversely, other potential users may have a more rigorous standard for accepting a drug than that offered by the results of a clinical trial. Thus, the level of benefit selected for statistical purposes might be lower than that needed to convince practitioners and patients of the clinical advantage of a drug. For example, a trial may successfully have shown that a drug decreases a disorder by 30%, but the potential users may be unwilling to take any agent that yields less than a 40% reduction.

Therefore, it would be reasonable to expect clinical trialists to make a judgment of "what difference would make a difference." In reality, this is already done. The design of clinical trials is based on input from clinicians as to the statistical component of clinical differences that are meaningful. The problem is that clinically meaningful may have a different connotation for clinical researchers involved in trial design than for clinicians practicing in the community and their patients. As a trial is designed, trialists could use input from the community perspective regarding clinically meaningful outcomes as they power the trial, and they should disclose the desired difference when the primary results of the trial are published. As an example, input from patients and clinicians in practice led to a shift in what was acceptable for FDA approval of cancer drugs, with the acceptance of tumor shrinkage, in addition to length of survival, as an end point.[1] Journal editors could also aid this cause by requiring the inclusion of these assumptions—that is, what difference makes a difference—at the time of manuscript submission.

Although this approach sounds appealing, there are several drawbacks. In some cases, community input might potentially require studies that are very expensive to carry out because they are powered using an assumption of an optimal outcome. In the extreme case, the optimal, and highly impractical, outcome would be 100% efficacy. A second issue that is particularly subject to input from the community perspective is that of the benefit/risk balance of a drug.

What Is a "Clinically Meaningful" Benefit/Risk Ratio for a Drug?

Benefit/risk ratios pose a difficult challenge in clinical trial design. Because people have individual differences in what they view as an acceptable balance of benefit and risk, a method for deciding what is a clinically meaningful result with respect to a benefit/risk ratio would be helpful. The example of tamoxifen for chemoprevention of breast cancer offers a case in point, demonstrating the complexities of this challenge. The Gail model[2] is a tool to help women decide if they are at high risk for developing breast cancer—information that may be used to determine if they would be good candidates for using tamoxifen as a chemopreventive agent. The Gail model identifies those women who, because of elevated breast cancer risk, are most likely to reap benefit from this agent. However, knowledge of the benefit to be gained from a drug does not automatically take into consideration the risk to be weighed against this benefit. This issue of weighing the risks versus the benefits of an intervention is critical to presenting a comprehensive picture to the patient.

In the case of tamoxifen, for example, some women view the possible development of vasomotor symptoms as a negative that outweighs the potential benefits of reduced breast cancer risk. Regarding more serious risks of tamoxifen, if we restrict our discussion to thromboembolic complications, only the risk of pulmonary emboli undergoes a statistically significant increase with drug use. However, all adverse thromboembolic events may be clinically meaningful to a patient. Conversely, for other women, almost any side effect would be tolerable in order to reduce breast cancer risk. In summary, data that are not statistically significant in a clinical trial may still be clinically meaningful to a patient and may be used by a patient in making decisions regarding a medical intervention.

Efforts have been made to statistically weigh the risks and benefits of preventive tamoxifen,[3] but they have met with criticism because of their failure to incorporate data from all population groups.[4] Decision-making regarding pharmacologic risk-reduction strategies for breast cancer, based on a patient's perception of risks and benefits, must incorporate multiple elements, including the psychological and sociological context of the patient.[3,5] These issues related to tamoxifen use in breast cancer prevention are clearly pertinent to drugs for other disease indications.

Head-to-Head Comparison of a New Drug with a Standard Agent in Trial Design and in Presentation to Patients

A second approach to expressing the magnitude of benefit and risk of a new drug in a clinically meaningful way is to make a direct comparison to an agent with which we are familiar. This is the way some drugs, such as antineoplastic agents and anti-infectives, are currently tested. Yet, the results are not always expressed against the comparator in the label, which is the information available for the practitioner and the patient. For instance, in the case of breast cancer, new hormone therapies should be compared to tamoxifen, the standard for chemoprevention based on results of the Breast Cancer Prevention Trial (BCPT).[6] Such a comparison is being done in the Study of Tamoxifen and Raloxifene (STAR).[7,8] Comparisons of new agents for treating menopausal symptoms have involved the pitting of such drugs against estrogen, which has traditionally been viewed as the "gold standard." However, these comparisons have not been in the form of rigorously designed "head-to-head" trials. Yet, as in the case of breast cancer prevention, new agents for the treatment of hot flashes should be compared directly to estrogen, with the type of estrogen, dose, formulation, and route of administration specified (e.g., conjugated equine estrogen, estrogen/progestin, transdermal estrogen). A practitioner could say to a woman, based on a head-to-head trial, that the use of one drug has less (or more) benefit compared to estrogen, with a similar (or different) risk profile. As an example, when phytoestrogens in the form of isoflavone extracts are prescribed for hot flashes, it would be helpful in terms of risks and benefits to know how these botanicals compare with estrogens.[9,10] Such head-to-head comparisons provide a context that allows physicians and patients to make informed decisions about treatment. This comparison approach is most useful if patients are already familiar with the effects of the gold standard drug. Even if patients are not knowledgeable in this respect, this approach would help health care providers who know the gold standard to make decisions about how to present benefits and risks to their patients.

How could an approach of head-to-head trials for assessing benefits and risks be implemented? Such comparator trials are being done, but the number needs to be increased and the quality needs to be improved. An example of such a trial is the recent Antihypertensive and Lipid-Lowering Treatment to Prevent Heart Attack Trial (ALLHAT), which compared chlorthalidone, amlodipine, lisinopril, and doxazosin.[11] The results of this study showed that chlorthalidone, a diuretic, was associated with an essentially equal risk of coronary death/nonfatal myocardial infarction, but with a significantly reduced risk of combined cardiovascular disease events relative to doxazosin, an alpha-blocker.[12] Similarly, the STAR trial is very important because it will provide this kind of direct comparison between raloxifene and tamoxifen for the prevention of breast cancer in high-risk postmenopausal women. Pharmaceutical companies, of course, typically do not have much incentive to pursue this sort of study. Therefore, the NIH could play an important catalytic role here by funding comparator trials.

Under some circumstances, it will not be possible to prospectively design a trial to compare a new intervention with an established agent. In such cases, an historical control may be necessary, that is, comparing the results from one trial against those from another. Where an historical control is viewed as the standard intervention, we need to make sure that this gold standard is truly the optimal therapy. A good example of the failure to verify the accuracy of an historical control is seen in the assumption that estrogen confers protection against coronary heart disease events in both healthy women and women with established coronary heart disease. This assumption is based on low-level evidence, such as data derived from observational studies and data involving surrogate markers of risk in response to drug intervention. This assumption of a cardioprotective effect for estrogen was extended to SERMs. Thus, because raloxifene and tamoxifen affect some cardiovascular risk factors, such as low-density lipoprotein cholesterol and total cholesterol, in a manner similar to estrogen, it was believed that these SERMs would confer this same protection. Instead, the estrogen cardioprotection hypothesis has been substantially weakened by high-level evidence from randomized controlled trials that employed clinical end points. These trials have shown that, among women with established coronary heart disease, estrogen actually increases the risk of coronary heart disease events immediately after the drug is started.[13,14] Although the effect in healthy women is not yet known, pending the outcome of the Women's Health Initiative, the American Heart Association has issued guidelines recommending that clinicians no longer prescribe estrogen for the sole purpose of preventing heart disease.[15]

The "Estrogen Dilemma"

The assumptions regarding estrogen's role as a standard for comparison of newer agents extend beyond clinical trials. Estrogen has been the gold standard in clinical practice as well. Even if other drugs are shown conclusively with data from randomized trials to be effective for an estrogen-like indication, it will be very difficult to dislodge estrogen from its current place as the most frequently prescribed treatment for postmenopausal symptoms. Hence, estrogen, and specifically conjugated equine estrogen, has achieved a dominant position for prevention and treatment of conditions associated with the menopause (www.pharmacytimes.com/top200.html). After giving a thorough presentation on osteoporosis, including all the new information about screening, therapy, and clinical trial results, to a group of practicing family doctors, one of us (S. Johnson) overheard someone asking one of the clinicians, "What do you do with all this new information?" He replied, "Well, you mostly do what you are used to doing." Thus, it is clear that changing physician prescribing behavior poses a major challenge.

The prescribing of estrogen is viewed by many practitioners as a moral imperative. While some readers may view this language as too strong, it just takes going out and talking to some practitioners and postmenopausal women who have seen these practitioners to understand the reality of this statement. Good reasons exist for this "estrogen dilemma," whereby estrogen has been widely prescribed to menopausal women. Estrogen was assumed to be effective not just for treating menopausal symptoms, but also for preventing many of the major causes of morbidity and mortality in older women: most prominently, osteoporosis, heart disease, colorectal cancer, and Alzheimer's disease. Clinical studies have confirmed the accuracy of some of these assumptions, such as the efficacy of estrogen in treating hot flashes and osteoporosis. In other cases, though, estrogen has not been shown to be effective and may even be harmful, such as in the cardiovascular system. Even if a practitioner does not share this strong proestrogen perspective, practical issues such as peer and patient pressure resulting from heavy marketing strategies by drug companies often prevail. Our point is not to encourage universal discontinuation of estrogen use, but rather to ensure that it will be prescribed in a calculated and thoughtful way and only where appropriate. Only in this way will other, newer drugs that are better suited for what have habitually been viewed as "estrogen" indications gain entry into these clinical niches and thereby improve the delivery of preventive interventions for conditions in older women. In order to unseat estrogen from its incontrovertible role of dominance in menopausal therapy, we are going to require high-level clinical evidence, and head-to-head comparisons would be a step in the right direction.

HOW CAN A PRACTITIONER COMMUNICATE THE "CLINICAL MEANINGFULNESS" OF TRIAL DATA TO THE PATIENT?

The clinician faces a daunting challenge in trying to incorporate the results of clinical trials into the decision-making process, especially in the area of preventive interventions for chronic conditions in postmenopausal women. Clinicians themselves (1) must be familiar with the "rules" of evidence-based decision-making and (2) need to become facile in explaining relevant aspects to patients. In this area, like many others, the literature is evolving at a rapid pace, and keeping up with the most recent trials is nearly impossible for the nonacademic generalist practitioner. Even if these first two potential barriers are overcome, it may be nearly impossible to find time in the typical clinic visit to adequately include meaningful clinical trial information in the discussion. Finally, in this area of chronic disease prevention among otherwise currently healthy women, determining how to deal with the high degree of uncertainty posed by the absence of definitive data makes both doctors and patients uncomfortable.

Despite these challenges, it is important for clinicians to do the best they can. There are now excellent resources available to assist in understanding how to use the evidence-based approach. We especially recommend the "Users' Guides to the Medical Literature," produced by the Evidence-Based Medicine Working Group, as they have appeared over the years in the *Journal of the American Medical Association*, in full text on the World Wide Web (http://www.cche.net/principles/), and in a new textbook, *Users' Guides to the Medical Literature* (2002).[16] Several of the individual guides are specifically relevant to the issue of incorporating clinical trial results into practice.[17–20]

In addition to understanding how to interpret the literature for herself, the clinician should be able to explain to patients how the validity of the different kinds of evidence varies—that is, why randomized trials are believed to be more accurate than observational studies and why anecdotal evidence (as in testimonials from the patient's friends and in books touting untested remedies) is virtually useless. This is actually easier than it sounds. One of us (S. Johnson) uses the example of the healthy user bias that is commonly found in cohort studies of hormone replacement therapy.[21] It is generally easy for patients to understand the following: if the group prescribed estrogen were healthier before they started taking estrogen than the group who never took estrogen, then it cannot be confidently assumed that an observed difference in heart attack rates between the two groups is due only (or even partially) to the estrogen. An explanation of the placebo effect can help in explaining why open trials, case series, and personal anecdotes often provide misleading conclusions.

The problem of the rapid pace of publication of new research results in the literature is harder to deal with. As an example, the 1998 United States Preventive Task Force recommendations are already out of date in areas of osteoporosis and breast cancer prevention.[22] They contain no mention of raloxifene and risedronate for osteoporosis prevention nor is there mention of tamoxifen for chemoprophylaxis for women at high risk for breast cancer. Certainly, the availability of web-based resources that can be immediately updated helps, but most practitioners, regardless of specialty, have to keep up in numerous areas of medicine. For now, clinicians simply need to be aware that the arena of prevention for postmenopausal women is in a state of rapid change and, therefore, clinicians need to get updated at least annually.

Finding time to provide relevant, up-to-date information to postmenopausal women about prevention issues and then to discuss this information adequately is more challenging in the new health care environment as reimbursement for cognitive services declines, and patient visit expectations are rising by the day. One response to this dilemma for some clinicians has been simply to direct women to take a preventive medication, such as hormone replacement therapy, with the advice, "this is best for you." However, given the complexities of the decisions that must be made and the widely varying values that women hold about the various risks and potential benefits to be achieved, this approach cannot be defended. Several approaches in combination can help. The use of "decision aids," such as videos, written materials, etc., to help patients make treatment decisions is common.[23] O'Connor et al. tested a written decision aid to assist women in making a decision about hormone replacement therapy; the material was individualized by including each woman's own risk for the various conditions being considered.[24] The group that received the decision aid had more realistic expectations of benefits and risks, felt less conflicted about their choices, and accepted their choices more readily than the comparison group that received a standard informational pamphlet. The two groups had similar knowledge of the issues and the same degree of uncertainty about their decisions. In a recent metanalysis of randomized trials of such aids, O'Connor et al. concluded that the use of decision aids resulted in higher knowledge scores, lower decisional conflict scores, and more active patient participation in decision-making, but no differences in anxiety, satisfaction with decisions (weighted mean difference = 0.6/100; −3 to 4), or satisfaction with the decision-making process.[25] Thus, while this approach is not perfect, it appears to have some clear benefits, especially for making complex decisions.

When discussing how the results of specific clinical trials relate to the individual patient, we have four suggestions:

- First, try to make sure the woman has a clear understanding of the condition(s) that is (are) the target of the preventive intervention, as well as potential risks and side effects. Here are two examples that one of us (S. Johnson) frequently encounters in her practice—(1) Unless they have a close friend or relative with the condition, women are often unclear about exactly what a vertebral fracture is and what its consequences are. (2) When women think about the possibility that their risk of breast cancer may increase with estrogen use, they generally assume (a) that the risk goes up immediately, rather than after several years, as seems to be the case; (b) that if they do develop breast cancer, they will certainly die from it, when in fact fewer than 25% of women with this disease die from it; and (c) that taking estrogen increases not only their risk of cancer, but also of dying from it, when most studies show that the mortality risk from cancer among estrogen users does not increase.

- Second, explain how the women who were participants in the trial are the same as or different from the woman who is your patient and how that may affect the generalizability of the results to her. For example, the BCPT trial enrolled only women at high risk for breast cancer[6] and, therefore, it is fair to assume that the results of the trial should apply to other women at high risk by the same (Gail model) criteria. Conversely, the MORE (Multiple Outcomes of Raloxifene Evaluation) trial enrolled women with osteoporosis, without regard to breast cancer risk; most of these women were probably at low risk for breast cancer.[26] Thus, the reduction in breast cancer risk that has been found in that trial with the use of up to 48 months of raloxifene does not necessarily apply to women at high risk for breast cancer. Furthermore, the observed reduction in breast cancer risk was merely a secondary end point in the MORE trial.

- Third, elicit the concerns of the woman and explain how her issues were or were not addressed in the trial. This is not always routinely done in clinical practice; in particular, clinicians often fail to address the issue of side effects, the concerns that friends and family have expressed to the woman about the intervention being considered, and the concerns that the woman may have about being on long-term medication.[27]

- Fourth, describe the benefit and risk estimates in the trial in terms of the woman's personal medical risk history. This approach is particularly important when dealing with long-term interventions that have multiple end point effects.[28] This approach was implemented effectively in the decision aid used in the O'Connor et al. study. Reasonable estimates can be made for most of the conditions relevant to postmenopausal prevention. The woman's Gail model breast cancer risk assessment score can be easily calculated and used to demonstrate the estimated reduction in five-year risk with chemoprevention or the estimated increase in risk with long-term estrogen use. Vertebral and hip fracture risk can be estimated using historical data, the woman's age, and her bone mineral density. Heart disease risk can be estimated according to the NCEP (National Cholesterol Education Program) guidelines.[29] The risk for adverse events and side effects can be based on age, past medical history, and other factors. For example, the risk of endometrial cancer with tamoxifen is, of course, restricted to women with a uterus, and this risk is low in premenopausal women. The vasomotor symptoms that can be associated with raloxifene are much less common in women over 60 compared to younger women. For hormone therapy, bleeding is more of a problem in younger women, whereas breast tenderness is more common in older women.

CONCLUSIONS

In summary, high-level clinical trial–derived evidence should serve as the practicing physician's source for recommendations to patients. The clinician should optimize both communication of such recommendations and their rationale to the patient. Also, the clinician should incorporate patient input in final decision-making for any proposed intervention. While true for all clinical settings, this approach is particularly pertinent to preventive interventions among healthy individuals for whom intervention-derived toxicities are especially unacceptable.

There are several layers of complexity that should be confronted in order to achieve these goals. First, we must present trial results that are "clinically meaningful" rather than merely statistically significant. This applies to assessing both the benefit of interventions as well as the benefit/risk ratio of interventions. Where possible, clinical trials should involve the head-to-head comparison of a new drug with a standard agent. Even though head-to-head comparisons have been routinely done with drugs for other indications, this approach has not been utilized to compare new menopausal agents with the prevailing standard, estrogen, in any of its formulations. The estrogen dilemma, the indisputable dominance of estrogen over the menopausal scene, must be thoughtfully challenged as new data emerge. Finally, as elaborated above, we must develop strategies to help practitioners adapt their practice to new scientific findings and communicate these findings effectively to their patients.

REFERENCES

1. NATIONAL PERFORMANCE REVIEW. 1996 (March). Reinventing the regulation of cancer drugs.
2. GAIL, M.H., L.A. BRINTON, D.P. BYAR et al. 1989. Projecting individualized probabilities of developing breast cancer for white females who are being examined annually. J. Natl. Cancer Inst. **81:** 1879–1886.
3. GAIL, M.H., J.P. COSTANTINO, J. BRYANT et al. 1999. Weighing the risks and benefits of tamoxifen treatment for preventing breast cancer. J. Natl. Cancer Inst. **91:** 1829–1846.
4. TAYLOR, A.L., L.L. ADAMS-CAMPBELL & J.T. WRIGHT, JR. 1999. Risk/benefit assessment of tamoxifen to prevent breast cancer—still a work in progress? J. Natl. Cancer Inst. **91:** 1792–1793.
5. CHLEBOWSKI, R.T., D. COLLYAR, M.R. SOMERFIELD et al. 1999. American Society of Clinical Oncology technology assessment on breast cancer risk reduction strategies: tamoxifen and raloxifene. J. Clin. Oncol. **17:** 1939–1955.
6. FISHER, B., J.P. COSTANTINO, D.L. WICKERHAM et al. 1998. Tamoxifen for prevention of breast cancer: report of the National Surgical Adjuvant Breast and Bowel Project P-1 Study. J. Natl. Cancer Inst. **90:** 1371–1378.

7. WOLMARK, N. 1999. The Breast Cancer Prevention Trial, and the woman at high risk for breast cancer. Primary Care Cancer **19**(suppl. 1): 11–16.
8. DUNN, B.K. & L. FORD. 2000. Prevention of breast cancer. Semin. Breast Dis. **3:** 90–99.
9. SCAMBIA, G., D. MANO, P.G. SIGNORILE et al. 2000. Clinical effects of a standardized soy extract in postmenopausal women: a pilot study. J. North Am. Menopause Soc. **7:** 105–111.
10. VINCENT, A. & L.A. FITZPATRICK. 2000. Soy isoflavones: are they useful in menopause? Mayo Clin. Proc. **75:** 1174–1184.
11. GRIMM, R.H., JR., K.L. MARGOLIS, V.V. PAPDEMETRIOU et al. 2001. Baseline characteristics of participants in the antihypertensive lipid-lowering treatment to prevent heart attack trial (ALLHAT). Hypertension **37:** 19–27.
12. ALLHAT COLLABORATIVE RESEARCH GROUP. 2000. Major cardiovascular events in hypertensive patients randomized to doxazosin vs. chlorthalidone: the antihypertensive and lipid-lowering treatment to prevent heart attack trial (ALLHAT). JAMA **283:** 1967–1975.
13. HULLEY, S., D. GRADY, T. BUSH et al. 1998. Randomized trial of estrogen plus progestin for secondary prevention of coronary heart disease in postmenopausal women. JAMA **280:** 605–613.
14. HERRINGTON, D.M., D.M. REBOUSSIN, K.B. BROSNIHAN et al. 2000. Effects of estrogen replacement on the progression of coronary-artery atherosclerosis. N. Engl. J. Med. **343:** 522–529.
15. MOSCA, L., P. COLLINS, D.M. HERRINGTON et al. 2001. Hormone replacement therapy and cardiovascular disease: a statement for health care professionals from the American Heart Association. Circulation **104:** 499–503.
16. GUYATT, G. & D. RENNIE, Eds. 2002. Users' Guides to the Medical Literature: Essentials of Evidence-Based Clinical Practice. The Evidence-Based Medicine Working Group. AMA Press. Chicago.
17. MCALISTER, F.A., S.E. STRAUS, G.H. GUYATT & R.B. HAYNES. 2000. Users' guides to the medical literature: XX. Integrating research evidence with the care of the individual patient—Evidence-Based Medicine Working Group. [See comments.] JAMA **283:** 2829–2836.
18. HUNT, D.L., R. JAESCHKE & K.A. MCKIBBON. 2000. Users' guides to the medical literature: XXI. Using electronic health information resources in evidence-based practice—Evidence-Based Medicine Working Group. JAMA **283:** 1875–1879.
19. BUCHER, H.C., G.H. GUYATT, D.J. COOK et al. 1999. Users' guides to the medical literature: XIX. Applying clinical trial results. A. How to use an article measuring the effect of an intervention on surrogate endpoints—Evidence-Based Medicine Working Group. JAMA **282:** 771–778.
20. GUYATT, G.H., J. SINCLAIR, D.J. COOK & P. GLASZIOU. 1999. Users' guides to the medical literature: XVI. How to use a treatment recommendation—Evidence-Based Medicine Working Group and the Cochrane Applicability Methods Working Group. JAMA **281:** 1836–1843.
21. DERBY, C.A., A.L. HUME, J.B. PHILLIPS et al. 1995. Prior and current health characteristics of postmenopausal estrogen replacement therapy users compared with nonusers. Am. J. Obstet. Gynecol. **173:** 544–550.
22. UNITED STATES PREVENTIVE TASK FORCE. 1998. Clinician's Handbook of Preventive Services. Second edition. U.S. Department of Health and Human Services, U.S. Government Printing Office Superintendent of Documents. Washington, D.C.
23. NEWTON, K.M., A.Z. LACROIX, S.G. LEVEILLE et al. 1998. The physician's role in women's decision making about hormone replacement therapy. Obstet. Gynecol. **92:** 580–584.
24. O'CONNOR, A.M., P. TUGWELL, G.A. WELLS et al. 1998. Randomized trial of a portable, self-administered decision aid for postmenopausal women considering long-term preventive hormone therapy. Med. Decision Making **18:** 295–303.
25. O'CONNOR, A.M., A. ROSTOM, V. FISET et al. 1999. Decision aids for patients facing health treatment or screening decisions: systematic review. Br. Med. J. **319:** 731–734.
26. CUMMINGS, S.R., S. ECKERT, K.A. KRUEGER et al. 1999. The effect of raloxifene on risk of breast cancer in postmenopausal women: results from the MORE randomized trial—Multiple Outcomes of Raloxifene Evaluation. JAMA **281:** 2189–2197.

27. CONNELLY, M.T., N. FERRARI, N. HAGEN & T.S. INUI. 1999. Patient-identified needs for hormone replacement therapy counseling: a qualitative study. Ann. Intern. Med. **131:** 265–268.
28. COL, N.F., S.G. PAUKER, R.J. GOLDBERG et al. 1999. Individualizing therapy to prevent long-term consequences of estrogen deficiency in postmenopausal women. Arch. Intern. Med. **159:** 1458–1466.
29. EXPERT PANEL ON DETECTION, EVALUATION, AND TREATMENT OF HIGH BLOOD CHOLESTEROL IN ADULTS. 2001. Executive summary of the third report of the National Cholesterol Education Program (NCEP) expert panel on detection, evaluation, and treatment of high blood cholesterol in adults (Adult Treatment Panel III). JAMA **285:** 2486–2497.

Roles of Industry, Government, and Academia in SERM Development

Introduction

MARIETTA ANTHONY[a] AND KAREN JOHNSON[b]

[a]Department of Pharmacology, Women's Health Research, Georgetown University Medical Center, Washington, District of Columbia 20007, USA

[b]Breast and Gynecologic Cancer Research Group, Division of Cancer Prevention, National Cancer Institute, Bethesda, Maryland 20892, USA

Successfully developing a SERM for a new indication involves a sophisticated effort to identify chemical candidates, perform extensive testing under diverse conditions, analyze the data, and assess opportunity. Members of industry and academia with partners from the National Institutes of Health (NIH) and Food and Drug Administration (FDA) as representatives of the public interest are major forces in this effort. While each entity has a different mission, there are specific and sometimes overlapping considerations in the development of new SERMs or the investigation of new uses for existing compounds.

While there are many SERM candidates with different profiles of selectivity, activity, and safety, the profile of estrogen agonist and antagonist effects in different tissues is usually a critical factor in the risk-to-benefit profile. In recent years, the research effort to identify SERMs that have a desirable risk-to-benefit ratio has expanded, following the classic developmental approach through preclinical testing involving molecular assays as well as studies in animals and proceeding on to clinical testing in humans. The purpose of preclinical research is to identify patterns of clinical activity and to establish a safety profile that will allow continued drug development in a clinical setting. For example, an *in vitro* assay for SERMs measures the expression of complement component 3 (C3) in rodent endometrial epithelial cells. Since estrogen must be present for C3 to be expressed, the C3 assay helps to predict which compounds would be considered estrogen agonists. Another example of predicting clinical activity is testing SERMs in the ovariectomized rat model to ascertain skeletal antiresorptive properties, stimulatory effects on the uterus, and serum cholesterol lowering. This animal model has been used to predict subsequent favorable and unfavorable response in clinical phases of testing. The focus of initial clinical development is to confirm the tissue-specific estrogen profile that was predicted in preclinical models by performing short-term studies with strict attention to safety issues. When considering the clinical value of SERMs for the prevention of

Address for correspondence: Marietta Anthony, Ph.D., Department of Pharmacology, Director, Women's Health Research, Georgetown University Medical Center, 3900 Reservoir Road, NW, SE 404, Washington, D.C. 20007. Voice: 202-687-1064; fax: 202-687-4872.
mma4@georgetown.edu

disease in healthy women, even relatively low frequency safety events, such as pelvic organ prolapse, may be sufficient to negate the benefits of therapy, particularly if therapeutic alternatives exist. The identification of toxicities that occur with low frequency is an outcome of careful drug development.

While industry has a major role in the development of SERMs, substantial support has been added by collaborations with NIH and academic institutions. Industry sponsorship of clinical research at academic institutions has been significant, but not without problems. Tension may evolve from a situation where the manufacturer's requirement for confidentiality of information related to proprietary drug development is juxtaposed against academia's need for access to data and publication rights in its mission for research, education, and patient care. The National Cancer Institute (NCI) has provided comprehensive support via its role in planning, reviewing, and coordinating all aspects of clinical trials for investigations of anticancer agents from inception to submission of an investigational new drug (IND) application to the FDA. As the FDA reviews data from the whole spectrum of research from preclinical testing through the late-phase clinical trials and performs surveillance of marketed products, this agency exercises its legal authority and responsibility to review the product for its safety relative to its intended use and effectiveness.

As an example of a successful three-way collaboration, AstraZeneca Pharmaceuticals, the National Surgical Adjuvant Breast and Bowel Project (NSABP), and the NCI have worked together in a series of trials to evaluate tamoxifen for treatment of invasive breast cancer or reduction in risk of its development. Data have been reported on over 50,000 women at high risk, with a history of atypical ductal hyperplasia (ADH) or lobular carcinoma *in situ* (LCIS), with ductal carcinoma *in situ* (DCIS), with invasive tumors of less than 1 cm, with node-negative or node-positive disease, and at risk of developing contralateral breast cancer. In all these trials, tamoxifen use is associated with a reduction of 42% to 49% in the occurrence/recurrence of invasive breast cancer at 5 years. When an application was submitted to the FDA for a new indication for tamoxifen in the setting of women at high risk for breast cancer, the FDA provided an efficient and rapid response with 30 reviewers from various disciplines so that this use was approved within 6 months of receiving the application. Cooperation on this scale has enabled research and accelerated findings that have tremendous implications for improving public health.

Developing a SERM: Stringent Preclinical Selection Criteria Leading to an Acceptable Candidate (WAY-140424) for Clinical Evaluation

BARRY S. KOMM AND C. RICHARD LYTTLE

Women's Health Research Institute, Wyeth-Ayerst Research, Collegeville, Pennsylvania 19426, USA

ABSTRACT: Estrogens are represented by a diverse group of compounds. Within this large family of molecules are tissue-selective estrogens that have been classified as selective estrogen receptor modulators (SERMs). These compounds are characterized by the fact that they exhibit both estrogen agonist and antagonist activity dependent upon the gene promoter and target tissue being examined. SERMs have been intensively studied over the past decade, especially since one, raloxifene, has been approved for the prevention and treatment of postmenopausal osteoporosis. While not a replacement for hormone replacement therapy (HRT), raloxifene can be an alternative to it and other treatments for osteoporosis. The ideal SERM would provide the positive benefits associated with HRT without the uterine and breast stimulation. Raloxifene does achieve some of the benefits of HRT, specifically on the skeleton and lipid metabolism with no apparent uterine effects, and a potential decreased risk of developing breast cancer associated with raloxifene therapy. However, there are a number of parameters that can be improved. A number of SERMs have been evaluated only to fail in development due to, for the most part, uterine safety issues. In order to develop an improved SERM, a stringent screening process was designed to select compounds that did not stimulate the uterus or breast. At the same time, these new compounds would have a positive impact on the skeleton and lipid metabolism with the additional improvement (over raloxifene) of a neutral effect on hot flashes. Under these strict conditions, WAY-140424 was developed and, to date, the preclinical pharmacology data have accurately predicted the clinical response demonstrated in phase I and II trials.

KEYWORDS: estrogens; SERMs; WAY-140424; raloxifene

Estrogens are represented by a diverse group of compounds (FIG. 1) whose role is associated with reproduction, sexual behavior, skeletal remodeling, lipid metabolism, and vasomotor function, and the list continues to grow. Classically, when discussing estrogens, the steroidal members of the group represented by 17β-estradiol (E2),

---

Address for correspondence: Dr. Barry S. Komm, Women's Health Research Institute, Wyeth-Ayerst Research, Collegeville, PA 19426. Voice: 484-865-2776; fax: 484-865-9368.
kommb@war.wyeth.com

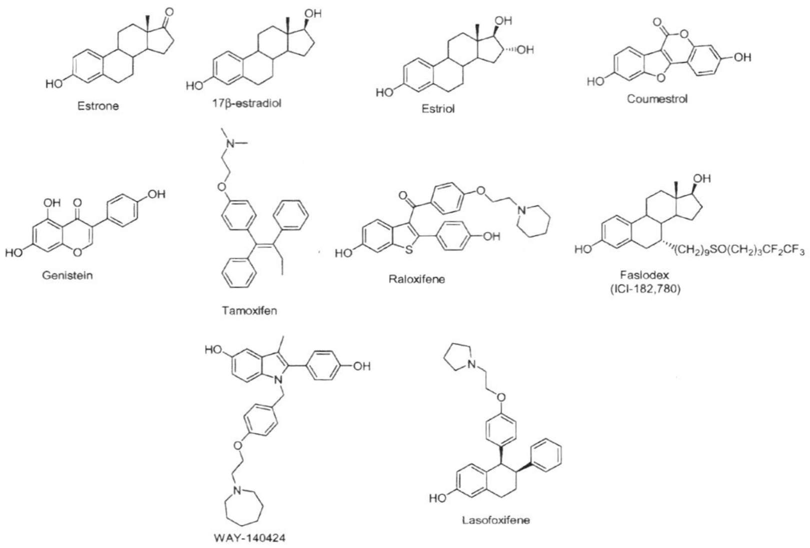

FIGURE 1. Estrogens: steroids, phytoestrogens, and SERMs. Representative members of the diverse group of compounds that make up the family of estrogens. Three steroidal estrogens are represented by estrone (E1), 17β-estradiol (E2), and estriol (E3). Coumestrol and genistein represent the nonsteroidal phytoestrogens. The SERMs are represented by the first-generation member, tamoxifen; the second generation by ICI-182,780 and raloxifene; and the third generation by lasofoxifene and WAY-140424. Note the diversity in structures, yet all function via binding to the estrogen receptors.

estrone (E1), and estriol (E3) come to mind. However, potent nonsteroidal estrogens like diethylstilbestrol (DES) also exhibit potent estrogenic effects. The true plant-derived estrogens, also nonsteroidal, such as genistein and coumestrol are estrogenic, but not as potent as E2 or DES. The newest members of the family, the so-called selective estrogen receptor modulators (SERMs),[1] distinguish themselves from the group by the fact that they exhibit mixed functional activity—that is, SERMs exhibit both estrogen agonist and antagonist function dependent upon the tissue and gene target.

What estrogens have in common is that their information is transduced by the estrogen receptors (estrogen receptor α and β, ERα and ERβ).[2,3] These proteins, which are members of a large group of nuclear receptors (progesterone, androgen, glucocorticoid, etc.), bind estrogens and, upon binding, a series of events ensue with the end result being transcriptional regulation of estrogen-target genes.[4] It is the biochemical and biophysical modifications to the ERs that permit mixed-function estrogen activity. Following ligand binding, the ERs undergo a conformational change in addition to other biochemical events such as phosphorylation.[5] Conceptually, the conformation of the receptor then dictates what other proteins, such as coregulators, it can efficiently interact with[6] and what amino acid residues are available for biochemical modification. It appears that some genes are more permissive than others in relation to what ER configuration will be tolerated to regulate or enhance transcription. Therein lies the fact that SERMs, dependent upon the gene and tissue in question, will demonstrate mixed functional activity.[7]

The development of the optimal SERM, or an improved SERM, compared to the marketed raloxifene (EVISTA®) is not a simple task. What would the ideal SERM do pharmacologically? This would be a molecule that protects the skeleton (i.e., maintains bone mass and bone quality; prevents osteoporosis), improves the lipid profile (lowers LDL, raises HDL cholesterol), reduces the incidence and severity of hot flashes, maintains vaginal lubrication, and maintains normal bladder function like conventional hormone replacement therapy (HRT). At the same time, this ideal SERM should not negatively affect the uterus [no endometrial hyperplasia or hypertrophy, no increased stromal fluid accumulation, no polyps, no bleeding (amenorrhea)] and should reduce the risk of developing breast cancer. This is quite a task for one compound to accomplish.

If we look at the effect of raloxifene, or any of the other SERMs that successfully entered into clinical evaluation, on these parameters, it becomes clear that this list is, at best, partially fulfilled, with room for improvement. Raloxifene's effect (at 60 mg/day) on bone mineral density compared to other antiresorbers such as HRT or bisphosphonates is a modest 1.5%–2.0% increase[8] measured at the spine compared to 4%–5% for HRT and up to 7%–9% for bisphosphonates.[9] Raloxifene does reduce the risk of vertebral fracture (~36%), but has no positive effect on nonvertebral fractures,[10] and does not appear to be as efficacious as bisphosphonates. Raloxifene does reduce LDL cholesterol by approximately 10%, which is comparable to HRT on this parameter; however, HRT also results in a significant increase in HDL cholesterol—an advantage since this can be a factor related to a reduced risk for the development of cardiovascular disease. The primary reason women choose to begin HRT is to alleviate menopausal symptoms, of which the most bothersome is the hot flash. Vasomotor instability is controlled in the vast majority of women who use HRT. On the other hand, raloxifene has been shown to increase the incidence of hot flashes. Raloxifene does not reestablish a normal vaginal environment, which is another clear advantage of HRT.[11,12] Thus, it would appear that an improved SERM profile is possible on one or more of a number of parameters.

Several candidate molecules have been developed to compete with raloxifene, only to fail. The reason for failure was, in general, unacceptable uterine changes. Thus, levormeloxifene, idoxifene, and droloxifene, all effective on the skeleton and LDL cholesterol lowering, had to be terminated for uterine safety reasons. Here are three good examples demonstrating that improving the SERM profile set by raloxifene was not going to be an easy task. To be successful in such an endeavor would require stringent selection at a preclinical level to develop a series of compounds that outperformed raloxifene in the appropriate *in vitro* and *in vivo* models.

A well-defined set of criteria have to be established to characterize compounds in order to assure (as well as possible) that the molecule is acceptable along every step of the preclinical development pathway. For the development of WAY-140424, a stringent selection process was implemented (FIG. 2). After demonstration of receptor binding affinity and activation, a series of *in vitro* transcription assays were performed in various cellular backgrounds to assess promoter and cell type activity. Endogenous gene activity was also measured via gene expression directly and by cell proliferation (i.e., more complex biological events). Finally, a series of *in vivo*

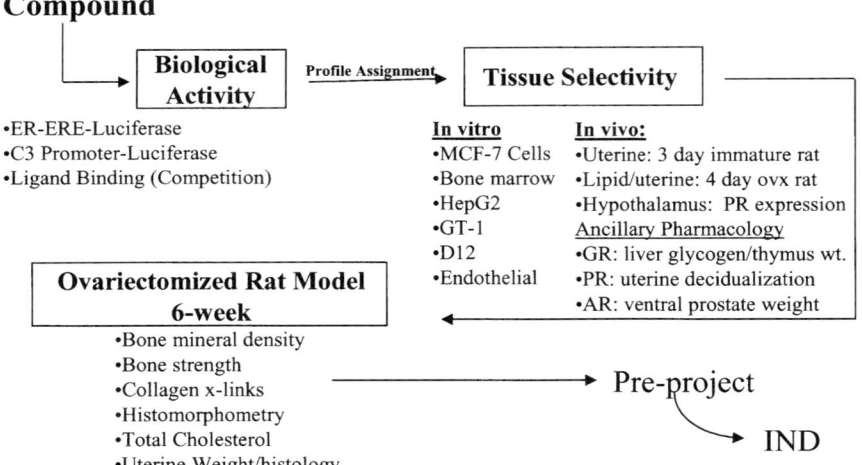

FIGURE 2. Multistep, stringent process for the development of third-generation SERMs. A complex and thorough screening paradigm to select novel, improved SERMs. This scheme starts by ensuring that the compounds bind to the estrogen receptors and that binding results in a functional receptor:ligand combination. Tissue and promoter selectivity were assessed in a number of cell lines using a variety of promoter constructs and endogenous genetic responses. If a compound passed the preset requirements of these *in vitro* tests, then it proceeded to the *in vivo* models, which assessed a compound's effect on the uterus, skeleton, lipid metabolism, and central nervous system. Abbreviations: ER = estrogen receptor; GR = glucocorticoid receptor; PR = progesterone receptor; AR = androgen receptor; ERE = estrogen response element; C3 = complement component 3; MCF-7 cells = human breast carcinoma cell line; HepG2 = human hepatoma cell line; GT-1 = human neuronal cell line; D12 = human neuronal cell line; ovx = ovariectomized; x-links = cross-links; IND = investigational new drug.

models were used to evaluate bioavailability and biologic activity on key end points, which included the uterus, lipid metabolism, bone remodeling, and central nervous system function. In all experimental paradigms, WAY-140424 was compared to raloxifene and, in many cases, other members of the SERM family.

It was first established that WAY-140424 was a high-affinity ligand for ERα (and subsequently for ERβ). WAY-140424 revealed a $K_i \cong 0.1$ nM (0.3 nM for ERβ) and no crossover binding to the other members of the steroid/retinoid family of nuclear receptors (e.g., androgen, progesterone, vitamin D, retinoid, rexinoid, etc.). In an effort to demonstrate that WAY-140424 binding to the ER resulted in a functionally active receptor, several *in vitro* transcription assays were performed. First, the simplest model was tested. A plasmid DNA construct containing a 2XERE (estrogen response element) linked to a weak promoter (thymidine kinase) driving luciferase was transfected into HepG2 cells treated for 24 hours and then luciferase activity measured. In this system, WAY-140424 was a relatively potent, E2 antagonist with an $IC_{50} \cong 5.0$ nM. Similarly, raloxifene was also a potent antagonist ($IC_{50} \cong 2.0$ nM). However, when the hepatic lipase (associated with HDL metabolism) promoter was substituted for the 2XERE-TK construct in the same cell line, WAY-140424 was an

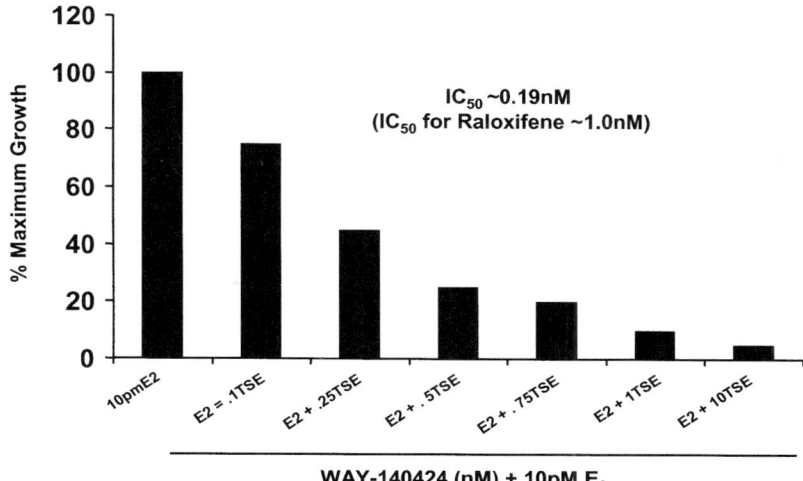

FIGURE 3. Inhibition of 17β-estradiol-stimulated proliferation in MCF-7 cells by WAY-140424. MCF-7 cell proliferation assay: MCF-7 cells treated with 10 pM E2 provide a positive control set to 100%, considered maximum proliferation. This concentration of E2 was combined with 0.1–10 nM WAY-140424. The WAY-140424 dose dependently inhibited E2-stimulated proliferation with an IC_{50} = 0.19 nM. In this assay, raloxifene also antagonized E2-stimulated proliferation with an $IC_{50} \cong 1$ nM. E2 = 17β-estradiol; WAY = WAY-140424.

agonist like E2 ($EC_{50} \cong 210$ nM vs. 100 nM). Interestingly, raloxifene tested at concentrations up to 10 μM did not activate this promoter and tamoxifen required at least 5 μM to detect minimal activation. These *in vitro* data support the concept of selective promoter activation and also the fact that all SERMs are not created equal. Other promoters such as TGF-β3 and quinone reductase have also been shown to respond to SERMs. Both are activated by raloxifene[13] and ICI-182,780 and, in fact, TGF-β3 activation by raloxifene is antagonized by 17β-estradiol.

Utilizing a more complex *in vitro* model, WAY-140424 was tested as an agonist and antagonist in an MCF-7 cell (human breast tumor cell line) proliferation assay (FIG. 3). These cells proliferate in response to some estrogens. WAY-140424 did not stimulate proliferation of these cells and potently antagonized E2-stimulated proliferation with an IC_{50} = 0.19 nM. This is an important assay in the development of any estrogen, especially SERMs, because of the perceived relationship of HRT and breast cancer. MCF-7 proliferation is quite sensitive to estrogen agonists and it serves as a complex *in vitro* model. An acceptable SERM should not demonstrate any type of stimulatory activity in this assay since an agonist response would suggest that such a compound may stimulate the breast and possibly increase the risk of developing breast cancer.

In addition to the breast, a key target where a SERM should not function as an agonist is the uterus. Based on current SERM history, it is this tissue's responsiveness where SERMs distinguish themselves most obviously in *in vivo* models. In order for a compound in the described screening process to clear the hurdle to *in vivo* evalua-

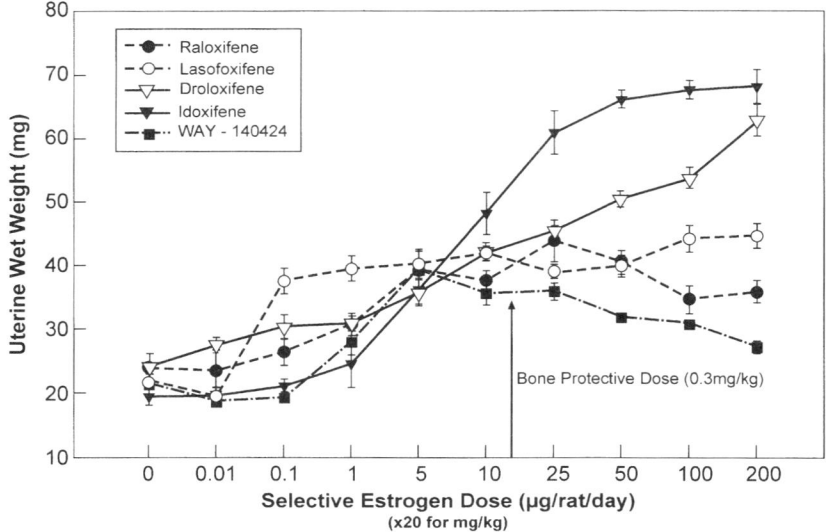

FIGURE 4. Comparison of SERMs on stimulating uterine wet weight increases in an immature rat model. Uterine wet weights obtained from the 3-day immature rat uterine model. Rats were treated for 3 days with compounds and uteri were collected 24 h following the last dose. WAY-140424 was compared to four other SERMs. From these data, the uterine stimulations by droloxifene and idoxifene clearly separate them from the other members of this group. WAY-140424 at its bone protective dose of 0.3 mg/kg and above (*arrow* on graph) reveals a wet weight lower than both raloxifene and lasofoxifene.

tion, it first had to demonstrate no agonist activity in an *in vitro* transcription assay utilizing the complement component 3 (C3) promoter. C3 has been demonstrated to require estrogen agonist stimulation to be expressed in rodent endometrial epithelial cells.[14]

In an immature or ovariectomized rat or mouse uterus, C3 cannot be detected. However, shortly after exposure to E2 or other estrogenic compounds, C3 expression is rapidly turned on and maintained for up to 36 hours following a single exposure event.[15] Interestingly, the isolated C3 promoter evaluated in an *in vitro* transcription model turned out to be quite accurate in predicting the *in vivo* responsiveness to SERM candidates. WAY-140424 does not exhibit any agonist activity on this promoter *in vitro*, while raloxifene minimally stimulates promoter function. However, tamoxifen, idoxifene, and droloxifene all act as agonists (tamoxifen > idoxifene > droloxifene) in this assay. The *in vitro* activity of these SERMs correlates quite nicely with wet weight stimulation in a 3-day immature rat model. In this model (3 days of treatment followed by removal of the uterus for wet weight measurement, histological evaluation, and C3 gene expression), WAY-140424 reveals a slight, but statistically insignificant increase in wet weight, although consistently less than the other SERMs tested including lasofoxifene (FIG. 4). Histologic analysis shows that WAY-140424 does not stimulate endometrial hypertrophy or hyperplasia, myometrial

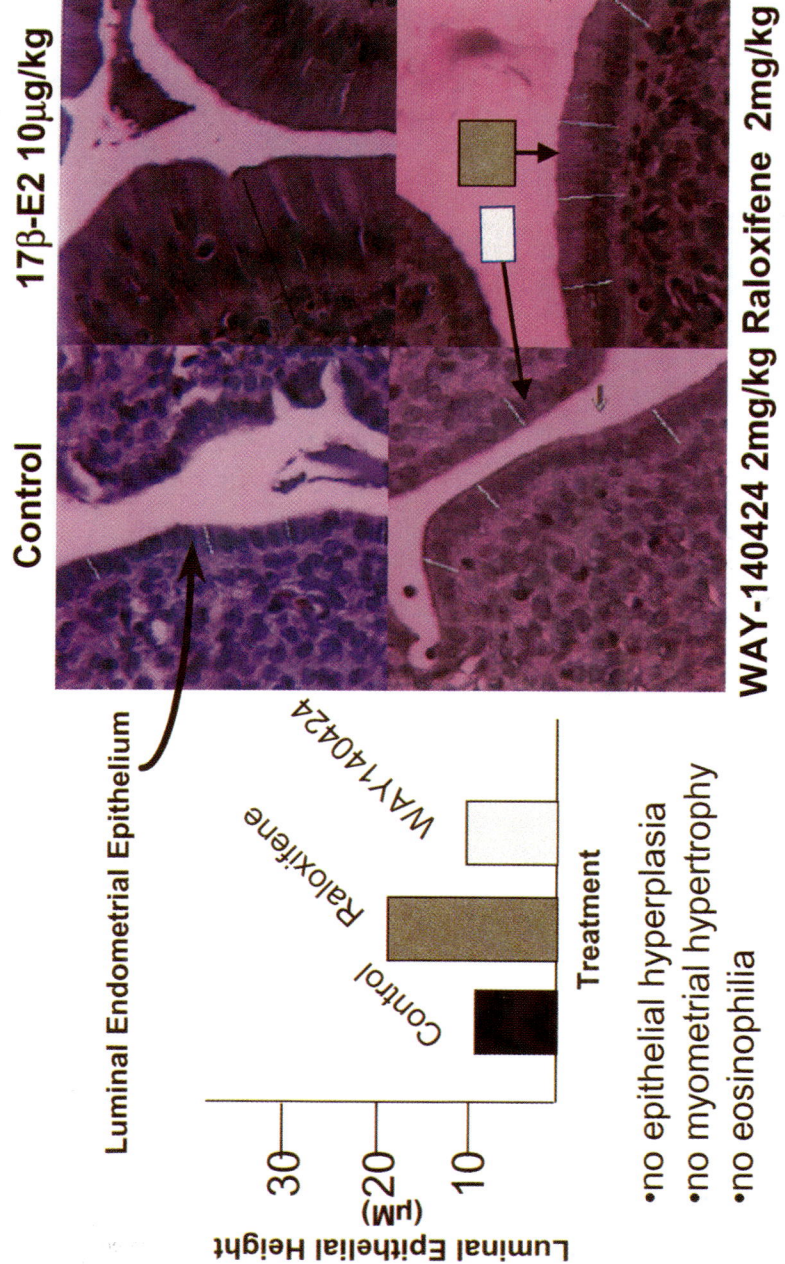

FIGURE 5. See following page for legend.

hypertrophy, or eosinophilia. Raloxifene at similar doses results in endometrial hypertrophy and a substantially greater increase in uterine wet weight (FIG. 5). In fact, when WAY-140424 is coadministered with raloxifene, it antagonizes raloxifene's stimulatory effect on wet weight, histologic parameters, and C3 gene expression (data not shown). To date, raloxifene has not demonstrated any clinically relevant changes to the uterus. WAY-140424 preclinical data also suggest that it will not affect the uterus, and it is unknown whether differences between the two compounds will be seen clinically.

As stated, the uterine assay is where most compounds failed in this screening paradigm. Idoxifene, droloxifene, and levormeloxifene—three compounds that were evaluated in clinical trials—would have been rejected by the criteria set in this screen. WAY-140424 passed and was subsequently tested in the remaining *in vivo* assays. While several assays are listed in FIGURE 2, two key models were used. One was the 6-week ovariectomized rat osteopenia model—a gold standard for analysis of a compound's effect on the skeleton. Additionally, this model allows uterine and lipid metabolism evaluation. The second model is a rat "hot flash" model,[16] which was used to assess the impact of WAY-140424 on vasomotor instability.

Like the other SERMs including raloxifene, WAY-140424 effectively maintains bone mass and reduces total cholesterol in the rat osteopenia model after 6 weeks of treatment. The efficacious dose of WAY-140424 in this model has been determined to be 0.3 mg/kg/day, which was approximately 10-fold less than the effective dose for raloxifene. This difference in efficacious dose to spare bone becomes important when discussing the results of the rat "hot flash" model. In this model, mature, ovariectomized female rats are addicted to morphine. When these rats are administered a bolus injection of naloxone, they exhibit an extreme vasomotor response that can be detected by a thermocouple attached to their tail. A 4–5°C increase in tail skin temperature is measured within 15–30 minutes of the naloxone injection. If these animals are treated with E2 or ethinyl estradiol, the vasomotor response is inhibited.[16] WAY-140424 and raloxifene do not behave as agonists in this model (FIG. 6). However, they both behave as E2 antagonists. WAY-140424 and raloxifene antagonism are detected at doses of ≥1.0 mg/kg. The dose of WAY-140424 to protect the skeleton is 0.3 mg/kg, which is below the dose required to antagonize E2's positive effect, while raloxifene's dose is 3.0 mg/kg. Thus, raloxifene's bone sparing dose in the rat model is above that required to antagonize E2's positive effect on reducing tail skin

---

FIGURE 5. Comparison of WAY-140424 and raloxifene in the immature rat uterine model: histologic evaluation. Histological comparison of WAY-140424 and raloxifene in the 3-day immature rat uterine model. While wet weights are not that dramatically different in rats treated with equivalent doses of WAY-140424 and raloxifene (100 µg/rat in FIG. 4), there are overt differences in morphological changes of the uterus between these two compounds. Comparing luminal endometrial epithelial cell (*arrows*) height, it can be seen that raloxifene at 2 mg/kg/day doubled the cell height compared to control, while WAY-140424 exhibited no stimulatory effect. Additionally, WAY-140424 did not cause myometrial hypertrophy or eosinophilia, which are both routinely increased in response to 17β-estradiol treatment. All micrographs are of identical magnification and stained with hemotoxylin and eosin. Luminal epithelial cell heights are the average of 10 measurements around the lumen of the uterus of 6 animals/group.

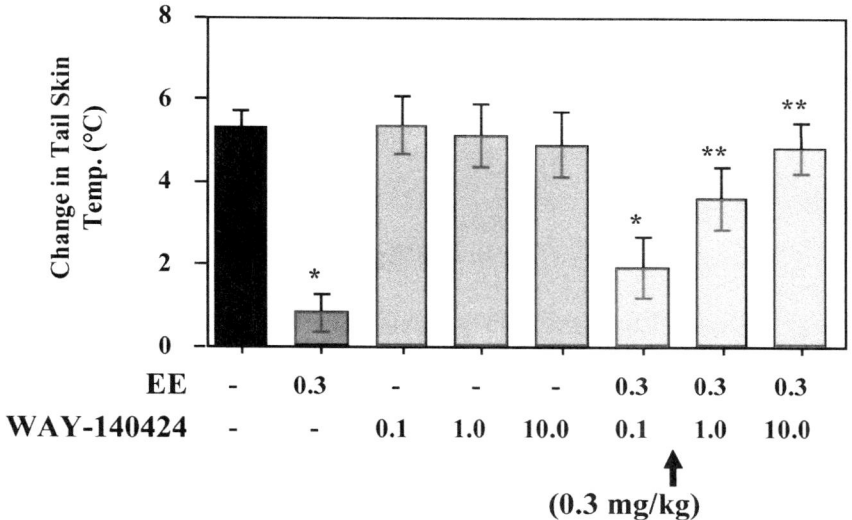

*Significantly Different from Vehicle ($P<0.05$)
**Significantly Different from EE ($P<0.05$)

FIGURE 6. Effect of WAY-140424 on vasomotor response in the rat "hot flash" model. Ovariectomized rats given a bolus injection of naloxone demonstrate an ~5°C increase in tail skin temperature. Treatment with 0.3 mg/kg ethinyl estradiol (EE) inhibited the vasomotor response. WAY-140424 dosed at 0.1, 1.0, and 10.0 mg/kg did not demonstrate estrogen agonist activity and antagonized EE at doses ≥ 1.0 mg/kg. Raloxifene functions similarly to WAY-140424 in this assay. The *arrow* at 0.3 mg/kg indicates the bone effective dose for WAY-140424 and it falls below the dose demonstrating antagonist activity in this assay.

temperature. Clinical data have confirmed that raloxifene does increase the incidence of hot flashes at its bone sparing dose in humans (60 mg/day).[8,11,12]

Stringent selection parameters, specifically enforced on the targets where SERM agonist activity is not desired, particularly in the breast and uterus, led to the selection of WAY-140424 for development. However, in the CNS where agonist activity is desired, no SERM tested to date has demonstrated to be effective. The acceptable alternative is to be neutral on vasomotor function and WAY-140424 achieves this goal at its bone sparing dose of 0.3 mg/kg. These preclinical data support the evaluation of WAY-140424 in the clinic and, based on the parameters described, would predict it to be superior to raloxifene. Thus far, in phase I and II clinical evaluation, WAY-140424 has exhibited no increase in hot flashes compared to placebo-treated women nor any significant changes in endometrial thickness assessed by transvaginal ultrasound. Bone marker data and LDL lowering are positive in phase II trials as predicted by *in vitro* and *in vivo* models in our screening pathway. We await longer-term, clinical data to conclusively determine if WAY-140424 is a superior SERM to those available today.

REFERENCES

1. GRIESE, T.A. & J.A. DODGE. 1998. Selective estrogen receptor modulators (SERMs). Curr. Pharm. Design **4:** 71–92.
2. GREEN, S., P. WALTER, G. GREENE *et al.* 1986. Cloning of the human oestrogen receptor cDNA. J. Steroid Biochem. **24:** 77–83.
3. KUIPER, G.J.M., E. ENMARK, M. PELTO-HUIKKO *et al.* 1996. Cloning of a novel estrogen receptor expressed in rat prostate and ovary. Proc. Natl. Acad. Sci. U.S.A. **93:** 5925–5930.
4. KLEIN-HITPASS, L., S.Y. TSAI, G.L. GREENE *et al.* 1989. Specific binding of estrogen receptor to the estrogen response element. Mol. Cell. Biol. **9:** 43–49.
5. AURICCHIO, F. 1989. Phosphorylation of steroid receptors. J. Steroid Biochem. **32:** 613–622.
6. SHIAU, A.K., D. BARSTAD, P.M. LORIA *et al.* 1998. The structural basis of estrogen receptor/coactivator recognition and the antagonism of this interaction by tamoxifen. Cell **95:** 927–937.
7. TZUKERMAN, M.T., A. ESTY, D. SANTISO-MERE *et al.* 1994. Human estrogen receptor transactivation capacity is determined by both cellular and promoter context and mediated by two functionally distinct intramolecular regions. Mol. Endocrinol. **8:** 21–30.
8. DELMAS, P.D., N.H. BJARNASON, B.H. MITLAK *et al.* 1997. Effects of raloxifene on bone mineral density, serum cholesterol concentrations, and uterine endometrium in postmenopausal women. N. Engl. J. Med. **337:** 1641–1647.
9. LIBERMAN, U.A., S.R. WEISS, J. BROLL *et al.* 1995. Effect of oral alendronate on bone mineral density and the incidence of fractures in postmenopausal osteoporosis. N. Engl. J. Med. **333:** 1437–1443.
10. NIH CONSENSUS CONFERENCE. 2001. Osteoporosis prevention, diagnosis, and therapy. JAMA **285:** 785–795.
11. CLEMETT, D. & C.M. SPENCER. 2000. Raloxifene—a review of its use in postmenopausal osteoporosis. Drugs **60:** 370–411.
12. DAVIES, G.C., W.J. HUSTER, L. YILI *et al.* 1999. Adverse events reported by postmenopausal women in controlled trials with raloxifene. Obstet. Gynecol. **93:** 558–565.
13. YANG, N.N., M. VENUGOPALAN, S. HARDIKAR *et al.* 1996. Identification of an estrogen response element activated by metabolites of 17β-estradiol and raloxifene. Science **273:** 1222–1225.
14. SUNDSTROM, S.A., B.S. KOMM, H. PONCE-DE-LEON *et al.* 1989. Estrogen regulation of tissue-specific expression of complement C3. J. Biol. Chem. **264:** 16941–16947.
15. KOMM, B.S., D.J. RUSLING & C.R. LYTTLE. 1986. Estrogen regulation of protein synthesis in the immature rat uterus: the analysis of proteins released into the medium during *in vitro* incubation. Endocrinology **118:** 2411–2416.
16. MERCHENTHALER, I., J.M. FUNKHOUSER, J.M. CARVER *et al.* 1998. The effect of estrogens and antiestrogens in a rat model for hot flush. Maturitas **30:** 307–316.

The Breast Cancer Continuum

Insights from the Tamoxifen Trials Impact Future Drug Development Strategies

JERRY P. LEWIS

AstraZeneca Pharmaceuticals, Wilmington, Delaware 19850, USA

> ABSTRACT: The Breast Cancer Continuum includes women at high risk, as in the Breast Cancer Prevention Trial; those with a history of atypical ductal hyperplasia (ADH) or lobular carcinoma *in situ* (LCIS); women with ductal carcinoma *in situ* (DCIS); those with <1 cm invasive disease or node-negative or node-positive disease; and those at risk of developing contralateral breast cancer. Women in all these categories benefit from therapeutic intervention with tamoxifen because each clinical state is associated with a certain probability of having early undiagnosed invasive breast cancer responsive to tamoxifen. This framework, relating these disorders to each other through their 5-year incidence of developing invasive breast cancer, leads to important conclusions relative to pharmaceutical drug development strategies, including chemoprevention investigations.
>
> KEYWORDS: tamoxifen; invasive and noninvasive breast cancer

Breast cancer trials are some of the largest and most replicated of all clinical investigations. As such, they lead to conclusions with strong statistical underpinnings. In 1998/1999, three seminal breast cancer trial analyses became available comparing tamoxifen with placebo in a variety of clinical settings. In total, data were reported on over 50,000 women, ranging from those without breast cancer, but with an increased risk of developing invasive breast cancer, to those diagnosed and treated for stage I and stage II breast cancer.[1-3] A critical assessment of these data offers a unique opportunity to compare the 5-year incidence of invasive breast cancer in various clinical settings and to document the impact of 5 years of tamoxifen on this incidence. These various clinical states represent a continuum, referred to here as the Breast Cancer Continuum, in which the particular clinical setting serves as a marker for the 5-year incidence of invasive breast cancer. These are shown schematically in FIGURE 1. These clinical states are potentially free of invasive breast cancer at the time of diagnosis or, in the case of women with early breast cancer, are rendered free of known disease following surgery. This Breast Cancer Continuum includes women at high risk, as in the Breast Cancer Prevention Trial; those with a history of atypical

---

Address for correspondence: Jerry P. Lewis, M.D., Senior Medical Director of Oncology, AstraZeneca Pharmaceuticals, 1800 Concord Pike, Wilmington, DE 19850-5437. Voice: 302-886-4646; fax: 302-886-7723.

Jerry.Lewis@astrazeneca.com

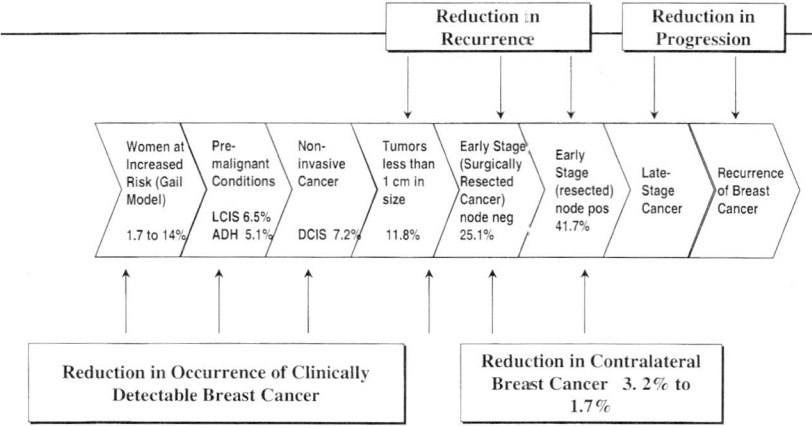

FIGURE 1. The various clinical entities within the Breast Cancer Continuum are arranged from the lowest to the highest risk of developing invasive breast cancer over a period of 5 years. This risk is reduced by about 40% to 50% with 5 years of tamoxifen. The ability of tamoxifen to reduce occurrence/recurrence and the effect on contralateral breast cancer are indicated.

ductal hyperplasia (ADH) or lobular carcinoma *in situ* (LCIS); women with ductal carcinoma *in situ* (DCIS); those with <1 cm invasive disease or node-negative or node-positive disease; and those at risk of developing contralateral breast cancer. Women in all these categories benefit from therapeutic intervention with tamoxifen because each clinical state is associated with a certain probability of having early undiagnosed invasive breast cancer responsive to tamoxifen. This framework, relating these disorders to each other through their 5-year incidence of developing invasive breast cancer, leads to important conclusions relative to pharmaceutical drug development strategies, including chemoprevention investigations.

In the three trials mentioned above,[1–3] the primary end point was occurrence/recurrence of invasive breast cancer over a 5-year period:

(1) The Early Breast Cancer Trialists' Collaborative Group published their metanalysis involving 55 adjuvant breast cancer trials representing over 37,000 women. This included 85% of the worldwide trials that began prior to 1990 and yielded data on women with both node-negative and node-positive early breast cancer who, following primary therapy, received 1, 2, or 5 years of tamoxifen or placebo. These women were followed for 10 years and the benefit of tamoxifen persisted after tamoxifen treatment was stopped. This analysis showed a 42% reduction in recurrence of breast cancer at 10 years for women assigned to 5 years of tamoxifen. In addition, there was a 47% reduction in occurrence of contralateral breast cancer at 10 years among women receiving 5 years of tamoxifen therapy.[1]

(2) The NSABP Breast Cancer Prevention Trial P-1 recruited women at increased risk of developing invasive breast cancer according to the Gail

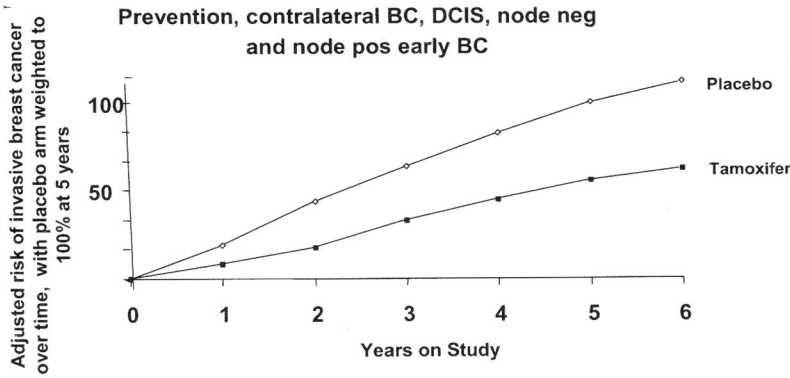

FIGURE 2. Combined data of 25,437 women in the Breast Cancer Continuum. The impact of tamoxifen given for 5 years is similar in the setting of the studies of treatment for breast cancer prevention (first primary breast cancers, second primary breast cancers in the contralateral breast), adjuvant treatment for early-stage breast cancer, and treatment for carcinoma *in situ* (DCIS, LCIS). This figure shows the weighted adjusted risk of invasive breast cancer occurrence using the data from these trials.[1–3] Since the percent of invasive breast cancer differs considerably in each setting (see FIG. 1), the figure has been normalized, with 100 representing 100% of invasive breast cancers seen on the placebo arm at 5 years. It is noted that the lines separate during the first year and continue to diverge through 5 years. Since the effect is immediate, the impact of tamoxifen is one of treatment of clinically unrecognized developing breast cancer.

model and showed that 5 years of tamoxifen reduced the occurrence of invasive breast cancer by 49% over 5 years.[2]

(3) The NSABP DCIS Trial B-24 recruited 1804 patients with DCIS treated with resection and ipsilateral radiation and then randomized to 5 years of tamoxifen or 5 years of placebo. This trial demonstrated that 5 years of tamoxifen reduced the occurrence of invasive breast cancer by 43%.[3]

In these trials, the reduction in occurrence/recurrence of invasive breast cancer at 5 years is essentially the same in each clinical setting and ranges from 42% to 49%. Furthermore, the benefit of tamoxifen was seen during the first year of tamoxifen administration regardless of the initial clinical state, and the benefit continued to accrue during the 5 years of drug therapy.[1–3] This is shown in FIGURE 2, which depicts the weighted adjusted benefit of tamoxifen as compared to placebo in these clinical settings. Moreover, the benefit, as shown in the adjuvant trials, is durable beyond 10 years even in women who only took tamoxifen for 1 year.[1] Although this could have occurred by chance alone, it is more likely that tamoxifen has a similar therapeutic effect in each of these clinical situations.

Thus, the impact of tamoxifen in women at high risk of breast cancer, with a history of LCIS or ADH, with DCIS or contralateral breast cancer, and with node-negative or node-positive early breast cancer is on early unrecognized breast cancer or on lesions destined to develop into invasive breast cancer. In chemoprevention, if the effect were on the very early cells (clusters of 8–32 cells perhaps) destined to

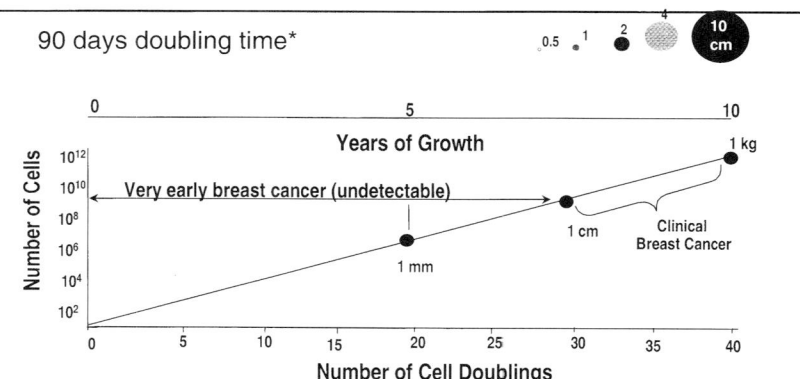

FIGURE 3. Detectable breast cancer is the result of years of neoplastic cell growth. For much of the tumor's development, it is clinically silent. It is in this "quiescent" period that tamoxifen acts to reduce the risk of invasive breast cancer in the different clinical entities of the Breast Cancer Continuum. Note: 90 days × 40 doublings = 3600 days (approx. 10 years).

develop into invasive breast cancer, the benefit would not have been apparent within the first year, or for that matter within the first 5 years, since breast cancer cells double slowly (approximately every 100 days) and take up to 5–10 years (20–30 doublings) to produce a clinically detectable tumor mass (see FIG. 3). Furthermore, these foci of early unrecognized breast cancer tissue, presumably ER-dependent cells, must regress and disappear under the influence of tamoxifen since they do not become clinically apparent later on, even with 9 years of follow-up, in women given only 1 year of tamoxifen.[1]

Early foci of invasive breast cancer have been identified in resected breast tissues of women thought to be without invasive breast cancer. Detailed sectioning of breast tissue in a variety of clinical situations, including women dying of causes other than breast cancer, confirm a surprisingly high incidence of malignant and premalignant lesions in clinically uninvolved breasts.[4–6] Foci of premalignant/malignant lesions increase as women progress from high risk of developing breast cancer to node-positive early breast cancer following primary therapy. Hence, the various clinical entities of the Breast Cancer Continuum serve as markers of the 5-year incidence of invasive breast cancer and these unrecognized foci respond similarly to therapeutic manipulation with tamoxifen.

The implications of this for future breast cancer drug development are profound. With tamoxifen, it took over 20 years to move from demonstrated efficacy in the advanced disease setting through proven efficacy in women with early breast cancer, women with DCIS, women with a history of ADH or LCIS, and finally to high-risk women with an increased incidence of developing invasive breast cancer. In the setting of the Breast Cancer Continuum, the effect of tamoxifen appears to be on similar targets in each of these clinical settings, supporting the thesis that it is early-unidentified estrogen-dependent premalignant/malignant cells whose growth is impacted by tamoxifen. This being the case, it is feasible to do one or two efficacy studies in any of the Breast Cancer Continuum segments and, having demonstrated that a new drug has equivalence to tamoxifen or, better yet, improved efficacy over tamoxifen, the experimental drug similarly will test equivalent to or better than tamoxifen in other settings. It is fully recognized that this would not likely meet regulatory muster; nevertheless, it will support clinical decisions to prescribe off-label where appropriate (for safety reasons, etc.) and will provide assurance to the pharmaceutical company that an investment in a clinical trial will lead to a successful outcome. In a similar tone, however, it is not likely that an agent that is inactive or weakly active in one setting, when compared to the standard agent, will be found to be more effective versus the standard agent in another setting.

In settings in which hormonal or chemotherapeutic agents are used, advanced breast cancer serves as a predictor of response for the various segments of the Continuum. This may not be the case, however, as we move into utilizing novel agents, such as signal transduction inhibitors or anti-angiogenic drugs. These new and potentially exciting agents may only affect very early developing tumors, while lacking significant efficacy in well-established advanced cancer.

An acceptance of the concept of the Breast Cancer Continuum expands our understanding of the pathobiology of breast cancer:

(1) The ratio of ER-dependent to ER-independent breast cancer appears to be relatively stable from women at increased risk of breast cancer to those with early breast cancer. The efficacy of tamoxifen is similar in women at increased risk of developing invasive breast cancer and those with stage II breast cancer.
(2) As little as 1 year of tamoxifen prevents some unrecognized breast cancers from developing into clinically recognized invasive breast cancer in women with early breast cancer treated with surgery and will have a similar effect in other segments of the Continuum. Women who are at high risk for developing breast cancer and who benefit from 5 years of tamoxifen have unrecognized premalignant/malignant lesions that are destined to develop into invasive breast cancer.
(3) With reference to the last point, if it were possible to identify women at high risk of developing invasive breast cancer who at that time had unrecognized very early foci of cells destined to develop into invasive breast cancer later, it would be feasible to treat only those with early unrecognized disease. This would negate the necessity to treat the many women who may be at high risk, but at that particular point in time do not have unrecognized lesions destined to develop into invasive breast cancer. For the present, this is not feasible. Considering the fact that breast cancer grows very slowly and that our techniques to diagnose very small breast cancers are improving, it raises hope that our future chemopreventive efforts can be more finely focused.

REFERENCES

1. EARLY BREAST CANCER TRIALISTS' COLLABORATIVE GROUP. 1998. Tamoxifen for early breast cancer: an overview of the randomised trials. Lancet **351**: 1451–1467.
2. FISHER, B., J.P. COSTANTINO, D.L. WICKERHAM *et al.* 1998. Tamoxifen for prevention of breast cancer: report of the National Surgical Adjuvant Breast and Bowel Project P-1 Study. J. Natl. Cancer Inst. **90**: 1371–1388.

3. FISHER, B., J. DIGNAM, N. WOLMARK et al. 1999. Tamoxifen in treatment of intraductal breast cancer: National Surgical Adjuvant Breast and Bowel Project B-24 randomised controlled trial. Lancet **353:** 1993–2000.
4. BARTOW, S.A., D.R. PATHAK, W.C. BLACK et al. 1987. Prevalence of benign, atypical, and malignant breast lesions in populations at different risk for breast cancer. Cancer **60:** 2751–2760.
5. RINGBERG, A., B. PALMER, F. LINELL et al. 1991. Bilateral and multifocal breast carcinoma—a clinical and autopsy study with special emphasis on carcinoma *in situ*: focal, occult *in situ*, and invasive carcinoma in 250 mastectomy specimens. Eur. J. Surg. Oncol. **17:** 20–29.
6. SKJORTEN, F., E. AMLIE & K. LARSEN. 1986. On the occurrence of focal, occult *in situ*, and invasive carcinoma in 250 mastectomy specimens. Eur. J. Surg. Oncol. **12:** 117–121.

The Cancer Therapy Evaluation Program (CTEP) at the National Cancer Institute

Industry Collaborations in New Agent Development

SHERRY S. ANSHER AND RAMI SCHARF

Regulatory Affairs Branch, Cancer Therapy Evaluation Program, Division of Cancer Treatment and Diagnosis, National Cancer Institute, National Institutes of Health, Rockville, Maryland 20852, USA

ABSTRACT: The mission of the Cancer Therapy Evaluation Program (CTEP), a clinical research program of the National Cancer Institute (NCI), is to reduce the burden of cancer. CTEP plans, reviews, and coordinates clinical trials for investigational anticancer agents, from the inception of protocols through the preparation and submission of Investigational New Drug Applications (INDs) to the Food and Drug Administration (FDA). CTEP also serves as a liaison to the FDA for the extramural clinical research community and industry collaborators. Other CTEP functions include managing, tracking, and reviewing clinical protocols as well as monitoring, planning, and maintaining regulatory compliance of the clinical trials. In addition, CTEP coordinates the distribution of the investigational agents from industry collaborators for use in all NCI-sponsored clinical trials. The advantages of collaborating with CTEP are described as well as details about the contractual framework, either a Clinical Trials Agreement (CTA) or a Cooperative Research and Development Agreement (CRADA), for such a collaboration. Many of the concerns raised by industry collaborators with respect to intellectual property, data access, and publications are also addressed.

KEYWORDS: NCI; DCTD; CTEP; CRADA; CTA; clinical trials; anticancer agents; industry collaboration; clinical trials cooperative groups; data access; intellectual property

INTRODUCTION

The mission of the National Cancer Institute's (NCI) clinical research program is to reduce the burden of cancer in the population. It does so by promoting preclinical as well as clinical research, the study of cancer prevention, treatment, and control, and the better understanding of basic cancer biology. The development of investigational anticancer agents by the NCI is a coordinated, collaborative effort. In the Division of Cancer Treatment and Diagnosis (DCTD) two programs are particularly

Address for correspondence: Dr. Sherry S. Ansher, Coordinator, Research and Development Agreements, Regulatory Affairs Branch, Cancer Therapy Evaluation Program, Division of Cancer Treatment and Diagnosis, National Cancer Institute, Executive Plaza North, Room 7111, 6130 Executive Boulevard, Rockville, MD 20852. Voice: 301-496-7912; fax: 301-402-1584.
anshers@ctep.nci.nih.gov

focused on this area. The Developmental Therapeutics Program (DTP) is responsible for preclinical investigations, including the screening of new agents in cell line panels for antitumor activity, and the pharmacology, toxicology, and formulation research for promising agents. More information on this program can be found on the web at http://www.dtp.nci.nih.gov/. The Cancer Therapy Evaluation Program (CTEP) plans, reviews, and coordinates clinical trials for investigational anticancer agents, through the establishment of a clinical development plan for each investigational agent, and the preparation and submission of an Investigational New Drug Application (IND) for each agent. CTEP also serves as the liaison to the Food and Drug Administration (FDA) for both the extramural clinical research community and industry collaborators. Other CTEP functions include managing, tracking, and reviewing clinical protocols as well as monitoring, planning, and maintaining regulatory compliance of clinical trials. In addition, CTEP coordinates the distribution of the investigational agents from industry collaborators for use in NCI-sponsored clinical trials.

ADVANTAGES OF COLLABORATION WITH THE CANCER THERAPY EVALUATION PROGRAM

CTEP provides expertise in the design of clinical development plans and a unique ability to evaluate investigational agents in a wide variety of tumor types and disease settings. As of January 2001, CTEP sponsored more than 1,000 active clinical protocols with an accrual rate of close to 25,000 patients per year. Furthermore, about 500 new clinical protocols are approved and activated by CTEP each year with a similar number of studies completed each year and leading to published results. These studies are accomplished by a cadre of investigators approaching 10,000 in number and located at 1,958 institutions. On the industry collaborator side, CTEP currently has 120 active collaborative agreements with pharmaceutical companies, including Clinical Supply Agreements (CSA), Clinical Trials Agreements (CTA), and Cooperative Research and Development Agreements (CRADA). These agreements define the interactions between NCI, the pharmaceutical industry collaborator, and the clinical investigators for the conduct of clinical trials. The CTEP clinical trials network is the most comprehensive in the world, sponsoring the cancer clinical trials cooperative groups as well as single institutions such as the comprehensive cancer centers. Development plans for investigational agents are coordinated between CTEP and the pharmaceutical or biotechnology company on a collaborative basis.

There are two major goals for industry collaborations. The first is to engage CTEP's assistance in expediting studies leading to agent registration and commercialization; the second is to facilitate investigations of relevant scientific questions concerning the agent. This includes the exploration of the activity of the agent in different disease settings and the optimization of formulations, schedules, and routes of administration for maximal activity. Collaborations with CTEP provide an efficient route to making the investigational agent more widely available to the public. These collaborations also ensure that the broadest range of disease settings is tested.

COLLABORATIVE CLINICAL DEVELOPMENT PATHWAY

Source of Agents

Investigational anticancer agents can originate from a number of sources; for example, they can be (1) agents that are discovered and/or developed at NCI; (2) agents developed through NCI-funded grants at extramural institutions; (3) agents developed independently of NCI by universities, academic or research institutions, or not-for-profit organizations; and (4) agents developed by pharmaceutical companies. Agents from pharmaceutical companies represent the largest portion of CTEP's portfolio.

Clinical Protocol Development and Agent Supply

For cancer treatment agents, the primary responsibility for the clinical development plan lies with one of the physicians in the Investigational Drug Branch (IDB) within CTEP. Following the formulation and finalization of a collaborative agreement with a collaborator, IDB prepares agent-specific solicitations for clinical investigators requesting the submission of protocol Letters of Intent (LOI) to conduct clinical trials. Once an LOI is approved by CTEP and the collaborator, investigators are asked to submit protocols. All protocols submitted to CTEP are evaluated and approved by both the CTEP Protocol Review Committee (PRC) and the collaborator. In addition, final approved versions of the protocol, as well as amendments and Adverse Event (AE) reports, are also sent to the industry collaborator at the same time that they are submitted to the FDA. The Pharmaceutical Management Branch (PMB) of CTEP is responsible for the registration of all clinical investigators participating in NCI-sponsored clinical studies. PMB is also responsible for the distribution, acquisition, and inventory management for all investigational agents.

Submission and Sponsorship of an Investigational New Drug Application

In the collaborative clinical development of investigational agents, the Regulatory Affairs Branch (RAB) of CTEP prepares and submits an Investigational New Drug (IND) Application to the FDA in order to conduct clinical trials with the investigational agent, which the NCI will sponsor. The collaborator may or may not hold or wish to hold its own IND for the agent (but always has the option to file its own IND for trials outside of the scope of the collaborative development with CTEP). If an IND and/or Master File (MF) is already held by the collaborator, CTEP will cross-reference the existing IND and/or MF. Likewise, the collaborator has the option to cross-reference the NCI-sponsored IND. All information in the NCI IND is made fully and exclusively available to the collaborator following the execution of an appropriate collaborative agreement such as a CTA or a CRADA. As of January 2001, CTEP held 160 active INDs.

CTEP, as an IND sponsor, can provide a myriad of functions ranging from attendance at pre-IND meetings to the preparation and sponsorship of INDs, the submission of subsequent protocols and protocol amendments, AE tracking, and the provision of pharmaceutical services for investigational agents. Moreover, CTEP can serve as liaison to the FDA for inquiries, meetings, and revisions requested by the FDA.

Clinical Studies Monitoring

Oversight of study monitoring is the responsibility of the Clinical Trials Monitoring Branch (CTMB) within CTEP. Special requests by the industry collaborator can be accommodated through the coordination of the RAB and CTMB, preferably in advance of protocol activation. There are two mechanisms for monitoring NCI-sponsored studies. Selected phase 1 studies are monitored by the Clinical Trials Monitoring Service (CTMS). Trial data from these studies are submitted on a biweekly basis to the CTMS contractor, who maintains the data for CTEP. Data summary tables are sent to the collaborator once a month. However, additional information and individual case report forms can be requested through separate arrangements between the collaborator and the CTMS contractor. The CTMS also conducts audits for data verification twice a year and site visits annually. CTMS routinely conducts a pharmacy inspection and reviews the NCI Drug Accountability Records for these trials.

All other clinical studies are monitored through the Clinical Data Update System (CDUS). CDUS reports are submitted to the NCI quarterly. The collaborator has the option of requesting copies of these reports. The CTMB conducts site visits for the CDUS-monitored studies at least once every three years. However, special response or for-cause audits may take place, if appropriate. If requested, arrangements may also be developed to provide special types of data collection to the collaborator.

CLINICAL TRIALS COOPERATIVE GROUPS AT THE NATIONAL CANCER INSTITUTE

The NCI's Clinical Trials Cooperative Groups (the Cooperative Groups) consist of researchers at institutions affiliated with the cooperative groups, who jointly develop and conduct cancer treatment clinical trials in multi-institutional settings. These groups, each of whom has a liaison in the Clinical Investigations Branch (CIB) of CTEP, are a major component of the extramural research effort of NCI. Each cooperative group is supported to continually generate new trials compatible with its particular areas of interest and expertise, as well as with national priorities for cancer treatment research.

The cooperative groups are heterogeneous in their research objectives and their structures. Research interests can be centered around disease orientation (e.g., gynecologic oncology), high technology, single modality studies (e.g., radiation therapy), an area in which the investigators have a particular expertise (e.g., pediatrics), or can encompass multiple center treatment areas. The common thread, however, is the development and the conduct of large-scale trials in a multi-institutional setting. Emphasis is placed on definitive, randomized phase 3 studies and the developmental efforts preliminary to them. This allows the rapid accrual of patients while reducing the possible introduction of statistical bias of studies due to small sample size carried out at a single or a few institutions.

Approximately 20,000 new patients are accrued onto group treatment studies each year. Some 12,000 new patients are evaluated annually on ancillary laboratory correlative studies, and many times the combined number is in follow-up. Thousands of individual investigators participate in cooperative group protocols.

Collaborative Clinical Development in Europe

The NCI interacts extensively with international organizations responsible for the conduct of clinical trials with investigational anticancer agents in Europe. The NCI maintains a liaison office, located in Brussels, Belgium, which helps to coordinate the NCI's interaction with cancer research and treatment programs in Europe, by working in close collaboration with the European Drug Discovery Network (EDDN), which comprises the European Organization for Research and Treatment of Cancer (EORTC), the Cancer Research Campaign (CRC) of the United Kingdom, and the recently organized Southern-Europe New Drugs Organization (SENDO).

Agents for development can be provided and distributed for clinical trials from either NCI or the EDDN. Co-development of these agents still requires the approval of the NCI Drug Discovery Group (DDG), as well as approval from the European committees. For agents approved for co-development in Europe, NCI will be responsible for the synthesis of the bulk agent and formulation of the final clinical product. European collaborators will be responsible for performing the preclinical toxicology required for IND approval. IND-equivalent filings for European trials are handled through the EDDN.

The NCI liaison office, in collaboration with the EDDN, has developed standard quality control procedures and common guidelines for both preclinical and clinical phases of investigational agent development. The guidelines ensure that procedures for formulation and preclinical toxicology studies use internationally accepted standards to meet regulatory requirements on both sides of the Atlantic. The EORTC and the CRC have filed MFs with the U.S. FDA so that the data collected from the clinical trials conducted by the participating institutions can be used in support of IND and licensing applications in the United States. The introduction of these common guidelines and standard procedures that fulfill U.S. regulatory requirements has facilitated the filing of IND applications, as well as the acceptance of European preclinical and clinical data by the U.S. FDA.

CONTRACTUAL FRAMEWORK FOR COLLABORATION WITH THE CANCER THERAPY EVALUATION PROGRAM

The mechanism for NCI–industry collaborations is primarily through the execution of collaborative agreements. The clinical co-development of an agent with the NCI can proceed under a CTA or a CRADA. The Confidential Disclosure (or Secrecy) Agreement (CDA) is also available to help facilitate the process. CDAs are appropriate when the information that is to be exchanged between the industry collaborator and CTEP is considered proprietary and confidential. When a CDA is executed between CTEP and the collaborator, the confidentiality relationship is equivalent to the relationship between the FDA and industry. The choice of the collaborative mechanism to be used is usually the collaborator's decision. Both the CTA and the CRADA have provisions for effective cooperative work with CTEP. Both address issues of clinical trial planning, IND filing, agent supply, data access, and adverse event reporting. The particular properties of each agreement should be considered when selecting the appropriate mechanism for collaboration.

Clinical Trials Agreements

NCI initiated the CTA to specify the interaction between the NCI and a collaborator for the clinical co-development of an agent. The CTA, unlike the CRADA, is not covered by congressional legislation and has no funding associated with its execution, but does address intellectual property disposition if a patent is filed as a result of the studies conducted. The CTA can be signed by the DCTD Director for rapid implementation, and is generally suitable when the collaborator has a strong intellectual property position; that is, the agent is owned and/or licensed by the biotechnology or pharmaceutical company. A CTA may also be appropriate when the collaborator has completed preclinical studies and IND-directed toxicology. In these cases, an IND has often been filed by the collaborator and phase 1 studies have been initiated or completed. Finally, a CTA is considered when the collaborator will be supplying the formulated agent only, and no funds will be provided to support the co-development of the agent.

Cooperative Research and Development Agreements

A mechanism created by congressional legislation (the Federal Technology Transfer Act, 1986), the CRADA is a more elaborate agreement that stipulates terms for a much broader scope of research than is usually performed under a CTA. This type of agreement also offers an option to the collaborator for the exclusive or nonexclusive licensing of intellectual property arising from intramural research supported by the CRADA. Intellectual property arising from a CRADA does not have to be offered as "fair access" (i.e., intellectual property may be licensed to the collaborator without advertisement of its availability). The CRADA offers the collaborator the broadest range of studies that can be conducted under the research plan, from preclinical laboratory studies through post-marketing clinical trials for supplemental indications. Furthermore, the CRADA is the only agreement under which the NIH can receive outside financial support for collaborative research conducted through intramural or extramural studies. Unlike the CTA, the CRADA requires full NIH subcommittee review and approval.

Finally, collaborative research for NCI-sponsored orphan agent development can be conducted only under a CRADA because this is the sole mechanism which allows NCI to provide data exclusively to a collaborator for the commercialization of a product.

ADDRESSING INDUSTRY CONCERNS ABOUT CANCER THERAPY EVALUATION PROGRAM INTERACTIONS AND COLLABORATIONS

Pharmaceutical and biotechnology companies spend vast resources in the development of therapeutic agents. It is only natural that these companies consider the protection of their scientific, technical, and commercial assets of utmost importance. The following approaches have been initiated to address some of the major concerns of the pharmaceutical and biotechnology industry when considering a collaboration with NCI in general, and with CTEP specifically.

Clinical Trial Data Access

All information from the CTEP-sponsored IND is made available exclusively to the collaborator. Data (including case report forms) held at the institutions where the clinical trials are conducted are available to the collaborator following a request made to the RAB. Collaborator on-site audit arrangements may also be facilitated by the RAB. Primary clinical trial data generated in NCI-sponsored clinical trials are made available exclusively to NCI, the FDA, and the collaborator. Provisions for this procedure are included in the terms of award of all extramural funding agreements, and the NCI standard protocol language required in all CTEP-reviewed and -approved protocols. Collaborators are given 30 days to review manuscripts prior to submission to assure that no collaborator's confidential or proprietary information is released. An additional 30 days can be requested for patent filings only. CTEP is implementing a new electronic web-based clinical trials reporting system, which will also improve the speed with which data are available to collaborators.

Control of Agent Development

All CTEP development plans are based on mutual agreement between CTEP and the collaborator. Areas of development are discussed to avoid duplication of effort or waste of resources. The collaborator is free to pursue areas outside the scope of the agreement with CTEP. All protocols are mutually approved by the collaborator and CTEP prior to activation.

Indemnification/Liability

The U.S. government is prohibited from indemnifying collaborators by federal statute (The Anti-Deficiency Act, Title 31, USC 3141). However, the collaborator is not expected to indemnify the government or assume liability for government activities. The government's liability for its own actions is limited by the Federal Tort Claims Act, 28 USC Chapter 171. Additionally, collaborators are not expected to indemnify the extramural investigators performing NCI-sponsored studies. Insurance is an allowable cost under funding agreements.

Intellectual Property and Extramural Inventions

One area of repeated concern to collaborators is access to intellectual property that might arise from an extramural investigator conducting an NCI-sponsored study using a collaborator's agent. Congressional legislation to promote academic inventions under government funding agreements prohibits the academic institutions from assigning those rights to another party. This approach has left many potential and actual collaborators especially concerned about the potential loss of intellectual property. This issue has recently been resolved by modifying the terms of award of the funding agreements supporting clinical trials to provide the first option to negotiate a license to the intellectual property to the collaborator who supplied the investigational agent to CTEP. Thus, the institution's right to own the intellectual property and the collaborator's need to license it are protected.

Furthermore, a statement restricting access to clinical data to the NCI, the FDA, and the collaborator is included to protect the collaborator's need for exclusive access to clinical data from trials of their investigational agents. The implementation of these terms is the responsibility of the Clinical Grants and Contracts Branch (CGCB) within CTEP.

ADDITIONAL INFORMATION

Additional information on the workings of CTEP and the collaborative development of novel anticancer agents can be obtained at the CTEP website: http://ctep.cancer.gov or by contacting Dr. Sherry S. Ansher.

[EDITOR'S NOTE: Within the National Cancer Institute, parallel programs and procedures for development of cancer prevention agents are located within the Division of Cancer Prevention. For instance, IDB finds its parallel in the Chemoprevention Agent Development Research Group (CADRG), and liaison to the Cooperative Groups is provided by the Community Oncology and Prevention Trials Group (COPTRG). Additional information about the collaborative development of cancer prevention agents can be found at http://dcp.nci.nih.gov]

FDA Review Practices and Priorities for Drugs Used in Cancer Treatment[a]

KEN KOBAYASHI[b] AND ROBERT J. DeLAP

Division of Oncology Drug Products, Center for Drug Evaluation and Research, United States Food and Drug Administration, Rockville, Maryland 20857, USA

> ABSTRACT: The Federal Food, Drug, and Cosmetic Act and related regulations (21 U.S.C. 301 *et seq.*) give FDA staff the legal authority and responsibility to review the safety and effectiveness of drugs and biological products (including products used in cancer treatment), from preclinical testing through all phases of clinical research and marketing. FDA review activities in the oncology arena can be divided into five major categories: (1) initial review of investigational new drug (IND) applications; (2) ongoing review of premarketing research (including new research protocols submitted to existing INDs and IND safety reports describing adverse events with the new drug); (3) discussions with commercial sponsors regarding their clinical development plans, including the design and conduct of key studies that are intended to support initial marketing approval for a new product or to support the addition of new indications to the prescribing information for currently marketed products; (4) review of submitted new drug applications (NDAs) or biological licensing applications (BLAs); and (5) continuing review of the safety and effectiveness of marketed products. Through these review activities, FDA staff work to ensure that products approved for marketing for cancer treatment are effective and adequately safe for their intended uses and to ensure that the quality, effectiveness, and safety of products on the market are preserved or enhanced, so patients and physicians may use these products with confidence and with adequate safety. Because these review activities generally fall into a chronologic sequence, the following discussion parallels the development course of a typical new drug.
>
> KEYWORDS: FDA review; investigational new drug (IND) application; cancer treatment

RESEARCH STUDIES OF INVESTIGATIONAL NEW DRUGS

A sponsor wishing to initiate studies of an investigational new drug or therapeutic biological product generally must submit an IND application. An open IND, formally termed an investigational new drug exemption, allows a research sponsor to legally put an investigational new drug or biological product into interstate commerce for

---

Address for correspondence: Robert J. DeLap, M.D., Ph.D., Director, Office of Drug Evaluation V, Center for Drug Evaluation and Research, U.S. Food and Drug Administration, 5600 Fishers Lane, Rockville, MD 20857. Voice: 301-827-2250; fax: 301-827-2317.
Delapr@cder.fda.gov
[a]A version of this paper was previously published in *Cancer Therapeutics* (1998, **1:** 146–148).
[b]Current address: Ken Kobayashi, M.D., Mike Mansfield Fellow, Mansfield Center for Pacific Affairs, No. 32 Kowa Building 2F, 5-2-32 Minami-Azabu, Minato-ku, Tokyo 106-0047, Japan.
kobayashi@attglobal.net

purposes of clinical research. A sponsor with an open IND is "exempted" from the requirement in the Federal Food, Drug, and Cosmetic Act for premarketing approval, based on adequate evidence of the product's effectiveness and safety, before a new drug or therapeutic biological product may be put into interstate commerce.

The primary question in an FDA review of a new IND application is whether or not the proposed study provides adequate safeguards for patients and volunteers. To assist in this evaluation, the sponsor must include the results of preclinical and other relevant studies supporting the use of the new drug according to the proposed dose, schedule, duration, and route of administration. For instance, when a sponsor proposes a phase I clinical study of a new product in patients with advanced cancer, the sponsor will usually have performed short-term animal toxicology studies to estimate a dose-toxicity relationship and to arrive at a qualitative picture of the adverse events that might occur in human use. Animal pharmacokinetic and *in vitro* metabolic (liver microsome and/or liver slice) studies may have also been performed to help predict product pharmacokinetics and potential drug interactions in humans. Additional preclinical studies to evaluate the product's mechanism of action may have been performed to help elucidate potential therapeutic targets and shed further light on potential toxicities and optimal uses of the drug. While all pertinent preclinical data are of interest to FDA staff, the primary focus of FDA review of a new IND is on safety. IND studies may proceed as long as sufficient data are provided to support the adequate safety of the proposed research. Studies beyond basic acute preclinical toxicology studies are not generally required to support initiation of clinical studies of new cancer treatment products in patients with advanced cancer. The FDA medical and pharmacology/toxicology reviews of a new IND application integrate all provided information and specifically evaluate the anticipated safety of the proposed starting dose, schedule, dose escalation scheme, monitoring plan, and overall study proposal. On occasion, FDA staff may determine that further preclinical toxicology studies are required. More frequently, FDA staff may suggest or require modifications in the initial clinical protocol to enhance the safety of the trial.

Subsequent IND clinical trials with the new agent are monitored to ensure that they are adequate in design to advance the clinical development of the product and to ensure that patient safety is adequately protected. New, unusual, or serious adverse events may require the modification of informed consent forms, protocol eligibility, patient monitoring, and/or the dose or schedule of administration of the investigational product. Sometimes, serious adverse events and a lack of evidence of major efficacy in early clinical trials lead to termination of product development. Reviewers typically work with the drug sponsor to identify and clarify any issues of substantial concern, to assess their overall significance, and to appropriately modify the protocols and/or development program when needed.

PLANNING KEY STUDIES TO SUPPORT PRODUCT MARKETING

After the new product has completed early clinical testing and the sponsor is ready to begin planning registration-directed trials, FDA staff routinely provide advice (as requested by the IND sponsor) on the planning of their development program. This support is provided in an effort to improve the efficiency of the drug development process and with the understanding that the FDA, the drug sponsor, prescribing physicians, patients, and the general public all have a shared interest in having well-designed, well-conducted clinical trials that target clinically useful end points in well-defined patient populations to support drug approvals for important indications. This advisory function usually takes the form of FDA-industry meetings at which preliminary data are reviewed and proposed clinical trials are discussed. These meetings typically involve 7 to 12 FDA reviewers from several disciplines (clinicians, pharmacology/toxicology specialists, biostatisticians, chemists or product manufacturing experts, and clinical pharmacokinetics/biopharmaceutics specialists). Research sponsors also typically bring a range of specialists to these meetings, appropriate to the stage of the product's development and the nature of the questions to be resolved. These discussions usually also include a representative of one of the FDA's technical advisory panels (the Oncologic Drugs Advisory Committee or the Biological Response Modifier Advisory Committee). Topics for discussion typically include the data obtained by the research sponsor in early clinical testing and plans for subsequent key clinical trials that will be intended to support a marketing application, and may include other issues such as orphan drug status, potential period of marketing exclusivity, and potential fast-track status (as described in the Food and Drug Administration Modernization Act of 1997 [PL 105–115]).

Although the FDA endeavors to give research sponsors the best possible advice on study designs and research strategies to support a marketing application, it is not possible for the FDA to guarantee that completion of a particular program of studies will be sufficient for marketing approval. The completed studies must yield results that clearly establish that a product provides a meaningful net clinical benefit for patients (or an effect on a surrogate marker that is very likely to correlate with meaningful patient benefit such as objective tumor shrinkage in patients with advanced cancer, with acceptable safety). Based on the study results, it must be possible to identify a clinical indication and a patient population for which the product can reasonably be used, considering the observed safety and effectiveness of the new product and its apparent value compared with other currently available products for the proposed patient group and indication.

THE PRODUCT MARKETING APPLICATION (NDA OR BLA)

Once the commercial sponsor has decided to submit a new drug application (NDA) for a drug, the review team usually meets at least once with company representatives to discuss the specific studies and data that will be submitted and how they should be formatted. The actual review of an NDA requires that a representative from each discipline (clinicians, biostatisticians, chemistry or product specialists, biopharmaceutics specialists, and pharmacology/toxicology specialists) should analyze the submitted data according to their specific expertise and make recommendations on the acceptability of the data to support marketing approval for the new product. For each patient entered on the key clinical trial(s), the volumes that document clinical information for an NDA typically contain the specific historic, physical examination, radiographic, and laboratory data that were used to determine patient eligibility, as well as details of the patient's treatment, adverse effects, tumor response, and final outcome. Detailed drug administration records and posttreatment follow-up data (when required) are also provided for each patient so that compliance and time-to-event parameters can be assessed. The application will also contain the original protocol and each amendment for all key studies. In the course of completing the medical review, the primary medical reviewer will typically verify patient eligibility, treatment, and major safety and effectiveness outcomes in a subset of patients (or in all patients enrolled in key clinical trials, in applications including data from small numbers of patients).

Product quality (chemistry and manufacturing controls, quality controls, impurity levels, etc.) is also continuously reviewed over the course of development of a new product, but is examined with particular care when sponsors begin to enroll large numbers of patients in advanced clinical trials or in treatment protocols, and when an NDA or BLA (biological licensing application) is filed.

MONITORING QUALITY OF MARKETED PRODUCTS

Following marketing approval, the FDA continues to monitor product safety and effectiveness, including literature surveillance and adverse experience surveillance; review of annual reports filed by the NDA/BLA holder; and monitoring of product production and quality, including issues of product stability and shelf life and periodic manufacturing plant inspections. Product manufacturers provide reports to the FDA at least annually regarding distribution of their product, any foreign regulatory or marketing developments significant to product safety or effectiveness, and any significant new information that they have obtained about the product (from sponsored studies, literature reviews, or other sources). Manufacturing procedures typically undergo continuing revision and improvement after marketing approval, and appropriate FDA staff review those changes. Product manufacturers occasionally encounter problems with failures of product batches to meet quality specifications and, in those cases, FDA staff will work with the manufacturer to identify solutions that will prevent or minimize any potential shortages of critical products. Finally, FDA staff monitor reports of product safety, effectiveness, or quality problems that are obtained from companies, health care professionals, patients, and others through the FDA's MedWatch program.

Tamoxifen for the Reduction in the Incidence of Breast Cancer in Women at High Risk for Breast Cancer[a]

SUSAN FLAMM HONIG

Division of Oncology Drug Products, United States Food and Drug Administration, Rockville, Maryland 20852, USA

ABSTRACT: Recent legislation, including the Prescription Drug User Fee Act (1992) and the FDA Modernization Act (FDAMA) (1997), has provided an environment in which new drug applications (NDA) can be efficiently reviewed, resulting in rapid access to new drugs or to new uses for approved drugs by the public. The recent submission of a supplemental NDA for tamoxifen for the reduction in the incidence of breast cancer in women at high risk for breast cancer is an excellent example of the application of this legislation. First, the application received expedited but thorough multidisciplinary and interdivisional review by the FDA. Second, it required collaboration between the manufacturer (AstraZeneca Pharmaceuticals), the National Surgical Adjuvant Breast and Bowel Project (NSABP), the National Cancer Institute (NCI), and the FDA. This process worked well and demonstrated that cooperative group data can be used effectively to support an application. Third, a single large adequate and well-controlled trial was sufficient to support the effectiveness of tamoxifen for this indication. The quantity of evidence required to support approval has been discussed in FDA guidances ("Providing Clinical Evidence of Effectiveness for Human Drug and Biological Products") and is part of FDAMA.

KEYWORDS: tamoxifen; breast cancer; high risk; prevention

SEQUENCE OF EVENTS

On April 2, 1998, the NSABP notified the NCI and FDA of significant efficacy results from the Breast Cancer Prevention Trial, NSABP P-1. A supplemental NDA (new drug application) for tamoxifen was submitted to the FDA on April 30, 1998. Data were submitted on a rolling basis and were complete by August 4, 1998. The review involved almost 30 reviewers from various disciplines and medical groups across the FDA. The application was presented to the Oncologic Drugs Advisory Committee (ODAC) on September 2, 1998, and the committee voted to recommend approval of tamoxifen for the reduction in the incidence of breast cancer. The FDA accepted the recommendation, and approval was granted on October 29, 1998.

Address for correspondence: Susan Flamm Honig, M.D., Division of Oncology Drug Products, HFD-150, U.S. Food and Drug Administration, 5600 Fishers Lane, Rockville, MD 20852. Voice: 301-594-2473; fax: 301-594-0499.
honigs@cder.fda.gov
[a]A version of this paper was previously published in *Cancer Therapeutics* (1999, **2**: 33–35).

STUDY DESIGN AND RESULTS

NSABP P-1 was a randomized double-blind placebo-controlled trial of tamoxifen with a planned duration of 5 years in 13,388 women at high risk for breast cancer. "High risk" was defined as women aged 35 or older with an absolute 5-year risk of breast cancer of 1.67% as calculated by the Gail model. The Gail model is a statistical program that calculates risk based on several factors, including current age, age at menarche, age at first pregnancy (or, conversely, nulliparity), number of breast biopsies, presence/absence of atypical hyperplasia, and family history of breast cancer in first-degree relatives. In addition, women with a history of lobular carcinoma *in situ* (LCIS) and any woman over the age of 60 were eligible for the study.

The trial showed a significant reduction in the number of cases of invasive breast cancer with tamoxifen therapy and a nonsignificant reduction in the number of cases of ductal carcinoma *in situ*. A nonsignificant reduction in hip fractures, but not in wrist fractures, was seen in women on tamoxifen. There was no difference in the overall death rate between treatments, for all causes or breast cancer–specific deaths.

Treatment with tamoxifen resulted in excess risk for endometrial cancer, deep vein thrombosis, pulmonary embolus (3 fatal), stroke (4 fatal), cataract formation, and the need for cataract surgery compared to placebo. Women diagnosed with endometrial cancer in some cases required radiation therapy in addition to surgery to treat the cancer. Fifteen percent of women on tamoxifen were asymptomatic at the time of diagnosis of endometrial cancer. Endometrial sampling did not increase the detection rate. For thromboembolic events, review of the data showed that women with an event remained at risk for a second event, and women with an event were also at risk for a complication of therapy. Hot flashes and vaginal discharge occurred more commonly and with greater severity in women on tamoxifen compared to women on placebo.

Women over age 60 with a 5-year breast cancer risk of less than 1.67% did not benefit from tamoxifen therapy and experienced significant adverse events. This population has been excluded from the "indications" section of the tamoxifen label.

INDICATION: RISK REDUCTION VERSUS PREVENTION

The original indication sought by the sponsor, AstraZeneca Pharmaceuticals, was for "prevention of breast cancer." This issue prompted lengthy discussion by the ODAC members and subsequently by the FDA. The term "prevention" has been sparingly used in previously approved labels. In considering when to use this indication, we believe the following points are relevant:

- Magnitude of the benefit: The product should cause a clinically meaningful and statistically significant reduction in the occurrence of the event of interest.
- Completeness of the benefit: The product should produce a benefit in a significant and clinically meaningful percentage of participants studied.
- Duration of the benefit: The product should convey long-term benefit.
- Number of participants treated: When a large number of participants has been treated in a variety of studies and settings, we feel more confident that the

magnitude, completeness, and duration of the benefit can be accurately estimated.

The data submitted in the supplemental NDA for tamoxifen do not meet the criteria for a "prevention" claim. Only 25% of participants completed 5 years of therapy. At the time the results were reported, the median follow-up on study was 4.2 years, a short period of time in which to evaluate a lifelong risk of breast cancer. Whether tamoxifen interferes with tumor initiation or instead treats microscopic, preexisting tumors has not been established. It is unknown whether tamoxifen will reduce breast cancer incidence after the drug is stopped. At present, there is no evidence that tamoxifen therapy causes an increase in tumors with poor prognostic features. However, long-term follow-up will be needed to evaluate this possibility. Finally, two European trials of tamoxifen compared to placebo for breast cancer risk reduction showed no benefit. While there are differences in the design and conduct of the European studies from those of P-1, the negative results warrant a cautious approach to labeling claims.

As a result of these discussions, the indication for tamoxifen is "... to reduce the incidence of breast cancer in women at high risk for breast cancer." It is important to communicate the limitations of the study results as well as the potential benefits and risks of the drug itself to physicians prescribing tamoxifen and to women considering tamoxifen for breast cancer risk reduction.

The "gold standard" for a prevention claim is a reduction in disease-specific mortality. For breast cancer, the large sample size and long follow-up required to demonstrate a difference in mortality preclude the ability to conduct such a trial.

MONITORING INFORMATION FOR WOMEN

Although there was a 44% reduction in invasive breast cancer with tamoxifen therapy, not all women benefited. Women considering therapy should understand that they may develop breast cancer despite drug treatment; that tamoxifen decreases the incidence of estrogen receptor–positive, but not estrogen receptor–negative breast cancer; and that breast cancer may not be diagnosed at an early stage. It is important that women continue routine monitoring for breast cancer, including regular breast examinations by a health care provider and yearly mammograms. A baseline gynecologic examination should be performed and should be repeated at regular intervals while on therapy. Women on tamoxifen or who have recently taken tamoxifen should seek prompt medical attention for new breast lumps, vaginal bleeding, gynecologic symptoms (menstrual irregularities, changes in vaginal discharge, pelvic pain/pressure), symptoms of leg swelling or tenderness, unexplained shortness of breath, or changes in vision. Women should inform all care providers, regardless of the reason for evaluation, that they take tamoxifen. Women with a history of deep vein thrombosis, pulmonary embolus, or coagulopathy should not take tamoxifen for this indication. Women with a family history of these problems should consider evaluation for a clotting disorder before taking tamoxifen. Coumarin-like anticoagulants may have a significant increase in anticoagulant effect when used with tamoxifen and are contraindicated in the setting of therapy for breast cancer risk reduction.

BENEFIT/RISK EVALUATION

Tamoxifen provides an important option for women at high risk of breast cancer. Because of its significant side effects, it should be used only in women at high risk. Risk should be formally calculated, not estimated using clinical judgment. Tools to calculate breast cancer risk using the Gail model are available through AstraZeneca; at the present time, these tools include a computer disk and a handheld calculator, for those providers who do not have access to a computer.

Women should have ample opportunity to learn about and discuss risks and benefits of therapy and make an informed decision. The NCI and AstraZeneca Pharmaceuticals provide educational materials. Providers should be prepared to discuss tamoxifen therapy in detail with women interested in therapy. It is likely that tamoxifen for breast cancer risk reduction will be prescribed predominantly by internists, family physicians, and gynecologists. It is particularly important to communicate information about tamoxifen to these providers, who have not commonly used the drug in their practices, as have medical oncologists.

SUMMARY

The approval of tamoxifen to reduce the incidence of breast cancer in women at high risk for breast cancer represents an important first step in clinical and regulatory medicine: tamoxifen is the first drug approved to reduce the incidence of cancer. Future steps may include more effective use of tamoxifen and development of new products that may offer additional benefits or reduced risks.

Negotiating Industry-Sponsored Clinical Trial Agreements

A View from the Trenches

NIKKI J. ZAPOL

Office of Corporate Sponsored Research and Licensing, Massachusetts General Hospital, Charlestown, Massachusetts 02129, USA

> ABSTRACT: A number of possible factors, including issues of cost, enrollment, and time, contribute to the decline in the percentage of industry-sponsored clinical trials conducted in academic institutions as opposed to those conducted at for-profit entities. This piece focuses on the agreement negotiation process. If negotiators were given easier access to the sponsor's decision makers, it is likely that the negotiations would proceed more efficiently. Also noted are reports by academic investigators of difficulty in getting access to unblinded trial data, which are needed for patient care and publication.
>
> KEYWORDS: industry-sponsored clinical trials

Industry sponsorship of clinical research at the Massachusetts General Hospital (MGH) represents a significant portion of the Hospital's total industry-sponsored research activity. In FY 2000, of MGH's $278 million sponsored research portfolio, $37 million was spent on industry-sponsored research, of which $12 million was in support of clinical trials. While the dollar expenditure on these trials has been increasing (from $7.7 million in FY 1996 to $12 million in FY 2000), the total number of agreements signed has declined in the past 2 years (from 176 in FY 1998 to 142 in FY 2000), a decline that is not surprising given the increasing percentage of industry-sponsored clinical trials conducted in nonacademic settings.[1]

In this short piece I will address aspects of the negotiation process that have made it difficult to execute clinical trial agreements in a timely manner and may well contribute to industry's lack of enthusiasm for using academic medical centers as sites for these trials. I will also mention concerns about these trials expressed by our own investigators. While there are a number of other factors that play a role in industry's increasing use of nonacademic centers for clinical trials, such as differentials in cost and patient enrollment between academic and nonacademic centers, these latter issues are not addressed here.

Present address: Nikki Zapol, J.D., Office of the General Counsel, Partners HealthCare System, Inc., 50 Staniford St., 10th Floor, Boston, MA 02114. Voice: 617-726-0783; fax: 617-726-1665.

nzapol@partners.org

Viewed from the trenches of a technology transfer office, there is good news and bad news about the negotiation of industry-sponsored clinical trial agreements. The good news is that we have been able to reach agreement and craft over a dozen master clinical trial agreements, mostly with major pharmaceutical companies, which enable us to enter into appropriate individual agreements rapidly. When the next proposed clinical trial for one of those companies comes to our office, so long as the investigator finds our master agreement acceptable and agrees to undertake the study, the study can commence as soon as we get budget approval and approval by the human studies committee.

The bad news is that the majority of our clinical trials do not fall under master agreements. For most companies, we do not have a master in place; further, even for those with which we do, there are a discouraging number of times when the company refuses to use that agreement. One of the most common circumstances in which we cannot use an already negotiated master agreement is when the study is run by a contract research organization (CRO), which acts as an agent for sponsors in setting up a trial and running it. CROs typically produce a document that is represented as the only agreement the sponsor has authorized the CRO to execute. Because the terms of those agreements are rarely acceptable as originally presented, further negotiations require additional time and energy from all parties. This is a pity because no one wins from the time wasted on needless negotiations—not the company, not the hospital, not the investigator, nor most importantly the patients.

What prevents negotiations from moving forward more quickly? There are the predictable stumbling blocks, such as human factors: a principal investigator who is out of town; a negotiator on either side who changes jobs; or financial issues such as a budget that needs to be worked out. However, most of the time, the problem comes down to the difference between two cultures—industry and academia—and the impact of that difference at the negotiating table. Industry performs clinical trials in order to get a drug to market as efficiently as possible. It seeks confidentiality and control over intellectual property. The academic medical center's participation in these trials must be consistent with its missions of research, education, and patient care. It seeks to publish and to use its findings to improve patient care.

All too often, a negotiator for a company or CRO receives instructions not to deviate from a form agreement and is given neither the background nor the authority to enable compromise. The negotiator from academia knows that there are a few key bottom-line academic protections that must be in the agreement if the institution is to sign it—the most important of which are a right for the academic center to use the data generated in the study for its mission of research, education, and patient care and a right to publish the study results. In addition, the academic institution's negotiator will seek parameters around intellectual property claims in order to prevent the agreement from casting a shadow over future research activities or research of other investigators. We estimate that 30% to 50% of all clinical trial agreements as initially written contain unacceptable data retention, publication, or intellectual property provisions, or a combination thereof. The negotiations will inevitably go on until these provisions are modified. If we cannot reach agreement on them, we will not sign the agreement and the study will not go forward. Do we lose studies because we will not give up these key rights? I am not aware of a single agreement negotiation in the last five years that ended without agreement because of academic freedom or intellectual property issues. Therefore, the end result is a good agreement that took an undue amount of time to reach—and, on some unfortunate occasions, so much time that the opportunity to enroll patients in the study had passed.

We believe that much of this delay would be obviated if the negotiators in industry were given easier access to decision makers in their companies. Our experience is that most senior people, be they in the business or legal office, or both, will understand the merit of our arguments regarding publication, data, and intellectual property and will be able to accept reasonable provisions that protect the academic center's interests in these areas. Even in phase III multicenter double-blind studies, they understand that academic investigators, if given access to their data, have the ability to produce valuable publications.

It is worth noting that many of our investigators are engaged in phase I and II trials and investigator-initiated trials. These studies generally come to us because of the reputation or expertise of a particular investigator or a department, and thus we may succeed in reaching agreement in a more timely manner than with phase III studies. This result does not occur because institutional negotiators have easier access to a company's decision makers, but because the company's own scientific and medical staff brings pressure to bear on those decision makers.

Turning to another area of concern, we have recently learned from our investigators about cases in which companies have failed to give the investigators access to the clinical trial data that they have generated in double-blind studies. The investigators point out that these data are important for the purpose of future treatment of patients as well as for publications that an investigator or a group of investigators might generate from the study. Experiences such as these may make investigators reluctant to engage in future industry-sponsored clinical trials in the absence of a clear contractual obligation by the company to give investigators access to their unblinded data. As with the other clauses discussed above, such provisions are likely to create further delays in the negotiation process. We can only hope that the delays will be lessened if negotiators from academia are given rapid access to decision makers at the sponsor who will address academic freedom and intellectual property concerns with an open mind.

REFERENCE

1. GETZ, A. 1999. CenterWatch Clinical Trials Listing Service. Boston. (www.centerwatch.com)

Conclusions

Considerations Regarding SERMs

BARBARA K. DUNN,[a] MARIETTA ANTHONY,[b] SHERRY SHERMAN,[c] AND JOSEPH P. COSTANTINO[d]

[a]*Division of Cancer Prevention, National Cancer Institute, National Institutes of Health, Bethesda, Maryland 20852, USA*

[b]*Department of Pharmacology, Georgetown University School of Medicine, Washington, District of Columbia 20007, USA*

[c]*National Institute of Aging, National Institutes of Health, Bethesda, Maryland 20892, USA*

[d]*Department of Biostatistics, Graduate School of Public Health, University of Pittsburgh, Pittsburgh, Pennsylvania 15213, USA*

> ABSTRACT: The "considerations" addressed in this section consist of a number of thought-provoking issues and unresolved questions that emerge from the papers in this volume. The evidence for tamoxifen carcinogenicity in animal models and, to a more restricted extent, in humans has led some investigators to question whether SERMs are ready or appropriate for clinical testing—specifically, in a disease prevention setting involving healthy but high-risk individuals. There is, however, inconsistency in both efficacy and toxicity—specifically, carcinogenicity—between animal models and humans, leading others to question the value of basing the decision to proceed with clinical studies on preclinical results in animals. Although the molecular basis for SERM action is rapidly being clarified, the cellular activity of these agents is still elusive. We discuss the view that the efficacy of tamoxifen in breast cancer is based on its treatment of "occult cancers," or small collections of cancer cells that are not clinically apparent, not only in the context of prevention but also in the treatment setting. As part of our approach that assumes estrogen activity to be the foundation upon which SERM development is being modeled, we discuss the inconsistency between the epidemiologic data and prospective randomized data with respect to the relationship between estrogen use and cardiovascular disease. The need to validate surrogate markers of SERM action is discussed in relation to bone but is clearly relevant to all disease sites. The semantics used in describing SERM action as agonistic or antagonistic in relation to estrogen at various target sites has been inconsistent, especially in the clinical context. We attempt to dissect out some of the inconsistencies in semantics in the hope that this will contribute to improved communication of data resulting from SERM research. In the clinical arena, we begin with the premise that the large, simple randomized trial offers the optimal design for the testing of SERMs. In view of limited resources, however, we counter this position with alternative, if less desirable, approaches to the clinical format for SERM testing. Finally, we

Address for correspondence: Barbara K. Dunn, Ph.D., M D., Division of Cancer Prevention, National Cancer Institute, EPN 2056, 1630 Executive Blvd., Bethesda, MD 20852. Voice: 301-402-1209; fax: 301-480-4110.

dunnb@mail.nih.gov

explore the process by which statistically meaningful results from clinical trials are extrapolated into the specific drug indications that apply to clinical practice.

KEYWORDS: clinical testing of SERMs; animal testing of SERMs; carcinogenesis of SERMs; tamoxifen; cellular basis of SERM action; cardiovascular system and SERMs; osteoporosis and SERMs; agonism/antagonism of SERM action

Our goals in this conclusion are to explore some of the key conceptual challenges, inconsistencies, and questions that have repeatedly been raised during our discussions about selective estrogen receptor modulator (SERM) research.

LINGERING CONCERNS AND QUESTIONS ABOUT SERM RESEARCH

Are SERMs Ready for Clinical Testing?

The view has been expressed by some basic researchers that SERMs are not yet ready for testing in the clinical arena. Clearly, this perspective is limited, since it fails to acknowledge the fact that tamoxifen has been used in clinical practice for over 20 years and that other SERMs are also approved for clinical use. Nevertheless, the concern embodied in this statement is well taken. The goal of the basic scientist is to elucidate thoroughly the mechanisms underlying drug action, in order to set the stage for the tailoring of clinical applications to these mechanisms. Insofar as the molecular basis of SERM action is proving to be far more complex than anticipated, this goal is still elusive. Furthermore, a paradox has emerged in the study of SERMs. More is known about the mechanism of action of these agents than of many other pharmaceutical drugs. Despite this wealth of knowledge, there have been many disappointments in predicting specific clinical outcomes in specific tissues based on established mechanisms. Although this apparent inconsistency between the basic and clinical science of SERMs has frustrated our expectations, it has also served as the motivating force behind the more current research into the molecular mechanisms of SERM action. This in turn has led to the blossoming field of coactivators and corepressors of transcription. What some may have regarded as premature testing in the clinical arena led to results that fed back to stimulate basic SERM research. Thus, we share the "Viewpoints" recently expressed by Dr. Richard Love in the *Oncology Times* that

> ... the goals of increasing cure rates, improving quality of life, decreasing costs, reducing side effects from therapies, and expanding biological knowledge are not mutually exclusive. Each is appropriate. We should pursue good ideas directed at any and all of these goals. It is how to pursue these goals that bedevils our endeavors. First, we should pursue good basic science and clinical research ideas simultaneously, without requiring complete and comprehensive biological data as a prerequisite. Good ideas may bear unexpected fruit.[1]

What is the Value of Animal Testing of SERMs?

One component of preclinical investigations of all drugs, not only SERMs, that is questioned by some investigators is the role of animal studies—specifically, the ability of animal studies to predict a response, either efficacy or toxicity, in humans. The response of animals to drugs often does not predict outcomes in humans. However, occasionally animal observations have pointed to forebodings of toxicities that were ultimately observed in humans. A case in point is that of the animal studies predicting teratogenicity with isotretinoin (Accutane®). Conversely, an example in which preclinical animal studies failed to predict specific toxicities later noted in humans is that of the SERM idoxifene.[2] Idoxifene was being developed in large part as a preventive agent for multiple diseases by measuring multiple end points (bone, lipid profile, coagulation markers, quality of life), the target population being healthy postmemopausal women. During clinical testing of idoxifene, endometrial thickening was observed in small phase 2 clinical trials, while additional adverse events, uterine prolapse and endometrial polyps, were revealed in larger phase 3 trials, leading ultimately to discontinuation of development of this agent. Preclinical studies involving rodents had not predicted any of these outcomes. Interestingly, subsequent to revelation of the human toxicities, idoxifene was noted to induce endometrial thickening in nonhuman primates. For animal work to be relevant to a specific end point in humans, it is critical to use the appropriate species. In this case, for an end point of the endometrium, nonhuman primates were better models than rodents.

The frequently observed inconsistencies between drug outcomes in animals and humans have prompted some clinical investigators to suggest that animal studies are not useful in drug development, despite the fact that animal research is required by the U.S. Food and Drug Administration (FDA). This viewpoint does not give enough credit to those cases in which there has been successful correlation between animal and human outcomes, particularly with regard to predicting human toxicities. Three compounds that went on to evaluation in clinical trials—idoxifene, droloxifene, and levormeloxifene—would have been rejected by a set of screening criteria that included preclinical *in vivo* models.[3] Furthermore, animal research may shed light on clinical activity by enabling us to better understand the mechanism of action of drugs.[4] Even though the outcomes in humans may not exactly mimic those in lower animals, drug development and patient care will benefit from this enhanced understanding of drug mechanism. Finally, a progressive hierarchy of research tools for drug development involves documentation of appropriate drug activity from molecular action through cellular response to animal outcomes and finally to clinical effects. As articulated by Drs. Komm and Lyttle in this volume, "A well-defined set of criteria have to be established to characterize compounds in order to assure (as well as possible) that the molecule is acceptable along every step of the preclinical development pathway."[3]

Are SERMs Carcinogenic?

Carcinogenicity represents one, and a particularly undesirable, toxicity that has been associated with SERM use. Specifically, tamoxifen causes cancer in both animals and humans. While these observations are not disputed, the details of its carcinogenicity have spawned different, often conflicting, views of whether (and under what circumstances) tamoxifen can safely be administered to humans.

In rats, tamoxifen induces liver cancer and, to a lesser degree, squamous cell cancers of the vagina/cervix.[5,6] The hepatocarcinogenicity of tamoxifen is limited to specific strains of rats and to doses that exceed those used for treatment and prevention of breast cancer.[7,8] In mice the data differ, with tamoxifen being associated with cancer of the testis, ovaries, and uterus, but not with liver cancer. Thus, in animals the target organ for carcinogenicity varies with the species and even with the strain in a given species. The presence of DNA adducts in the livers of rats treated with tamoxifen[9] has suggested that this agent may act as a direct genotoxic carcinogen, rather than acting via the estrogen receptor.

These observations in animals have raised concern about similar effects in humans.[10] On the one hand, in humans there has not been evidence for an increased incidence of liver cancer with tamoxifen use.[6,11] In agreement with this, tamoxifen does not appear to induce DNA adducts in the human liver.[5,12] Therefore, one cannot simply extrapolate from positive carcinogenic data in rats (moreover, in only certain strains) to humans in attempting to decide whether this drug is safe for clinical use. In summary, the best argument against the relevance of the animal data to humans is that there are decades of tamoxifen use in the adjuvant breast cancer setting that have failed to demonstrate a comparable hepatocarcinogenicity in humans.[7]

However, tamoxifen has been shown in treatment and prevention breast cancer studies to increase the incidence of endometrial cancer, yielding a relative risk of 2.3 to as high as 7 compared to nonusers.[6,11,13,14] Although certain observations point to the association of tamoxifen use with cancers that have a less favorable histology and more dire prognosis,[15,16] most studies suggest that the endometrial cancers resulting from tamoxifen are no more aggressive in terms of stage, grade, histology, or biology than those occurring in its absence.[13, 17–20]

Despite the negative data just cited, the undisputed evidence for its association with human endometrial cancer places the issue of the clinical applicability of tamoxifen in the realm of the risk/benefit question that has been discussed extensively in several papers in this volume.[21–23] Most investigators would concur that the increased risk of endometrial cancer is acceptable in the treatment setting (either metastatic or adjuvant) where the progression of breast cancer has been shown to be slowed or arrested by tamoxifen. In contrast, the preventive use of tamoxifen in healthy women to decrease breast cancer risk, although supported by the results of the National Surgical Adjuvant Breast and Bowel Project's (NSABP) Breast Cancer Prevention Trial (BCPT)[14] and approved by the FDA, is disputed by some, in part because of the increased risk of endometrial cancer. Furthermore, additional opposition arises from the position that the animal data on nonuterine cancer—specifically, liver cancer—should elicit concern that tamoxifen may in fact cause such cancers in humans, despite the fact that the studies to date do not show this. For specific categories of women who are at very high risk according to Gail model criteria, the risk of cancer, both documented (endometrial) and undocumented (liver, etc.), appears far outweighed by the benefit to be gained in terms of decreased risk for breast cancer.[24] However, two points must be emphasized. First, any decision to implement the use of tamoxifen in the prevention (also, the treatment) setting must be preceded by a discrete, interactive decision-making process involving the patient, the physician, and other relevant parties, as discussed earlier in this volume.[23,24] Second, investigators must continue to record adverse events associated with tamoxifen use, particularly as part of long-term follow-up, so that the unanswered questions that underlie the controversy over whether animal toxicity data apply to humans can be definitively answered.

What is the Cellular (in Contrast to the Molecular) Basis for SERM Action on Cancer Cells?

Despite the growing knowledge about the action of SERMs at the molecular level, in the case of cancer, uncertainty exists regarding the effects of these drugs at the cellular level. Two questions have been addressed in this volume relating to the action of tamoxifen at the cellular level.

First, in the breast cancer prevention setting, is tamoxifen treating existing occult clusters of cancer cells, or is it preventing the emergence of brand-new cancer cells? Furthermore, if tamoxifen is actually "treating" occult cancers in the preventive setting, is it not working in the same manner in the treatment setting? In this volume, Dr. Jerry Lewis elaborates a "Breast Cancer Continuum" showing a similar pattern of response to tamoxifen for all stages from the prevention setting (no clinically apparent cancer) through early-stage breast cancer.[25] At all stages, tamoxifen elicits a reduction in occurrence/recurrence of invasive breast cancer ranging from 42% to 49%. In addition, for all clinical stages the benefit of tamoxifen relative to placebo is seen during the first year of its use and continues to increase through five years of therapy. The comparable benefit to women with all these stages of breast cancer could be attributable to association of each stage with a certain probability of having early undiagnosed invasive breast cancer that is responsive to tamoxifen. In essence, this interpretation of the data supports the view that even in the prevention setting, where no disease is clinically apparent, occult breast cancer exists and responds to tamoxifen in a manner resembling the response of similarly occult disease that accompanies diagnosed disease.

A second question emerges from the assumption that in a clinically healthy breast tamoxifen is actually treating occult cancers. Is tamoxifen effective in reducing cancer risk because it is eradicating all the cancer cells, or is it just cytoreducing the number of cells or slowing the growth of these cells so that it takes longer for the initial cluster of malignant cells to grow to a size that is clinically detectable? If the latter is true, a longer follow-up would be required to confirm the reduction in breast cancer incidence that has been observed in the Breast Cancer Prevention Trial.

This notion that the "anticarcinogenic" action of tamoxifen in the prevention setting is due to either cytoreduction or growth inhibition of occult cancer cells leads one to predict that the time-to-diagnosis curve will be pushed to the right. In this volume Drs. Dickler and Norton point out the relevance of this model to diagnosed breast cancer in either the adjuvant or metastatic setting as well as to the prevention setting.[26]

What Effects Do SERMs Have on the Cardiovascular System?

Based on observational studies using biomarkers as end points, estrogen was thought to provide benefit to the cardiovascular system. Estrogen has been reported to raise serum high-density lipids and lower serum total cholesterol and low-density lipids. However, results of an attenuated response were reported when estrogen was combined with medroxyprogesterone acetate.[27] Observational studies in postmenopausal women without established coronary heart disease (CHD) have reported a reduction in CHD events among estrogen replacement therapy (ERT)/hormone replacement therapy (HRT) users versus nonusers.[28–31] In contrast to the epidemiologic data, the Heart and Estrogen Replacement Study (HERS)[32] and the Estrogen Replacement and Atherosclerosis (ERA)[33] trial reported an increase in the rate of coronary events in women who had existing coronary heart disease and were receiving ERT or HRT. Similarly, an increase in the rate of coronary events in women on ERT or HRT was reported from the Women's Health Initiative, whose participants were predominantly without existing coronary heart disease.[34]

Thus, the role of estrogen in the cardiovascular system needs to be clarified as to its molecular basis of action as well as in terms of clinical outcomes to be able to determine what effect SERMs will have on this system. So far, raloxifene appears to lower low-density lipoprotieins but not to change high-density liproprotiens, triglycerides, or plasminogen activitator inhibitor–1.[35] Raloxifene is being evaluated for cardiovascular end points in the Raloxifene Use for the Heart Trial (RUTH).[36] Results of the Breast Cancer Prevention Trial (BCPT) showed that tamoxifen had no beneficial or adverse cardiovascular effects; however, this was a secondary end point in this trial.[37]

What Is the Fidelity of Current Surrogate Markers for Osteoporotic Fractures?

An osteoporotic fracture is a stochastic event that is driven by a multiplicity of factors, including bone strength and the experience of trauma. Bone strength, which represents the amalgamation of bone density and bone quality, is one of the key determinants of the propensity to fracture. Bone quality encompasses bone geometry and the distribution of bone mineral, architecture and connectivity, remodeling status, and the accumulation of microdamage. For fractures of the hip and other sites in the appendicular skeleton, the increased propensity to fall (due to impairments in physical function, balance, muscle strength, reflexes, cognition, and vision) as well as the specifics of fall biomechanics become highly important. Consequently, it is not surprising that the risk of fracture cannot be fully explained by even the most promising of surrogate markers, either alone or in combination. However, a number of highly informative and reasonably well validated surrogate markers exist to estimate changes in fracture risk.

Bone mineral density (BMD) is commonly used as a surrogate in assessing the risk of fracture. BMD has been estimated to account for approximately 70% of bone strength and can be reliably assessed by bone densitometry technologies, such as dual-energy X-ray absorptiometry (DEXA). For this reason, BMD is accepted by the FDA for the approval of estrogen-like drugs in the prevention of osteoporosis. However, as discussed earlier in this volume,[38,39] the magnitude of the BMD response does not parallel the magnitude of the reduction in fracture risk with different classes of antiresorptive therapies (e.g., the bisphosphonates and SERMs such as raloxifene). New SERMs need to be compared with raloxifene with respect to their impact on the relationship between the magnitude of increases in BMD and the reductions of fracture risk.

Recent innovations, such as quantitative ultrasound (QUS), computerized tomography (CT), and magnetic resonance imaging (MRI) promise great sensitivity in assessing structural aspects of bone, in addition to quantifying bone density or mass. In population studies, fracture risk based on QUS compares favorably with that determined by DEXA. However, QUS needs to be validated in clinical trials to ensure that changes in fracture risk in response to treatment are accurately and reliably predicted by changes in QUS measurements. Further studies using CT and MRI are needed to test the potential of these technologies to elucidate the mechanisms of pathophysiological processes[40] and their reversal by pharmacologic agents at the level of the basic multicellular unit (BMU), the structure that carries out bone remodeling.

Biochemical markers of bone resorption and formation offer great potential to predict fractures in population studies. As discussed previously in this volume,[38,39] in untreated postmenopausal women, elevated levels of a number of biochemical indices of bone turnover are associated with an increased risk of fractures. And after antiresorptive therapy, reductions in the levels of these "bone markers" have been associated with significant treatment-induced reductions in vertebral and nonvertebral fracture risk. However, the relationship(s) between the levels of a given biochemical marker at baseline or the magnitude of marker change (after treatment) with the reduction in fracture risk may be dependent on the specific pharmacologic agent tested. Thus, acceptance of biochemical markers of bone turnover as surrogates for fractures in clinical trials awaits the identification of markers that are considerably more sensitive and specific in predicting the magnitude of the risk reduction for fracture in response to various SERMs and other agents.

Keeping Our Terminology Consistent in Describing SERM Action

SERM action has generally been defined in terms of being "agonistic" or "antagonistic" when compared to estrogen. Issues of semantics revolving around the use of these terms are important to recognize. The actions of SERMs are complex and can vary depending on the organ system and disease in question (see Action of SERMs in Target Tissues, p. 383). In a nondisease setting, an agent may have a net neutral effect, allowing the natural history of the tissue to evolve; it may induce disease (adverse effect such as endometrial cancer); or it may prevent a disease (breast cancer, osteoporosis). In a disease setting, the SERM may treat—that is, reduce the burden of—the disease (breast cancer, osteoporosis). Thus, when ascribing an action to a SERM, it is important to clarify the nature of the effect in terms of both the organ system and the disease setting to which the action is being attributed.

In practice, the semantics of expressing agonistic or antagonistic SERM action has varied. For example, Dr. Dhingra[41] states that "... SERMs which are devoid of estrogen-agonist effects on the uterus or breast cancer cells but retain potentially beneficial effects on bones and lipids, have been described as 'ideal' SERMs." In actuality the "ideal" SERMs might more precisely be viewed as having an antagonistic effect on the breast, since SERMs have been used to obliterate or prevent (i.e., antagonize) likely breast cancers, rather than merely not to cause (i.e., agonize) breast cancers. The distinction between *antagonism* and the *absence of agonism* has also been alluded to in this volume by Drs. Komm and Lyttle in describing the goals set out for the development of the SERM WAY-140424.[3] The maintenance of semantic consistency is important if there is to be a universal understanding among researchers of what the goals are during the quest for a better SERM.

Even with such clarification of these activities at the clinical level, we still do not know how these definitions relate to activity at the molecular level. The notion of whether an agent acts in an *actively* antagonistic fashion or merely is not agonistic in relation to a given end point is complex and not yet understood for the SERMs at the molecular level. A tendency exists to classify SERMs as agonistic or antagonistic, with the absence of agonism being subsumed in the antagonism class.[42,43] This approach emphasizes that a given ligand antagonizes the effect that estrogen would have had (i.e., an estrogenic, or agonistic, effect) in a specific tissue. The distinction between antagonism and absence of agonism will reside in part in an understanding of whether coactivators or corepressors predominate in a given tissue and disease setting and exactly how the corepressors modulate transcription. In order to avert misunderstandings, it is also important that the relationship between the molecular basis for agonistic/antagonistic/neutral action and the clinical manifestation be clarified.

ISSUES IN CLINICAL TRIALS OF SERMs

The Statistician's Dream Trial: Optimizing Clinical Trial Design

Optimization of clinical trial design was discussed by Dr. Richard Peto at the NIH Workshop on Selective Estrogen Receptor Modulators (SERMs);[44] he emphasized the value of the *large, simple, randomized* trial. Because the effects of an intervention on key clinical end points such as mortality and disease incidence are generally not very big, a very *large*–scale randomized trial is needed to get the right answer. This argument applies both to treatment as well as prevention interventions. Dr. Peto also stressed the importance of looking at all the randomized evidence from a large trial, rather than focusing on subgroups, an approach that can generate false negative and false positive results. Similarly, small trials yield irreproducible results, since the play of chance with small numbers can produce effects that are bigger than the quantity one is trying to measure. Even metanalyses bringing together all randomized trials addressing the same clinical question can yield wrong answers by overemphasis on selected bits of evidence. The key point here is that rare clinical outcomes, which are generally the outcomes of greatest importance from a public health perspective, can be evaluated statistically only by randomizing very large numbers, often in the tens of thousands, of trial participants.

As a complement to large size, *simplicity* of clinical trials was noted to be essential in order to ensure that accrual is adequate to get the answers to the questions that are posed. Yet, the recent trend has been toward trials with multiple end points. The complexity of such trials often makes it difficult to accrue adequate numbers of participants. Furthermore, the added end points are often molecular or genetic in nature, requiring specimen collection and therefore implying additional obstacles to accrual. Trials are also made more complicated by having an overabundance of rules, such as elaborate eligibility requirements, which also impede participant recruitment. Dr. Peto argued for "defining eligibility by the uncertainty principle," whereby less precise eligibility criteria would be compensated for by randomization. This approach should maximize the size of the trial as well as yield a heterogeneous mixture of randomized participants. Additional logistical difficulties have resulted from extensive regulatory requirements, again impeding the large-scale accrual that would yield optimal clinical results. In recent years regulatory requirements have come to play a major role in trials that involve genetic cohorts and tissue acquisition for molecular genetic end points.

Finally, Dr. Peto emphasized that trials must be *randomized*, since wrong answers often emerge from nonrandomized evidence. A good illustration is the difference in conclusions from randomized and nonrandomized studies with hormone replacement therapy and its effect on the cardiovascular system. Consistent with this perspective, randomized trials have been recommended to address specific unanswered questions relating to adjuvant therapy for breast cancer, including the risks and benefits of continuing tamoxifen therapy beyond five years; the risks and benefits of new agents, such as SERMs and aromatase inhibitors, in the adjuvant setting; and the relative risks and benefits of hormonal therapy versus chemotherapy or combinations of the two.[45]

Alternatives to the Large Simple Trial: How to Deal with Limited Resources

Available resources are too limited to carry out full-fledged prevention trials with clinical end points for every SERM individually and then in combination with other agents (aromatase inhibitors). Such trials target infrequent clinical end points, requiring huge numbers of participants, implying long recruitment times and long periods of follow-up. These obstacles may discourage pharmaceutical companies from investing in the development of these agents.[2,46] In addition, government agencies, such as the National Institutes of Health, have only limited resources, which are able to support only a finite number of such trials.

What are the alternatives? As discussed by Drs. Dickler and Norton in this volume, new trial designs will be necessary if rapid progress in drug development is to be made.[26] This need is especially relevant to the area of SERMs, since many agents in this class are currently in preclinical development. If it is required that each new agent be tested against a standard drug in trials targeting clinical end points, as is currently being done in the STAR (Study of Tamoxifen and Raloxifene) trial, enormous numbers of participants and years would be necessary to make substantial progress. The following approaches are being explored to accommodate the limitations of monetary and human resources that prevent our undertaking the large trial format for every new agent in development.

One approach to the problem of finite resources is to improve the efficiency of large trials by designing trials with multiple disease end points. An example of such an effort is seen in the attempt to model development of the SERM idoxifene by means of multi-end point studies.[2] This undertaking did not work because of the number of women experiencing the target disease entities and the complexity that multiple end points introduced into the study. This negative experience with multi-end point trial design bears out the views expressed by Dr. Peto in his support of the "simple" trial. If clinical trials with multiple end points fail to yield meaningful data, another potential answer to the resource dilemma would be multiple smaller trials with single, or at least a limited number of, clinical end points.

At the forefront of alternative trial designs are those that utilize end points that serve as surrogates for clinical outcomes—specifically, end points based on biochemical, or molecular, modulation at the tissue level.[26] In theory the use of such surrogate end point biomarkers would obviate the need to wait for long time periods until rare clinical end points emerge. Unfortunately, few or no proposed biomarkers have been validated as appropriate surrogates for their respective clinical end points. One major function of the Early Detection Research Network (http://edrn.nci.nih.gov/), funded by the National Cancer Institute's Division of Cancer Prevention, is to provide such validation of surrogate biomarkers for clinical cancer end points. This will require the observation of modulation of the proposed surrogates in parallel with clinical outcome data, in the context of long, large randomized trials. But, once validated, biomarkers could serve as surrogates for the clinical end points, avoiding the need for repeated large trials for every agent.

A natural corollary of biomarker validation would be the acceptance of a "group effect" as evidence for the activity of a given agent.[46] Thus, if one member of a drug class displays a clinically acceptable efficacy/toxicity profile in the ideal large, simple trial, preclinical data combined with data from smaller, biomarker-based trials might suffice to permit approval of additional agents in this class. An analogous application of a group effect would be the extrapolation from data supporting the intervention with a given agent for one stage of a disease to its use in another stage. The "Breast Cancer Continuum" elaborated by Dr. Jerry Lewis [25] is based on the premise that "each clinical state [stage] is associated with a certain probability of having early undiagnosed invasive breast cancer responsive to tamoxifen." This model implies that identical targets exist in all stages of breast cancer. Therefore, in comparing a new drug to tamoxifen, only a few studies demonstrating equivalent or superior efficacy over tamoxifen need to be done in any of the Breast Cancer Continuum segments for the experimental drug to merit approval. Overall, however, this approach would have to be validated, as it is known that drugs in the same class, such as benzodiazapenes, can have different effects.

THE JOURNEY FROM THE DATA TO THE INDICATION

The extrapolation of drug indications from published clinical trial results to clinical practice is a complex process. Once the evidence is deemed sufficient to warrant the conclusion that a drug should be approved, decisions must be made to define the approval in terms of the specific indications for the drug use and the exact cohort in which the drug should be administered as a therapy for the indication. The drug approval process focuses primarily on the scientific data that is presented. In terms of the weight of the scientific evidence, the optimal information base for drug approval is that derived from a prospective, randomized clinical trial addressing predefined clinical end points. In this respect, the optimal trial described above[44] is also the type of trial that yields data ideally suited to justify a clinical indication. However, due to the nature of trial design and restrictions of resource availability, even the "optimal" trial will be limited in that it cannot provide an all-encompassing database sufficient to answer all possible treatment effect questions. For example, although a clinical trial database will be sufficient to provide statistically significant evidence to support the use of an approved agent in a population similar to the trial cohort as a whole, it is likely that the database will be insufficient to provide statistically significant evidence for particular subgroups of the cohort. As such, if there is concern regarding an acceptable therapeutic benefit/risk ratio among a specific subgroup of the trial cohort, limitations circumscribing the cohort to which FDA-approved indications apply may be based on the absence of a statistically verifiable effect in the subgroup.

The BCPT is a good example of how a randomized clinical trial can be used as the basis for drug approval. The results provided a strong weight of scientific evidence that tamoxifen has a "prevention" effect; and in general the approved indication of tamoxifen for "prevention" (formally, "risk reduction") applies to the cohort of women who are at increased risk for breast cancer by virtue of possessing attributes that would have made them eligible for entry into the BCPT. The trial is also a good example of how the absence of statistical evidence for a particular subgroup of individuals may come into play to circumscribe the cohort approved for drug administration. In the BCPT, all participants were required to be at least 60 years of age or, if less than 60 years of age, to have a five-year risk of developing breast cancer that was at least 1.67%. The level of 1.67% was chosen because it represented the *average* risk among 60-year-old women at that time.[24] As a result of these dual eligibility criteria, a small subgroup of women ≥60 years old but with a five-year risk of breast cancer <1.67% were eligible to participate in the trial. Despite belonging to the eligible cohort for the BCPT, women who fall into this category of eligibility are excluded from the FDA indication for tamoxifen. This omission is understandable because: (1) women with a five-year breast cancer risk <1.67% are a group of individuals (all ≥60 years old) for whom the potential side effects of tamoxifen (thromboembolic events and endometrial cancer) may outweigh the potential breast cancer risk reduction benefits; and (2) when analyzed as a separate entity, the sample size of participants who fall into this subgroup is too small to draw any statistically definitive conclusions regarding the presence or absence of any tamoxifen effect.

In summary, the extrapolation of drug indications from published clinical trial results to clinical practice involves a series of evaluations and decisions based on several factors. Data from randomized clinical trials are essential sources of information upon which to base the decision making and the definition of the cohort in which the drug is approved for use. In some instances, a drug indication may be restricted from use in a subgroup of the cohort who would be eligible for the trial. This may be due to the presence of statistically significant evidence demonstrating a contraindication in a subgroup, or it may be due to the absence of statistically significant evidence supporting a treatment effect in a subgroup of interest. Such distinctions are important to note when involved in physician-patient discussions leading to clinical decisions to use the drug.

ACKNOWLEDGMENT

The authors are grateful to Dr. Ronald Lubet, with whom we had many stimulating and informative discussions relating to portions of this manuscript.

REFERENCES

1. LOVE, R.R. 2001. Viewpoints: controlling breast cancer: the goals are clear—it's how to get there that's in dispute. Oncol. Times **23:** 2–4.
2. MACDONALD, B. 2000. Clinical assessment of the risk-to-benefit profile of idoxifene. Presentation at the NIH Workshop on Selective Estrogen Receptor Modulators (SERMs). April 26–28, 2000.

3. KOMM, B.S. & C.R. LYTTLE. 2001. Developing a SERM: stringent preclinical selection criteria leading to an acceptable candidate (WAY-140424) for clinical evaluation. Ann. N.Y. Acad. Sci. **949:** this volume.
4. WEINSHILBOUM, R. 1999. Presentation at the NIH Workshop on Molecular and Biological Mechanisms of Sex Differences in Pharmacokinetics, Pharmacodynamics and Pharmacogenetics. May 5–6, 1999.
5. INTERNATIONAL AGENCY FOR RESEARCH ON CANCER (IARC). WORLD HEALTH ORGANIZATION. 1996. Tamoxifen. *In* IARC Monographs on the Evaluation of Carcinogenic Risks to Humans, Vol. 66. Some Pharmaceutical Drugs: 253–365. IARC. Lyon, France.
6. PHILLIPS, D.H. 2001. Understanding the genotoxicity of tamoxifen? Carcinogenesis **22:** 839–849.
7. GUZELIAN, P.S. 1997. Relevance of rat liver tumors to human hepatic and endometrial cancer. Semin. Oncol. **24** (Suppl. 1): S1-105–S1-121.
8. STANLEY, L.A., P. CARTHEW, R. DAVIES, *et al.* 2001. Delayed effects of tamoxifen in hepatocarcinogenesis-resistant Fischer 344 rats as compared with susceptible strains. Cancer Lett. **171:** 27–35.
9. HARD, G.C., M.J. IATROPOULOS, K. JORDAN, *et al.* 1993. Major difference in the hepatocarcinogenicity and DNA adduct forming ability between toremifene and tamoxifen in female Crl:CD(BR) rats. Cancer Res. **53:** 4534–4541.
10. WHITE, I.N. 1999. The tamoxifen dilemma. Carcinogenesis **20:** 1153–1160.
11. RUTQVIST, L.E., H. JOHANSSON & T. SIGNOMKLAO. 1995. Adjuvant tamoxifen therapy for early stage breast cancer and second primary malignancies. J. Natl. Cancer Inst. **87:** 645–651.
12. PHILLIPS, D.H., P.L. CARMICHAEL, A. HEWER, *et al.* 1996. Activation of tamoxifen and its metabolite alpha-hydroxytamoxifen to DNA-binding products: comparisons between human, rat and mouse hepatocytes. Carcinogenesis **17:** 89–94.
13. FISHER, B., J.P. COSTANTINO, C.K. REDMOND, *et al.* 1994. Endometrial cancer in tamoxifen-treated breast cancer patients: findings from the National Surgical Adjuvant Breast and Bowel Project (NSABP) B-14. J. Natl. Cancer Inst. **86:** 527–537.
14. FISHER, B., J.P. COSTANTINO, D.L. WICKERHAM, *et al.* 1998. Tamoxifen for prevention of breast cancer: Report of the National Surgical Adjuvant Breast and Bowel Project P-1 Study. J. Natl. Cancer Inst. **90:** 1371–1378.
15. MARGRIPLES, U., F. NAFTOLIN, P.E. SCHWARTZ & M.L. CARCANGIU. 1993. High-grade endometrial carcinoma in tamoxifen-treated breast cancer patients. J. Clin. Oncol. **11:** 485–490.
16. BERGMAN, L., M.L. BEELEN, M.P. GALLEE, *et al.* 2000. Risk and prognosis of endometrial cancer after tamoxifen for breast cancer. Comprehensive Cancer Centres' ALERT Group. Assessment of liver and endometrial cancer risk following tamoxifen. Lancet: **356:** 881–887.
17. FORNANDER, T., A.-C. HELLSTRÖM & B. MOBERGER. 1993. Descriptive clinicopathologic study of 17 patients with endometrial cancer during or after adjuvant tamoxifen in early breast cancer. J. Natl. Cancer Inst. **85:** 1850–1855.
18. BARAKAT, R.R., G. WONG, J.P. CURTIN, *et al.* 1994. Tamoxifen use in breast cancer patients who subsequently develop corpus cancer is not associated with a higher incidence of adverse histologic features. Gynecol. Oncol. **55:** 1614–168.
19. JORDAN, V.C. & V.J. ASSIKIS. 1995. Endometrial carcinoma and tamoxifen: clearing up a controversy. Clin. Cancer Res. **1:** 467–472.
20. AMERICAN COLLEGE OF OBSTETRICIANS AND GYNECOLOGISTS (ACOG). 1996. ACOG committee opinion. Tamoxifen and endometrial cancer. Int. J. Gynecol. Obstet. **53:** 197–199.
21. COSTANTINO, J. 2001. Benefit/risk assessment of SERM therapy: clinical trial versus clinical practice settings. Ann. N.Y. Acad. Sci. **949:** this volume.
22. GAIL, M.H. 2001. The estimation and use of absolute risk for weighing the risks and benefits of selective estrogen receptor modulators for preventing breast cancer. Ann. N.Y. Acad. Sci. **949:** this volume.
23. JOHNSON, S.R., B.K. DUNN & M. ANTHONY. 2001. Defining benefits and risks for SERMs in clinical trials and clinical practice. Ann. N.Y. Acad. Sci. **949:** this volume.

24. GAIL, M.H., J.P COSTANTINO, J. BRYANT, et al. 1999. Weighing the risks and benefits of tamoxifen treatment for preventing breast cancer. J. Natl. Cancer Inst. **91:** 1829–1846.
25. LEWIS, J.P. 2001. The Breast Cancer Continuum: insights from the tamoxifen trials impact future drug development strategies. Ann. N.Y Acad. Sci. **949:** this volume.
26. DICKLER, M.N. & L. NORTON. 2001. The MORE trial: Multiple Outcomes of Raloxifene Evaluation. Breast cancer as a secondary end point: implications for prevention. Ann. N.Y Acad. Sci. **949:** this volume.
27. THE WRITING GROUP FOR THE PEPI TRIAL. 1995. Effects of estrogen or estrogen/progestin regimens on heart disease risk factors in postmenopausal women: The Postmenopausal Estrogen/Progestin Interventions (PEPI) Trial. JAMA **273:** 199–208.
28. STAMPFER, M.J. & G.A. COLDITZ.. 1991. Estrogen replacement therapy and coronary heart disease: a quantitative assessment of the epidemiologic evidence. Prev. Med. **20:** 47–63.
29. GRADY, D., S.M. RUBIN, D.B. PETITTI, et al. 1992. Hormone therapy to prevent disease and prolong life in post-menopausal women. Ann. Intern. Med. **117:** 1016–1037.
30. PSATY, B.M., S.R. HECKBERT, D. ATKINS, et al. 1994. The risk of myocardial infarction associated with the combined use of estrogens and progestins in postmenopausal women. Arch. Intern. Med. **154:** 1333–1339.
31. SIDNEY, S., D.B. PETITTI & C.P. QUESENBERRY, JR. 1997. Myocardial infarction and the use of estrogen and estrogen-progestogen in postmenopausal women. Ann. Intern. Med. **127:** 501–508.
32. HULLEY, S., D. GRADY, T. BUSH, et al. 1998. Randomized trial of estrogen plus progestin for secondary prevention of coronary heart disease in postmenopausal women. JAMA **280:** 605–613.
33. HERRINGTON, D.M., D.M. REBOUSSIN, K.B. BROSNIHAN, et al. 2000. Effects of estrogen replacement on the progression of coronary-artery atherosclerosis. N. Engl. J. Med. **343:** 522–529.
34. NATIONAL INSTITUTES OF HEALTH. NATIONAL HEART LUNG AND BLOOD INSTITUTE. 2000. http://www.NHLBI.NIH.GOV/WHI/HRT-EN.HTM.
35. WALSH, B.W., L.H. KULLER, R.A. WILD, et al. 1998. Effects of raloxifene on serum lipids and coagulation factors in healthy postmenopausal women. JAMA **279:** 1445–1451.
36. MOSCA, L.E., E. BARRETT-CONNOR, N. WENGER, et al. 2001. Design and methods of the Raloxifene Use for The Heart (RUTH) Study. Am. J. Cardiol. In press.
37. REIS, S.E., J.P. COSTANTINO, D.L. WICKERHAM, et al. FOR THE NATIONAL SURGICAL ADJUVANT BREAST AND BOWEL PROJECT BREAST CANCER PREVENTION TRIAL INVESTIGATORS. 2001. Cardiovascular effects of tamoxifen in women with and without heart disease: Breast Cancer Prevention Trial. J. Natl. Cancer Inst. **93:** 16–21.
38. SHERMAN, S. 2001. Preventing and treating osteoporosis: strategies at the millennium. Ann. N.Y Acad. Sci. **949:** this volume.
39. CUMMINGS, S.R. 2001. The paradox of small changes in bone density and reductions in risk of fracture with raloxifene. Ann. N.Y Acad. Sci. **949:** this volume.
40. CUMMINGS, S.R., S. SHERMAN & J. MCGOWAN. 2000. Biomarkers of osteoporosis. In Biomarkers of Osteoporosis: 275–289. Elsevier Science. Amsterdam.
41. DHINGRA, K. 2001. Selective estrogen receptor modulation: the search for an ideal hormonal therapy for breast cancer. Cancer Invest. **19:** 649–659.
42. KATZENELLENBOGEN, B.S., J. SUN, W.R. HARRINGTON, et al. 2001. Structure-function relationships in estrogen receptors and the characterization of novel selective estrogen receptor modulators with unique pharmacological profiles. Ann. N.Y Acad. Sci. **949:** this volume.
43. MCKENNA, N.J. & B.W. O'MALLEY. 2001. Nuclear receptors, co-regulators, ligands and selective receptor modulators: making sense of the patchwork quilt. Ann. N.Y Acad. Sci. **949:** this volume.
44. PETO, R. 2000. Synthesis of key issues in clinical trial design. Presented at the NIH Workshop on Selective Estrogen Receptor Modulators (SERMs), April 26–28, 2000, Bethesda, MD.

45. NATIONAL INSTITUTES OF HEALTH. 2000. National Institutes of Health Consensus Development Conference Statement. Adjuvant therapy for breast cancer. November 1–3, 2000. http://odp.od.nih.gov/consensus/cons/114/114_statement.htm
46. KOMM, B. 2000. Developing a SERM: stringent preclinical selection criteria leading to appropriate clinical trials. Presented at the NIH Workshop on Selective Estrogen Receptor Modulators (SERMs), April 26–28, 2000, Bethesda, MD.

Opportunities for Future Research

SHERRY SHERMAN[a] AND BARBARA K. DUNN[b]

[a]*National Institute on Aging, National Institutes of Health, Bethesda, Maryland 20892, USA*

[b]*Divison of Cancer Prevention, National Cancer Institute, National Institutes of Health, Bethesda, Maryland 20852, USA*

ABSTRACT: Remarkable progress has been made in SERM development. Profiles of new SERMs indicate great potential for efficacy in the prevention and treatment settings, in more than one physiological system, and with improved risk/benefit ratios. The concept of what is achievable with respect to broad-spectrum disease prevention and what constitutes an "ideal" SERM is likely to undergo considerable reevaluation over time. The development of new, more broadly efficacious SERMs will require continued exploration of the effects of estrogen at the cellular and molecular level in tissues and physiologic systems throughout the body. A better understanding is needed of the mechanisms of the biological actions that are mediated through major forms of the estrogen receptor. High priority must be placed on elucidation of the role of the coregulators of estrogen receptor (ER) action. The quest for a SERM(s) with the "optimal clinical profile" also constitutes a major research challenge with respect to designing clinical trials that are simultaneously parsimonious with respect to time, monetary, and human resources and yet capable of delivering unequivocal outcomes with respect to primary end points. A vigorous research effort is needed to identify highly sensitive and specific surrogate measures to facilitate future clinical studies. Research to identify and validate relevant measures of safety is also essential to inform the risk/benefit balance and, thus, the ultimate usefulness of SERMs and their potential for long-term use. Future advances in the modulation of ER action are likely to have profound effects—not only on diseases and conditions known (or later discovered) to be related to estrogen action, but on the development of paradigms for understanding and modifying the action of other nuclear hormone receptors in the prevention and treatment of additional age- and disease-related pathologies.

KEYWORDS: selective estrogen receptors; bone; osteoporosis; risk factors; menopause; randomized controlled trials (RCTs)

The closing decade of the 20th century witnessed an extraordinary burgeoning in the magnitude and sophistication of research efforts and research advances on the effects of estrogen at the cellular and molecular level, in animal models of menopause and

Address for correspondence: Sherry Sherman, Ph.D., Director, Clinical Endocrinology and Osteoporosis Research, National Institute on Aging, NIH, Gateway Building, Suite 3E327, 7201 Wisconsin Ave., Bethesda, MD 20892-9205. Courier/express mail ZIP 20814. Voice: 301-435-3048; fax: 301-402-1784.

shermans@nia.nih.gov

in epidemiological and clinical studies of postmenopausal women. Well-established effects of estrogen (ERT) or estrogen/progestin (HRT in women with a uterus) include symptomatic relief of menopause-related hot flashes, night sweats, and dry vagina and the prevention and amelioration of bone loss. However, the stimulus to the expansion of research on estrogen has arisen primarily from the growing belief that estrogen could be "the magic bullet," the "antiaging" panacea that could even "turn back the clock." Widespread belief in this global hypothesis was nurtured by the abundance of positive findings emerging from observational studies comparing estrogen users to nonusers vis-à-vis incidence or prevalence rates of a variety of diseases. These findings were interpreted as indicative of the beneficial "effects" of estrogen on risk reduction for a large variety of common conditions, disorders, and chronic diseases of aging (e.g., osteoporotic fractures, cardiovascular disease, heart attacks, stroke, colon cancer, urinary incontinence, depression, dementia, and Alzheimer's disease) and even mortality. However, as discussed earlier, despite the potentially profound benefits indicated in epidemiologic studies, recent randomized controlled trials (RCTs) have found an absence of benefit in reducing the risk of myocardial infarctions and stroke and in preventing or reversing Alzheimer's disease. Importantly, ERT/HRT use has been associated with serious adverse events in the cardiovascular/hemostasis systems in both primary and secondary cardiovascular disease prevention studies. Nevertheless, hopes for the realization of an agent that, if not a "magic bullet," could at least produce benefits in more than one physiologic system have been fueled by observations of specific SERM effects. Thus raloxifene, although developed to protect bone, can promote positive risk factor profiles in the skeletal and cardiovascular systems and potentially benefit the breast without detrimental effects in the uterus. Further SERM development and refinement could lead to innovations that provide greater benefits in multiple systems or at least maximize risk/benefit profiles for those SERMs that are associated with marked efficacy and effectiveness in fewer physiologic systems.

One important goal of the April 2000 NIH Workshop on the SERMs was the identification of opportunities for future basic, translational, and clinical research that is aimed at promoting disease prevention and healthy aging through strategies related to the modulation of estrogen receptor action. The recommendations provided below were gleaned from transcripts of the individual workshop sessions and from the papers in this volume.

BASIC RESEARCH

The development of new, more broadly efficacious SERMs will require continued exploration of the effects of estrogen at the cellular and molecular level in tissues and physiologic systems throughout the body. A better understanding is needed of the mechanisms of the biological actions that are mediated through major forms of the estrogen receptor (ER)—that is, ERα and ERβ, the recently identified putative estrogen receptor gamma (ERγ), and new ER subtypes yet to be discovered. High priority must be placed on elucidation of the role of the coregulators of ER action. This should include studies of the qualitative and quantitative responses (structure, distribution, specificity, and function) of ER coactivators and corepressors in the presence of estrogen and other SERMs in a variety of target tissues. This knowledge in conjunction with the development of appropriate biological models and peptidomimetic agents will be critical to gaining new insights into pathological processes and to defining and maximizing the desired biological actions in the design of improved pharmaceutical agents.

Importantly, the exploration of such new possibilities involving the ER can be extended to research into disease prevention and treatment through the modulation of the action of receptors for steroid hormones other than estrogen. Lessons learned from intensified basic, translational, and clinical research on the ER can inform the development of optimal research paradigms for the selective modulation of other nuclear hormone receptors. Thus, the development and testing of new ligands that agonize/antagonize classical effects of hormones such as the progestins, androgens, aldosterone, and glucocorticoids, could capitalize on the advantageous aspects of these hormones while minimizing their associated deleterious effects. With respect to the glucocorticoid receptor, for example, success in realizing future goals, such as the separation of the antiinflammatory effects of glucocorticoids from those resulting in tissue destruction, could have vast potential in the prevention of many of the chronic diseases of the elderly and in the promotion of healthy aging.

CANCER

Strategies for Clinical Trial Design

The abundance of SERMs currently in preclinical development offers great opportunities for clinical testing for efficacy in breast cancer prevention and treatment. Yet, a dilemma remains as to the best strategy to use in designing clinical trials of these agents. The optimal approach would be to test each new agent in a *large, simple randomized* trial focused on the important, rare *clinical end points* of *mortality* and *disease incidence*, as discussed in detail earlier in this volume.[1] Such an undertaking is simply not feasible for every new agent, however, because resources (monetary and human) and time are limited. Therefore, compromise approaches will have to be employed. One such approach would be to carry out a single, or a limited number of, large randomized clinical trials testing one SERM in each chemical *class* of agents. Other agents belonging to this class ("same-class" SERMs) would then be tested by alternative trial designs. For example, these same-class SERMs could be evaluated in smaller trials that focus primarily on measuring the modulation of potential biomarkers. Success in a biomarker trial implies that a candidate SERM causes a change in expression of a candidate marker (molecular, biochemical, histologic) in a direction that is expected to correlate with a desirable clinical outcome. In this manner, small trials could serve as stepping stones for the selection of promising same-class SERMs and biomarkers for testing in subsequent higher level trials. The definitive evaluation of SERM efficacy together with the validation of promising biomarkers would occur in the next step, which consists of studies of biomarker modulation and important clinical end points in parallel in a large randomized trial. If and when such validation is successful, the *surrogate end point biomarkers* would then have potential to be used in trials testing newer same-class SERMs.

What is needed, therefore, is a multipronged approach to the clinical testing of SERMs for cancer outcomes:

(1) A limited number of large randomized clinical trials should be designed to test selected, highly promising SERMs from different chemical classes for efficacy with respect to key clinical outcomes. This will establish the SERM in each class that, in light of having an acceptable risk/benefit ratio, can now serve as the prototype SERM for that class.

(2) Additional SERMs (same-class SERMs) in the same chemical classes represented in the large trials of (1) should then be tested in smaller clinical trials targeting the modulation of highly selected biomarkers as the primary end point. Biomarkers are chosen as "highly selective" because they have shown promise as being predictive of important clinical outcomes in prior, more preliminary studies.

(3) Highly selected biomarkers that appear extremely promising as surrogates for clinical end points in trials described in (2) will next be tested in parallel with clinical end points in large randomized clinical trials. Only those same-class SERMs that are most promising in the small trials in (2) will go on for testing in (3). These trials will serve to validate the ability of the selected biomarkers to act as surrogates for the clinical end points that are being measured in parallel. These trials will also allow statistically powered comparisons of the efficacy of candidate same-class SERMs versus established prototype SERMs with regard to these important clinical end points.

(4) For the large randomized trials described in (1), the inclusion of secondary clinical end points (i.e., clinical end points pertaining to other diseases) should be considered. The importance of testing drug efficacy in other diseases (osteoporosis, cardiovascular disease, etc.) is most relevant to cancer prevention, in contrast to cancer treatment trials, which generally emphasize only cancer-related clinical end points.

Agents with Improved SERM Profiles: Aim for the "Ideal SERM"

The "ideal SERM" has yet to be developed (see Action of SERMs in Target Tissues, p. 383).[2] The quest for a SERM with the *optimal clinical profile* should constitute a central part of the clinical testing of SERMs by cancer researchers. The emphasis should be on the testing of new SERMs for clinical efficacy with regard to breast cancer and for absence of toxicity relative to endometrial cancer and thromboembolic disease. Concomitant efficacy in the realm of bone and cardiovascular disease would be desirable. However, the inability thus far to demonstrate the ideal profile (coexisting disease efficacies, no toxicities) in any SERM supports a more realistic approach in which the emphasis should be on achieving efficacy in a single, designated target end point (in this case, breast cancer) and avoiding life-threatening toxicities. Outcomes related to other diseases should be evaluated as secondary end points.

COGNITIVE FUNCTION

In animal models, the demonstration of seemingly beneficial neuromodulatory and neurotrophic effects, as well as improvements in behavioral functions in response to estrogen, supports the hypothesis that estrogen has a neuroprotective effect in the central nervous system and on memory. A neuroprotective potential for estrogen is also suggested by observational studies demonstrating that normal postmenopausal women who take estrogen appear to be protected from age-related declines in memory and are at reduced risk for Alzheimer's disease. However, these observational studies, like those in other disciplines, are confounded by multiple biases that favor estrogen users and their preexisting better health status. Given these biases, it is not surprising that prospective randomized controlled trials, which have not revealed clinically significant protective effects on cognitive function in normal women or benefits for those with varying degrees of cognitive impairment, have failed to confirm the observational data.

Because the effects of estrogen on structures in the central nervous system and on cognitive function and brain aging are poorly understood, a comprehensive research focus on the neurobiology of estrogen is essential. Such a research approach is required if the effects of currently approved and future SERMs on cognition and memory are to be appropriately categorized as protective or detrimental. Methodological confounders and/or issues related to the concurrent use of progestins (to reduce the risk of endometrial cancer in women with a uterus) need to be addressed in order to disentangle the effects of estrogens from those of progestins, which may produce dysphoric effects that are independent of those resulting from estrogen. Research needs to be conducted to characterize the differential effect of aging on the response to treatment; that is, the effects of estrogen and SERMs on cognitive function need to be compared in younger and older postmenopausal women. In normal, healthy (and, particularly, early) postmenopausal women, new instruments with greater sensitivity and specificity in assessing mild cognitive impairment and/or small decrements in cognitive function must be developed in order to improve the feasibility of conducting intervention studies in middle-aged women (and men). Finally, large randomized controlled trials (RCTs) are necessary to determine if estrogen therapy or SERMs can preserve cognitive function and reduce the risk of developing Alzheimer's disease.

CARDIOVASCULAR AND THROMBOEMBOLIC DISEASE.

By analogy to studies indicating a reduced risk of Alzheimer's disease, prospective observational studies in postmenopausal women have shown that estrogen users (generally of oral conjugated equine estrogens, with addition of the progestin medroxyprogesterone acetate in women with a uterus) compared to nonusers have a reduced risk of cardiovascular disease and mortality. Controlled interventions with estrogen in animal models and in humans have demonstrated a salutary effect on cardiovascular risk factors including high-density and low-density lipoprotein cholesterol, vascular endothelial function and parameters of hemostasis such as fibrinogen. However, RCTs of ERT or HRT have not demonstrated a significant benefit on clinically important coronary heart disease end points or on the progression of atherosclerosis. Indeed, adverse experiences (in the cardiovascular system and on hemostasis) in the Heart and Estrogen/Progestin Study (HERS) and similar early indications from the NIH-funded Women's Health Initiative (WHI) provide a sobering reminder of the absolute need to confirm epidemiological findings by adequately powered RCTs.

RCTs testing the efficacy of SERMs (like raloxifene) in preventing osteoporotic fractures or breast cancer (as single or multiple end points) also need to be adequately powered to evaluate safety—that is, to detect meaningful effects (or changes in surrogate markers) on hemostasis and in other systems, such as the cardiovascular system. Research to identify and validate relevant measures of safety is essential when considering the risk/benefit balance and thus the ultimate usefulness of SERMs and their potential for long-term use. Serious adverse events such as deep venous thrombosis and pulmonary embolism are increased in treatment regimens using estrogen and SERMs such as tamoxifen and raloxifene. Therefore, new studies or secondary analyses of data from previous trials of these agents need to be conducted to identify susceptible populations in order that treatment be more appropriately targeted. Studies of the associations of adverse outcomes in these systems with baseline values (in relation to treatment-induced changes) in relevant inflammation markers and hemostasis factors could be of great value in identifying women who are particularly vulnerable to early adverse effects of estrogen or the SERMs. Clearly, an important goal is the design of new SERMs that are at least neutral if not protective with respect to the risk of venous thromboembolism.

REPRODUCTIVE AND RELATED ENDOCRINE CONSIDERATIONS

Estrogen manifests its most striking impact in reproductive tissue, where it is associated with a variety of short- and long-term effects leading to cellular growth, differentiation, maturation, and specialization in target tissues. Similar to the effects of estrogen (without concurrent or sequential progestin) in the uterus, tamoxifen also has a stimulatory effect on the endometrium and increases the risk of endometrial cancer. In contrast, raloxifene appears to be neutral, or at least not associated with stimulatory effects in this tissue.

Because SERMs have the potential to exhibit varying degrees of agonism or antagonism in estrogen-sensitive tissues, the inclusion of protocols (in RCTs testing new SERMs) to monitor potentially vulnerable structures involved in reproductive function is key to ensuring the health of reproductive tissues. Given the increased risk of endometrial cancer with tamoxifen treatment, future research must address the optimal technology and frequency of endometrial surveillance so that timely recognition of pathological conditions in women on tamoxifen therapy can be ensured. Furthermore, because some women appear to be more vulnerable than others to tamoxifen-induced endometrial cancer, research to determine the relevance of existing reproductive tissue abnormalities is necessary to identify groups that are at high and low risk for the development of tamoxifen-induced endometrial pathologies in order to inform potential screening strategies or guidelines before initiation of therapy.

Although recent research efforts have been more diligent in addressing gaps in our knowledge on the effects of SERMs on the endometrium (and the consensus is that all studies of new SERMs should include assessments of endometrial effects), little is known regarding SERM action on estrogen-sensitive reproductive tissues beyond the endometrium. Given that long-term treatment with SERMs may be recommended, particularly in the prevention setting, the long-term consequences of SERMs on other potentially responsive reproductive structures and functions need to be evaluated. Safety studies of SERMs need to focus on effects on the pelvic floor and on other genital tissues to clarify the role, if any, of SERMs in the development of polyps, vaginal bleeding, urinary incontinence, uterine prolapse, ovarian cysts, vaginal dryness or excessive secretion, and pathologies involving the ovaries and fallopian tubes.

Since the clinical profile of SERMs may be influenced by the prevailing hormonal environment, future research efforts need to evaluate the effects of SERMs on a wide range of hormonal parameters and functions, particularly those involving the hypothalamic-pituitary-gonadal axis in women (both pre- and postmenopausal) and in men. Last, it is essential to understand the potential impact of SERMs on fertility and teratogenicity when these agents are used by premenopausal women.

THE SKELETAL SYSTEM

Although the skeletal system is exquisitely sensitive to estrogen, and estrogen therapy is remarkably effective in preserving bone mass in postmenopausal women, the antifracture efficacy of estrogen remains to be convincingly demonstrated in RCTs. Nevertheless, estrogen therapy continues to be the mainstay for the prevention and treatment of postmenopausal osteoporosis because of its proved benefits in reducing excessive bone turnover and impeding or reversing bone loss at all skeletal sites studied in both younger and older postmenopausal women. Other approved agents for the prevention and treatment of osteoporosis include raloxifene and the bisphosphonates alendronate and risedronate; however, raloxifene is the only SERM approved for this indication.

Because estrogen is the only agent approved as efficacious in relieving menopause-related symptoms, initiation of estrogen therapy is largely driven by this indication. However, troublesome side effects such as bleeding, breast tenderness, bloating, weight gain, and concerns over increased risks of breast cancer and venous thromboembolic events continue to limit acceptability and the long-term adherence apparently needed for enduring skeletal protection. Although the improved profile of raloxifene appears to circumvent many of the side effects associated with estrogen, the risk of venous thromboembolism is comparable to that for estrogen; and the increased likelihood of hot flashes with raloxifene treatment represents a step backward. Further efforts to develop SERMs with improved efficacy in fracture prevention should simultaneously focus on ameliorating (or preventing) menopause-related symptoms while avoiding the untoward side effects/adverse events of estrogen. SERMs displaying a profile of this nature are likely to meet with much better acceptability and compliance than ERT/HRT. Enhanced acceptance is especially likely for those SERMs with profiles associated with positive cardiovascular health outcomes and clinically significant reductions in breast cancer risk.

Although large-scale studies have demonstrated the efficacy of raloxifene and the bisphosphonates alendronate and risedronate in preventing new vertebral fractures in osteoporotic women, only the bisphosphonates are effective in reducing nonvertebral fractures; and this benefit appears to be limited to the context of secondary prevention. Research is needed to elucidate the mechanisms mediating the broader-spectrum antifracture efficacy of the bisphosphonates (in osteoporotic women) and to guide selection of new SERMs for preventing fractures in the appendicular skeleton and in the primary prevention setting. Also, a substantial research effort should focus on the establishment of the optimal agent, timing, and duration of therapy for the primary prevention of bone loss and fractures in women who have low bone mass but are not osteoporotic.

Of high priority are prospective intervention studies with new and existing SERMs (as well as with other alternatives to estrogen) to protect bone in women prior to, or during, the transition from pre- to postmenopause—that is, before the skeleton becomes compromised by excessive bone turnover and bone loss. Thus, new and existing strategies need to be tested in middle-aged women for their long-term efficacy in preserving bone mass and preventing fractures. Importantly, it should be recalled that compared to its positive effects on BMD in postmenopausal women, tamoxifen is associated with paradoxical deleterious effects on BMD in premenopausal women. Hence, SERM testing for indications like breast cancer risk reduction must also evaluate (at least for safety) changes in BMD. A negative effect on bone mass observed in the breast cancer prevention setting would signal the need to consider adding an antiosteoporotic agent or some other strategy to protect the skeleton.

Because men have been understudied in the SERM arena and the effect of SERMs in men have not been well described, clinical investigations in men that are aimed at identifying the potential value of current and future SERMs on the prevention and treatment of osteoporosis, prostate cancer, and other chronic diseases of aging are highly desirable. Studies on SERM efficacy and safety also need to be conducted in non-Caucasian populations to assess potential differences in responses to treatment and to determine the predictors of, and mechanisms underlying, both positive and negative outcomes.

Last, research is needed to identify promising new markers of bone metabolism and new parameters reflecting bone strength as surrogates for fractures in clinical trials. Currently, there is little consistency between the responses (i.e., timing, magnitude, and/or duration) of any given biochemical marker of bone turnover and the magnitude of the fracture reduction achieved upon treatment. The relationships between the magnitude of change in higher-order surrogates, such as bone mineral density (BMD), and the magnitude of the change in fracture risk are also highly variable and treatment dependent. Thus, the search for new surrogate makers that have significantly increased sensitivity and specificity in predicting changes in fracture risk is urgently needed in order to better identify appropriate target populations and predict fracture outcomes in clinical trials. High-quality surrogate markers will also be of inestimable value in predicting the potential responsiveness of a given patient to a given therapeutic strategy in both the primary and secondary prevention settings.

QUALITY OF LIFE

The effect of SERMs on users' quality of life (QOL) has been examined in the context of SERM testing for efficacy in various diseases. The measurements of QOL encompass both objective (as manifest by specific symptoms) and subjective scales. The commonly used SERMs tamoxifen and raloxifene have objective toxicities (hot flashes, vaginal discharge, etc.) that might be expected to negatively influence more subjective QOL measurements. Yet, despite the association of such symptoms with tamoxifen use in the Breast Cancer Prevention Trial, QOL measurements in this trial suggest that QOL is not adversely affected by this SERM.[3] Future clinical trials testing SERM efficacy for all disease end points should include QOL studies of at least subgroups of participants. This is especially true for trials addressing disease end points that occur in healthy individuals—for example, in the prevention of breast cancer, osteoporosis, and other diseases. SERMs as a class tend to be applied more frequently to disease prevention than do agents belonging to many other drug classes, reinforcing the need to include well-run QOL substudies as part of larger SERM trials.

SUMMARY

The great promise of estrogen to serve as an effective overall antiaging strategy, or as the magic bullet, is rapidly fading as new findings showing little or no benefit in some domains (such as on cognition and stroke occurrence) and, problematically, deleterious effects in others (e.g., cardiovascular and thromboembolic events) continue to mount. Remarkable progress has been made in SERM development; and profiles of new SERMs indicate great potential for efficacy in more than one system and with improved risk/benefit ratios. However, it is hard to imagine that even the most creative and successful schemes for ER modulation will lead to a single agent that can simultaneously prevent cancer and all the chronic diseases of aging while improving or maintaining quality of life. Thus the concept of what is achievable with respect to broad-spectrum disease prevention and what constitutes an ideal SERM is likely to undergo considerable reevaluation over time. Nevertheless, continuing advances in SERM development and in our understanding of ER biology are to be strongly encouraged. Future advances in the modulation of ER action are likely to have profound effects—not only on diseases and conditions known (or later discovered) to be related to estrogen action, but on the development of paradigms for understanding and modifying the action of other nuclear hormone receptors in the prevention and treatment of additional age and disease-related pathologies.

REFERENCES

1. DUNN, B.K., M. ANTHONY, S. SHERMAN & J.P. COSTANTINO. 2001. Conclusions: considerations regarding SERMs. Ann. N.Y. Acad. Sci. **949:** this volume.
2. ANTHONY, M.. J.K. WILLIAMS & B.K. DUNN. 2001. What would be the properties of an ideal SERM? Ann. N.Y. Acad. Sci. **949:** this volume.
3. DAY, R. 2001. Quality of life and tamoxifen in a breast cancer prevention trial: a summary of findings from the NSABP P-1 study. Ann. N.Y. Acad. Sci. **949:** this volume.

Everything You Wanted to Know about SERMs

Timeline of Key Events in SERM Development

Date	Event	Investigator
1896 1900	Oophorectomy (estrogen deprivation) observed to have potential benefits in advanced breast cancer	Beatson, Boyd
1936	Antiestrogenic drugs proposed as a concept to prevent breast cancer	Lacassagne
1941	Orchiectomy/castration (testosterone deprivation), high-dose estrogen have benefits for advanced prostate cancer	Huggins
1944	High-dose estrogen and DES (diethylstilbestrol) (first chemotherapeutic agent to treat cancer) used for palliation in advanced breast cancer	Dodds, Haddow
1958	First nonsteroidal antiestrogen, MER25, developed - too toxic for clinical use	Lerner
1960	First clinically useful antiestrogen, clomiphene - short-term use for ovulation induction - too toxic for long-term use	Lerner, Holtkamp
1962	Tamoxifen (TAM)/ ICI 46,474 discovery	Richardson, Walpole
1966	Estrogen receptor discovery	Jensen, Gorski
1967	TAM - fertility control in rats	Harper, Walpole
1971	TAM - first shown to confer benefit in palliation of advanced breast cancer	Cole
1973-UK 1977-US	TAM - approved for advanced breast cancer in postmenopausal women	
1977-1979	TAM - breast cancer prevention in animals	Jordan
early 1980s	TAM - first shown to confer survival advantage to postmenopausal women in the adjuvant breast cancer setting	Baum/NATO trial
1982	Raloxifene (RAL) discovery	
1980s	RAL in animals: inhibits breast cancer, preserves bone, benefits lipid profile, does not stimulate endometrium	Clemens, Black, Jordan, others

MER25

Tamoxifen
(Nolvadex®)

Raloxifene
(Evista®)

Date	Event	Investigator
1988–90	TAM - benefits lipid profile	Love/Wisconsin group
1989	TAM - benefits both premenopausal and postmenopausal women with node-negative ER+ breast cancer in the adjuvant setting	Fisher/NSABP
1985–1992	TAM - decreased contralateral breast cancer 39% in the adjuvant setting	Baum/NATO, Fisher/NSABP, Early Breast Cancer Trialists' Collaborative Group, others
1992	TAM benefits bone: increases bone mineral density (BMD)	Love/Wisconsin group
1996	TAM for >5 years has no advantage versus 5 years in adjuvant treatment of breast cancer	Fisher/NSABP
1996	Estrogen receptor beta is cloned	Gustafsson
1996	RAL does not stimulate endometrium	Draper
1997	RAL benefits bone: increases BMD, lowers cholesterol in postmenopausal women	Delmas
1997	FDA approves RAL to prevent osteoporosis in postmenopausal women	
BPCT 1992-1998	Breast Cancer Prevention Trial (BCPT) P-1: TAM reduces breast cancer risk 49% versus placebo in Gail model high-risk women	Fisher/NSABP
Royal Marsden TAMO-PLAC 1998	Royal Marsden Hospital Randomized Chemoprevention Trial: TAM does not reduce breast cancer risk versus placebo in family history-based high-risk women	Powles
Italian Study 1998	Italian Tamoxifen Prevention Study: TAM does not reduce breast cancer risk versus placebo in hysterectomized women	Veronesi, Decensi
1998	FDA approves TAM for breast cancer risk reduction in high-risk women	
1998	Phase I trials show SERM-III is well tolerated	Hudis

Date	Event	Investigator
1998	RAL benefits lipid/cardiovascular profile and coagulation factors in postmenopausal women	Walsh
MORE 1999	Multiple Outcomes of Raloxifene Evaluation (MORE) Study: RAL reduces breast cancer risk 76% versus placebo in osteoporotic postmenopausal women	Cummings, Norton
1999	MORE Study: RAL benefits bone: increases BMD, decreases vertebral fracture risk	Ettinger, Cummings
CORE 2000 ongoing	MORE extended to >8 years as Continued Outcomes of Raloxifene Evaluation (CORE): to observe long-term effects of RAL on breast cancer risk	Cummings
RUTH 2000 ongoing	Raloxifene Use for The Heart (RUTH) Trial: RAL's cardioprotection versus placebo in postmenopausal women	Barrett-Connor, Wenger
STAR 2000 ongoing Study of Tamoxifen And Raloxifene	Study of Tamoxifen and Raloxifene (STAR): Trial of breast cancer prevention in postmenopausal Gail model-based high-risk women	NSABP
2001 ongoing	TAM - 20 years of clinical testing, more than IO million woman-years of clinical experience, 400,000 women alive today because of tamoxifen development	
Fulvestrant 2001 ongoing (ICI182,780) (Faslodex®)	Newer SERMs and related drugs: Fulvestrant (Faslodex®)/ICI 182,780) shows efficacy at least equivalent to Anastrozole in advanced breast cancer. Scheduled for presentation before FDA Advisory Committee December 2001	Osborne, Howell, others
	SERM III/Arzoxifene (LY353381·HCl) testing in metastatic breast cancer	Hudis, others
	EM800 and its active metabolite EM652 (SCH57050) testing in phase 2 studies in advanced breast cancer	Labrie, others
	Lasofoxifene (CP-336,156) is being developed for osteoporosis prevention; in preclinical studies prevents bone loss in rats	Thompson
	GW 5638 in preclinical studies is being developed for breast cancer treatment and prevention	McDonnell

Recent SERM Review References

Osborne, C.K., H. Zhao, S.A.W. Fuqua. 2000. Selective estrogen receptor modulators: Structure, function, and clinical use. J. Clin. Oncol. 18: 3172-3186.

Goldstein, S.R., S. Siddhanti, A.V. Ciaccia, L. Plouffe Jr. 2000. A pharmacological review of selective oestrogen receptor modulators. Human Reproduction Update 6: 212-224.

O'Regan, R.M. & W.J. Gradishar. 2001. Selective estrogen-receptor modulators in 2001. Oncology 15: 1177-1190.

Dhingra, K. 2001. Selective estrogen receptor modulation: The search for an ideal hormonal therapy for breast cancer. Cancer Investigation 19: 649-659.

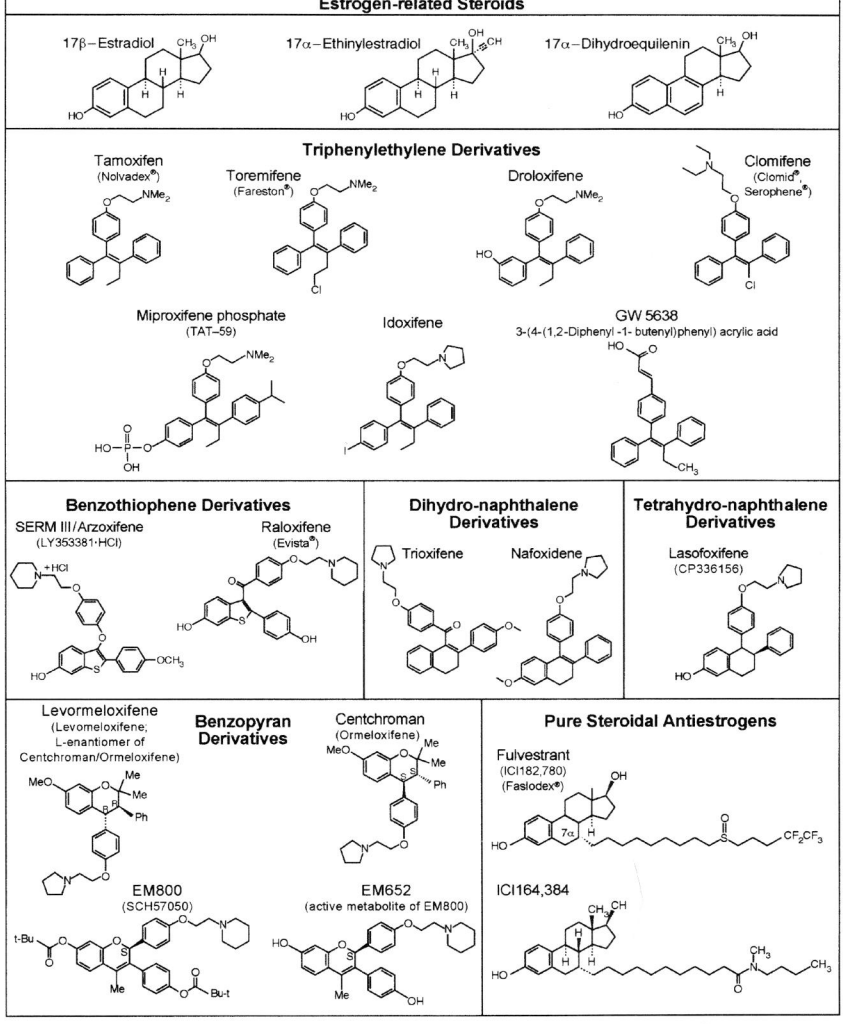

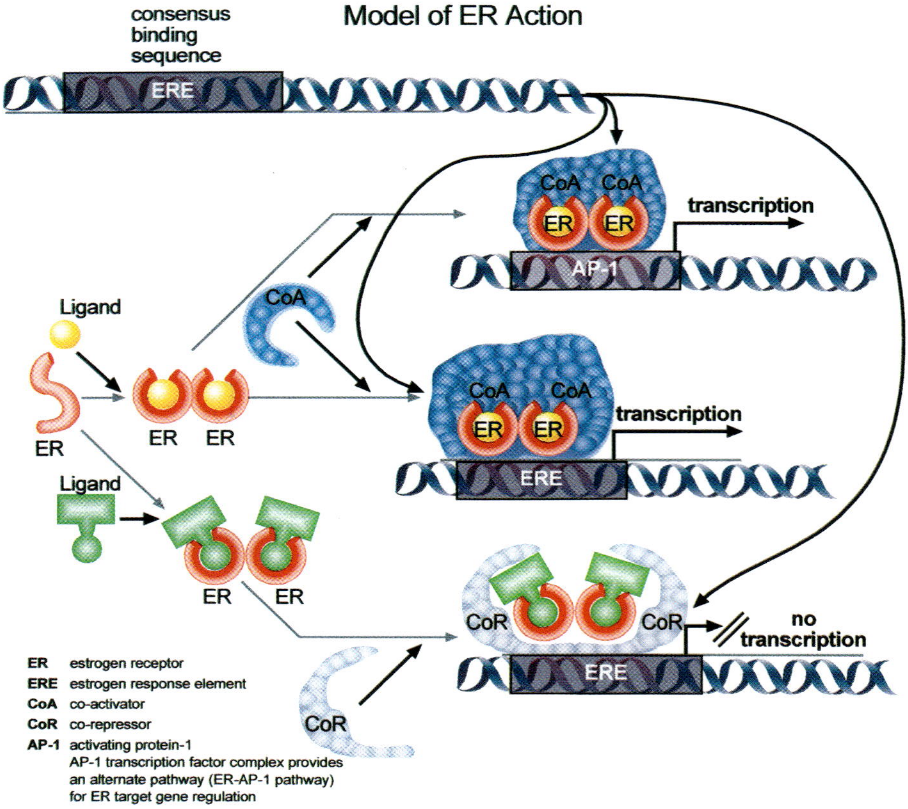

Model of ER Action
consensus binding sequence
ERE
CoA
CoA
ER
ER
transcription
AP-1
Ligand
CoA
ER
ER ER
CoA
CoA
ER
ER
transcription
ERE
Ligand
ER ER
CoR
CoR
no transcription
ERE
CoR
ER estrogen receptor
ERE estrogen response element
CoA co-activator
CoR co-repressor
AP-1 activating protein-1
AP-1 transcription factor complex provides an alternate pathway (ER-AP-1 pathway) for ER target gene regulation

Adapted from McDonnell, Trends Endocrinol Metab 10:301-310, Figure 5, 1999

Structure of Estrogen Receptor (ER) and Models of ER Action
DNA–binding domain
Ligand–binding domain
NH2
COOH
ERα
AF1
AF2
NH2
COOH
ERβ
AF1
AF2
AF1 activation function 1
AF2 activation function 2
ER estrogen receptor

Adapted from McDonnell, this Proceedings

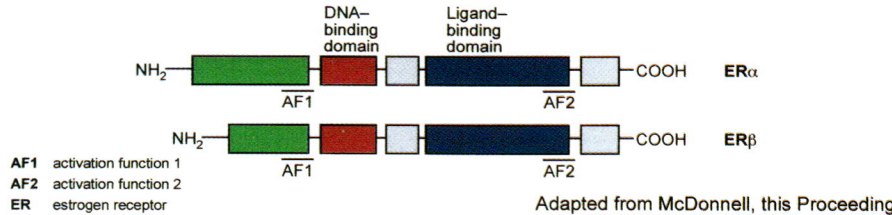

Action of SERMs in Target Tissues**

SITE	ESTROGENS	1ST GENERATION	2ND GENERATION	PURE ANTI-ESTROGENS	IDEAL SERM
Prototype compound	17β-Estradiol	Tamoxifen	Raloxifene	ICI 164384	
Breast	Agonist*	Antagonist	Antagonist	Antagonist	Antagonist
Bone	Agonist	Agonist	Agonist	Antagonist	Agonist
Cholesterol metabolism	Agonist	Agonist	Agonist	?	Agonist
Coagulation (DVT, PE)	Agonist	Agonist	Agonist	?	Antagonist
Endometrium	Agonist	Partial agonist	Antagonist	Antagonist	Antagonist
Hot flashes	Agonist	Antagonist	Antagonist	?	Agonist
Vagina	Agonist	Antagonist	Antagonist	?	Agonist

DVT, deep vein thromboses; PE, pulmonary emboli; ?, not known or not reported

*Agonist and Antagonist are defined in relation to the action of estrogen, such that "Agonist" = estrogenic and "Antagonist" = anti-estrogenic. "?" indicates that the SERM action is not established.

**Table adapted from references:
    Kauffman, R.F. & H.U. Bryant. J 1995. Drug News & Perspectives 8:531-539.
    Osborne, C.K. 1999. Primary Care & Cancer (March/Supplement No. 2).
    Fuqua, S.A.W., J. Russo, S.E. Shackney, ME. Stearns. 2001. March. Postgrad. Med. Special Report. No:3-10.

Glossary of Abbreviations

ACE, angiotensin-converting enzyme
ACOG, American College of Obstetricians and Gynecologists
ACTR, acetyl transferase, a coactivator of nuclear receptors
AD, Alzheimer's disease
ADH, atypical ductal hyperplasia
AE, adverse event
AF-1, N-terminal constitutive activation function–1 domain of a nuclear receptor; transactivating function–1
AF-2, C-terminal second activation function domain–2 of a nuclear receptor; transactivating function–2
AF-36, Medical Outcomes Study short form
AH, atypical hyperplasia
AI, aromatase inhibitor
AIB-1, amplified in breast cancer–1
ALLHAT, Antihypertensive and Lipid Lowering Treatment to Prevent Heart Attack Trial
AP-1, activator protein–1, a transcription factor consisting of either a Jun-Jun homodimer or a Jun-Fos heterodimer
APC, activated protein C
ApoE, apolipoprotein E
APP, amyloid precursor protein
AR, androgen receptor
ArKO, aromatase knockout mouse
ATAC, Anastrazole and Tamoxifen Alone or in Combination Trial; Arimidex, Tamoxifen Alone, and in Combination Adjuvant Trial
ATLAS, Adjuvant Tamoxifen Longer Against Shorter
aTTom, Adjuvant Tamoxifen Treatment, Offer More?

B/rA, benefit/risk assessment
BCDDP, Breast Cancer Detection Demonstration Project
BCPT, Breast Cancer Prevention Trial
BLA, Biologics Licensing Application
BLSA, Baltimore Longitudinal Study of Aging
BMD, bone mineral density
BMI, body mass index
BMU, basic multicellular unit
BVRT, Benton Visual Retention Test

C_3, complement component 3
CADRG, Chemoprevention Agent Development Research Group, NCI
CAF, CGP-associated factor
CBP, CREB-binding protein
CC, clomiphene citrate
CDUS, Clinical Data Update System
CEE, conjugated equine estrogen
CES-D, Center for Epidemiological Studies–Depression Scale
CGCB, Clinical Grants and Contracts Branch, CTEP, NCI
CHD, coronary heart disease
CI, confidence interval
CIB, Clinical Investigations Branch, CTEP, NCI
CIP, CBP cointegrator–associated protein
CLOM, clomiphene
CNS, central nervous system
CoA, coactivator
COPTRG, Community Oncology and Prevention Trials Group, NCI
CORE, Continuing Outcomes Relevant to Evista
COUP-TF, chicken ovalbumin upstream promoter-transcription factor
CRADA, Cooperative Research and Development Agreement
CRC, Cancer Research Campaign (UK)
CREB, cAMP regulatory element binding protein
CRO, contract research organization
CRP, C-reactive protein
CSA, Clinical Supply Agreement

CT, computerized tomography
CTA, Clinical Trials Agreement
CTEP, Cancer Therapy Evaluation Program, NCI
CTMB, Clinical Trials Monitoring Branch, CTEP, NCI
CTMS, Clinical Trials Monitoring Service
CTx, collagen T–telopeptide
CV1, monkey kidney–derived cells
CVD, cardiovascular disease
CVLT, California Verbal Learning Test
CWR-22, prostate cancer–derived cells
CYP19, cytochrome P450 19 (aromatase)

DCIS, ductal carcinoma *in situ*
DCTD, Division of Cancer Treatment and Diagnosis, NCI
DDG, Drug Discovery Group, NCI
DDT, dichloro-diphenyl-trichloro-ethane (an insecticide)
DES, diethylstilbestrol
DEXA, dual-energy X-ray absorptiometry
DHT, dihydrotestosterone
DRIP, vitamin D receptor–interacting protein
DTP, Developmental Therapeutics Program
DVT, deep-vein thrombosis

E1, estrone
E2, estradiol
E3, estriol
E4, isoform e4 of apolipoprotein E (ApoE)
EAGAR, Estrogen and Graft Atherosclerosis Research
EBCTCG, Early Breast Cancer Trialists' Collaborative Group
ECOG, Eastern Cooperative Oncology Group
EDDN, European Drug Discovery Network
EORTC, European Organization for Research and Treatment of Cancer

EPAT, Estrogen and Prevention of Atherosclerosis Trial
ER, estrogen receptor
ERA, Estrogen Replacement and Atherosclerosis trial
ERE, estrogen response element
ERKO, estrogen receptor knockout mouse
ERT, estrogen replacement therapy

FDA, Food and Drug Administration
FDAMA, FDA Modernization Act
FIGO, Federation of Gynecology and Obstetrics
FIT, Fracture Intervention Trial
FSH, follicle-stimulating hormone

GFP-AR, jellyfish green fluorescent protein–androgen receptor
GnRH, gonadotropin-releasing hormone
GR, glucocorticoid receptor
GRIP-1, glucocorticoid receptor interacting protein–1

HAT, histone acetylase
HBD, hormone binding domain
HDL, high-density lipoprotein
HDS, Hasegawa Dementia Scale
HeLa, uterine/cervical cancer–derived cells
HERS, Heart and Estrogen/Progestin Replacement Study
HPG, hypothalamic-pituitary-gonadal
HPO, hypothalamic-pituitary-ovarian
HRQL, health-related quality of life
HRT, hormone replacement therapy

IBIS, International Breast Cancer Intervention Study
ICAM-1, intercellular adhesion molecule–1
ICI 182,780, fulvestrant, Faslodex
IDB, Investigational Drug Branch, NCI

GLOSSARY OF ABBREVIATIONS

IGF, insulin-like growth factor
IGFBP, IGF-binding protein
IHC, immunohistochemistry
IL-6, interleukin-6
IND, Investigational New Drug application

JAK, Janus kinases—i.e., tyrosine kinases that participate in signaling from cell-surface receptors, especially members of the cytokine receptor superfamily

LBA, ligand-binding assay
LBD, ligand-binding domain
LCIS, lobular carcinoma *in situ*
LDL, low-density lipoprotein
LH, luteinizing hormone
LHRH, luteinizing hormone–releasing hormone
LIF, leukemia inhibitory factor
LOI, Letter of Intent

MAP kinase, mitogen-activated protein kinase
MCS, mental component score
MF, Master File
MGH, Massachusetts General Hospital
MI, myocardial infarction
mMMSE, modified Mini-Mental Status Exam
MMP-9, matrix metalloproteinase–9
MORE, Multiple Outcomes of Raloxifene Evaluation trial
MOS, Medical Outcomes Study
MPA, medroxyprogesterone acetate
MRC, Medical Research Council (UK)
MRI, magnetic resonance imaging

NCI, National Cancer Institute
NCoA, nuclear receptor coactivator
NCoR, nuclear receptor corepressor
NDA, New Drug Application

NHLBI, National Heart, Lung, and Blood Institute
NIA, National Institute on Aging
NIH, National Institutes of Health
NINDS, National Institute of Neurological Diseases and Stroke
NLS, nuclear localization signal
NNT, number needed to treat
NR, nuclear receptor
NSABP, National Surgical Adjuvant Breast and Bowel Project

ODAC, Oncologic Drugs Advisory Committee
OR, odds ratio

P-1, Breast Cancer Prevention Trial (BCPT)
PAI-1, plasminogen activation (activator) inhibitor–1
PBP, PPARγ-binding protein
PC3, prostate cancer–derived cells
PCOS, polycystic ovary syndrome
PCS, physical component score
PE, pulmonary embolism
PEPI, Postmenopausal Estrogen/ Progestin Interventions trial
PET, positron emission tomography
PGE2, prostaglandin E2
PHASE, Papworth HRT Atherosclerosis Study Enquiry
PHOREA, Postmenopausal Hormone Replacement against Atherosclerosis
PMB, Pharmaceutical Management Branch, NCI
PPAR, peroxisome proliferator–activated receptor
PR, progesterone receptor
PRC, Protocol Review Committee
PRL, prolactin
PTH, parathyroid hormone

QCT, quantitative computed tomography
QOL, quality of life
QUS, quantitative ultrasound

RAB, Regulatory Affairs Branch, CTEP, NCI
RAC-3, receptor associated coactivator–3
RAL, raloxifene
RCBF, regional cerebral blood flow
RCT, randomized controlled trial
RMH, Royal Marsden Hospital
RR, relative risk
RT-PCR, reverse transcription–polymerase chain reaction
RUTH, Raloxifene Use for the Heart trial

SAM, selective aromatase modulator
SARM, selective androgen receptor modulator
SCL, symptom checklist
SEB, surrogate end point biomarker
SEER, Surveillance, Epidemiology, and End Results
SENDO, Southern Europe New Drugs Organization
SERM, selective estrogen receptor modulator
SF1, steroidogenic factor–1
SHBG, sex hormone–binding globulin
SMRT, silencing mediator for retinoid and thyroid hormone receptor
SRC, histone acetyl transferase steroid receptor coactivator
SRM, selective receptor modulator
STAR, Study of Tamoxifen and Raloxifene
STAT, signal transducers and activators of transcription—i.e., latent cytoplasmic transcription factors that become activated after recruitment to an activated receptor complex

T, testosterone
TAM/Tam, tamoxifen
TGF-β, transforming growth factor–β
TIA, transient ischemic attack
TIF2, transcription intermediary factor–2
TNF-α, tumor necrosis factor–α
TOR, toremifene
TR, thyroid hormone receptor
TRAP, thyroid hormone receptor–associated protein

UKCCCR, United Kingdom Coordinating Committee for Cancer Research
UTR, untranslated region

VCAM-1, vascular cell adhesion molecule–1
VTE, venous thromboembolism; venous thromboembolic event

WAVE, Women's Angiographic Vitamin and Estrogen trial
WELL-HART, Women's Estrogen-Progestin Lipid Lowering Hormone Atherosclerosis Regression Trial
WEST, Women's Estrogen for Stroke Trial
WHI, Women's Health Initiative
WHISCA, Women's Health Initiative Study of Cognitive Aging
WHO, World Health Organization
WISDOM, Women's International Study of Long-Duration Oestrogen after the Menopause

Index of Contributors

Ahn, S.C., 44–57
Ansher, S.S., 333–340
Anthony, M., 261–278, 304–314, 315–316, 352–365

Barrett-Connor, E., 295–303
Bellino, F.L., 259–260
Blum, A., 168–174
Buckholtz, N.S., 223–234
Bulun, S., 58–67

Cannon, R.O., III, 168–174
Chang, C.-Y., 16–35
Chatterjee, B., 44–57
Clyne, C., 58–67
Costantino, J.P., 280–285, 352–365
Cummings, S.R., 198–201
Cushman, M., 175–180
Cuzick, J., 123–133

Davidson, N.E., 80–88
Day, R., 143–150
Decensi, A., 113–122
DeLap, R.J., 341–344
Dickler, M.N., 134–142
Dunn, B.K., 68–71, 99–108, 261–278, 304–314, 352–365, 366–374

Emmen, J.M.A., 36–43

Finnegan, L., 259–260

Gail, M.H., 286–291
Galli, A., 113–122
Ganessunker, D., 6–15
Goldstein, S.R., 237–242
Gordon, D.J., 151–152
Guerrieri-Gonzaga, A., 113–122

Gupta, J., 186–187

Harrington, W.R., 6–15
Hendrix, S.L., 243–250
Herrington, D.M., 153–162
Honig, S.F., 345–348

Johnson, K., 315–316
Johnson, S.R., 304–314
Jordan, V.C., 72–79

Katzenellenbogen, B.S., 6–15
Katzenellenbogen, J.A., 6–15
Klein, K.P., 153–162
Kobayashi, K., 341–344
Komm, B.S., 317–326
Korach, K.S., 36–43
Kraichely, D.M., 6–15
Kramer, B., 68–71

Lavrovsky, Y., 44–57
Lewis, J.P., 327–332
Lyttle, C.R., 317–326

Maki, P.M., 203–214
Margolis, R., 1–2
Mark, S., 186–187
McCaskill-Stevens, W., 279
McDonnell, D.P., 16–35
McKenna, N.J., 3–5
McNeeley, S.G., 243–250
Miller, M.M., 223–234
Monjan, A.A., 202, 223–234
Mosca, L., 181–185

Norris, J.D., 16–35
Norton, L., 134–142

O'Malley, B.W., 3–5

Oh, T.-S., 44–57

Parrott, E.C., 235–236
Plouffe, L., Jr., 251–258
Powles, T.J., 109–112
Pritchard, K.I., 89–98

Resnick, S.M., 203–214
Rotmensz, N., 113–122
Roy, A.K., 44–57
Rubin, G., 58–67

Scharf, R., 333–340
Sherman, S., xi–xiii, 188–197, 352–365, 366–374
Siddhanti, S., 251–258
Simpson, E.R., 58–67

Song, C.S., 44–57
Speed, C., 58–67
Sun, J., 6–15

Taylor, A.L., 292–294
Tyagi, R.K., 44–57

Walsh, B.W., 163–167
Williams, J.K., 261–278
Wolff, A.C., 80–88
Wolmark, N., 99–108

Yaffe, K., 215–222

Zapol, N.J., 349–351

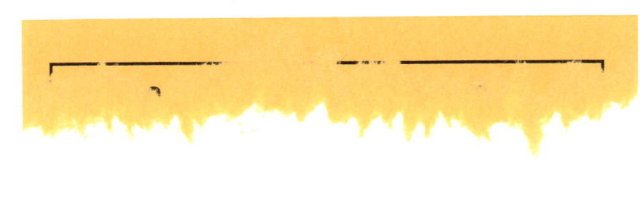